Praise for *The Myth of Normal*

"In *The Myth of Normal*, Gabor Maté takes us on an epic journey of discovery about how our emotional well-being and our social connectivity (in short, how we live) are intimately intertwined with health, disease, and addictions. Chronic mental and physical illnesses may not be separate and distinct diseases but intricate, multilayered processes that reflect (mal)adaptations to the cultural context that we live in and the values we live by. This riveting and beautifully written tale has profound implications for all of our lives, including the practice of medicine and mental health."

—Bessel A. van der Kolk, MD, president, Trauma Research Foundation, professor of psychiatry, Boston University School of Medicine, and author of the #1 *New York Times* bestseller *The Body Keeps the Score: Brain, Mind, and Body in the Healing of Trauma*

"Gabor and Daniel Maté have created a magnificent resource for us all in *The Myth of Normal*, a powerful, in-depth, science-packed, inspiring story–filled opus that helps us see how stress within our culture shapes our well-being in all its facets. By carefully reviewing medical and mental health through a wide lens of inquiry, they challenge simplistic views of disease and disorder to offer instead a wider perspective on human flourishing that has direct implications for how we live individually, at home, and as a larger human family. A thorough and inspiring work of the heart, this book urges us to question our assumptions and think deeply about who we are and how we can live more fully and freely, harnessing the power of the mind to bring healing and wholeness into our shared lives on Earth."

—Daniel J. Siegel, MD, clinical professor, UCLA School of Medicine, executive director, Mindsight Institute, and *New York Times* bestselling author of *IntraConnected: MWe (Me + We) as the Integration of Self, Identity, and Belonging*

"Wise, sophisticated, rigorous, and creative: an intellectual and compassionate investigation of who we are and who we may become. Essential reading for anyone with a past and a future."

—Tara Westover, *New York Times* bestselling author of *Educated*

"Gabor and Daniel Maté have delivered a book in which readers can seek refuge and solace during moments of profound personal and social crisis. *The Myth of Normal* is an essential compass during disorienting times."

—Esther Perel, psychotherapist, author, and host of *Where Should We Begin?*

"Gabor Maté articulates bluntly, brilliantly, and passionately what all of us instinctively know but none of us really want to face: The entire social construct of the world we're living in is deeply flawed, with toxicities on every level. Yet though the book makes clear what's so terribly wrong, it also points to how we can make it right. Maté is a guide through the dangerous forest of our minds and our society, not letting us ignore the darkness but ultimately showing us the light. *The Myth of Normal* is exactly what we need."

—Marianne Williamson, *New York Times* bestselling author of *A Return to Love*

of and physician for it than Gabor Maté. This book contains a prescription that, if we have the courage to follow it, will heal us all."

—Richard Schwartz, PhD, creator of the Internal Family Systems model of psychotherapy

The Myth of Normal is a book literally everyone will be enriched by—a wise, profound, and healing work that is the culmination of Dr. Maté's many years of deep and painfully accumulated wisdom."

—Johann Hari, *New York Times* bestselling author of *Stolen Focus*

"This gripping book builds upon two key truths for our time—that everything is connected, including psychic wounds and physical illnesses, and that these are not anomalies but ordinary, even epidemic, in the society we've built. *The Myth of Normal* is a powerful call for change in how we live with, love, understand, treat, and think about one another, by someone ideally situated to map the terrain and to give us some valuable tools with which to navigate it."

—Rebecca Solnit, author of *Men Explain Things to Me*

"In this wide-ranging and beautifully written book, Gabor Maté and his co-writer son Daniel offer an acute diagnosis of what ails our culture and a blueprint for personal healing, while pointing the way to what is required to create a more hospitable, human-friendly world for ourselves and our children."

—Dr. Shefali, *New York Times* bestselling author and clinical psychologist

"Gabor Maté's latest book is a guide to self-awareness, social insight, and healing that is deeply personal and utterly transparent. Written with fluid, crystalline prose, profound wisdom, great humor, and hard-won humility, it merits becoming this generation's *The Road Less Traveled*. In my two-word summation, *The Myth of Normal* is Fiercely Tender."

—William M. Watson, SJ, DMin, president and founder, Sacred Story Institute

"*The Myth of Normal* is a detailed and wide-ranging look at what we all need to know—but all too often fail to live up to—when it comes to human health, sanity, maturation, and happiness. It's also a clear-eyed examination of the benefits, triumphs, limitations, and blind spots of our health and mental health care system."

—Resmaa Menakem, bestselling author of *My Grandmother's Hands*, *The Quaking of America*, and *Monsters in Love*

"*The Myth of Normal* is a tour de force journey into the dissonant experience of being human in our aberrant and toxic modern culture. The journey is both heartrending and exalted in its underlying purpose—to heal the rift from our authentic selves and the collective trauma that stifles our natural expression and joy. If you are ready to do the brave and life-shaking work of examining the truth of your life and the culture that we are literally in the death grips of—this is your read."

—Rachel Carlton Abrams, MD, MHS, ABoIM

"*The Myth of Normal* presents a unique perspective in viewing what we see as 'normal' and opens up a way to wake up to what is real and authentic in our lives. Gabor and Daniel Maté have written a compelling book that will challenge your views and help lift the veil of illusion to what is truly happening in your mind and in your body."

—Sharon Salzberg, author of *Lovingkindness* and *Real Happiness*

"With rigorous research and painstaking detail, this book by esteemed physician Gabor Maté is a tour de force manifesto of how trauma impacts not just our individual bodies and psyches but our whole society. *The Myth of Normal* plants seeds for revitalizing what we consider 'normal' and giving ourselves permission to say no to what is making us unnecessarily sick."

—Lissa Rankin, MD, *New York Times* bestselling author of *Mind Over Medicine* and *Sacred Medicine*

"This, Gabor Maté's magnum opus, is essential reading for us all. A genius writer, he gives it to us straight: From the mindbody to the body politic, we learn how loss of authenticity takes its toll psychologically, physically, spiritually, and socially."

—Julie Holland, MD, author of *Good Chemistry: The Science of Connection, from Soul to Psychedelics*

"Every once in a rare while a book comes along creating a new vision of the world, illuminating for us that which until now has been invisible, yet as vital to our health and well-being as water is to fish, oxygen is for our bodies, and love is for our souls. This work is such a tour de force, a humbling and brilliantly written exposition of what deeper healing requires."

—Jeffrey D. Rediger, MD, MDiv, assistant professor, Harvard Medical School, and author of *Cured: Strengthen Your Immune System and Heal Your Life*

"Gabor Mate is brilliant and passionate, tender and fierce, writing with an urgent honesty. His analysis is comprehensive and penetrating, combining deep scholarship, hard-earned clinical wisdom, personal trauma, and practical suggestions. This is a masterwork that reads like an intelligent thriller, highlighting our challenges with dramatic clarity while showing the way to their solutions. A must-have book for anyone interested in their own mind, in how our world got so crazy, and in the better future we can forge together."

—Rick Hanson, PhD, author of *Resilient: How to Grow an Unshakable Core of Calm, Strength, and Happiness*

the Myth of Normal

Trauma, Illness & Healing in a Toxic Culture

Gabor Maté, MD,

with Daniel Maté

Avery

an imprint of Penguin Random House

New York

AVERY

an imprint of Penguin Random House LLC
penguinrandomhouse.com

Most Avery books are available at special quantity discounts for bulk purchase
for sales promotions, premiums, fund-raising, and educational needs. Special
books or book excerpts also can be created to fit specific needs. For details,
write SpecialMarkets@penguinrandomhouse.com.

Library of Congress Cataloging-in-Publication Data

Names: Maté, Gabor, author. | Maté, Daniel, author.
Title: The myth of normal: trauma, illness, and healing in a toxic culture /
    Gabor Maté, with Daniel Maté.
Description: New York: Avery, 2022. | Includes bibliographical
    references and index.
Identifiers: LCCN 2022005936 (print) | LCCN 2022005937 (ebook) |
    ISBN 9780593083888 (hardcover) | ISBN 9780593083895 (epub)
Subjects: LCSH: Health—Social aspects. | Diseases—Social aspects. |
    Social medicine. | Civilization, Modern—21st century—Health aspects.
Classification: LCC RA418 .M3272 2022 (print) | LCC RA418 (ebook) |
    DDC 362.1—dc23/eng/20220609
LC record available at https://lccn.loc.gov/2022005936
LC ebook record available at https://lccn.loc.gov/2022005937

Printed in the United States of America
4th Printing

Book design by Shannon Nicole Plunkett

To dearest Rae, my life partner, who saw me before I could see myself and who loved all of me long before I could love myself at all. None of my work would exist without her. And to the children we brought forth together—Daniel, Aaron, and Hannah—who light up our world.

The best physician is also a philosopher.

—Aelius Galenus (Galen of Pergamon)

For if medicine is really to accomplish its great task,
it must intervene in political and social life. It must point
out the hindrances that impede the normal social functioning
of vital processes, and effect their removal.

—Rudolf Virchow, nineteenth-century German physician

When you're trying to survive, you turn malady into
a coping strategy, and loss into culture.

—Stephen Jenkinson

Author's Note

There are no composite or fictional characters in this book. Each story told is that of a real person whose words, from transcribed interviews, are reproduced accurately with occasional editing for purposes of clarity. When only a given name is used, it is a pseudonym to protect privacy, at the interviewee's request. In such cases, some biographical data may also be slightly altered. Where both names are given, the identity is real.

Unless otherwise stated, all italics are mine.

A word about authorship. This book was co-written with my son Daniel. Usually the word "with" in identifying authors is meant to denote a ghostwriter, one who actually renders the main author's ideas into written form. That wasn't the case here: on most chapters I was the primary author, with Daniel following up with a particular eye to style, tone, clarity of argument, and accessibility, and often contributing his own thoughts. Occasionally, when I found myself stuck on what to say or how to say it, he would take the writing reins for a while, crafting a particular section or chapter based on material I had collated and penned. In all cases, we would pass the chapters back and forth until we were both satisfied. The structure and flow of the book was also very much an ongoing collaboration between us, from the preparation of the book proposal through the final draft.

So while the book's *authorship* is unequally distributed, in that it reflects my work, research, analysis, and experience, it was very much *co-written*. I truly could not have accomplished the task without Daniel's brilliant partnership.

Gabor Maté
Vancouver, B.C.

Contents

Why Normal Is a Myth
(And Why That Matters)

*The fact that millions of people share the same vices does not
make these vices virtues, the fact that they share so many errors
does not make the errors to be truths, and the fact that millions
of people share the same forms of mental pathology does not
make these people sane.*

—Erich Fromm, *The Sane Society*

In the most health-obsessed society ever, all is not well.

Health and wellness have become a modern fixation. Multibillion-dollar industries bank on people's ongoing investment—mental and emotional, not to mention financial—in endless quests to eat better, look younger, live longer, or feel livelier, or simply to suffer fewer symptoms. We encounter would-be bombshells of "breaking health news" on magazine covers, in TV news stories, omnipresent advertising, and the daily deluge of viral online content, all pushing this or that mode of self-betterment. We do our best to keep up: we take supplements, join yoga studios, serially switch diets, shell out for genetic testing, strategize to prevent cancer or dementia, and seek medical advice or alternative therapies for maladies of the body, psyche, and soul.

And yet our collective health is deteriorating.

What is happening? How are we to understand that in our modern world, at the pinnacle of medical ingenuity and sophistication, we are seeing more and more chronic physical disease as well as afflictions such as mental illness and addiction? Moreover, how is it that we're not more alarmed, if we notice at all? And how are we to find our way to preventing and healing the many ailments that assail us, even putting aside acute catastrophes such as the COVID-19 pandemic?

As a physician for over three decades, in work ranging from delivering infants to running a palliative care ward, I was always struck by the links between the individual and the social and emotional contexts in which our lives unfold and health or illness ensue. This curiosity, or should I say fascination, led me in time to look deeply into the cutting-edge science that has elegantly delineated such links. My previous books have explored some of these connections as they manifest in particular ailments such as attention deficit hyperactivity disorder (ADHD), cancer and autoimmune disease of all types, and addiction. I have also written about child development, the most decisively formative period of our lives.[1]

This book, *The Myth of Normal*, sets its sights on something far more encompassing. I have come to believe that behind the entire epidemic of chronic afflictions, mental and physical, that beset our current moment, something is amiss in our culture itself, generating both the rash of ailments we are suffering *and,* crucially, the ideological blind spots that keep us from seeing our predicament clearly, the better to do something about it. These blind spots—prevalent throughout the culture but endemic to a tragic extent in my own profession—keep us ignorant of the connections that bind our health to our social-emotional lives.

Another way of saying it: chronic illness—mental or physical—is to a large extent a *function* or *feature* of the way things are and not a *glitch*; a consequence of how we live, not a mysterious aberration.

The phrase "a toxic culture" in this book's subtitle may suggest things like environmental pollutants, so prevalent since the dawn of the industrial age and so antagonistic to human health. From asbestos particles to carbon dioxide run amok, there is indeed no shortage of real, physical toxins in our midst. We could also understand "toxic" in its more contemporary, pop-psychological sense, as in the spread of negativity, distrust, hostility, and polarization that, no question, typify the present sociopolitical moment.

We can certainly fold these two meanings into our discussion, but I am using "toxic culture" to characterize something even broader and more deeply rooted: *the entire context of social structures, belief systems, assumptions, and values that surround us and necessarily pervade every aspect of our lives.*

That social life bears upon health is not a new discovery, but the recognition of it has never been more urgent. I see it as the most important and consequential health concern of our time, driven by the effects of burgeoning stress, inequality, and climate catastrophe, to name a few salient factors. Our concept of well-being must move from the individual to the global in every sense of that word. That is particularly so in this era of globalized capitalism, which, in the words of the cultural historian Morris Berman, has become the "total commercial environment that circumscribes an entire mental world."[2] Given the mind-body unity to be highlighted in this book, I would add that it constitutes a total physiological environment as well.

It is my contention that by its very nature our social and economic culture generates chronic stressors that undermine well-being in the most serious of ways, as they have done with increasing force over the past several decades.

Here's an analogy I find helpful. In a laboratory, a culture is a biochemical broth custom-made to promote the development of this or that organism. Assuming the microbes in question start out with a clean bill of health and genetic fitness, a suitable and well-maintained culture should allow for their happy, healthy growth and proliferation. If the same organisms begin showing pathologies at unprecedented rates, or fail to thrive, it's either because the culture has become contaminated or because it was the wrong mixture in the first place. Whichever the case, we could rightly call this a *toxic culture*—unsuitable for the creatures it is meant to support. Or worse: dangerous to their existence. It is the same with human societies. As the broadcaster, activist, and author Thom Hartmann asserts, "Culture can be healthy or toxic, nurturing or murderous."[3]

From a wellness perspective, our current culture, viewed as a laboratory experiment, is an ever-more globalized demonstration of what can go awry. Amid spectacular economic, technological, and medical resources, it induces countless humans to suffer illness born of stress, ignorance, inequality, environmental degradation, climate change, poverty, and social isolation. It allows millions to die prematurely of diseases we know how to prevent or of deprivations we have more than enough resources to eliminate.

In the United States, the richest country in history and the epicenter of the globalized economic system, 60 percent of adults have a chronic disorder such as high blood pressure or diabetes, and over 40 percent have two or more such conditions.[4] Nearly 70 percent of Americans are on at least one prescription drug; more than half take two.[5] In my own country, Canada, up to half of all baby boomers are on track for hypertension within a few years if current trends continue.[6] Among women there is a disproportionate elevation in diagnoses of potentially disabling autoimmune conditions like multiple sclerosis (MS).[7] Among the young, non-smoking-related cancers seem to be on the rise. Rates of obesity, along with the multiple health risks it poses, are going up in many countries, including in Canada, Australia, and notably the United States, where over 30 percent of the adult population meet the criteria. Recently Mexico has surpassed its northern neighbor in that unenviable category, with the result that thirty-eight Mexicans are diagnosed with diabetes every hour. Thanks to globalization, Asia is catching up. "China has entered the era of obesity," Ji Chengye, a child health researcher in Beijing, reported. "The speed of growth is shocking."[8]

Throughout the Western world, mental health diagnoses are escalating among the young, in adults, and among the elderly. In Canada, depression and anxiety are the fastest-growing diagnoses; and in 2019 more than fifty million Americans, over 20 percent of U.S. adults, suffered an episode of mental illness.[9] In Europe, according to the authors of a recent international survey, mental disorders have become "the largest health challenge of the 21st century."[10] Millions of North American children and youths are being medicated with stimulants, antidepressants, and even antipsychotic drugs whose long-term effects on the developing brain are yet to be established—a perilous social experiment in the chemical control of young people's brains and behavior. A chilling 2019 headline on the online news site ScienceAlert speaks for itself: "Child Suicide Attempts Are Skyrocketing in the US, and Nobody Knows Why."[11] The picture is similarly stark in the U.K., where the *Guardian* recently reported, "British universities are experiencing a surge in student anxiety, mental breakdowns and depression."[12] As globalization envelops the world, conditions hitherto found in "developed" countries are finding their way into new venues. ADHD among children, for example, has become "an increasing public health concern" in China.[13]

The climate catastrophe already afflicting us has introduced an entirely new health hazard, a magnified version—if that is possible—of the existential threat that nuclear war has posed since Hiroshima. "Distress about climate change is associated with young people perceiving that they have no future, that humanity is doomed," found the authors of a 2021 survey of the attitudes of over ten thousand individuals in forty-two countries. Along with a sense of betrayal and abandonment by governments and adults, such despondence and hopelessness "are chronic stressors which will have significant, long-lasting and incremental negative implications on the mental health of children and young people."[14]

Casting ourselves as the organisms in the laboratory analogy, these and other metrics indicate unmistakably that ours is a toxic culture. Worse yet, we have become accustomed—or perhaps better to say *acculturated*—to so much of what plagues us. It has become, for lack of a better word, normal.

In medical practice, the word "normal" denotes, among other things, the state of affairs we doctors aim for, setting the boundaries delineating health from disease. "Normal levels" and "normal functioning" are our goal when we apply treatments or remedies. We also gauge success or failure against "statistical norms"; we reassure worried patients that this symptom or that side effect is completely normal, as in "to be expected." These are all specific and legitimate uses of the word, enabling us to assess situations realistically so that we can aim our efforts appropriately.

It is not in these senses that this book's title refers to "normal," but rather in a more insidious one that, far from helping us progress toward a healthier future, cuts such an endeavor off at the pass.

For better or worse, we humans have a genius for getting used to things, especially when the changes are incremental. The newfangled verb "to normalize" refers to the mechanism by which something previously aberrant becomes normal enough that it passes beneath our radar. On a societal level, then, "normal" often means "nothing to see here": all systems are functioning as they should, no further inquiry needed.

The truth as I see it is quite different.

The late David Foster Wallace, master wordsmith, author, and essayist, once opened a commencement speech with a droll parable that well illustrates the trouble with normality. The story concerns two fish crossing aquatic paths with an elder of their species, who greets them jovially: " 'Morning, boys. How's the water?' And the two young fish swim on for a bit, and then eventually one of them looks over at the other and goes, 'What the hell is water?' " The point Wallace wanted to leave his audience pondering was that "the most obvious, ubiquitous, important realities are often the ones hardest to see and talk about." On its surface, he allowed, that might sound like "a banal platitude" but "in the day-to-day trenches of adult existence, banal platitudes *can have a life-or-death importance.*"

He could have been articulating this book's thesis. Indeed, the lives, and the deaths, of individual human beings—their quality and in many cases their duration—are intimately bound up with the aspects of modern society that are "hardest to see and talk about"; phenomena that are, like water to fish, both too vast and too near to be appreciated. In other words, those features of daily life that appear to us now as normal are the ones crying out the loudest for our scrutiny. That is my central contention. My core intention, accordingly, is to offer a new way of seeing and talking about these phenomena, bringing them from the background to the foreground so we might more swiftly find their much-needed remedies.

I will make the case that much of what passes for normal in our society is neither healthy nor natural, and that to meet modern society's criteria for normality is, in many ways, to conform to requirements that are profoundly *abnormal* in regard to our

Nature-given needs—which is to say, unhealthy and harmful on the physiological, mental, and even spiritual levels.

If we could begin to see much illness itself not as a cruel twist of fate or some nefarious mystery but rather as an *expected and therefore normal consequence of abnormal, unnatural circumstances,* it would have revolutionary implications for how we approach everything health related. The ailing bodies and minds among us would no longer be regarded as expressions of individual pathology but as living alarms directing our attention toward where our society has gone askew, and where our prevailing certainties and assumptions around health are, in fact, fictions. Seen clearly, they might also give us clues as to what it would take to reverse course and build a healthier world.

Far more than a lack of technological acumen, sufficient funds, or new discoveries, our culture's skewed idea of normality is the single biggest impediment to fostering a healthier world, even keeping us from acting on what we already know. Its occluding effects are particularly dominant in the field where clear sight is most called for: medicine.

The current medical paradigm, owing to an ostensibly scientific bent that in some ways bears more resemblance to an ideology than to empirical knowledge, commits a double fault. It reduces complex events to their biology, and it separates mind from body, concerning itself almost exclusively with one or the other without appreciating their essential unity. This shortcoming does not invalidate medicine's indisputably miraculous achievements, nor sully the good intentions of so many people practicing it, but it does severely constrain the good that medical science could be doing.

One of the most persistent and calamitous failures handicapping our health systems is an ignorance—in the sense either of not knowing or of actual, active ignoring—of *what science has already established.* Case in point: the ample and growing evidence that living people cannot be dissected into separate organs and systems, not even into "minds" and "bodies." Overall, the medical world has been unwilling or unable to metabolize this evidence and to adjust its ways accordingly. The new science—much of which isn't all that conceptually new—has yet to have significant impact on medical school training, leaving well-meaning health providers to toil in the dark. Many end up having to connect the dots for themselves.

For me, the process of putting the pieces together began several decades ago when, on a hunch, I went beyond the standard repertoire of dry doctorly questions about symptom presentation and medical history to ask my patients about the larger context for their illnesses: their lives. I am grateful for what these men and women taught me through how they lived and died, suffered and recovered, and through the stories they shared with me. The core of it, which accords entirely with what the science shows, is this: health and illness are not random states in a particular body or body part. They are, in fact, an expression of an entire life lived, one that cannot, in turn, be understood in isolation: it is influenced by—or better yet, it arises from—a web of circumstances, relationships, events, and experiences.

Of course, we have cause to celebrate the past two centuries' astonishing medical advances and the tireless fortitude and intellectual brilliance of those whose work has led to giant strides in many different fields of human health. To take just one example, the incidence of polio—an awful illness that killed or maimed countless children only two or three generations back—has dropped by more than 99 percent since 1988, according to the U.S. Centers for Disease Control and Prevention; most kids today probably have never heard of the disease.[15] Even the more recent epidemic of HIV has been downgraded in a relatively short period of time from a death sentence to a manageable chronic condition—at least for those with access to the right kinds of treatment. And as destructive as the COVID-19 pandemic has been, the rapid development of vaccines may be counted among the triumphs of modern science and medicine.

The problem with good news stories like these—and they are very good news—is that they stoke the reassuring conviction that we are, overall, making advances toward a healthier standard of life, lulling us into a false passivity. The actual picture is quite different. Far from being on the verge of curbing the contemporary health challenges facing us, we are barely keeping pace with most of them. Often the best we can do is mitigate symptoms, whether surgically or pharmacologically, or both. As welcome as medical breakthroughs are, and as fruitful as research can be, the crux of the problem is not a dearth of facts, not a lack of technology or techniques, but an impoverished, out-of-date perspective that cannot account for what we are seeing. My aim here is to offer a fresh one that I believe brings with it enormous possibilities for a healthier paradigm: a new vision of normal that nurtures the best in who we are.

This book's arc follows the concentric circles of cause, connection, and consequence that influence how healthy or unhealthy we are. Beginning from the inside at the level of human biology, and then examining the close relationships within which our bodies, brains, and personalities develop, we will make our way outward to the most macro dimensions of our collective existence, namely the socioeconomic and the political. Along the path I will show how our physical and mental health is intricately interwoven with how we feel, what we perceive or believe about ourselves and the world, and the ways that life does or does not satisfy our nonnegotiable human needs. Because trauma is a foundational layer of experience in modern life, but one largely ignored or misapprehended, I will begin with a working definition to set up everything that follows.

At each stage, my task is to lift the veil of common knowledge and received wisdom, considering what science and watchful observation tell us, with the aim of unfastening the myths that keep the status quo locked in place. As in my previous books, the science and its health implications will be brought home via real-life stories and case studies of people who have generously shared something of their journeys through illness and health with me. These range from the mildly surprising to the truly incredible, the heartbreaking to the inspiring.

Yes, inspiring. For there is a heartening corollary to all the difficult news. When we can look soberly at what we as a culture have normalized about health and illness, and realize that it is not, in fact, the way things are meant or fated to be, there arises the possibility of returning to what Nature has always intended for us. Hence the "healing" in our subtitle: once we resolve to see clearly how things are, the process of healing—a word that, at its root, means "returning to wholeness"—can begin. That statement contains no promise of miracle cures but simply the recognition that each of us contains as-yet-unimagined possibilities for wellness, possibilities that reveal themselves only when we face and debunk the misleading myths† about normality to which we have become passively accustomed. If that is true for us as individuals, it must also be true for us as a species.

Healing is not guaranteed, but it is available. It is no exaggeration to say at this point in Earth's history that it is also required. Everything I have seen and learned over the years gives me confidence that we have it in us.

---

†   Although I'll mostly be using "myth" in its contemporary meaning of "fictional" or "misleading," I will have occasion much later in the book to acknowledge the healing power of genuine *mythic thinking*, in the ancient sense of the word.

Part I

Our Interconnected Nature

Because we think in a fragmentary way, we see fragments. And this way of seeing leads us to make actual fragments of the world.

—Susan Griffin, *A Chorus of Stones*

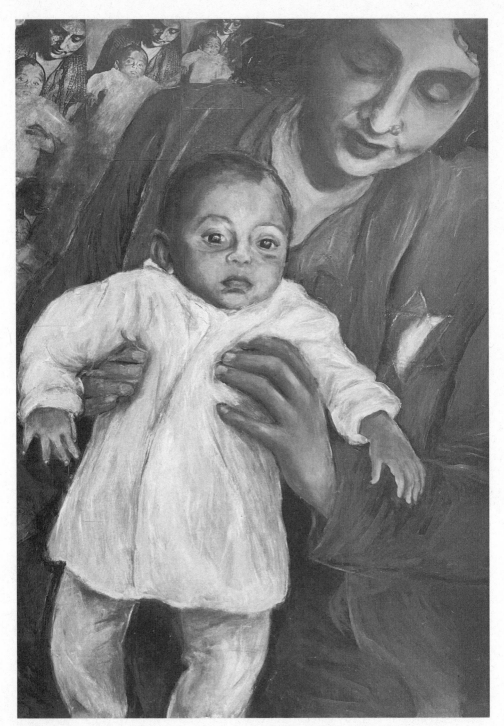

A painting by my wife, Rae, based on a 1944 photograph (seen in the upper left corner) of me at three months, held by my mother, Judith. The yellow star she wears is the badge of shame mandated for Hungarian Jews, as in other Nazi-occupied territories. Rae well captures the haunted look and fear in my infant eyes. Acrylic on canvas, 40 × 30 inches, 1997. www.raemate.com

Chapter 1

The Last Place You Want to Be:
Facets of Trauma

It is hard to imagine the scope of an individual life without
envisioning some kind of trauma, and it is hard for
most people to know what to do about it.

—Mark Epstein, *The Trauma of Everyday Life*[†]

Picture this: At the tender age of seventy-one, six years before this writing, your author arrives back in Vancouver from a
speaking jaunt to Philadelphia. The talk was successful, the audience enthusiastic, my message about addiction and trauma's
impact on people's lives warmly received. I have traveled in unexpected comfort, having been upgraded to the business-class
cabin, thanks to a courtesy from Air Canada. Descending over
Vancouver's pristine sea-to-sky panorama, I am a regular Little
Jack Horner in my corner of the plane, suffused with a "What a
good boy am I" glow. As we touch down and begin to taxi to the
gate, the text from my wife, Rae, lights up the tiny screen: "Sorry.
I haven't left home yet. Do you still want me to come?" I stiffen,
satisfaction displaced by rage. "Never mind," I dictate tersely
into the phone. Embittered, I disembark, clear customs, and take
a taxi home, all of a twenty-minute ride door-to-door. (I trust the
reader is already gripping the pages in empathetic outrage at the

---

†   Mark Epstein is a psychiatrist, Buddhist meditation teacher, and author.

indignity suffered by your author.) Seeing Rae, I growl a hello that is more accusation than greeting, and scarcely look at her. In fact, I barely make eye contact for the next twenty-four hours. When addressed, I utter little more than brief, monotone grunts. My gaze is averted, the upper part of my face tense and rigid, and my jaw in a perma-clench.

What is happening with me? Is this the response of a mature adult in his eighth decade? Only superficially. At times like this, there is very little grown-up Gabor in the mix. Most of me is in the grips of the distant past, near the beginnings of my life. This kind of physio-emotional time warp, preventing me from inhabiting the present moment, is one of the imprints of trauma, an underlying theme for many people in this culture. In fact, it is so deeply "underlying" that many of us don't know it's there.

The meaning of the word "trauma," in its Greek origin, is "wound." Whether we realize it or not, it is our woundedness, or how we cope with it, that dictates much of our behavior, shapes our social habits, and informs our ways of thinking about the world. It can even determine whether or not we are *capable* of rational thought at all in matters of the greatest importance to our lives. For many of us, it rears its head in our closest partnerships, causing all kinds of relational mischief.

It was in 1889 that the pioneering French psychologist Pierre Janet first depicted traumatic memory as being held in "automatic actions and reactions, sensations and attitudes . . . replayed and reenacted in visceral sensations."[1] In the present century, the leading trauma psychologist and healer Peter Levine has written that certain shocks to the organism "can alter a person's biological, psychological, and social equilibrium to such a degree that the memory of one particular event comes to taint, and dominate, all other experiences, spoiling an appreciation of the present moment."[2] Levine calls this "the tyranny of the past."

In my case, the template for my hostility to Rae's message is to be found in the diary my mother kept, in a nearly illegible scrawl and only intermittently, during my first years in wartime and post–World War II Budapest. The following, translated by me from the Hungarian, is her entry on April 8, 1945, when I was fourteen months old:

> My dear little man, only after many long months do I take in hand again the pen, so that I may briefly sketch for you the unspeakable horrors of those times, the details of which I do not wish you to know . . . It was on December 12 that the Crossed-Arrows[†] forced us into the fenced-in Budapest ghetto, from which, with extreme difficulty, we found refuge in a Swiss-protected house. From there, after two days, I sent you by a complete stranger to your Aunt Viola's because I saw that your little organism could not possibly endure the living conditions in that building. Now began the most dreadful five or six weeks of my life, when I couldn't see you.

I survived, thanks to the kindness and courage of the unknown Christian woman to whom my mother entrusted me in the street and who conveyed me to relatives living in hiding under relatively safer circumstances. Reunited with my mother after the Soviet army had put the Germans to flight, I did not so much as look at her for several days.

The great twentieth-century British psychiatrist and psychologist John Bowlby was familiar with such behavior: he called it detachment. At his clinic he observed ten small children who had to endure prolonged separation from their parents due to uncontrollable circumstances. "On meeting mother for the first time

---

†   The viciously anti-Semitic fascist Hungarian political movement and paramilitary allied with the Nazi occupiers.

after days or weeks away every one of the children showed some degree of detachment," Bowlby observed. "Two seemed not to recognize mother. The other eight turned away or even walked away from her. Most of them either cried or came close to tears; a number alternated between a tearful and expressionless face."[3] It may seem counterintuitive, but this reflexive rejection of the loving mother is an adaptation: "I was so hurt when you abandoned me," says the young child's mind, "that I will not reconnect with you. I don't dare open myself to that pain again." In many children—and I was certainly one—early reactions like these become embedded in the nervous system, mind, and body, playing havoc with future relationships. They show up throughout the lifetime in response to any incident even vaguely resembling the original imprint—often without any recall of the inciting circumstances. My petulant and defensive reaction to Rae signaled that old, deep-brain emotional circuits, programmed in infancy, had taken over while the rational, calming, self-regulating parts of my brain went offline.

"All trauma is preverbal," the psychiatrist Bessel van der Kolk has written.[4] His statement is true in two senses. First, the psychic wounds we sustain are often inflicted upon us before our brain is capable of formulating any kind of a verbal narrative, as in my case. Second, even after we become language-endowed, some wounds are imprinted on regions of our nervous systems having nothing to do with language or concepts; this includes brain areas, of course, but the rest of the body, too. They are stored in parts of us that words and thoughts cannot directly access—we might even call this level of traumatic encoding "subverbal." As Peter Levine explains, "Conscious, *explicit* memory is only the proverbial tip of a very deep and mighty iceberg. It barely hints at the submerged strata of *primal implicit experience* that moves us in ways the conscious mind can only begin to imagine."[5]

To her credit, my wife will not allow me to get away with pinning the entire blame for my arrivals-gate hissy fit on Nazis and fascists and infant trauma. Yes, the backstory merits compassion and understanding—and she has given me an abundance of both—but there comes a point when "Hitler made me do it" won't fly. Responsibility can and must be taken. After twenty-four hours of the silent treatment, Rae had had enough. "Oh, knock it off already," she said. And so I did—a measure of progress and relative maturation on my part. In times past, it would have taken me days or longer to "knock it off": to drop my resentment, and for my core to unfreeze, my face to relax, my voice to soften, and my head to turn willingly and with love toward my life partner.

"My problem is that I am married to someone who understands me," I have often grumbled, only partly in jest. Really, of course, my great blessing is to be married to someone with healthy boundaries, who sees me as I am now and who will no longer bear the brunt of my prolonged and unplanned visits to the distant past.

What Trauma Is and What It Does

Trauma's imprint is more endemic than we realize. That may seem a puzzling statement, as "trauma" has become something of a catchword in our society. To boot, the word has taken on a number of colloquial valences that confuse and dilute its meaning. A clear and comprehensive reckoning is warranted, especially in the field of health—and, since everything is connected, in virtually all other societal domains as well.

The usual conception of trauma conjures up notions of catastrophic events: hurricanes, abuse, egregious neglect, and war. This has the unintended and misleading effect of relegating trauma to the realm of the abnormal, the unusual, the exceptional. If there exists a class of people we call "traumatized," that must mean that most of us are not. Here we miss the mark by a wide margin. Trauma pervades our culture, from personal functioning through social relationships, parenting, education, popular culture, economics, and politics. In fact, someone *without* the marks of trauma would be an outlier in our society. We are closer to the truth when we ask: Where do we each fit on the broad and surprisingly inclusive trauma spectrum? Which of its many marks has each of us carried all (or most) of our lives, and what have the impacts been? And what possibilities would open up were we to become more familiar, even intimate, with them?

A more basic question comes first: What is trauma? As I use the word, "trauma" is an inner injury, a lasting rupture or split within the self due to difficult or hurtful events. By this definition, trauma is primarily what happens within someone as a result of the difficult or hurtful events that befall them; it is not the events themselves. "Trauma is not what happens *to* you but what happens *inside* you" is how I formulate it. Think of a car accident where someone sustains a concussion: the accident is what happened; the injury is what lasts. Likewise, trauma is a psychic injury, lodged in our nervous system, mind, and body, lasting long past the originating incident(s), triggerable at any moment. It is a constellation of hardships, composed of the wound itself and the residual burdens that our woundedness imposes on our bodies and souls: the unresolved emotions they visit upon us; the coping dynamics they dictate; the tragic or melodramatic or neurotic scripts we unwittingly but inexorably live out; and, not least, the toll these take on our bodies.

When a wound doesn't mend on its own, one of two things will happen: it can either remain raw or, more commonly, be replaced by a thick layer of scar tissue. As an open sore, it is an ongoing source of pain and a place where we can be hurt over and over again by even the slightest stimulus. It compels us to be ever vigilant—always nursing our wounds, as it were—and leaves us limited in our capacity to move flexibly and act confidently lest we be harmed again. The scar is preferable, providing protection and holding tissues together, but it has its drawbacks: it is tight, hard, inflexible, unable to grow, a zone of numbness. The original healthy, alive flesh is not regenerated.

Raw wound or scar, unresolved trauma is a constriction of the self, both physical and psychological. It constrains our inborn capacities and generates an enduring distortion of our view of the world and of other people. Trauma, until we work it through, keeps us stuck in the past, robbing us of the present moment's riches, limiting who we can be. By impelling us to suppress hurt and unwanted parts of the psyche, it fragments the self. Until seen and acknowledged, it is also a barrier to growth. In many cases, as in mine, it blights a person's sense of worth, poisons relationships, and undermines appreciation for life itself. Early in childhood it may even interfere with healthy brain development. And, as we will witness, trauma is an antecedent and a contributor to illness of all kinds throughout the lifespan.

Taken together, these impacts constitute a major and foundational impediment to flourishing for many, many people. To quote Peter Levine once more, "Trauma is perhaps the most avoided, ignored, belittled, denied, misunderstood, and untreated cause of human suffering."[6]

Two Types of Trauma

Before we go on, let's distinguish two forms of trauma. The first—the sense in which clinicians and teachers like Levine and van der Kolk usually employ the word—involves automatic responses and mind-body adaptations to specific, identifiable hurtful and overwhelming events, whether in childhood or later. As my medical work taught me and as research has amply shown, painful things happen to many children, from outright abuse or severe neglect in the family of origin to the poverty or racism or oppression that are daily features of many societies. The consequences can be terrible. Far more common than usually acknowledged, such traumas give rise to multiple symptoms and syndromes and to conditions diagnosed as pathology, physical or mental—a linkage that remains almost invisible to the eyes of mainstream medicine and psychiatry, except in specific "diseases" like post-traumatic stress disorder. This kind of injury has been called by some "capital-*T* trauma." It underlies much of what gets labeled as mental illness. It also creates a predisposition to physical illness by driving inflammation, elevating physiological stress, and impairing the healthy functioning of genes, among many other mechanisms. To sum up, then, capital-*T* trauma occurs when things happen to vulnerable people that should *not* have happened, as, for example, a child being abused, or violence in the family, or a rancorous divorce, or the loss of a parent. All these are among the criteria for childhood affliction in the well-known adverse childhood experiences (ACE) studies. Once again, the traumatic events themselves are not identical to the trauma—the injury to self—that occurs in their immediate wake within the person.

There is another form of trauma—and this is the kind I am calling nearly universal in our culture—that has sometimes been termed "small-*t* trauma." I have often witnessed what long-lasting marks seemingly ordinary events—what a seminal researcher poignantly called the "less memorable but hurtful and far more prevalent misfortunes of childhood"—can leave on the psyches of children.[7] These might include bullying by peers, the casual but repeated harsh comments of a well-meaning parent, or even just a lack of sufficient emotional connection with the nurturing adults.

Children, especially highly sensitive children, can be wounded in multiple ways: by bad things happening, yes, but also by good things not happening, such as their emotional needs for attunement not being met, or the experience of not being seen and accepted, even by loving parents. Trauma of this kind does not require overt distress or misfortune of the sort mentioned above and can also lead to the pain of disconnection from the self, occurring as a result of core needs not being satisfied. Such non-events are what the British pediatrician D. W. Winnicott referred to as "nothing happening when something might profitably have happened"—a subject we will return to when we consider human development. "The traumas of everyday life can easily make us feel like a motherless child," writes the psychiatrist Mark Epstein.[8]

If, despite decades of evidence, "big-*T* trauma" has barely registered on the medical radar screen, small-*t* trauma does not even cause a blip.

Even as we make this distinction between big-*T* and small-*t* traumas, given the continuum and broad spectrum of human experience, let's keep in mind that in real life the lines are fluid, are not easily drawn, and should not be rigidly maintained. What the two types share is succinctly summarized by Bessel van der Kolk: "Trauma is when we are not seen and known."

Although there are dramatic differences in the way the two forms of trauma can affect people's lives and functioning— the big-*T* variety, in general, being far more distressing and disabling—there is also much overlap. They both represent a fracturing of the self and of one's relationship to the world. *That fracturing is the essence of trauma.* As Peter Levine writes, trauma "is about a loss of connection—to ourselves, our families, and the world around us. This loss is hard to recognize, because it happens slowly, over time. We adapt to these subtle changes;

sometimes without noticing them."[9] As the lost connection gets internalized, it forges our view of reality: we come to believe in the world we see through its cracked lens. It is sobering to realize that who we take ourselves to be and the ways we habitually act, including many of our seeming "strengths"—the least and the most functional aspects of our "normal" selves—are often, in part, the wages of traumatic loss. It may also be disconcerting for many of us to consider that, as happy and well adjusted as we think ourselves to be, we may fall somewhere on the trauma spectrum, even if far from the capital-*T* pole. Ultimately, comparisons fail. It doesn't matter whether we can point to other people who seem more traumatized than we are, for there is no comparing suffering. Nor is it appropriate to use our own trauma as a way of placing ourselves above others—"You haven't suffered like I have"—or as a cudgel to beat back others' legitimate grievances when we behave destructively. We each carry our wounds in our own way; there is neither sense nor value in gauging them against those of others.

What Trauma Is Not

Most of us have heard someone, perhaps ourselves, say something like "Oh my God, that movie last night was so disturbing, I left the theater traumatized." Or we've read a (typically dismissive) news story about university students agitating for "content warnings" lest they be "retraumatized" by what they hear. In all these cases, the usage is understandable but misplaced; what people are actually referring to in these cases is *stress,* physical and/or emotional. As Peter Levine aptly points out, "Certainly, all traumatic events are stressful, but not all stressful events are traumatic."[10]

An event is traumatizing, or retraumatizing, only if it renders one *diminished,* which is to say psychically (or physically) *more limited* than before in a way that *persists*. Much in life, including in art and/or social intercourse or politics, may be upsetting, distressing, even very painful without being newly traumatic. That is not to say that old traumatic reactions, having nothing to do with whatever's going on, cannot be triggered by present-day stresses—see, for example, a certain author arriving home from a speaking gig. That is not the same as being retraumatized, unless over time it leaves us even more constricted than before.

Here's a fairly reliable process-of-elimination checklist. It is *not* trauma if the following remain true over the long term:

– It does not limit you, constrict you, diminish your capacity to feel or think or to trust or assert yourself, to experience suffering without succumbing to despair or to witness it with compassion.
– It does not keep you from holding your pain and sorrow and fear without being overwhelmed and without having to escape habitually into work or compulsive self-soothing or self-stimulating by whatever means.
– You are not left compelled either to aggrandize yourself or to efface yourself for the sake of gaining acceptance or to justify your existence.
– It does not impair your capacity to experience gratitude for the beauty and wonder of life.

If, on the other hand, you *do* recognize these chronic constraints in yourself, they might well represent trauma's shadow on your psyche, the presence of an unhealed emotional wound, no matter the size of the *t*.

Trauma Separates Us from Our Bodies

"Once somebody has invaded you and entered you, your body is no longer yours," the writer V, formerly known as Eve Ensler, told me, recalling her sexual abuse by her father as a young girl.[†] "It's a landscape of dread and betrayal and sorrow and cruelty. The last place you want to be is in your body. And so, you begin to live in your head, you begin to live up here without any ability to protect your body, to know your body. Look, I had a tumor the size of an avocado inside me, and I didn't know it— that's how separated I was from myself." Although the details of my past diverge wildly from V's, I know whereof she speaks. For many years the most difficult question that could be put to me was "What are you feeling?" My customary response was an irritated "How should I know?" I faced no such problem on being asked what my thoughts were: on those I am a tenured expert. Not knowing how or what one feels, on the other hand, is a sure sign of disconnect from the body.

What causes such a disconnect? In my case, the answer requires no speculation. As an infant in wartime Hungary, I endured chronic hunger and dysentery, states of acute discomfort threatening and distressing to adults, let alone to a one-year-old. I also absorbed the terrors and unrelenting emotional distress of my mother. In the absence of relief, a young person's natural response—their only response, really—is to repress and disconnect from the feeling-states associated with suffering. One no longer knows one's body. Oddly, this self-estrangement can show up later in life in the form of an apparent *strength*, such as my ability to perform at a high level when hungry or stressed or fatigued, pushing on without awareness of my need for pause, nutrition, or rest. Alternatively, some people's disconnection from their bodies manifests as not knowing when to stop eating or drinking—the "enough" signal doesn't get through.

In whatever form, disconnection is prominent in the life

[†]   See chapter 6, first paragraph and footnote.

experience of traumatized people and is an essential aspect of the trauma constellation. As was the case for V, it begins as a natural coping mechanism on the organism's part, and a mandatory one. She could not have survived her childhood horrors had she stayed present in and aware of her moment-by-moment experience of physical and emotional torment, fully taking in what was happening. And so these coping mechanisms ride in on the wings of grace, as it were, to save our lives in the short term. Over time, though, if untended to, they become stamped on the psyche and soma, indelibly so, as conditioned responses harden into fixed mechanisms that no longer suit the situation. The result is chronic suffering and frequently, as we will proceed to explore, even disease.

"What was so remarkable about my encounter with cancer," V told me, "was that the whole journey from waking up after a nine-hour surgery and losing several organs and seventy nodes—I woke up with bags and tubes and everything coming out of me, but for the first time in my life, I was a body . . . It was painful, but it was also exhilarating. It was like, 'I'm a body. Oh my God, I'm here. *I'm inside this body.*'" Her account of a sudden at-home-ness in her physical self is emblematic of how healing works: when trauma's shackles begin to loosen, we gladly reunite with the severed parts of ourselves.

Trauma Splits Us Off from Gut Feelings

For the average person in V's early predicament, Nature's best recommendations would be to escape or to fight back against the misuse of her body and the assault on her soul. But therein lies the rub: neither option is available to a small child, for to attempt either would be to put herself in further jeopardy. Therefore, Nature defaults to plan C: both impulses are suppressed by tuning out the emotions that would propel such responses. This suppression would seem to be akin to the *freeze* response that creatures often display when *fight* and *flight* are both impossible. The crucial difference is this: once the hawk is gone, the possum is free to go about his business, his survival strategy having succeeded. A traumatized nervous system, on the other hand, never gets to *un*freeze.

"We have feelings because they tell us what supports our survival and what detracts from our survival," the late neuroscientist Jaak Panksepp once said. Emotions, he stressed, emerge not from the thinking brain but from ancient brain structures associated with survival. They are drivers and guarantors of life and development. Intense rage activates the fight response; intense fear mobilizes flight. Therefore, if the circumstances dictate that these natural, healthy impulses (to defend or run away) must be quelled, their gut-level cues—the feelings themselves—will have to be suppressed as well. No alarm, no mobilization. If this seems self-defeating, it is so only in a limited sense: on an existential level, it is the "least worst" option, being the only available one that reduces risk of further harm.

The result is a tamping down of one's feeling-world and often, for extra protection, the hardening of one's psychic shell. A vivid example is given by the writer Tara Westover in her bestselling memoir, *Educated*. Here she recalls the impact of abuse at the hands of a sibling, willfully ignored by her parents:

> I saw myself as unbreakable, tender as stone. At first I merely believed this, until one day it became the truth. Then I was able to tell myself, without lying, that it didn't affect me, that *he* didn't affect me, because nothing affected me. I didn't understand how morbidly right I was. How I had hollowed myself out. For all my obsessing over the consequences of that night, I had misunderstood the vital truth: that its not affecting me, that *was* its effect.[11] [Italics in original.]

Trauma Limits Response Flexibility

A flashback to our chapter's tragic opening scene, only this time set in a parallel universe where my trauma imprints don't rule the day: The plane lands and Rae's text pops up on my screen. "Hmm, that's not what I expected," I say to myself. "But I get it: she's probably immersed in her painting. Nothing new there, nor anything personal. Actually, I can empathize: How many times have *I* gotten so absorbed in work that the clock got away from me? Okay, taxi it is." I might well notice some disappointed feelings, in which case I allow myself to feel them until they pass; in effect, I choose vulnerability over victimhood. Arriving home, there is no upset, no emotional detaching, no sulking—maybe some gentle teasing, but all within the bounds of loving humor and with affinity intact.

I would have thus exhibited what is called *response flexibility*: the ability to choose how we address life's inevitable ups and downs, its disappointments, triumphs, and challenges. "Human freedom involves our capacity to pause between stimulus and response and, in that pause, to choose the one response toward which we wish to throw our weight," wrote the psychologist Rollo May.[12] Trauma robs us of that freedom.

Response flexibility is a function of the midfrontal portion of our cerebral cortex. No infant is born with any such capacity: babies' behavior is governed by instinct and reflex, not conscious selection. The freedom to choose develops as the brain develops. The more severe and the earlier the trauma, the less opportunity response flexibility has to become encoded in the appropriate brain circuits, and the faster it becomes disabled. One becomes stuck in predictable, automatic defensive reactions, especially to stressful stimuli. Emotionally and cognitively, our range of movement becomes well-nigh sclerotic—and the greater the trauma, the more stringent the constraints. The past hijacks and co-opts the present, again and again.

Trauma Fosters a Shame-Based View of the Self

One of the saddest letters I have ever received was from a Seattle man who had read my book on addiction, *In the Realm of Hungry Ghosts*, in which I show that addiction is an outcome—not the only one possible, but a prevalent one—of childhood trauma. Nine years sober, he was still struggling, had not worked for a decade, and was being treated for obsessive-compulsive disorder (OCD). Although he found the book fascinating, he wrote, "I resist the opportunity to blame my mother. I'm a piece of shit because of me." I could only sigh: self-assaulting shame so easily moonlights as personal responsibility. Moreover, he had missed the point: there is nothing in my book that blamed parents or advocated doing so—in fact, I explain over several pages why parent-blaming is inappropriate, inaccurate, and unscientific. This man's impulse to protect his mother was not a defense against anything I had said or implied but against his own unacknowledged anger. Stored away in deep-freeze and finding no healthy outlet, the emotion had turned against him in the form of self-hatred.

"Contained in the experience of shame," writes the psychologist Gershen Kaufman, "is a piercing awareness of ourselves as fundamentally deficient in some vital way as a human being."[3] People bearing trauma's scars almost uniformly develop a shame-based view of themselves at the core, a negative self-perception most of them are all too conscious of. Among the most poisonous consequences of shame is the loss of compassion for oneself. The more severe the trauma, the more total that loss.

The negative view of self may not always penetrate conscious awareness and may even masquerade as its opposite: high self-regard. Some people encase themselves in an armored coat of grandiosity and denial of any shortcomings so as not to feel that enervating shame. That self-puffery is as sure a manifestation of self-loathing as is abject self-deprecation, albeit a much more normalized one. It is a marker of our culture's insanity that certain individuals who flee from shame into a shameless narcissism may even achieve great social, economic, and political status and success. Our culture grinds many of the most traumatized into the mud but may also—depending on class background, economic resources, race, and other variables—raise a few to the highest positions of power.

The most common form shame assumes in this culture is the belief that "I am not enough." The writer Elizabeth Wurtzel, who died of breast cancer at age fifty-two in 2020, suffered depression from an early age. Her childhood was traumatic, beginning with a secret deliberately kept from her about who her actual father was. "I was intensely downcast," she chronicled in an autobiographical piece for *New York* magazine, "with a chronic depression that began when I was about 10, but instead of killing my will, it motivated me: I thought if I could be good enough at whatever task, great or small, that was before me, I might have a few minutes of happiness."[14] That conviction of one's inadequacy has fueled a great many glittering careers and instigated many instances of illness, often both in the same individual.

Trauma Distorts Our View of the World

"Everything has mind in the lead, has mind in the forefront, is made by the mind." Thus opens the *Dhammapada*, the Buddha's timeless collection of sayings.[15] Put another way, the world we believe in becomes the world we live in. If I see the world as a hostile place where only winners thrive, I may well become aggressive, selfish, and grandiose to survive in such a milieu. Later in life I will gravitate to competitive environments and endeavors that can only confirm that view and reinforce its validity. Our beliefs are not only self-fulfilling; they are world-building.

Here's what the Buddha left out, if I may be so bold: before the mind can create the world, the world creates our minds. Trauma, especially severe trauma, imposes a worldview tinged with pain, fear, and suspicion: a lens that both distorts and determines our view of how things are. Or it may, through the sheer force of denial, engender a naively rosy perspective that blinds us to real and present dangers—a veneer concealing fears we dare not acknowledge. One may also come to dismiss painful realities by habitually lying to oneself and others.

Trauma Alienates Us from the Present

I once shared a meal in an Oslo restaurant with the German psychologist Franz Ruppert. The noise was overwhelming: loud pop music pumping through several speakers and multiple TV channels blaring from bright screens mounted high on the walls. I have to think that when the great Norwegian playwright Henrik Ibsen used to hold court in that same establishment a little over a century before, the ambience was much more serene. "What's this all about?" I shouted to my companion over the cacophony, shaking my head in exasperation. "Trauma," he replied as he shrugged his shoulders. Ruppert meant, simply, that people were desperately seeking an escape from themselves.

If trauma entails a disconnection from the self, then it makes sense to say that we are being collectively flooded with influences that both exploit and reinforce trauma. Work pressures, multitasking, social media, news updates, multiplicities of entertainment sources—these all induce us to become lost in thoughts, frantic activities, gadgets, meaningless conversations. We are caught up in pursuits of all kinds that draw us on not because they are necessary or inspiring or uplifting, or because they enrich or add meaning to our lives, but simply because they obliterate the present. In an absurd twist, we save up to buy the latest "time-saving" devices, the better to "kill" time. Awareness of the moment has become something to fear. Late-stage capitalism is expert in catering to this sense of present-moment dread—in fact, much of its success depends on the chasm between us and the present, our greatest gift, getting ever wider, the false products and artificial distractions of consumer culture designed to fill in the gap.

What is lost is well described by the Polish-born writer[†] Eva Hoffman as "*nothing more or less than the experience of experience itself. And what is that? Perhaps something like the capacity to enter into the textures or sensations of the moment; to relax enough so as to give oneself over to the rhythms of an episode or a personal encounter, to follow the thread of feeling or thought without knowing where it leads, or to pause long enough for reflection or contemplation.*"[16] Ultimately, what we are distracted from is living.

It Didn't Start with You

Jessica, a sixty-seven-year-old resident of Regina, Saskatchewan, is caring for her two grandchildren, their father—her son—having died of an overdose. Her other son suffered the same fate. As I interviewed her, it occurred to me that Jessica even being willing to speak with me was remarkable, knowing my view that addiction originates in childhood trauma, most often in the family of origin. "When I go back and look at my sons' lives, I understand that there was a lot of trauma," she explained. "I was living with them, so I was part of that. I was a single parent from the time they were two and three until I remarried, when they were six and seven. I understand that how I lived, what I was doing, what I knew and what I didn't know, affected them."

After the birth father abandoned the family early, a stepfather abused the boys both physically and emotionally. "I was very

---

† And fellow 1950s émigré to Vancouver, now a longtime London resident.

lonely and scared and feeling trapped," Jessica recalled. That she would lack the gut-sense not to choose such men and that she would not assert herself and protect her sons in the face of abuse were the marks of a wounding sustained in Jessica's own childhood. Though aware she was loved, she was also left alone with deep emotional distress that, over time, she was forced to disconnect from. "I was ashamed a lot for my feelings as a child," she recalled. "I was very sensitive, and I cried a lot."

Trauma is in most cases multigenerational. The chain of transmission goes from parent to child, stretching from the past into the future. We pass on to our offspring what we haven't resolved in ourselves. The home becomes a place where we unwittingly re-create, as I did, scenarios reminiscent of those that wounded us when we were small. "Traumas affect mothers and mothering and fathers and fathering and husbanding and wifeing," the family constellations therapist Mark Wolynn told me. "The repeated traumas continue to proliferate from that—as a result, they never get healed." Wolynn is the author of the aptly titled *It Didn't Start with You: How Inherited Family Trauma Shapes Who We Are and How to End the Cycle*. Trauma may even affect gene activity across generations, as we will see.[†]

It is no surprise, then, that Jessica's eldest grandchild has faced problems with substance use and behavior and learning difficulties. Because of all she has learned and despite her unfathomable losses, she is able to be present for him much more warmly and effectively than she ever could be for her own sons. Note, too, the absence of self-judgment in Jessica's description of the situation: she speaks of "understanding" rather than castigating herself for what she didn't—nay, couldn't—understand way back when. The act of blaming herself, its gravitational center planted

---

†   Chapter 4.

permanently in the past, would only divert her from showing up for her loved one in the here and now.

Blame becomes a meaningless concept the moment one understands how suffering in a family system or even in a community extends back through the generations. "Recognition of this quickly dispels any disposition to see the parent as villain," wrote John Bowlby, the British psychiatrist who showed the decisive importance of adult-child relationships in shaping the psyche. No matter how far back we look in the chain of consequence— great-grandparents, pre-modern ancestors, Adam and Eve, the first single-celled amoeba—the accusing finger can find no fixed target. That should come as a relief.

The news gets better: seeing trauma as an internal dynamic grants us much-needed agency. If we treat trauma as an external event, something that happens *to* or around us, then it becomes a piece of history we can never dislodge. If, on the other hand, trauma is what took place *inside* us as a result of what happened, in the sense of wounding or disconnection, then healing and reconnection become tangible possibilities. Trying to keep awareness of trauma at bay hobbles our capacity to know ourselves. Conversely, fashioning from it a rock-hard identity— whether the attitude is defiance, cynicism, or self-pity—is to miss both the point and the opportunity of healing, since by definition trauma represents a distortion and limitation of who we were born to be. Facing it directly without either denial or over-identification becomes a doorway to health and balance.

"It's those adversities that open up your mind and your curiosity to see if there are new ways of doing things," Bessel van der Kolk told me. He then cited Socrates: "An unexamined life is not worth living. As long as one doesn't examine oneself, one is completely subject to whatever one is wired to do, but once you become aware that you have choices, you can exercise those choices." Notice that he didn't say "once you spend decades in therapy." As I will present later, we can access liberation via even modest self-examination: a willingness to question "many of the truths we cling to" and the "certain point of view" that makes them seem so real—as a famous Jedi master's Force ghost told his dispirited young apprentice at a pivotal moment in a galaxy far, far away.[†]

Although this chapter has focused on its personal dimensions, trauma exists in the collective sphere, too, affecting entire nations and peoples at different moments in history. To this day it is visited upon some groups with disproportionate force, as on Canada's Indigenous people. Their multigenerational deprivation and persecution at the hands of colonialism and especially the hundred-year agony of their children, abducted from their families and reared in church-run residential schools where physical, sexual, and emotional abuse were rampant, has left them with tragic legacies of addiction, mental and physical illness, suicide, and the ongoing transmission of trauma to new generations. The traumatic legacy of slavery and racism in the United States is another salient example. I will have more to say about this painful subject in Part IV.

[†]   Obi-Wan Kenobi to Luke Skywalker in 1983's *Return of the Jedi.*

Chapter 2

Living in an Immaterial World: Emotions, Health, and the Body-Mind Unity

Unless we can measure something, science won't concede
it exists, which is why science refuses to deal with such
"nonthings" as the emotions, the mind, the soul, or the spirit.
—Candace Pert, Ph.D., *Molecules of Emotion*

"I was thirty-six when they told me it was a very early breast cancer," said Caroline, a resident of the Pocono Mountains of Pennsylvania. That diagnosis occurred more than three decades ago, in 1988. The tumor was treated with surgery and radiation. A few years later, when a new malignancy showed up in her left hip and femur, Caroline required emergency joint replacement; the surgeons had to remove a large part of her thigh bone as well. "At that time, they gave me a timeline of one to two years," she recalled. "My boys were very young, only eight and nine. I've just turned fifty-six, so I've beaten all their records."

Caroline had multiple courses of chemotherapy over the intervening years. By the time of our conversation, the cancer had reached the palliative stage, having spread to her right hip and thigh. As we spoke, she could not expect to outpace her current prognosis by much;‡ still, this mother of two radiated deep satis-

---

‡   I was saddened to learn of her death, about a year after our interview.

faction with how things had gone. She had, after all, gained two unforeseen decades to raise her kids. "You know," she mused, "looking at my own mortality, and them telling me I had twelve to twenty-four months . . . I got extremely profane with the doctor and said, you know, sorry, I need ten years to raise them to be men. I will do anything in my power to raise them to be men."

" 'Profane,' " I repeated. "What exactly did you say?"

"I used the f-word. I said, 'Fuck your statistics.' "

"Good for you," I offered. "That probably helped extend your life."

"Well, that's what I said to him." Caroline laughed. "I said, 'Fuck your statistics. I need those years to raise them to be men.' He walked out of the room. He didn't appreciate my language. He thought I was a crazy, vulgar woman. I've often wanted to look for that doctor—he has since moved to California—and tell him that my boys are now twenty-four and twenty-five. One's in grad school at Princeton. The other one went through a difficult period, pulled himself up, and will be graduating with three degrees, on the dean's list."

Caroline's outburst at the unsuspecting physician was out of character. All her life she had fit the profile of the nice person who avoids confrontation. "My way was always being the caretaker, being needed, always coming to somebody's rescue, a lot of the time to my own detriment," she told me. "I never wanted to have conflict with anyone. And I always had to be in charge, making sure everything was okay." Caroline had exhibited what has been called "superautonomous self-sufficiency,"[†] which means exactly what it sounds like: an exaggerated and outsize aversion to asking anything of anyone.

A quick note: Nobody is born with such traits. They invariably stem from coping reactions to developmental trauma, beginning

---

†   A phrase coined in 1982 by researchers at Heidelberg University, Germany.

with self-abnegation in early childhood. Such suppression takes a lasting toll, a process we'll explore more fully in chapter 7.

"I've come to believe that virtually all illness, if not psychosomatic in foundation, has a definite psychosomatic component," the pioneering neuroscientist Candace Pert wrote in her 1997 book, *Molecules of Emotion.* By "psychosomatic," Pert did not imply the modern, often derisive dismissal of disease as a neurotic figment. Instead she meant the word's strict scientific connotation: having to do with the oneness of the human *psyche* (mind and spirit) and the *soma* (the body), a oneness she did much to measure and record in the laboratory. Her discoveries, as she justly claimed, would help fuel "a synthesis of behavior, psychology, and biology."[1]

There is nothing novel about the notion of the mind and body being intricately linked; if anything, what is new is the belief, tacitly held and overtly enacted by many well-meaning doctors, that they are separable. Traditional healing practices the world over, while lacking the wondrous technology and scientific know-how developed in the West, have long understood this unity implicitly. Despite Western medicine's artificial cleaving of the two, most people still know—if only on a gut level—that what they think and how they feel have everything to do with each other. It is run-of-the-mill, for instance, to speculate about which life stresses have contributed to one's ulcer, what mental strain is behind a headache, or what unprocessed fears lead one to experience panic attacks. The same principle applies when we look not just at individual symptoms but at most types of diseases. Emotional perturbances stemming from relationship troubles, financial worries, or any other source of chronic upset impose physiological burdens that can result in illness.

Pert coined the term "bodymind" to describe this oneness. The official website dedicated to her work and legacy takes care to note that this expression was "intentionally written without a hyphen *in order to emphasize unity of its component parts.*" Body and mind, while not identical, cannot be understood separately from each other. We can ignore or deny this paradox, but we cannot escape it. Since Pert's groundbreaking work, the biological impacts of emotions—those "nonthings" whose non-recognition she lamented—have been extensively researched and documented in many thousands upon thousands of ingenious studies. It's worth looking at a few of these, bearing in mind that each is only the tip of an iceberg of similarly compelling findings.

A 1982 German study presented at the fourth international Symposium on the Prevention and Detection of Cancer in London found certain personality traits to have a strong association with breast cancer. Fifty-six women admitted to hospital for biopsy were evaluated for characteristics such as emotional suppression, rationalization, altruistic behavior, the avoidance of conflict, and the superautonomous self-sufficiency we saw embodied by Caroline. Based on the interview results alone, both the interviewers and "blind" raters who had no direct contact with the women were able to predict the correct diagnosis in up to 94 percent of all cancer patients, and in about 70 percent of the benign cases.[2] In a previous British study at King's College Hospital in London, it had also been shown that women with cancerous breast lumps characteristically exhibited "extreme suppression of anger and of other feelings" in "a significantly higher proportion" than the control group, which was made up of women admitted for biopsy at the same time but found to have benign breast tumors.[3]

In 2000 the publication *Cancer Nursing* surveyed the relationship of anger repression and cancer, often noted by, among others, the cancer nurses themselves: "Somehow, nurses had an intuitive understanding that this 'niceness' was deleterious.

[This] view now is being supported by research."[4] The nurses' insight reminded me of a paper on amyotrophic lateral sclerosis (ALS)[†] presented by two Cleveland Clinic neurologists at an international congress in Bavaria in the 1990s.[5] Their staff, too, found that their ALS patients were extraordinarily nice—so much so, that the staff could in most cases accurately predict who would be diagnosed with the condition and who would not. "I'm afraid this person has ALS, she is too nice," they would jot on the patient's file. Or, "This person cannot have ALS, he is not nice enough." The neurologists were dumbfounded. "In spite of the briefness of [the staff's] contact with the patients, and the obvious unscientific method by which they form their opinions, almost invariably they prove to be correct," they remarked.

I interviewed Dr. Asa J. Wilbourn, senior author of the paper. "It's almost universal," he told me. "It becomes common knowledge in the laboratory where you evaluate a lot of patients with ALS—and we do an enormous number of cases. I think that anyone who deals with ALS knows that this is a definite phenomenon." Such anecdotal observations have since been reaffirmed by more formal research, as seen in the title of a recent paper from a neurological journal: " 'Patients with Amyotrophic Lateral Sclerosis (ALS) Are Usually Nice Persons'—How Physicians Experienced in ALS See the Personality Characteristics of Their Patients."[6]

In a study of men with prostate cancer, anger suppression was associated with a diminished effectiveness of natural killer (NK) cells—a frontline immune system defense against malignancy and foreign invaders. These cells play a key role in tumor resistance.[7] In previous research, NK cell activity was reduced in healthy young people in response to even relatively minor

---

†   A degenerative and nearly always fatal disease of the nervous system, it is known in Britain as motor neuron disease and in the United States also as Lou Gehrig's disease.

stresses—especially for those who were emotionally isolated, a significant source of chronic stress.

Grief, too, has a powerful physiological dimension. An illuminating study from the British journal *Lancet Oncology* described the impact of psychological factors on the intricate pathways linking the immune system, the hormones, and the nervous system in, for example, bereavement. Among parents who lost an adult son to an accident or military conflict, the authors reported increased occurrence of lymphatic and hematological malignancy—cancers of the blood, bone marrow, and lymph nodes—along with skin and lung cancer.[8] War kills, and so, it seems, can deep emotional loss. As for cancer, so with other illnesses. In a Danish nationwide study, grieving parents had double the risk of multiple sclerosis.[9]

(Despite such compelling evidence, I do not believe the loss of a loved one, howsoever tragic, by itself necessarily poses a health risk. I believe the latter depends on how people are able to process their loss, including what support they may reach out for and receive. It's not only events as such but also our emotional responses and how we process them that affect our physiology.)

One 2019 study alone in *Cancer Research* should set every clinician on a fast-track exploration of bodymind medicine. Women with severe post-traumatic stress disorder (PTSD) were found to have twice the risk of ovarian cancer as women with no known trauma exposure.[10] The *Daily Gazette*, published by Harvard University, where the study was done, reported, "The findings indicate that having higher levels of PTSD symptoms, such as being easily startled by ordinary noises or avoiding reminders of the traumatic experience, can be associated with increased risks of ovarian cancer even decades after women experience a traumatic event." The more severe the trauma symptoms, the more aggressive the cancer proved to be.

This Harvard research provided further striking evidence that emotional stresses are inseparable from the physical states of our bodies, in illness and health. Already in previous work, depression had been associated with elevated ovarian cancer risk. The impact of stress had also been studied: among lab mice with ovarian cancer cells injected into their abdominal cavities, those subjected to emotional aggravation such as being physically restrained or isolated had much greater incidence of tumor growth and spread than socially housed animals that were not restrained.[11] The Harvard scientists theorized that stress can "promote ovarian cancer development by inhibiting key defenses against unrestrained cell growth." In other words, stress may disable our immune systems' capacity to control and eliminate malignancy.

The implications extend far beyond PTSD, since, in our culture, stress and trauma affect many people who do not qualify for that diagnosis. Finnish researchers, writing in the *British Journal of Psychiatry* in 2005, found, quite remarkably, that people undergoing "life events"—relatively ordinary stresses and emotional losses such as relationship issues and work problems that would not qualify them for a formal diagnosis—suffered more PTSD-like symptoms such as bad dreams or emotional numbing than more obviously traumatized people who had endured war or disaster.[12]

The Harvard paper on ovarian cancer pointed to some promising possibilities for treatment, suggesting that women whose PTSD symptoms had abated, perhaps due to effective psychotherapy, had less risk for malignancy than women with active symptoms. It is exciting to contemplate the preventive and healing potentials, as well as the social implications, of a wellness perspective that treats emotions like the real and relevant "things" they are.

While all this is timely and the science freshly minted, the principles are not new. In a 1939 lecture to a graduating medical class, published in the *Journal of the American Medical Association* (*JAMA*), Dr. Soma Weiss informed his audience that "social and psychic factors play a role in every disease, *but in many conditions, they represent dominant influences.*"[13] The revered Hungarian-American clinician added that "mental factors represent as active a force in the treatment of patients as chemical and physical agents." He made these comments not as a psychoanalytic theoretician, but as a respected practitioner of pathophysiology and pharmacotherapy—the use of medications in treating illness. At Harvard Medical School, Weiss's memory is kept alive by a yearly research day in his honor, yet his integrative perspective, and the extensive scientific literature now supporting it, still elude conventional medical thinking. "The mind-body stuff is historically something that one pursues at great peril to their career at Harvard," a leading physician and academic at that hallowed institution told me recently. "That's starting to change, but it's a very difficult thing."[14]

Difficult indeed. When I give talks, I often ask audience members to raise their hands if, in the past five years, they have visited a neurologist, cardiologist, respirologist, rheumatologist, gastroenterologist, dermatologist, immunologist—"any kind of a medical ologist," I say. Many hands shoot up. "Now keep your hands up," I continue, "if these specialists asked you about your childhood stresses or traumas, your relationship with your parents, the quality of your current relationships, your degree of loneliness or companionship, your job satisfaction and how you relate to work, how you feel about your boss or how your boss treats you, your experience of joy or anger, any present stresses, or how you feel about yourself as a person." In rooms packed with hundreds of people, the number of hands remaining elevated can most often be counted on the fingers of one of them. "And yet," I add, "those unasked questions had everything to do with why most of you had reason to seek medical help."

For all that, a clear picture is emerging as modern research confirms traditional wisdom. A (relatively) new science, psychoneuroimmunology maps the myriad pathways of the body-mind unity; its field of study includes the connections between emotions and our nervous and immune systems, and how stress might instigate disease. Even "connection" is a misleading word: only entities distinct from each other can be connected, whereas reality knows only oneness. Sometimes referred to even more tongue-twistingly as psychoneuroimmunoendocrinology, this new discipline is predicated on the unity between *all* our constituent parts: mind, brain, nervous and immune systems, and the hormonal apparatus (that's the "endocrine" part). The pieces can be studied separately, but we cannot fully understand any of them without grasping the whole picture. From the cerebral cortex to the brain's emotional nuclei to the autonomic nervous system, from the solid or fluid aspects of the immune apparatus to the hormonal organs and secretions, from the stress-response system to the viscera . . . it's all one.

That evolution has furnished us with instincts, emotions, complex behaviors, and individuated organs and systems does not, in the slightest way, diminish this unity. No matter how sophisticated our minds may be, the fact remains that their basic contents—what we think, believe consciously or unconsciously, feel or are prevented from feeling—powerfully affect our bodies, for better or worse. Conversely, what our bodies experience from conception onward cannot but affect how we think, feel, perceive, and behave. This, in a nutshell, is psychoneuroimmunology's core lesson.

One fascinating example is the demonstrated link between

the brain's fear center, the amygdala, and cardiovascular disease. The more stress someone perceives or experiences, the higher the resting activity of the amygdala and the greater the risk of heart ailments. The pathway from amygdala overactivation to heart problems runs through increased bone-marrow activity and arterial inflammation.[15] Emotional stress affects the heart more generally as well. In 2012, a study from Harvard Medical School showed that women with high job strain are 67 percent more likely to experience a heart attack than women in less stressful jobs.[16] A Canadian study from the University of Toronto in the same year found that men sexually abused as children had a tripled rate of heart attacks.[17] The researchers' natural assumption was that abused men would be more prone to high-risk behavior, such as smoking and drinking, which would account for their higher rate of heart attacks. To the team's surprise, the impacts of abuse were more direct, quite independent of behavioral factors.

The Machinery of Stress

Understanding stress and its mechanics can give us a finer appreciation for how the bodymind unity plays itself out in real time and real tissue.

Like its cousin, the pain response, stress is a mandatory survival function for any living being. When activated, our stress apparatus immediately empowers us to confront or escape threats to our existence or to the existence or well-being of those we care for. It's an impressive whole-body event involving virtually every organ and system.

Stress can show up in two forms: as an immediate reaction to a threat or as a prolonged state induced by external pressures or internal emotional factors. While *acute* stress is a necessary reaction that helps maintain our physical and mental integrity, *chronic stress,* ongoing and unrelieved, undermines both. Situational anger, for example, is an instance of acute stress being marshaled for a positive purpose—think self-defense or setting interpersonal boundaries. It makes us more alert of mind, quicker, and stronger of limb. Chronic rage, by contrast, floods the system with stress hormones long past the allotted time. Over the long term, such a hormonal surplus, whatever may have instigated it, can

- make us anxious or depressed;
- suppress immunity;
- promote inflammation;
- narrow blood vessels, promoting vascular disease throughout the body;
- encourage cancer growth;
- thin the bones;
- make us resistant to our own insulin, inducing diabetes;
- contribute to abdominal obesity, elevating the risk of cardiovascular and metabolic problems;
- impair essential cognitive and emotional circuits in the brain; and
- elevate blood pressure and increase blood clotting, raising the risk of heart attacks or strokes.

The hub of our body's system for handling stress smoothly and economically is called the "HPA axis." This acronymic term describes the pathways and feedback loops linking the *hypothalamus*—the small, crucial area in the center of our brain whose role is to keep our body in a healthful, balanced state—with the *pituitary gland* at the top of our brain stem and the *adrenal gland* that sits atop our kidneys. Think of a busy transportation corridor connecting three major urban centers, replete with on-ramps, exits, and interchanges, and you start to get a picture.

Although our species can survive in a broad range of *external* environments—far more than almost any other animal—our *internal* milieu must stay within a relatively narrow range of physiological states. Our temperature, blood acidity or pressure, and heart rate, along with many other bodily metrics, are all obliged by Nature, on pain of death, to stay within definite and nonnegotiable limits.

The renowned American stress researcher Bruce McEwen[†] popularized the word "allostasis" to capture the body's attempt to maintain inner equilibrium in the face of changing circumstances. The term is a combination of the Greek words *allo,* for "variable," and *stasis*, for "standing" or "stoppage"; combined, we have something like "staying the same amid change." We cannot do without it, and so our bodies will go to great lengths to maintain it—even to the point of long-term wear and tear if stresses do not abate. Such strain on our body's regulatory mechanisms, which McEwen dubs "allostatic load," leads to an excessive and prolonged release of the stress hormones adrenaline and cortisol, nervous tension, immune dysfunction, and, in many cases, exhaustion of the stress apparatus itself.

We now know that the infrastructure of the HPA axis is set early in life, starting in utero and on through the young childhood years. Stress or abuse incurred during this delicate period can distort the stress-hormonal apparatus for a lifetime. Again and again, we see supposedly immaterial "nonthings" such as emotions having a material impact, decidedly and decisively.

Reducing stress where possible, attending to emotions, overt or repressed, and taking care of our psychic well-being can have profound effects on physical health—this is intuitively obvious to many people. Yet for all their dazzling physiological and technical

---

†   Longtime head of the Harold and Margaret Milliken Hatch Laboratory of Neuroendocrinology at Rockefeller University (d. 2020).

expertise, doctors by and large are not initiated by their training into the ancient wisdom and new science of the bodymind unity. Medical professionals often do little to encourage—and may even resist—people trusting their own hunches, which tend to synthesize signals from both mind and body.

Memories Aflame: Glenda's Story

Such was the case with Glenda, a Montreal woman, now fifty-eight, who thirty years ago underwent removal of parts of her intestine for severe Crohn's disease, an ulcerative, painful inflammatory disease of the bowel. In 2010 Glenda got some more bad news when she was diagnosed with stage 2 aggressive breast cancer. It was during the healing journey from the latter that she recovered repressed memories of being raped as a young girl. "Through the process of journaling and dreaming," she told me, "subconscious memories of my childhood began to emerge along with feelings of sheer panic and terror." Afraid to know the truth, she tried to keep the memories at bay, but they would not be deterred. "Every time the memories of the trauma surfaced," she continued, "they were accompanied with very visceral emotional feelings and physical digestive symptoms including indigestion, nausea, and gut aches."

The memories are harrowing enough to roil even an outside listener's guts. Eight-year-old Glenda and a younger friend were gang-raped by four teenage boys from the neighborhood. The first responder was her mother, who rushed Glenda into the house, she said, "and put me right into the bath. She told me that we were never going to tell anyone about this or ever speak of it again. My mom said it would always be 'our little secret,' and put me to bed."

When the memories returned at age fifty-three, they came as "this intense clear visual" of her young self in the bathtub, with her mother crouched on the floor beside her "trying to wash away the rape." I asked Glenda, gently, whether she had any independent evidence for these recovered memories. She nodded. "My older sister recalls that she actually came into the bathroom that day. Arriving home and hearing my mother bawling her eyes out, she came and opened the door. My back was to her; she said, 'What's wrong with Glenda?' My mother said, 'Nothing, she'll be fine. Get out.' [My sister] told me that I looked very disheveled—my mother never let us go out disheveled—and that my whole body was shaking."

As if that scene weren't intense enough, Glenda's intuitive understanding, now emerging into awareness after a lifetime of self-protective submersion, produced an additional visual layer. "As soon as I recovered the memory of being in the bathroom," she said, "I saw my body, I was transparent . . . I saw my entire digestive system from mouth to rectum. There were red blistering ulcers throughout my entire digestive system. There was a flaming, flowing hot lava, adding fuel to the fire. It was just raging, and that to me was a guide telling me that these two things are connected, the rape and my Crohn's." It doesn't take a psychoanalyst or a poetry professor to see the image of the "raging" fire as a powerful analogue for the rage and pain Glenda had to bury away in the deepest parts of herself, given her mother's utter inability to be there for her emotionally.

Glenda's "visual" is apt not only metaphorically but scientifically as well. To quote just one survey of research among an ever-growing trove, there is "strong evidence that childhood traumatic events significantly impact the inflammatory immune system . . . offering a potential molecular pathway by which early trauma confers vulnerability to developing psychiatric and physical disorders later in life."[18] None of Glenda's many physicians, nor even her psychiatrist—in her depiction, "very science-and-medicine"—ever once asked her about the possible childhood antecedents of her psychic turmoil.

Candace Pert envisioned the mind as involving the unconscious flow of information "among the cells, organs and systems of the body . . . occurring below the level of awareness." Thus, she asserted, "the mind as we experience it is immaterial, yet it has a physical substrate, which is both the body and the brain." By "immaterial" she did not mean the word's usual connotation of insignificant or irrelevant but—on the contrary—that the mind, unlike the brain, is not a material thing: we cannot get a hold of it, put it in a test tube or petri dish, or even "see" it directly. Its impacts and consequences, however, are material indeed.

The opportunity we have today is to create a multivalent health care approach that appreciates the impact of "nonthings" on the "thinglike" bodies we've come to be so marvelously expert in. The "immaterial" mind and its "physical substrate," the brain and body, are in a constant dance, as intimate as it is intricate.

On closer examination, we see that this choreography of psyche and soma involves far more than two "partners" contained within one person: there is also a vital and underappreciated *interpersonal* component. After all, the mind and body exist inescapably in the context of relationships, social circumstances, history, and culture. If we want a clear and accurate view of human health, we will have to broaden our understanding of "bodymind" to include the myriad roles that *other* minds and *other* bodies play in shaping our well-being, indeed our very sense of self. Unity, it turns out, extends well beyond the unitary individual.

Chapter 3

You Rattle My Brain:
Our Highly Interpersonal Biology

For every atom belonging to me as good belongs to you.
—Walt Whitman, "Song of Myself," in *Leaves of Grass*

"All my relations." I have often heard this greeting when visiting Native communities in Canada. These are the places where my country, to its shame, sees the highest levels of physical and mental illness, addictions, and early death—a tragic situation analogous with that of similarly colonized aboriginal populations in the United States and Australia. The phrase, as I understand it, refers to the individual's multidimensional bond with the entire world, including people—from close relatives to strangers, from the living to ancestors who lived long before—and also the rocks, the plants, the earth, the sky, and all creatures. Ancient cultures have long understood that we exist in relationship to all, are affected by all, and affect all.

In the Hindu scripture the Bhagavad Gita, the divine avatar Krishna declares, "They live in wisdom who see themselves in all and all in them." And the early seventeenth-century cleric and poet John Donne famously mused, "No man is an island, entire of itself." He composed this line, perhaps not coincidentally, during a period of illness and convalescence. Walt Whitman, writing in mid-nineteenth-century America, could have cribbed the verse cited in the above epigraph from today's quantum physics.

Then we have the man born 2,500 years ago as Gautama. "Contemplate the nature of interdependent co-arising during every moment," the Buddha said. "When you look at a leaf or a raindrop, meditate on the conditions, near and distant, that contributed to the presence of that leaf or raindrop. Know that the world is woven of interconnected threads. This is because that is. This is not because that is not. This is born because that is born. This dies because that dies." The leaf, as the Buddha implied, is both a discrete entity—a thing—*and* a process that derives from sun, sky, and earth: light, photosynthesis, rain, organic matter, and minerals and perhaps even the activity of humans and animals. "The one contains the many and the many contains the one. Without the one, there cannot be the many. Without the many, there cannot be the one." These are not merely esoteric wisdom teachings; they accurately describe the physical and organic universe, including health and pathology. Indeed, Friedrich Nietzsche once called the Buddha "that profoundest physiologist."

The pioneering U.S. internist and psychiatrist George Engel argued nearly half a century ago that the "crippling flaw" of modern medicine "is that it does not include the patient and his attributes as a person. Yet in the everyday work of the physician the prime object of study is a person." We must make provision for the whole person in their full "psychological and social nature,"[1] he said, calling for a *biopsychosocial* approach: one that recognizes the unity of emotions and physiology, knowing both to be dynamic processes unfolding in a context of relationships, from the personal to the cultural.[2]

The great traumatologist Dr. Bessel van der Kolk has noted that "our culture teaches us to focus on our personal uniqueness, but at a deeper level we barely exist as individual organisms."[3] This will certainly be news to the average ego. The word "ego," as I use it here, refers not to the trait of arrogance or conceit in certain "egotistical" people but to the internally perceived separate self with which we each identify: the "me," "myself," and "I" we mean when we use these personal pronouns, as we do hundreds of times a day. Even a healthy ego is convinced of its separateness, an entirely reasonable perception: the capacity to experience individual selfhood in all its facets (physical, psychological, biographical, etc.) is part and parcel of being human. Our difficulties begin when we lose sight of the other side of the equation, which is just as real, if less apparent.

The interrelatedness of seemingly isolated organisms has now been discovered even in the lives of trees that form living networks, communicating through electrical impulses akin to animal and human nervous systems, hormones, chemical signals, and scents. As an article in *Smithsonian* magazine reports, "Trees of the same species are communal, and will often form alliances with trees of other species." Peter Wohlleben, the German forester who has become well known for popularizing such information, wittily calls it "the wood-wide web."[4]

That our own individual minds and bodies are intimately linked is fairly simple to grasp. Less obvious but no less true is the fact that those same bodyminds are in many ways shaped, in the first place and throughout our lives, by factors *external* to us. Although modern medicine's focus on the individual organism and its internal processes isn't wrong as such, it misses something vital: the pivotal influence of the mental, emotional, social, and natural environments in which we live. Our biology itself is interpersonal.

The concept of *interpersonal neurobiology* was introduced some years ago by Dr. Daniel Siegel,[†] a psychiatrist, researcher, and prolific author. Like myself and many of our colleagues, Dr.

---

†   Clinical professor at the University of California, Los Angeles (UCLA), School of Medicine and executive director of the Mindsight Institute.

Siegel had become uncomfortable with the limitations of his education. "When I was in medical school," he writes, "many of the fine teachers we had approached their patients, and their students, as if they had no center of inner experience—no subjective internal core we might call our mental life. It was as if we were just bags of chemicals and bodily organs without a self, without a mind."[5] He sensed that both research and practice lacked a consensus definition of "health" and, startlingly, in the mental health field lacked even a shared agreement of what "mind" is, let alone a shared view of the relationship of mind and brain. Recruiting co-workers in medicine, neurology, psychiatry, psychology, anthropology, sociology, history, physiology, biology, physics, and related disciplines that study the human experience, he set out to explore what such a consensus might look like. The team's findings confirmed that our brains and minds are not independent operators, functioning in isolation from other brains and minds. In fact, nothing about us, mental or physical, can be comprehended apart from the many-faceted milieu in which we exist. We can perhaps treat human biology as strictly self-contained in an artificial setting like a medical laboratory or pathology theater, but not in real life. "Interpersonal neurobiology is both a way of understanding the world through many disciplines and it is also the reality of our interconnected nature," Dan told me in an interview. My amendment is to remove the "neuro-" prefix— leaving us with the broader "interpersonal biology," which places not only the brain and nervous system under the interpersonal banner but our entire mental-physical makeup.

The brain itself is the central organ of a supersystem that extends throughout the body and influences every aspect of physiological functioning, from the caliber of blood vessels to the contractions of our intestines, the beating of our heart, the manufacture of immune cells in our bone marrow, the secretions of hormones from our sex glands, and the functioning of our kidneys. Again, it's all one: emotions affect nerves and vice versa; nerves act on hormones; hormones on the immune system; the immune system on the brain; the brain on the gut; the gut on the brain; and all of these act on the heart, and vice versa. In turn, our bodies influence our brains and minds and, necessarily, the brains, minds, and bodies of others.

We all know the power of interpersonal biology from a lifetime of personal experience. Think of the effect that other people can have on you: it can be quite literally visceral. Poets and songwriters tell of being weak in the knees, shot through the heart, or even, in Bruce Springsteen's vivid image, stabbed in the brain by a dull, serrated blade.† Jerry Lee Lewis was right: we really do shake each other's nerves and rattle each other's brains.‡

Unsurprisingly, the closer we are to someone, the more our physiology interacts with theirs. Accordingly, the phenomenon of interpersonal biology has been well studied in the case of intimate relationships. Married people have lower rates of mortality than their age-matched single contemporaries, whether the latter were separated, divorced, widowed, or had never married.[6] Single people showed an elevated risk for heart disease and cancer, for infectious diseases such as pneumonia and influenza, and for such life-habit-related conditions as cirrhosis of the liver and lung disease. Tellingly, the degree of protection offered by married status was five times as great for men as for women, a finding that speaks to the relative roles of the genders in this culture, with profound implications for health—a topic I will circle back to in chapter 23. Interestingly, "unhappily married persons are worse off in well-being than unmarried persons."[7]

---

†   "I'm on Fire" (1984), third verse.

‡   As in his rock-and-roll classic "Great Balls of Fire."

In other studies, perfectly healthy married couples' stress hormone levels were elevated in those exhibiting higher degrees of hostility during conflict, and their immune functioning was diminished. The results were the same for newlyweds as for septuagenarians.[8]

Given their vulnerability and dependence, children's physiology is especially susceptible to the emotional states of their caregivers. Young kids' stress hormone levels, for example, are heavily influenced by the emotional atmosphere in the home, whether outright conflict or bristling tension.[9] Asthma is a well-studied example: the inflammation of the child's lungs is directly affected by the mother's or father's emotions.[10] In the words of a recent review: "It has been consistently shown that parents in an unfavorable mental health state such as 'depression,' 'anxiety,' 'stress,' or 'chronic irritation' may predict a poorer status for the child's asthma."[11]

Racism is another risk factor for asthma. In a large cohort of Black American women, experiences of racial discrimination were associated with the adult onset of the disease.[12] And that raises an inescapable question we should all ponder: Is the inflammation and airway constriction of these women a case of individual pathology or the manifestation of a social malaise?

The more we learn, the more we realize that our health is a complex consequence of "all our relations," and not just the ones close at hand (family, friends, intimate others, etc.). Leading U.S. stress researchers Teresa Seeman and Bruce McEwen noted in 1996 that human biology "seem[s] to be highly sensitive" also to factors like one's social status relative to others, and even how stable or precarious the social order happens to be at a given time.[13] In a British study, unemployed people had higher markers of inflammation in their bodies, and hence were at higher risk for illness; the longer the unemployment, the greater the risk. The most severe inflammation levels were recorded in Scotland, the part of the U.K. where unemployment was most endemic and chronic.[14] Even the gainfully employed can experience physiological blowback. In a study of the British civil service, a lower ranking on the ladder of authority was a greater predictor of death from heart disease than commonly listed risk factors such as smoking, cholesterol, or hypertension. Along similar lines, Australian researchers found that a bad job is worse for mental health than being out of work.[15] So the next time a co-worker complains to you, "This job is killing me," you can tell them they may be right.

Interpersonal biology also accounts for why loneliness can kill, especially in older people separated from pleasures, social connections, or support. A vast review of multiple studies encompassing more than three hundred thousand participants concluded that the lethal effect of deficient interpersonal relationships is comparable to such risk factors as smoking and alcohol, and even exceeds the dangers posed by physical inactivity and obesity.[16]

The recently deceased Buddhist monk and renowned spiritual leader Thich Nhat Hanh long taught the concept of "inter-being." It's not merely that we are, he said: we "inter-are." "There are no separate entities," he wrote, "only manifestations that rely on each other to be possible."[17] Again, we would be quite mistaken to relegate these observations to the realm of mystical belief. A scientist lacking a spiritual bone in his body, yet conversant with the growing body of evidence, would nod in agreement: "Yup, that about covers it."

Chapter 4

Everything I'm Surrounded By: Dispatches from the New Science

So much of what makes people either well or not is not coming
from within themselves, it's coming from their circumstances.
It makes me think much more about social justice and the
bigger issues that go beyond individuals.

—Elizabeth Blackburn, Ph.D.[†]

In 2009 Dr. Elizabeth Blackburn shared the Nobel Prize in Physiology or Medicine for her work on telomeres—minuscule DNA structures at the end of chromosomes. Not unlike the plastic aglets placed at the end of shoelaces to keep them from fraying, these tiny sheaths help protect chromosomal integrity. Good thing, too, since as chromosomes unravel, so do we. Tracking the length and stability of telomeres throughout the lifespan, it turns out, can tell us a great deal about health and longevity.

You wouldn't think it to look at them, but what has been discovered about these tiny biological structures also has huge social implications. One of Dr. Blackburn's discoveries was that telomeres bear the actual marks—or rather, the markers—of the circumstances in which we live our lives. Amazingly, she found that factors such as poverty, racism, and urban blight can directly impact our genetic and molecular functioning. As the psychologist

---

[†] Professor emerita, Department of Biochemistry and Biophysics, University of California San Francisco.

Elissa Epel, who is Dr. Blackburn's research collaborator and co-author of the bestselling volume *The Telomere Effect: A Revolutionary Approach to Living Younger, Healthier, Longer*, told me in an interview, "These effects are not small."

The neuroscientist Candace Lewis, whose own research is in epigenetics, the growing field that investigates the impact of life experience on the activity of our genes, sees things the same way. "More and more the science is demonstrating this holistic model of who we are," she told me. "It's more than just what's enclosed in my skin—it's everything I'm surrounded by. Not to see that is to remove healing from medicine." As Dr. Lewis has peered at molecules and strands of DNA, she, too, has found herself lifting her gaze to the whole person and from the individual to broader social issues. "As a specialist in the complexity of brain and behavior, I know it's not just brain and behavior," said the former Fulbright scholar. "One of the biggest take-home messages from my work is how malleable we are as an organism, how responsive to environmental cues throughout the lifespan."

The dominant assumption in our culture is that genetic inheritance determines the better part of our destiny, who we are, what we suffer from, and what we are capable of. In 2000, at a White House briefing, Bill Clinton proclaimed the findings of the Human Genome Project "the most wondrous map ever produced by humankind," adding that "today we are learning the language in which God created life." The new science, the soon-to-be ex-president predicted, "will revolutionize the diagnosis, prevention and treatment of most, if not all, human disease," leading to cures for conditions like Alzheimer's, Parkinson's, and cancer "by attacking their genetic roots."[†]

[†] There are a few diseases that are determined purely by genes, such as Huntington's and one that runs in my family, muscular dystrophy. If one has the gene, one is almost 100 percent certain to get the disease. Such conditions are exceedingly rare. There is, for example, a gene for breast cancer, but only about 7 percent of women with the disease have the gene. And far from all the ones with the gene will necessarily get the disease, though their risk, to be sure, is significantly elevated.

Two decades later, we know that little of the sort has happened.[1] And for good reason: genes are not, in fact, life's language, any more than a scrambled alphabet or a randomly arranged dictionary is a Shakespeare play, or a musical scale is equivalent to a John Coltrane solo. For letters or words to become language, they must be arranged, enunciated, inflected, punctuated with pauses, EMPHASIZED or softened. Like all building blocks, genes help make up the language of existence, but it is through the workings of epigenetics that they are activated, accented, or quieted. The mechanisms of epigenetics include, among myriad others, adding certain molecules to DNA sequences so as to change gene function, modifying the numbers of receptors for certain messenger chemicals, and influencing the interactions between genes.[‡]

Experience, in other words, determines how our genetic potential expresses itself in the end. This is what the field of epigenetics—meaning "on top of" genes—is all about. Epigenetic processes act on chromosomes, delivering and translating messages from the environment that "tell" the genes what to do. All this takes place without in any way altering the genes themselves. As the BBC's Martha Henriques explains, epigenetics offers "a way of adapting to changing conditions without inflicting a more permanent shift in our genomes."[2]

It isn't that genes don't matter—they certainly do—only that they cannot dictate even the simplest behaviors, let alone account for most illnesses or address possible cures for them. Far from being the autonomous arbiters of our destinies, genes answer to their environment; without environmental signals, they could not function. In fact, life for us would be impossible if not

---

‡   Receptor molecules embedded in the membranes of cells receive and bind with chemical messengers such as opiates and hormones. Their interaction with these messenger substances induces the DNA in the cell's nucleus to manufacture proteins that instigate life processes. By such mechanisms, the environment instructs the cell what to do and when.

for the epigenetic mechanisms that "turn" genes "on" or "off" in response to signals from within and from outside the body.[†]

Epigenetics revamps our understanding of human development from embryo to adult, and even how our species got to be here. I spoke with one of the foremost researchers in the field, Dr. Moshe Szyf, at McGill University's storied medical school. "Evolutionary theory is a difficult one to change because it became almost religion, a religion of science," he said. "And any questioning of it seems to be a heretical question of the whole system, which obviously it isn't. Epigenetics doesn't deny evolution. Epigenetics is part of evolution, but it demands a new look at how evolution works." The new biology improves upon the standard Darwinian view of spontaneous mutations and random selection as the motors of species adaptations; it demonstrates that circumstances themselves can shape how genes adjust to the environment.

Said another way, our lives are what happens when life acts upon life.

Dr. Szyf and his team in Montreal performed one of the most cited epigenetic studies, with major implications for how we view development, behavior, and health. Working with laboratory rats, they examined the effect of the mother's interactions with the infant in the first days after birth on how the offspring, for the rest of their lives, respond to stress—whether appropriately and confidently or with anxiety and over-reactivity. The focus was the HPA axis, the stress-regulating feedback loop between the hypothalamus and the pituitary and adrenal glands.[‡] In particular, the researchers looked at receptor molecules in the

---

[†] How a gene acts—that is, what protein messengers it will produce, if any—is called *gene expression*. Gene expression is determined by inputs from the environment that reach the DNA by means of receptors on the cell membrane, and also by complex intracellular mechanisms programmed by experience.

[‡] The hypothalamic-pituitary-adrenal axis is discussed in chapter 2.

brain whose task it is to modulate stress, which is to say, to ensure the appropriate behavior when stress is present. Creatures with poorly self-regulated stress reactions will be more anxious, less capable of confronting ordinary environmental challenges, and overstressed even under normal circumstances.

The study showed the quality of early maternal care to have a causal impact on the offspring's brains' biochemical capacity to respond to stress in a healthy way into adulthood. Key epigenetic markers—the ways certain genes expressed themselves—were different in the brains of rats who had received either more, or less, nurturing contact from their mothers.[3] Strikingly, the offspring in turn passed on to their *own* infants the type of mothering they had been given. Szyf and his colleagues have also shown that the quality of maternal care affects the receptor activity for estrogen—a key female hormone—in daughters, with ramifications for mothering patterns down the generations.[4] Through ingenious manipulation of the rat population studied—inconceivable in human research—both the physiological and behavioral effects of early nurturing patterns were found to be *nongenetic*: that is, not transmitted through the so-called genetic code, which remained unchanged. Rather, they were *epigenetic*—in other words, determined by how the various kinds of maternal nurturing influenced gene activity in the offspring's brain. (The specific maternal behavior tracked by these researchers was how "lovingly" the moms "groomed," or licked, their infants.)

"Okay, but these are rodents in a lab," you might find yourself saying. "What do these findings mean for people in the real world?" A reasonable question, to which Nature provided an eloquent answer in the form of a devastating ice storm in January 1998—in the same province, no less, where Dr. Szyf and his team did their work.[5] Considered one of Canada's worst-ever natural disasters, the storm left many Quebecers without heat or electricity. The more "objective stress" that pregnant women had to live through during those trying days—as in concrete, measurable factors like darkness, cold, and home damage[†]—the more their kids' physiology was marked by that adversity even near puberty. (The participants were of a similar socioeconomic, cultural, and ethnic background, and lived in the same suburban area.) "Over the years [of tracking the children]," Suzanne King, a professor of psychiatry at McGill University said, "we found that that objective stress explained how kids varied one from another in a whole host of things: language, BMI [body mass index] and obesity, insulin secretion, their immune system."[6] Even IQ was affected. "We also saw increased asthma," Dr. Szyf added, "as well as increased inflammatory genes and immune genes that are connected with autoimmunity."

I should emphasize that mothers aren't alone in transmitting chronic disturbances of the body's stress apparatus to their young. In one experiment, healthy male mice were vexed by a series of stressors: frequent cage changes, constant light or white noise, exposure to fox odor, being restrained in a small tube, and so on. They were then mated with non-stressed females who provided their pups with perfectly good mothering. Their young showed impaired stress-response behaviors and blunted stress hormone patterns. In other words, despite the mothers' best efforts, the fathers had transmitted the disturbing effects through their sperm.[7] In humans, paternal stress early in a child's life can also have long-term effects, into adolescence at the least. Adversity among *both* mothers and fathers bear "reliable linkages" to the epigenetic profiles of the children, a group of researchers concluded.[8]

Socioeconomic circumstances, too, can alter the epigenome— the web of epigenetic influences on genes. The indefatigable

---

[†]   The impact of "subjective" stress—fear, loss, emotional pain, etc.—is no less physiologically impactful.

Dr. Szyf teamed with scientists from Canada and the U.K. to study the epigenetic workings of a broad range of genes in blood samples of middle-aged British males. The study subjects had begun life at opposite ends of the wealth-to-poverty spectrum, some poor and others rich. Gene expression in those who were born well-off was markedly different from that observed in their counterparts who grew up disadvantaged.[9]

Another study observed higher rates of inflammation in African Americans than in Caucasians, an epigenetic effect that remained even when comparing those of the same socioeconomic level.[10] "We found that experiences with racism and discrimination accounted for more than 50% of the black/white difference in the activity of genes that increase inflammation," wrote the lead author, Dr. April Thames, in an article titled "Racism Shortens Lives and Hurts Health of Blacks by Promoting Genes That Lead to Inflammation and Illness."[11]

Much like gene expression, telomeres manifest the vagaries of fate and history, class and race, stress and trauma. How? At birth, telomeres have many "units"—the DNA base pairs of which they are constituted—and by old age, far fewer. "We start out with about ten thousand when we're a baby, and we get down to four thousand when we die," Elissa Epel told me. Every time a cell in our body divides, telomeres shorten; when they get too short, their host cell dies or may deteriorate and become dysfunctional. As they shrink, immune function is impaired, inflammation rises, and we fall more prone to illness.

Telomeres have been called "cellular clocks," in that they are a measure of biological rather than chronological age. Two people, even identical twins, could be the same age as computed in years, months, weeks, and days, yet one may be biologically older than the other, depending on how much stress, adversity, or trauma they have endured. That's because stress shortens telomeres.

(Doctors should take special heed: the telomeres of medical residents suffer greater attrition than those of other young adults in their age group.)[12] One of Dr. Epel's studies found that caregiving mothers of chronically ill children had shorter telomeres than their counterparts of the same age. This biological age differential was proportionate to both the number of years of caregiving *and* the degree of stress as perceived by the moms.[13] Similar results were seen in caregivers of people with dementia: shortened telomeres and impaired immunity, reinforcing the idea that "chronic psychological stress has a negative impact on immune cell function and may accelerate their aging."[14] In other words, stress ages our chromosomes, and therefore ages us.

Just as poverty and racism affect epigenetic functioning, so do these factors also shorten telomeres, and therefore lives. This sobering linkage was brought home vividly by a study of Black American men in 2014. "Our findings literally suggest that racism makes people old," the lead author commented.[15] The same holds true for women. As part of the U.S.-based Study of Women's Health Across the Nation (SWAN), the telomeres of Black and white middle-aged women were compared. The results were shocking: Black women were found, on average, to be over seven years more biologically aged than their white counterparts, consistent with higher rates of poverty, stress, hypertension, obesity, and related health conditions.[16]

As Dr. Epel told me, the effects of our socioeconomic environment are visible within our cells, if one knows what to look for. "The neighborhood deprivation, the crime, the income of the zip code," she said, "all of that is associated with aging of the cells. That is to me one of the biggest demonstrations that our health is outside of our body." Dr. Szyf spoke in similar tones: "For a century we've been obsessed with chemical changes, thinking anything that is chemical is true and anything that is not chemical is not true. What epigenetics taught us is that social changes are really not different than chemical changes." The one is manifested in the other.

Fortunately, the door of environmental effects swings both ways: it turns out that experiences that build stress resilience can *lengthen* our telomeres, even in the face of illness or adversity. This has been shown by the work of Dr. Epel and colleagues with meditators, by Dr. Gene Brody's work with deprived Black American teenagers, and in other research on men with prostate cancer.[17] This will be a recurring theme as we proceed: the seemingly bad news giving way to something empowering, if we approach it wisely. By learning about the impacts of adversity, we can also find pathways toward healing.

Chapter 5

Mutiny on the Body:
The Mystery of the Rebellious
Immune System

A lot of times I've had to pretend I felt good when I felt terrible.

—Venus Williams

"I kind of injured myself," Mee Ok[†] told me recently, "because I was doing very well and then I tripped, running up a flight of stairs. So I stubbed my toe." Her warm, impish humor radiates in the telling, as does a certain sense of pride. For most of us that would be an odd reaction to a painful mishap like that. But to the Mee Ok of seven years ago, such an injury, incurred while moving vigorously against gravity, would have seemed like an impossible dream. Diagnosed at age twenty-seven with scleroderma, she had become completely disabled in a short time despite all that mainstream medicine had to offer. She lives in the Boston area and was assessed and treated at one of Western medical science's most hallowed venues.

From the Greek for "hard skin," scleroderma is an autoimmune disorder that manifests in debilitating joint inflammation and painful tightening of the connective tissues. A more inclusive

---

† Her Korean given name, pronounced "Mee Oak." For much of her life, growing up in the United States, she went by "Mandy." Her full name now is Mee Ok Icaro, for reasons I'll explain when we return to her remarkable story in chapter 31 (see footnote, p. 458).

name for the condition is systemic sclerosis, as the buildup of hardened tissue can occur in many organs, including the esophagus, blood vessels, and lungs. In Mee Ok's case, it showed up in agonizing swelling of her hands, shoulders, and knees. "The pain was everywhere," she recalls. "It flooded my whole body." She soon had to leave her job at Harvard as an assistant to a prominent academic. Formerly a 120-word-per-minute typist, she now found her hands becoming rigid and clawlike, stiffening into near paralysis. Merely touching the keyboard was agony. When I first interviewed her in 2014, her physiognomy was grim, her face a rigid mask, her taut lips barely able to cover her teeth. She was unrecognizable to herself—and wholly incongruous with the person one encounters now, her smile quick and responsive.

Within a few years of the onset of her disease, still in her early thirties, Mee Ok wanted only to end her life. Facing a death-sentence diagnosis, needing a wheelchair to mobilize, unable even to get out of bed without assistance, and anticipating that her torments would only intensify the longer she lived, she investigated the possibility of medically assisted suicide. "If I had been in a country where euthanasia was legalized, I would have fit all the criteria. The pain was unbelievable," she told me. "There was no prognosis that really gave me a reason to stick around. I was losing my body so quickly, I knew that if I waited much longer, I was going to be trapped and I wouldn't have even been able to push a button."

Today, in defiance of all conventional medical logic, Mee Ok—completely off all medications—walks, travels, and hikes independently. She is currently writing her memoir, albeit at the speed of fifty words per minute: relative to the shape she was in not long ago, a true victory.

Scleroderma is among eighty or more related conditions dubbed autoimmune, each representing a virtual civil war inside the body. In effect, autoimmunity amounts to an assault by one's immune system against the body it ought to defend. The particular form of the disease depends on which tissues or organs become the targets of this ruinous internal rebellion. If the nervous system is under fire, the result may show up as multiple sclerosis; if the gut, celiac disease or inflammatory bowel disease (IBD) such as Crohn's or ulcerative colitis; if the joints and connective tissues, systemic lupus erythematosus (SLE) or rheumatoid arthritis (RA) or scleroderma; if the skin, psoriasis or autoimmune eczema; if the pancreas, type 1 diabetes; if the lungs, pulmonary fibrosis; if the brain, perhaps Alzheimer's. In many of these conditions, several regions of the body are affected at once. Chronic fatigue syndrome—also known as myalgic encephalomyelitis (ME)—which affects millions worldwide, is among the best known of the recent additions to this roster.

Virtually all autoimmune diseases are characterized by inflammation of the afflicted tissues, organs, and body parts— which explains why frontline medical measures often begin with anti-inflammatory drugs. When nonsteroidal anti-inflammatories like ibuprofen or heavier artillery such as steroids themselves prove inadequate, physicians may prescribe medications to suppress the body's immune activity.

Because the disease had first affected Mee Ok's joints, the doctors believed it was rheumatoid arthritis. Their prescription was steroids: lab-made analogues of the natural stress hormone cortisol, a secretion of the adrenal gland in response to a threat. Ultimately it was the failure of both steroids and immunosuppressants that drove Mee Ok to suicidal despair. Her doctors had nothing left to prescribe. (I should add that Mee Ok's illness was so extreme that her recovery is entirely unexpected, indeed unexplainable, according to standard medical thinking. I contacted her family physician in Boston, who verified the details.)

Although often disruptive and highly distressing, autoimmune symptoms can be nebulous and hard to pinpoint at first—not so much to the patient suffering them and seeking validation and support as to the physician in search of precise findings. Hence, it is not unusual for such diseases, which not infrequently overlap with each other, to fly under the diagnostic radar. Such was the experience of the tennis star Venus Williams, whose illness expressed itself in swollen hands, persistent fatigue, and misshapen joints: symptoms that would be alarming for anyone, even more so for an elite athlete. "I'd go to doctors, but never get any answers, so there was nothing I could do but keep going," she told a newspaper reporter. "You almost get used to having all these symptoms," she said. "You tell yourself to shake it off. Just keep going. Over time, you do start to wonder what's happening and if you're going crazy."[1] She was eventually found to have Sjögren's syndrome, a condition that primarily affects moisture-producing glands so that people suffer dry mouth and dry eyes, but which can also cause dysfunction in many organs such as the lungs, kidneys, pancreas, and blood vessels. Like many others, Williams was relieved to finally learn there was some objective reason, and even a name, for her physical tribulations.

In Mee Ok's case it fell to the patient herself to make the diagnosis: a not-unusual role reversal in the internet age, particularly in cases where doctors have already thrown up their hands. "My body just continued to stiffen," she recalled. "It was like it was undergoing mummification, like a self-mummification over time. It kept spreading and spreading throughout my body, and the pain was just unbelievable . . . They were giving me steroids and telling me that it was something that I would have to maintain, that the arthritis would never be cured—it wasn't curable. I insisted on being tested for scleroderma, and that was when I found out my diagnosis: six months after the symptoms started."

Autoimmune diseases are among the great unsolved mysteries of the medical profession. Most are considered "idiopathic" in nature, which simply means "of unknown origin." Naturally, if we cannot identify the *cause* of a condition, we will be stymied in our efforts to cure or reverse it. In many cases symptom suppression or, sometimes, surgical repair or removal of damaged tissue is the most modern medicine can offer. Such measures do afford welcome relief to many, but they cannot reverse the course of disease and, as with Mee Ok, leave a great number of people consigned to prolonged deterioration and disability.

Troubling as this lack of clarity is for doctors and patients alike, these illnesses also present a number of other head-scratchers, scientifically speaking.

The first mystery is why they are becoming more frequent. Across many Western countries, rates of everything from celiac disease to IBD, from lupus to type 1 diabetes, and even allergies, are steadily rising, stymieing researchers.[2] "In the last half-century, the prevalence of autoimmune disease . . . has increased sharply in the developed world," a 2016 *New York Times* article noted. "An estimated one in 13 Americans has one of these often debilitating, generally lifelong conditions."[3] In the U.K., the diagnosis of Crohn's disease increased more than threefold between 1994 and 2014,[4] while in Canada the rate of IBD in children grew by over 7 percent a year between 1999 and 2010, giving my country among the highest rates of this disease in the world.[5]

Such trends immediately rule out that go-to of medical explanations, genetic causes. Whatever effect genetics may exert—and no doubt they figure in some cases—logically they cannot account for the rise in prevalence of autoimmune disorders. "Genes do not change in such a short period of time," Virginia Ladd, chief executive of the American Autoimmune Related Diseases Association, told

Medical News Today in 2012. "The rapid increase in autoimmune diseases . . . clearly suggests that environmental factors are at play."[6] In other words, something in our environment—or a combination of somethings—is inflaming our bodies.

For most of us, when we hear "environmental factors" in conjunction with disease, our minds tend to go to well-publicized, material factors such as air pollution, lead paint, and cell phone radiation. One interesting but unproven theory has it that the rise in junk food consumption is responsible for the globally increasing prevalence of autoimmunity.[7] Studies have not yet identified such a link.[8] Either way, a complete understanding of health and disease requires a far more encompassing view of the word "environment": a biopsychosocial one.

The second mystery is the highly skewed gender distribution of autoimmune diseases. About 70 to 80 percent of sufferers are women, among whom such conditions are a leading cause of disability and death. Rheumatoid arthritis, for example, is three times more likely to strike women than men; lupus affects women by a disproportionate factor of nine. Mee Ok's condition, systemic sclerosis, is three times more common among females.[9] Even more of a puzzle is why the gender imbalance is *increasing* in, for example, multiple sclerosis, a chronic, highly debilitating, potentially lifelong disease of the nervous system.

In 1930s Canada, the gender ratio was about equal; nowadays more than three women are diagnosed with MS for every man.[10] The trend is reflected internationally. "There is an increasing incidence of multiple sclerosis in women in Denmark. Danish women's risk of developing MS has more than doubled in twenty-five years, while it has remained virtually unchanged for men," noted a recent article in the *Danish Medical Journal*. Then, right in line with Dr. Ladd's observations: "The explanation for these epidemiological changes *should be sought in the environment*, as genetics only explain a small part of the MS risk. The changes are too rapid to be explained by gene alterations."[11]

None of the specialists who looked after Mee Ok inquired about the conditions—physical and emotional—that preceded her life-blighting illness. This, despite the voluminous research that links stress, trauma, and inflammation, and despite the multiple studies that over many decades have explored such connections in rheumatoid arthritis, in MS, and in other autoimmune conditions. Not only are such possible lines of inquiry not pursued, but they seem to be verboten in mainstream circles. "I've come to feel a little bit off the wall when talking about these issues," a specialist in rheumatic diseases at one of the best-known U.S. teaching hospitals told me. "Since my graduation I have markedly changed the way I practice, because I started observing in my patients the relation between stress and the onset of their disease, and how great a role trauma, psychological and physical, plays in their disease." This doctor, who requested anonymity for fear of alienating her colleagues (!), has observed firsthand what she calls "remarkable results" among her patients, both in terms of recovery and even, in some cases, getting off medications altogether. Yet she feels like a renegade in her own profession. "I'm surrounded by all my, you know, esteemed colleagues at the university who are investigators, and nobody is looking at these things." Hearing this, I recalled the Harvard physician who told me that doctors follow these sorts of threads "at their own peril"—though he did think it was changing.

If even doctors who stray beyond medical orthodoxy can feel intimidated and misunderstood, what do patients experience? Another lamentable feature of Western medical practice—not universal, but all too often seen—is a power hierarchy that casts physicians as the exalted experts and patients as the passive recipients of care. For all doctors' dedication and goodwill, the imbalance compromises patients' agency over their own health and healing process. Essential questions about their lives go un-asked, while patients in turn lack the confidence to insist that their intuitions and insights about themselves contribute to the process, much less guide it.

Had Mee Ok's doctors inquired along these lines when she presented her distressing symptoms, they would have learned that she had sustained two major abandonments by the end of her first year. She was born in Korea to a single mom who placed her in an orphanage when Mee Ok was six months old. At one year of age, she was adopted and brought to the United States by an evangelical couple who reared her according to the strictest fundamentalist principles. Before Mee Ok was ten, her adoptive mother suffered a nervous breakdown. Sometime in her teenage years, her father, in a fit of religious remorse, confessed to her that he had sexually abused her for much of her early childhood, from age two onward. She had completely repressed these mem-ories, secreted them and all associated feelings—pain, terror, rage—deep beneath the surface of her awareness. As we will see later when we discuss healing, Mee Ok's improbable recovery, veritably a deathbed resurrection, owed everything to her con-fronting this long-buried trove of hurt.

Upon the emotional graveyard of what she could not afford to feel, Mee Ok erected an impressive edifice: a positive, can-do persona that not only kept her from experiencing her despair and impelled her to ignore her own needs, but also helped her achieve success beyond what she really believed was her due. In her job as assistant to the world-renowned professor, the grown-up Mee Ok found her work stressful and would habitually bear the tensions and pressures of everyone around her. "I was re-ally not myself while I was there," she said. "I was always hav-ing to operate as a more highly functioning person than I really was." Such hyperfunctioning on top of hidden inner distress is a recurring theme among the many autoimmune patients I've encountered in my years of practice and teaching.

Just prior to the onset of her agonizing joint inflammation, Mee Ok was in a complicated romantic partnership whose many ups and downs took a psychic toll and culminated in a wrenching breakup. All the lifelong hurt she could not allow herself to experience, all her terror of abandonment, showed up in her reactions to the loss of the relationship. It was a full-body grief response. Once more, none of her history, from childhood to the present day, was considered as admissible evidence by the highly trained experts who treated her scleroderma. "My body was really like a battleground, and I was losing," Mee Ok told me. Her language resonated with me: I've long pictured autoimmune disease as resembling a powerful army invading its own motherland, a violent mutiny against the body. In effect, with no conscious outlet and lacking resolution, Mee Ok's inflamed emotions rebelled, manifesting in the inflammation of her tissues.

Microbiologists these days speak of "neurogenic inflammation," stress-induced inflammation triggered by discharges of the nervous system—a system we now understand to be powerfully influenced by emotions.[12] And there is elegant research connecting early adversity, such as the traumas Mee Ok endured in childhood, to inflammation in adult life. A recent American study found that emotional and physical abuse in childhood more than doubles the risk of systemic lupus erythematosus, with inflammation being one of the likely pathways.[13] Yet more connections between stress and compromised autoimmunity have been found in other studies.[14] In 2007, British scientists found that adults who had been maltreated in childhood had higher blood levels of certain inflammation-signaling substances† produced in the liver,

---

†   For example, the C-reactive protein (CRP).

independent of personal behaviors and lifestyle considerations. "Childhood maltreatment is a previously undescribed, independent, and preventable risk factor for inflammation in adulthood," wrote the researchers.[15] "Inflammation *may be* an important developmental mediator linking adverse experiences in early life to poor adult health," they added cautiously. Many studies since attest that there is no "may be" about it.

Some clinicians have noted a relationship between rheumatoid arthritis and certain types or features of personality. We will have much more to say about personality in chapter 7, but, to avoid misunderstanding, a quick clarification is in order here. What we call the personality traits, in addition to reflecting genuine inborn temperaments and qualities, also express the ways that people, as children, had to accommodate their emotional environment. They reflect much that is neither inherent nor immutable about a person, no matter how closely identified he or she is with them. Nor are they character faults; though they may cause us difficulty now, they began as modes of survival.

As far as back as 1892 the great Canadian-born Johns Hopkins physician William Osler—later knighted by Queen Victoria for his contributions to British medicine—had already noted "the association of the disease with shock, worry, and grief." Many years later, a 1965 survey reported the prevalence in rheumatoid arthritis–prone individuals of an array of self-abnegating traits: a "compulsive and self-sacrificing doing for others, suppression of anger, and excessive concern about social acceptability."[16] An unusually perceptive Canadian specialist in autoimmune disease, Dr. C. E. G. Robinson, wrote in 1957 that his patients with RA "usually tried very hard to please both in professional and personal contacts, and either concealed hostility or expressed it indirectly. Many of them were perfectionistic." The onset of disease was often preceded by stress. He added, sagely, "Frequently as much time is needed for dealing with the emotional problems of the patient with chronic rheumatoid arthritis as with the joint or systemic disorders . . . I think the emotional and psychological aspect of many rheumatoid patients is of first importance."[17] Four decades after Dr. Robinson published his comments, American researchers likewise found that the degree of interpersonal stress was correlated with disease severity among a group of women with rheumatoid arthritis.[18]

A case in point is forty-two-year-old Julia, from one of Canada's prairie provinces, diagnosed with rheumatoid arthritis at age twenty-nine. She had been rear-ended in a motor vehicle accident and the next day felt some pain in her left shoulder, which quickly resolved—only to flare up again and again in various joints throughout her body, migrating with bewildering unpredictability. "It would show up in a joint and then leave," she told me. "Then all at once I ended up with twenty-six joints that were all inflamed simultaneously." Blood tests found one of the indicators of rheumatoid arthritis highly elevated, clinching the diagnosis. Her emotional profile aligned with the hyper-responsible, anger-suppressing personae described in the literature, traits she developed in a family of origin with an alcoholic father and an emotionally dependent mother to whom she could not divulge her sexual abuse at the hands of a family friend who also victimized the younger sister Julia tried to protect.

None of Julia's treating physicians ever asked about her inner life. Why does that matter? Because such personality patterns as Dr. Robinson and others have observed are reversible and, with them, so may be the disease. Despite having been told the illness would inevitably progress, Julia is now symptom-free and medication-free. "I have beautiful conversations with my rheumatoid arthritis these days—it makes me want to cry telling you," she said to me. "I'm great." What could such a statement mean, and why so deeply felt in Julia's case? We will return to these "beautiful conversations" later, when we look at healing.[†]

Grief and Vexation: Miray, Bianca, and Multiple Sclerosis

Miray is a fifty-one-year-old physician from Turkey, now working as a clinical trial coordinator at a Canadian hospital. She first experienced diplopia—double vision—at age eighteen, but without the advanced imaging techniques now available, she remained at first undiagnosed. "I saw an ophthalmologist, and he said, oh, this is just a temporary thing," she recalled. "So I went on corticosteroids for six weeks, and it went away. At twenty-two I had multiple attacks. *Whenever I would see my mom, I would see double.* I studied in another city and was perfectly okay, but when I would go back to Istanbul, I would have another attack every time I saw my mom." At age twenty-four, Miray had an MRI that confirmed the diagnosis of multiple sclerosis. After she immigrated to Canada, she was symptom-free for years. But during her pregnancy, her husband, in the midst of some business woes, became abusive. "He had this rage and hatred toward women," she said, "and he would project it on me." One stress begat another. "He wasn't making enough money to hire people, so I would work in the hospital from morning to afternoon, then I had to go and mind the store from four until midnight. When I gave birth, things got worse. He was shouting, extremely angry. He was always demeaning me, mocking me, ridiculing me." Finally, Miray left the marriage and, after many years, saw her parents again. When she did, she was soon unable to walk—a pattern that has persisted ever since. The emotional triggers of suppressed fear and anger instilled in her in childhood were activated around her family, and that, in turn, would inflame her nervous system.

---

† See chapter 27.

Multiple sclerosis is another autoimmune condition for which personal histories, childhood adversity, and the decisive influence of stress have been extensively studied. The first to describe this illness, the French physician Jean-Martin Charcot, sometimes called the father of modern neurology, proposed in 1872 that MS resulted from "long-continued grief and vexation." As with his younger contemporary and fellow medical giant William Osler's insights about rheumatoid arthritis, much information has since accrued to support Charcot's pioneering formulation. "A majority of the MS patients had grown up against an unhappy family background," found a 1958 study at two Montreal hospitals. "Marital discord, broken homes, alcoholism, and lack of parental love and affection were given as reasons for unhappiness." The vast majority had suffered prolonged emotional stress prior to the onset of their disease. Also salient in triggering relapses were such stresses as "worry over financial matters, unhappy home life, increased responsibility, either alone or in combination with such other factors as fatigue, overexertion, overwork, accidents, injuries, and childbirth."[19] A decade later, another study (in which Dr. George Engel, of the "biopsychosocial" coinage, participated) also concluded that "the majority of patients . . . reported psychologically stressful experiences to have preceded the onset of the symptoms that ultimately led to the diagnosis of multiple sclerosis, findings corroborated by family members when available."[20]

The evidence just keeps coming. MS patients experiencing significant life stresses were seen to have a nearly quadrupled incidence of disease flare-ups.[21] Finally, a major review of the literature presented at an international conference in Portugal in 2013 found a host of patterns among MS patients, including

- more unwanted stress or traumatic events occurring between six months to two years before onset;

- a cumulative correlation between stress and relapse: after one stressful life event, the relapse risk doubles or triples; after three or more, the risk increases by five- to nearly sevenfold;
- histories of childhood trauma, which are double or triple those of the general population;
- physical and sexual abuse histories correlated with higher relapse rates;
- being less in touch with their emotions, in general, and therefore less able to protect themselves from stress; and
- social support mitigating the effect of life stresses.[22]

Over the years I have interviewed dozens of people with MS, many of them long before I was aware of such studies. I have yet to find an exception to these general findings. The "long-continued grief and vexation" of which Jean-Martin Charcot spoke a century and a half ago factor mightily in the presence and severity of the illness. As in the other autoimmune conditions, in virtually every case the childhood patterning that led people to be overconscientious, hyper-responsible, and emotionally stoic about their own needs was evident—as were stresses preceding the illness, such as interpersonal conflict, family crisis, loss of a relationship, or added duties at work.

Bianca—like Miray, a physician—also had double vision (diplopia) as her first symptom of MS. Now thirty-seven, she first experienced it in her twenties while she was stressing herself over her school examinations. "Through the years," she told me as we spoke online, she from her home in Bucharest and I in Vancouver, "all the time that I had the symptom of double vision I was preparing for exams or a lot of stress in work—professional stress. The other symptoms, I make the connection, like numbness and tingling or pins-and-needles sensations or paralysis, happen usually when I have personal problems and emotional problems." Contrary to medical expectation, Bianca has made the disease work for her. She has learned to make friends with and allow herself to be instructed by a condition most of us would naturally regard as pure misfortune. "I was overcompensating all my life, and working hard, and trying to please people," she told me. "With MS, I finally had a reason to relax and focus on myself."

Why the Rise of Autoimmune Diseases?

Genetic explanations missing the mark, the hunt for elusive "environmental factors" continues; in the modern world, there are bound to be many.[23] I believe, however, that one such factor is salient, ubiquitous, and, for the most part, woefully overlooked. Here the very treatment of inflammatory conditions offers an essential, even obvious clue about their origins, a hint that may help resolve the mystery of where in the world these illnesses come from. We physicians frequently dole out large doses of synthesized stress hormones for inflammations of the skin, joints, brain, intestines, lungs, kidneys, and so on. We do so for a good reason: hormones often alleviate or ameliorate symptoms, albeit with many potentially hazardous side effects. Yet we rarely think to ask ourselves—or our patients—whether stress itself may, just may, have something to do with the condition we are treating.

There is plenty of evidence for such a view. A recent Swedish study in the *Journal of the American Medical Association* showed that people with stress-related disorders had significantly greater risk of autoimmune disease.[24] Tellingly, those who had been treated for their stress-related mental conditions with SSRI-type medication—the most widely prescribed class of antidepressants,† of which Prozac is probably the most famous—

†   SSRI stands for "selective serotonin uptake inhibitor," meaning that these medications block the uptake of the neural messenger chemical serotonin into nerve cells.

had lower risk for autoimmunity: a clear indication of the *body-mind*, to use Dr. Candace Pert's phrasing for the interflow of psychology and physiology in humans, and of the role of emotions in illness.

Not only in humans, either. Laboratory mice in a 2013 study were subjected to three weeks' stress, meant to mimic "the diversity of stressful events in daily human life." That meant immersing the creatures in cold water, wafting predator odors in their direction, making them endure bright lights or restraint or isolation—unpredictable stresses of variable duration they could not easily adapt to. The researchers called this "chronic variable stress." Mice so exposed were found to be at an elevated risk for pathogenic autoimmunity—in other words, for immune activity directed against the physical self.[25]

Life in our current culture, I believe, makes many of us experimental mice subject to "chronic variable stress" beyond our control.‡

A necessary caveat: in foregrounding the role of biographical factors in disease, we must be mindful to avoid blame or guilt. "Some people see lupus as an external attacker," a British woman with lupus has written. "But I prefer to think I did it to myself . . . Too much striving, too much living on the edge, too much stress. Yet despite the consequences, I wouldn't change how I lived my life. It is who I am, so this disease is who I am too."[26]

There is wisdom in that view, but I also hear an unwarranted self-accusation and an all-too-characteristic lack of self-compassion. No person *is* their disease, and no one *did* it to themselves—not in any conscious, deliberate, or culpable sense. Disease is an outcome of generations of suffering, of social conditions, of cultural conditioning, of childhood trauma, of physiology bearing the brunt of

---

‡   The striking gender differences in autoimmune disease as well as the racial disparities are addressed in chapters 22 and 23.

people's stresses and emotional histories, all interacting with the physical and psychological environment. It is often a manifestation of ingrained personality traits, yes—but that personality is not who we are any more than are the illnesses to which it may predispose us.

Yet if our British writer errs in identifying entirely with her disease, she is still skillfully directing us to a profound and fruitful set of questions. Could it be that illness as "external attacker" does not even exist when it comes to such chronic, auto-mutinous conditions as we have looked at in this chapter?[†] What if disease is not, in fact, a fixed entity but a *dynamic process* expressive of real lives in concrete situations? What new (or old) pathways to healing, unthinkable within the prevailing medical view, might follow from such a paradigmatic shift in perspective?

---

†   Obviously, with an external agent such as the novel coronavirus, we are facing an entirely different challenge. But even there, internal factors and social conditions play a major role in people's vulnerability to the infection.

Chapter 6

It Ain't a Thing:
Disease as Process

*Cancer is no more a disease of cells than a traffic jam is a
disease of cars. A lifetime study of the internal-combustion
engine would not help anyone to understand our traffic
problems . . . A traffic jam is due to a failure of the normal
relationship between driven cars and their environment and can
occur whether they themselves are running normally or not.*

—Sir David Smithers, *Lancet*, 1962

V, formerly known as Eve Ensler,‡ rose to fame in the 1990s as
the author of the *Vagina Monologues*, the play the *New York Times*
called "probably the most important piece of political theater of
the last decade." Her blockbuster stage success has given rise to a
life of activism. A fearless advocate for and defender of women's
rights, she has traveled worldwide, witnessing the bloody aftermath of mass rape and misogynist brutality in Bosnia and the
war-torn Democratic Republic of the Congo.

The political is personal for V. In her heartrending yet triumphant memoir of surviving life-threatening stage IV uterine cancer, *In the Body of the World*, she poses a question of stunning
frankness and insight: "Do I have rape cancer?" From an early

‡   Since our original interview, the writer and activist has changed her name to V, eschewing
the names—personal and familial—given to her by her rapist father, by whose legacy
she does not wish to be defined. Throughout this book, we honor that self-affirming
designation.

age and over many years, her father sexually violated her—a chronic assault on which was superimposed severe emotional abuse and, later, terrifying physical violence. All the while, her mother, hobbled by the legacy of her own childhood suffering, remained oblivious and/or silent. The child Eve felt she was "betraying" her mom by having an affair with her own father. "As a child when your father incests you, you feel you were the betrayer," she told me in an online interview. "And my mother hated me for it. She hated me for how much he adored me." Toxic self-blame is one of the torments imposed on the traumatized child. For much of her life V loathed herself, as so many victims of early abuse end up doing.

"How did I get it?" she writes about the onset of her cancer. "Was it worry every day for fifty-seven years that I wasn't good enough? . . . Was it the pressure to fill Madison Square Garden with eighteen thousand or the Superdome with forty thousand? . . . Was it the line of two hundred women repeated in hundreds of small towns for many years after each performance, after each speech, women lined up to show me their scars, wounds, warrior tattoos? Was it suburban lawn pesticides? . . . Was it my first husband sleeping with my close friend? . . . Was it sleeping with men who were married? . . . Was it not enough boundaries? Was it too many walls?"

When I asked her what she thinks now, V prefaced her answer with a laugh, perhaps sardonic. "I think it's a combination of all of the above," she said. "But I think that if there were one underlying reason why I got sick, it was unreckoned—I hadn't gone deep enough in processing my trauma." She then made a profound observation about the nature of illness itself: "A disease *is not like a thing*. It is energy flow, it's a current; it is evolution or devolution that occurs when you're not awake and connected, and trauma is essentially ruling your life. I think it's such a mistake to identify it as a thing, because that makes it hard matter when it's in fact a much more psychological, spiritual, emotional condition."

This hard-won perspective raises some unfamiliar, potentially fruitful questions. What if, she writes, "when you got sick, you weren't a stage [of a disease] *but in a process*? And cancer, just like having your heart broken, or getting a new job, or going to school, were a teacher? What if, rather than being cast out and defined by some terminal category, you were identified as someone in the middle of a transformation that could deepen your soul, open your heart?"

V's survival of a near-terminal diagnosis owed much to the heroic efforts and skills of modern medicine, including multiple complex surgeries and chemotherapy. But that's not all that saved her, as she sees it. V herself generated a powerful complement to these interventions in the way she approached healing: a willingness to experience disease not as a "thing," an external enemy, but as a process that encompasses all of her life—present, past, and future—and, ultimately, even as a teacher.

Beyond the War Metaphor

We are used to seeing disease as a thing to get rid of or a foe to battle against—as, for example, in the "war on cancer." (Which "war," for the record, has been far from victorious.)[1] Someday, we tell ourselves, with enough research, we as a society will "beat" cancer and wipe it out; in the meantime, we maintain a tenaciously defiant attitude, as expressed in the viral hashtag #FuckCancer. Our everyday language gives voice to our combative stance: we hear of a friend or a family member courageously "battling MS" or some other illness; they will either prevail in the struggle or else "succumb."

It may be that these martial metaphors are so appealing because their force matches our feelings of anger and despair; that does not, however, make them helpful. In a previous work I quoted the Canadian oncologist Karen Gelman, a leading breast cancer specialist, who looks askance at the military depiction of cancer care and research. "What happens in the body is a matter of flow—there is input and there is output," she said, "and you can't control every aspect of it. We need to understand that flow, know there are things you can influence and things you can't. It's not a battle, it's a push-pull phenomenon of finding balance and harmony, of kneading the conflicting forces into one dough."[2] I noticed how closely her use of "flow" mirrors V's language—one woman speaking from medical expertise, the other from hard-earned, subjectively sourced insight.

Beyond the declarations of war, there is another, even more popular class of misapprehensions that cloud our view of disease: "I *have* cancer." "She *has* MS." "My nephew *has* ADD." Embedded in each phrase is the unexamined assumption that there is an *I* (or a *someone*) distinct and independent from the *thing* called disease, which the "I" *has*—as in the statement "I have a flat-screen TV." Here is my life, and over there is the disease that has encroached upon it. Seen this way, disease is something external with its own nature, existing independently of the person in whom it shows up. Given where that perspective has gotten us, it is time to consider a new one.

We have already glimpsed the countless hormonal, immunological, neurological, molecular, intracellular, and epigenetic pathways that make our physiology inseparable from our emotional, psychological, spiritual, and social lives. V's understanding of trauma and stress as major founts of the process that ultimately came close to killing her is completely aligned with modern science. In a five-decades-long British study that followed nearly ten thousand people from birth until the age of fifty, it was found that early-life adversity—abuse, socioeconomic disadvantage, family strife, for example—greatly increased the risk of cancer before the mid-century mark. Women who experienced two or more such adversities had a doubled risk by midlife.[3]

"These findings suggest that cancer risk may be influenced by exposure to stressful conditions and events early on in life," wrote the researchers, once more employing the carefully reticent language of "suggest" and "may." To my clinical sensibilities, concerned as I am with how people fall ill and/or find healing, such results, mirrored over and over in multiple other studies, do not *suggest*: they scream for attention. The disorganizing impact of stress hormones on the immune system as a risk for cancer is far from a scientific secret. We have also seen how stress and trauma are prime drivers of inflammation, another central gear in the cancer-causing apparatus. Along parallel lines, girls who are sexually and physically abused have far greater risk in adulthood of endometriosis, a painful and often disabling condition that heightens the risk of ovarian cancer and whose origins perplex conventional medical thinking.[4] Considered from the mind-body psychoneuroimmunological perspective, the puzzle becomes rather less puzzling.[†]

To restate a question essential to our theme: What if we saw illness as an imbalance in the entire organism, not just as a manifestation of molecules, cells, or organs invaded or denatured by pathology? What if we applied the findings of Western research and medical science in a systems framework, seeking all the connections and conditions that contribute to illness and health?

Such a reframing would revolutionize how we practice medicine. Rather than treating disease as a solid entity that imposes its ill will on the body, we would be dealing with a *process*, one that can't be extricated from our personal histories and the context and culture in which we live. This change in approach has much

---

[†] Recall, too, the connection between PTSD symptoms and ovarian cancer (chapter 2).

to recommend it, and not only because it takes interpersonal biology into account. When we cease to view illness as a concrete, autonomous thing with a predetermined trajectory—and when we have the proper help and a willingness to look both within and without—we can start to exercise agency in the matter. After all, if disease is a manifestation of something in our lives rather than merely their cruel disruptor, we have options: we can pursue new understandings, ask new questions, perhaps make new choices. We can take our rightful place as *active participants in the process,* rather than remain its victims, helpless but for our reliance on medical miracle workers.

Disease itself is both a culmination of what came before and a pointer to how things might unfold in the future. Our emotional dynamics, including our relationship to ourselves, can be among the powerful determinants of that future. An attitude of helplessness and hopelessness at the time of diagnosis, for example, has been shown to exert a marked adverse effect on survival in women with breast cancer even ten years later.[5] Conversely, a decrease in depressive symptoms is associated with longer survival.[6] Even in a study of women requiring biopsies for cervical abnormalities identified on routine Pap smears, those with a dejected view of life *before* diagnosis were much more likely to find that they received a diagnosis of cancer.[7] In men, the immune system's capacity to react to prostate cancer was diminished in those with a tendency to suppress anger.[8] Another prostate study found that social support reduced the risk.[9]

Dr. Steven Cole[†] is a prolific researcher whose work has cast bright light on the disease process. "We now know that *disease is a long-term process,*" he told me, "a physiological process taking place in our bodies, and how we live influences how quickly

---

[†] Professor of medicine and psychiatry and biobehavioral sciences at the UCLA School of Medicine.

that's going to get us at a clinical level . . . The more we understand about disease, the less clear it becomes when you have it and when you don't." Within the myth of normal, of course, this kind of nuance is barely comprehensible: you're either "sick" or you're "well," and it should be obvious which camp you're in. But really, there are no clear dividing lines between illness and health. Nobody all of a sudden "gets" an autoimmune disease, or "gets" cancer—though it may, perhaps, make itself known suddenly and with tremendous impact.

A few years ago, the *New Yorker* featured an article titled "What's Wrong with Me?," a poignant first-person account of yet another "idiopathic" autoimmune condition.[10] The piece was also a perfect depiction of disease as a long-term process rather than a distinct entity. "I got sick," the author writes with a pained humor, "the way Hemingway says you go broke: 'gradually and then suddenly.' One way to tell the story is to say that I was ill for a long time—at least half a dozen years—before any doctor I saw believed I had a disease. Another is to say that it took hold in 2009, the stressful year after my mother died, when a debilitating fatigue overcame me, my lymph nodes ached for months, and a test suggested that I had recently had Epstein-Barr virus."

The telltale hallmarks of the disease process are there: the prolonged course; the professional befuddlement at the lack of specific markers on physical examination, blood tests, or imaging studies; and the sudden interpersonal stress that finally brings on the full-blown manifestations of illness. Toward the end of the article the writer reports a revealing clue as to the source of her devitalizing malady, one that should have been a signal to her treating physicians: "In May, my endocrinologist speculated, after various M.R.I.s, that I had an 'idiopathic' disorder in the hypothalamus which is probably untreatable."

The clue? We've seen it already: the hypothalamus is the hub of the body's and brain's stress apparatus, a key modulator of immune activity, and the apex of the autonomic nervous system. It is the transducer into physiological data of our emotional functioning and, therefore, of our interpersonal relationships and of our relationship to ourselves. It translates fear, loss, grief, and stress into responses in our bloodstream, organs, cells, nerves, lymph nodes, messenger chemicals, and molecules throughout the entire organism. Thus, from a broader interpersonal biology point of view, her illness may not be so idiopathic after all, but the understandable outcome of chronic and acute stress. Even if untreatable by present-day medical techniques, it need not be beyond healing, especially if we bring in a wiser, science-based appreciation of the interconnected complexity of the disease process and the bodymind unity.

Returning to cancer, the work of Dr. Cole and colleagues has shown that activation of the body's stress response can promote tumor growth and spread. It is important to note, as they warned, "that stress *per se* does not cause cancer; however, clinical and experimental data indicate that stress and other factors such as mood, coping mechanisms, and social support can significantly influence the underlying cellular and molecular processes that facilitate malignant cell growth."[11]

This raises a key point. Stress cannot "cause" cancer, for the simple reason that our bodies naturally harbor potentially malignant cells at all times. The body contains over thirty-seven trillion cells, in all various stages of development, maturity, and decay. Malignant transformation happens regularly, as an accidental by-product of natural cell division. Under normal conditions the organism's defenses can eliminate such threats to well-being. We know from autopsies, for example, that many women have breast cancer cells, just as many men have prostate cancer cells, without ever developing the disease of cancer. The question is, What drives the progression of these cells into clinical illness? What keeps the immune system from successfully confronting the internal menace? This is where stress plays its incendiary role: for example, through the release of inflammatory proteins into the circulation—proteins that can instigate damage to DNA and impede DNA repair in the face of malignant transformation. These proteins, called cytokines, can also inactivate genes that would normally suppress tumor growth, enable chemical messengers that support the growth and survival of tumor cells, stimulate the branching of blood vessels that bring nutrients to feed the tumor, and undermine the immune system. Even at the cellular and molecular levels, the generation of ill health is a multifaceted, multistep process.

In 1962 the leading British cancer physician David Smithers published a paper of prophetic force. He explored cancer as process: not a disease of individual cells gone rogue but a manifestation of an imbalanced environment, "merely the terminal [event] in a much longer progressive chain of circumstances with no distinctive starting-point." Doctors and researchers, he wrote, do not experience cancer's "essential dynamic quality; they see its static effects, not the process in action."[12] The activity of cells, Smithers pointed out, "is possible only in relation to their environment, and none of their actions can be explained by laws governing intracellularly initiated events alone." That prescient assertion has been more than validated by the half century of research since.

"I now have a much more complex view of causation," Steve Cole told me. "If you get a disease, a whole series of things had to have gone wrong. Some of that may be related to your genes; some of that may be related to pathogen exposure. Some of it is related to hard lives—the way that can wreak wear and tear on the body and on what would otherwise be resilient tissues. It's better to think of it as a multistep causation . . . One of the things many diseases have in common is inflammation, acting as kind of a fertilizer for the development of illness. We've discovered that when people feel threatened, insecure—especially over an extended period of time—our bodies are programmed to turn on inflammatory genes."

A Physician Heals Herself

Threatened and insecure over an extended period of time is precisely how the obstetrician-gynecologist Lissa Rankin felt since childhood, an emotional state her medical training only exacerbated. Her book *The Anatomy of a Calling* begins with a nightmarish recounting of how she, as a medical resident, had to rush all night from one delivery room to another, dealing with one difficult delivery in the wake of another, supporting parents after the death of four babies, and all the while being berated by her superiors to suppress her own grief, even in the privacy of the women's changing room. "Doctors," she writes, "become masters at stuffing their emotions. We can't cry when we're grieving or when someone has hurt our feelings, or when we are sad." I recently spoke with the California-based physician. "In medical school," she told me, "I was being sexually harassed by my surgery professors all the time. All the time. I just had to tolerate it . . . I never went to the medical school director, I never told anybody, or asked for protection, because that was part of my wounding: I wasn't allowed to ask for help, to be 'needy,' to complain."

When she was twenty-seven, Dr. Rankin was admitted to the coronary care unit at her hospital for an episode of distressingly rapid heartbeat that did not respond to the usual noninvasive measures. After receiving electrical shock treatment to restore her normal heart rate, she was sent directly back to work. By age thirty-three, she was taking multiple medications for a number of conditions, including three drugs for high blood pressure and palpitations, antihistamines, and a steroid—which, again, is a stress hormone—and weekly injections for allergies, which, she was told, she'd have to stay on for the rest of her life. She was also treated for a cervical abnormality, a precancerous state that reappeared soon after the procedure. All the while—and this will sound familiar—no physician asked her what stresses might be weighing on her, promoting immune problems, and potentiating malignancy.

Today Dr. Rankin is fully healthy and taking no drugs at all. In her case, healing owed nothing to conventional medical treatment and everything to the personal transformation she was guided to undertake—a journey she began when, at age thirty-five, she was nearly suicidal. "Within six months of quitting my job I was off all my medications," she reports. She is now a mother, a healer, a seminar leader, and the author of several books. Her key insight was to recognize her entire life as the ground for her several illnesses, physical and mental; not separate entities but dynamic processes expressing her interactions with her world. "I had been a stereotypical good girl, overachiever, top of my class, always pushing to develop my talent and intellect, not to satisfy me but to be accepted by others," she told me. That relentless pressure, she learned, manifested in her medical conditions. She had to let it go.

As Lissa Rankin realized, much good can come from an open-minded engagement with the process that disease represents. It may not be the guest we ever desire to see, but a modicum of hospitality—welcoming the unwelcome, so to speak—costs us nothing. It may even lead to an opportunity to find out why this particular visitor has come to call, and what it might tell us about our lives.

Chapter 7

A Traumatic Tension:
Attachment vs. Authenticity

Most of our tensions and frustrations stem from compulsive
needs to act the role of someone we are not.

—János (Hans) Selye, M.D., *The Stress of Life*

To hear Anita Moorjani tell it, the disease that nearly killed her was no random misfortune. "The person I was before I got cancer," the bestselling author told me, "was afraid of disappointing other people. I was a pleaser. I completely lost myself in satisfying other people, I became so drained. I was someone who could not say no; I was a rescuer, and I would be the one who was there for everyone. I didn't even learn that it's okay to be me when I had cancer. It took being in a coma to learn that." Now a vibrant sixty-year-old, Moorjani is convinced that chronic stress induced by the compulsive suppression of her own needs was one of the roots of her metastatic lymphoma, thought to be terminal when she was diagnosed at age forty-three. "My personality was such that I needed something as drastic as cancer to give me reason to take care of myself."

Many of us have heard such sentiments: the notion of "finding the gold" in catastrophe is not at all unfamiliar, nor limited to the sphere of health crises. But the idea that features of our personality may contribute to the onset of pathology is anathema to many. In her still-influential 1978 essay "Illness as Metaphor," the late filmmaker, activist, and brilliant woman of letters Susan Sontag—then a forty-five-year-old cancer survivor—flatly and forcefully rejected the possibility that ill health might signify anything beyond bodily calamity. "Theories that diseases are caused by mental states . . . are always an index of how much is not understood about the physical terrain of a disease," she wrote.[1] To assert that emotions contribute to disease was, for her, to promote "punitive or sentimental fantasies," to traffic in "lurid metaphors" and their "trappings." She found this view especially distasteful because she perceived it as a way of blaming the patient. "I decided that I was not going to be culpabilized."[2]

Sontag's acerbic rejection of the mind-body connection resonated not only in intellectual circles but also in some of the most hallowed centers of medical thinking. A few years later, the *New England Journal of Medicine*'s future first woman editor, Dr. Marcia Angell, cited it approvingly, deriding as "folklore" the idea that "mental state is a factor in the causing and curing of specific diseases," a "myth" for which the evidence is at best "anecdotal." Like Sontag, Dr. Angell espied in this line of thinking an insidious patient-blaming tendency: "At a time when patients are already burdened by disease, they should not be further burdened by having to accept responsibility for the outcome."[3]

I agree wholeheartedly that no one, ever, ought to be made to feel guilty for whatever transpires with or within their body, whether that guilt arises from the self or is imposed from without. As I stated earlier, blame is inappropriate, unmerited, and cruel; it is also unscientific. But we have to take care not to fall into an easy fallacy. Asserting that features of the personality contribute to the onset of illness, and more generally perceiving connections between traits, emotions, developmental histories, and disease *is not* to lay blame. It is to understand the bigger picture for the purposes of prevention and healing—and ultimately for the sake of self-acceptance and self-forgiveness.

My intent in reframing Sontag's perspective, then, is to offer a more helpful view. I empathize with her apprehension about being blamed for becoming ill, even as I see her refutation of the mind-body confluence as misguided and scientifically untenable. A clear and honest look at the biographical factors that can disrupt our biological well-being helps us respond intelligently and effectively to illness—or preferably, to mitigate the risks in the first place. This is as true for individuals as for society.

There is nothing radical about the idea that certain personality traits can pose risks for illness; in fact, it is a restatement in modern scientific terms of insights that date far back. The physiological pathways connecting an irascible temper and heart disease, for instance, have long been well understood: they include increased blood pressure and heart rate, intensified clotting, and tightening of blood vessels, among others.[4, 5, 6] Already in ancient times Hippocrates spoke of the "choleric" temperament, believed to result from an excess of choler (yellow bile). In English we still speak of people who are habitually grumpy as "bilious." And in traditional Chinese medicine, the liver—the source of bile—is associated with anger, bitterness, and resentment. In 1896, the renowned internist and medical teacher Sir William Osler, often called the father of modern medicine, asserted to graduate students at Baltimore's Johns Hopkins Hospital that "it is not the delicate, neurotic person who is prone to angina [a cardinal symptom of coronary artery disease], but the robust, the vigorous in mind and body, the keen and ambitious man . . . whose engine is always at full speed ahead." He was foreshadowing the modern concept of the driven, compulsively preoccupied, impatient, readily upset, and heart-disease-prone type

A personality—a biopsychosocial dynamic, which, both scientifically and "anecdotally," is easy to grasp.

In 1987 the psychologist Dr. Lydia Temoshok[†] proposed what became known as the "type C personality," referring to traits strongly associated with the onset of malignancy.[‡] These couldn't have been further from the type A traits on the temperamental spectrum; they included being "cooperative and appeasing, unassertive, patient, unexpressive of negative emotions (particularly anger) and compliant with external authorities." She had interviewed 150 people with melanoma and found these patients to be "excessively nice, pleasant to a fault, uncomplaining and unassertive." They were identified "pleasers": while anxious about their disease progression, their worries were focused in a specifically outward direction, away from themselves and toward the effect that their illness was having on their families. Such self-abnegation was too well typified in an article I once read in the *Globe and Mail*, written by a woman just diagnosed with breast cancer. "I'm worried about my husband," she immediately told her physician. "I won't have the strength to support him."[7]

Around the same time, about ten years into my medical practice, I was beginning to notice similar patterns in the lives of many of my patients, folks with all manner of illnesses. This, despite my lack of familiarity at the time with the voluminous research that in the past half century has shed light on how stress, including the stress of self-suppression, may disturb our physiology, including the immune system. Not knowing then of Dr. Temoshok's work, I came to alike conclusions because they virtually urged themselves upon me: I couldn't help seeing what I saw. Time after time it was

†   At that time, director of the Behavioral Medicine Program at the University of Maryland Medical School.

‡   In fact, Temoshok was describing character traits, not a complete "personality"—more below on this misperception of her ideas.

the "nice" people, the ones who compulsively put other's expectations and needs ahead of their own and who repressed their so-called negative emotions, who showed up with chronic illness in my family practice, or who came under my care at the hospital palliative ward I directed. It struck me that these patients had a higher likelihood of cancer and poorer prognoses.

The reason, I believe, is straightforward: repression disarms one's ability to protect oneself from stress. In one study, the physiological stress responses of participants were measured by how their skin reacted electrically to unpleasant emotional stimuli, while the patients reported how much these stimuli bothered them. Flashed on a screen were insulting or demeaning statements, such as "You deserve to suffer," "You are ugly," "No one loves you," and "You have only yourself to blame." Three groups of participants were assessed in this way: people with melanoma, people with heart disease, and a healthy control group. Among the melanoma group there was a consistently large gap between what they reported—that is, to what degree they *consciously* felt upset by these scornful and disparaging messages—and the level of bodily stress their skin reactions betrayed. In other words, they had pushed their emotions below conscious awareness. This cannot help affecting the body: after all, if you go through life being stressed *while not knowing you are stressed*, there is little you can do to protect yourself from the long-term physiological consequences. Accordingly, the scientists concluded that repressiveness ought to be seen "as a mind-body, rather than as just a mental, construct."[8]

Some years later, psychologists at the University of California, Berkeley, investigated the physiological effects not of repression, a largely unconscious process, but of *suppression*, defined as "the *conscious* inhibition of one's own emotional expressive behavior while emotionally aroused." If I know I'm afraid but choose to conceal that from a rabid dog who can "smell fear," I am suppressing my feelings—as opposed to repressing them, as in compulsively pretending to agree with opinions one finds repellent and not realizing it until later. In the Berkeley study, participants were shown films normally expected to elicit disgust, such as burn patients being treated or an arm being surgically amputated. Some participants were specifically instructed not to reveal emotions when watching, while the control group was free to express emotion by means of facial or body movements. On a number of physiological measurements, the suppression group showed heightened activation of their sympathetic, or fight-or-flight, nervous system: in other words, a stress response.[9] There may be certain situations where a person, for perfectly valid reasons, deliberately chooses not to express how he feels; if one does it habitually or under compulsion, the impact is more than likely to be toxic.

I have distilled my own list of the personality features most often present in people with chronic illness, as observed by myself and many others. They may remind you of some of the personal stories I've included thus far. Whether a person exhibits one, a few, or every one of these features, they all, each in their own way, speak to self-suppression and/or repression. I have found them not only present but *prominent* among people with all manner of chronic illnesses, from cancer to autoimmune disease to persistent skin conditions, through a gamut of maladies including migraine headaches, fibromyalgia, endometriosis, myalgic encephalomyelitis (ME), also known as chronic fatigue syndrome, and many others.

In no particular order, these traits are

- an automatic and compulsive concern for the emotional needs of others, while ignoring one's own;

- rigid identification with social role, duty, and responsibility (which is closely related to the next point);
- overdriven, externally focused multitasking hyper-responsibility, based on the conviction that one must justify one's existence by doing and giving;
- repression of healthy, self-protective aggression and anger; and
- harboring and compulsively acting out two beliefs: "I am responsible for how other people feel" and "I must never disappoint anyone."

These characteristics have nothing to do with will or conscious choice. No one wakes up in the morning and decides, "Today I'll put the needs of the whole world foremost, disregarding my own," or "I can't wait to stuff down my anger and frustration and put on a happy face instead." Nor is anyone born with such traits: if you've ever met a newborn infant, you know they have zero compunction about expressing their feelings, nor do they think twice before crying lest they inconvenience someone else. The reasons these habits of personality, as we might call them, develop and grow to prominence in some people are both fascinating and sobering. At root they are coping patterns, adaptations originally formed to preserve something essential and nonnegotiable.

Why these features and their striking prevalence in the personalities of chronically ill people are so often overlooked—or missed entirely—goes to the heart of our theme: they are among the most *normalized* ways of being in this culture. Normalized how? Largely by being regarded as admirable strengths rather than potential liabilities. These dangerously self-denying traits tend to fly under our radar because they are easily conflated with their healthy analogues: compassion, honor, diligence, loving kindness, generosity, temperance, conscience, and so forth. Note that the qualities on the latter list, while perhaps superficially resembling those of the first, do *not* imply or require that a person overstep, ignore, or suppress who they are and what they feel and need. True compassion, for example, is an equal-opportunity offering, granted to others precisely because we know and honor what we ourselves feel. We might well admire someone who puts another's needs before their own in a crisis, or the leader of a struggle for the rights of many, but such sacrifices are undertaken in a conscious and time-bound manner, appropriate to the situation at hand and with full awareness of the risks.

I have a rather unusual habit when it comes to reading the newspaper: I've long been taken with reading obituaries in which friends and relatives pay homage to deceased loved ones. I frequently note in these a certain poignant paradox. Composed with affection and sorrow, these moving tributes often reveal and unwittingly celebrate their dearly departed's self-abnegating traits, without recognizing that these may have played a central role in the illness that ended the life being remembered. Consider, for instance, the case of an Ontario physician—we'll call him Stanley—who died of cancer. Stanley's closeness with his mother was approvingly lauded in his obituary in Canada's national newspaper, the *Globe and Mail,* in its daily "Lives Lived" section:[†] "Stanley and his mother had an incredibly special relationship, a bond that was apparent in all aspects of their lives until her death. As a married man with young children, Stanley made a point to have dinner with his parents every day, as his wife Lisa and their four kids waited for him at home. He would walk in, greeted by yet another dinner to eat and to enjoy. Never wanting to disappoint either woman in his life, Stanley kept having

---

[†]   I used to write the *Globe and Mail's* medical column and often contributed to the op-ed pages.

two dinners a day for years, until gradual weight gain began to raise suspicions."[†]

Another column memorializes a woman who, despite her metastatic cancer, "did not give up any of her roles," including "several hockey practices, school board, orchestra and other extracurricular activities," and even took on new ones—all directed toward helping others—as the disease spread throughout her body. I am all for enthusiastic engagement with one's community. But there is such a thing as a lust for life, and then there is being driven to derive one's sense of self from constant activity, even to the point of not being able to pause for self-care when disaster strikes.

As a final example, we have a widower remembering his wife (dead of breast cancer at age fifty-five) in these terms: "In her entire life she never got into a fight with anyone . . . She had no ego, she just blended in with the environment in an unassuming manner." The phrase "no ego" should give us pause. Intended to lovingly convey an admirable lack of arrogance or conceit, those two little words reveal, to me, a deeper story. A healthy ego—not in the sense of superiority, but as in a stable identity, the ground of self-respect, self-regulation, capacity for good decision making, a working memory, and more—is a vital asset of a thriving human being. Unbeknownst to the grieving spouse, what he was describing was the same lifelong repression of one's feelings— particularly healthy anger—which undermines the immune system and poses a risk for malignancy and other illness.

Where does such forsaking of the self come from? "Type C," Lydia Temoshok pointed out, "is not a personality, but rather a behavior pattern that can be modified."[10] I completely agree with her view. Precisely because no one is born with such traits ingrained,

---

[†] The original names appeared in the column; I've changed them here to further protect privacy. Otherwise, the obituary is cited verbatim.

we can unlearn them. That's a pathway toward healing—not an easy road by any means, and one we will take up later in detail. But first, let's see if we can trace the origins of these patterns.

A recurring theme—maybe the core theme—in every talk or workshop I give is the inescapable tension, and for most of us an eventual clash, between two essential needs: *attachment* and *authenticity*. This clash is ground zero for the most widespread form of trauma in our society: namely, the "small-*t*" trauma expressed in a disconnection from the self even in the absence of abuse or overwhelming threat.

Attachment, as defined by my colleague and previous co-author, the psychologist Dr. Gordon Neufeld, is the drive for closeness—proximity to others, in not only the physical but the emotional sense as well. Its primary purpose is to facilitate either caretaking or being taken care of. For mammals and even birds, it is indispensable for life. For the human infant especially—at birth among the most immature, dependent, and helpless animals, and remaining that way for by far the longest period of time—the need for attachment is mandatory. Without reliable adults moved to take care of us, and without our impulse to be close to these caregivers, we simply could not survive—not for a day. As we'll see in the next chapter, we each arrive in the world "expecting" attachment, just as our lungs expect oxygen. Hardwired into our brains, our drive for attachment is mediated by vast and complex neural circuits governing and promoting behaviors designed to keep us close to those without whom we cannot live. For many people, these attachment circuits powerfully override the ones that grant us rationality, objective decision-making, or conscious will—a fact that explains much about our behavior across multiple realms.

In infancy our dependence is an obligatory and long-haul proposition. Everything from crying to cuteness—two unignorable cues babies transmit—is an inbuilt behavior tailored by Nature to keep our caregivers giving and caring. But the need for attachment does not expire once we're out of diapers: it continues to motivate us throughout our lifespan. As we saw in chapter 3, unsatisfactory attachments can wreak havoc even with adult physiology. What distinguishes our earliest attachment relationships—and, crucially, the coping styles we develop to maintain them—is that they form the template for how we approach *all* our significant relationships, long after we have grown out of the do-or-die phase. We carry them into interactions with spouses, partners, employers, friends, colleagues: into all aspects of our personal, professional, social, and even political lives. It follows that attachment is a major concern of the culture—as we see, in a trivial form, in popular media gossip about who loves, leaves, or lies to whom. Attachment—along with attachment frustration, as in the "satisfaction" that we, along with Mick Jagger, can't get none of—is never far from our minds.

Our other core need is *authenticity*. Definitions vary, but here's one that I think applies best to this discussion: the quality of being true to oneself, and the capacity to shape one's own life from a deep knowledge of that self. What may not be apparent is that authenticity is not some abstract aspiration, no mere luxury for New Agers dabbling in self-improvement. Like attachment, it is a drive rooted in survival instincts. At its most concrete and pragmatic, it means simply this: knowing our gut feelings when they arise and honoring them. Imagine our African ancestor on the savanna, sensing the presence of some natural predator: Just how long will she survive if her gut feelings warning of danger are suppressed?

The elemental root of "authenticity" is the Greek *autos*, or "self," closely related to "author" and "authority." To be authentic is to be true to a sense of self arising from one's own unique and genuine essence, to be plugged into this inner GPS and to navigate from it. A healthy sense of self does not preclude caring for others, or being affected or influenced by them. It is not rigid but expansive and inclusive. Authenticity's only dictate is that we, not externally imposed expectations, be the true author of and authority on our own life.

The seed of woe does not lie in our having these two needs, but in the fact that life too often orchestrates a face-off between them. The dilemma is this: *What happens if our needs for attachment are imperiled by our authenticity, our connection to what we truly feel?* What happens, in other words, when one nonnegotiable need is pitted by circumstance against the other? These circumstances might include parental addiction, mental illness, family violence and poverty, overt conflict, or profound unhappiness—the stresses imposed by society, on children as well as adults. Even without these, the tragic tension between attachment and authenticity can arise. Not being seen and accepted for who we are is sufficient.

Children often receive the message that certain parts of them are acceptable while others are not—a dichotomy that, if internalized, leads ineluctably to a split in one's sense of self. The statement "Good children don't yell," spoken with annoyance, carries an unintended but most effective threat: "Angry children don't get loved." Being "nice" (read: burying one's anger) and working to be acceptable to the parent may become a child's way of survival. Or a child may internalize the idea that "I'm lovable only when I'm doing things well," setting herself up for a life of perfectionism and rigid role identification, cut off from the vulnerable part of herself that needs to know there is room to fail—or even to just be unspectacularly ordinary—and still get the love she needs.

Although both needs are essential, there is a pecking order: in the first phase of life, attachment unfailingly tops the bill. So when the two come into conflict in a child's life, the outcome is well-nigh predetermined. If the choice is between "hiding my feelings, even from myself, and getting the basic care I need" and "being myself and going without," I'm going to pick that first option every single time. Thus our real selves are leveraged bit by bit in a tragic transaction where we secure our physical or emotional survival by relinquishing who we are and how we feel.

The fact that we don't consciously choose such coping mechanisms makes them all the more tenacious. We cannot will them away when they no longer serve us precisely because we have no memory of them *not* being there, no notion of ourselves without them. Like wallpaper, they blend into the background; they are our "new normal," our literal *second* nature, as distinct from our original or authentic nature. As these patterns get wired into our nervous system, the perceived need to be what the world demands becomes entangled with our sense of who we are and how to seek love. Inauthenticity is thereafter misidentified with survival because the two were synonymous during the formative years—or, at least, seemed so to our young selves.

Here we see the perilous downside of our much-vaunted and wondrous capacity to adapt to diverse and challenging circumstances. After all, most adaptations are meant for specific situations, not as eternally applicable responses in every possible case. Here's an analogy plucked from the headlines: At the time of this writing, freezing weather has enveloped Texas.[†] People are adapting by wearing extra clothing, heating their homes when power is available, wrapping themselves in warm blankets—all necessary strategies for surviving inclement winter conditions. Those same adaptations, meant to be temporary, would jeopardize health and life if not discarded by the time of summer's

---

† February 2021.

blazing heat. The internal adaptations we make to our own personalities in order to survive adversity early in life carry the same risks as conditions shift, but we are far less wise to the danger. No matter how the weather changes, the protective gear, welded as it is onto the personality, never comes off.

It is sobering to realize that many of the personality traits we have come to believe *are us,* and perhaps even take pride in, actually bear the scars of where we lost connection to ourselves, way back when. The sources of these scars are most often evident in their shape, so to speak: in many cases, specific traits can be traced to particular kinds of wounding. For example, if we don't receive the agenda-free, unconditional attention we all require, one way to guard against that deprivation is to become concerned with physical attractiveness or other attention-getting attributes or accomplishments. A child who does not experience himself as consistently and unconditionally *lovable* may well grow to be preternaturally likable or charming, as with many a politician or media personality. Someone who is not *valued* or *recognized* for who she is early in life may develop an outsize appetite for status or wealth. If we are not made to feel important for just who we are, we may seek significance by becoming compulsive helpers—a syndrome I know intimately.

And here's the final part of the disappearing act: as mentioned, in our culture, many of these compensations for what we lost are seen as not only normal but even admirable. Valued as "strong suits," they too often encase and wall off the authentic self by assuming its guise.

These traits and the behaviors that follow are "runaway addictive," in Gordon Neufeld's phrasing. Funny enough, this tractor-beam pull exists precisely because they do *not* work—or to be more accurate, they work only temporarily. I am fond of the physician and trauma researcher Vincent Felitti's astute remark about addiction that "it's hard to get enough of something that almost works." Much like the rush an addict experiences immediately after using, the relief we buy with our compensatory pseudo-strengths does not last: we crave more and more, again and again and again. In fact, the analogy is entirely appropriate physiologically, since among the brain chemicals released when we have moments of feeling loved or valued or accepted are our own internal opiates, or endorphins. And just as an opiate like heroin does not satiate, so the temporary endorphin hit of valuation or appreciation or approval or success cannot possibly resolve the ache in the soul. We are compelled to persevere in seeking those external sources of fleeting relief, only to have to replenish them once the thrill is gone. Hence the seeming sturdiness of the personality: we keep experiencing the same emotions and associated body states, and we persist in performing the same behaviors. But it is closer to the truth to think of the personality as a *recurring* phenomenon than a *fixed* or *permanent* one, much like the way individual movie frames projected at rapid speed create the optical illusion of a single, continuous narrative.

For most of us it may require a crisis of some kind before we question the veracity and solidity of the self-concept we act from, before it even occurs to us that it might conceal something truer about us. Such crises might take the form of some relational catastrophe such as a divorce or near divorce; a debilitating addiction that disrupts our functioning, such that we can no longer ignore or tolerate it; the midlife bewilderment that may befog our forties or fifties; a sudden depression that ensnares us as we go along what we thought was our merry way; or a medical affliction, such as Anita Moorjani endured. All these can—and often seem uncannily as if they were designed to—point toward the need for a fundamental reassessment of who we think we are.

Strikingly, in her private musings Susan Sontag unwittingly pinpointed the emotional dynamics for which her cancer stood as a perfect metaphor. "I'm being wasted by self-pity and self-contempt," she wrote in her journal.¹¹ Cancer, of course, is a wasting disease—it devastates the body from the inside. She also located the source of her self-loathing in her anguished childhood. "Everyone who has had a bad childhood is angry. I must have felt angry at first (early). Then I 'did' something with it. Turned it into—what? Self-hatred." Eerily, Sontag touched upon the forbidden link just after her original diagnosis with breast cancer in 1971—some eight years before she wrote "Illness as Metaphor." "The first thing I thought was: What did I do to deserve this? I've led the wrong life, I've been too repressed." The word "wrong" there is a delicate thing, of course, resting very much on the spirit in which it is used. Sontag did not lead an *incorrect* life—that would be a harsh and blaming view—but neither, the word implies, did she get to live the life she might have wanted for herself.

Rereading "Illness as Metaphor" now, knowing what I know, I am saddened. Sontag spurned the connection between emotion, personality, and illness more forcefully and articulately than anyone—and, too, with bitter and unintended irony. The life and death of this powerful thinker, etched with tragedy, has much to tell us.

Abandoned as an infant by her mother and deserted again a few years later after a brief reunion, Sontag learned early to repress her rage: "I've always made excuses for her. I've never allowed my anger, my outrage." As an adult she reported herself "seething with resentment. But I dare not show it." "Profoundly neglected, ignored, unperceived as a child," she compensated by developing character features that promoted her success in the world. "One of the healthiest things about me—my capacity to 'take it,' to survive, to bounce back, to do, to prosper—is intimately connected with my biggest neurotic liability: *my facility in disconnecting from my feelings* . . . When a small child, I felt abandoned and unloved. My response to this was to want to be very good."

"Guilt is awful," Sontag said, poignantly—and yes, it is. But there *is* no culpability where there is no choice. No conceivable condition exists under which a human being has less agency or fewer options than in infancy and early childhood. The imperative to survive overrides everything, and that survival depends on the maintenance of attachment, at whatever cost to authenticity. This is why so many childhoods, particularly in a culture that both breeds stress and feeds on it, are marked by a tense standoff between the two, where the outcome is predictable and the consequences are lifelong.

Here's something else I've come to know, which I hope will be heartening for you as it is for me: it is not only necessary to leave blame and guilt behind on the road to healing, to move from self-accusation to curiosity, from shame to "response ability"—it is also and always possible. "What changed for me is that I realized that I had a choice," Anita Moorjani says. "When you are conditioned to do something, you're not even aware you're doing it. Not even aware that you're suppressing yourself, because you're in survival mode."

The onset of inauthenticity may not be a choice, but with awareness and self-compassion, authenticity can be.

Part II

The Distortion of Human Development

*If our society were truly to appreciate the significance of children's
emotional ties throughout the first years of life,
it would no longer tolerate children growing up, or
parents having to struggle, in situations that cannot
possibly nourish healthy growth.*

—Stanley Greenspan, M.D., *The Growth of the Mind*[†]

[†]   Stanley Greenspan (1941–2010), former director of the Clinical Infant Development
Program, U.S. National Institute of Mental Health.

Chapter 8

Who Are We Really?
Human Nature, Human Needs

There is always some conception of human nature, implicit or
explicit, underlying a doctrine of social order or social change.
—Noam Chomsky, *The Chomsky-Foucault Debate:*
On Human Nature

What is our nature? The query is age-old, in part because it is so hard to get a handle on. Taking in the vast horizon of deeds and accomplishments, from the life-affirming to the murderous, it certainly seems as if "being human" is a rather plastic, malleable thing.

Though it may not be obvious why a book about health in the twenty-first century should concern itself with so broad and elusive a topic, I believe the question is central, with far-ranging implications. The relative health of any life-form is a function of its essential needs being met, or not met. Thus, to know what kind of beings we are is to know what we need in order to *be* those beings to the fullest. Who we take ourselves to be dictates how we set up our lives, individually and as a collective, and determines the extent to which a culture does or doesn't meet the requirements for optimal health and functioning.

Every society makes assumptions about human nature, and ours is no exception. "It's human nature," we say, shrugging our shoulders at someone's—often our own—manipulative, self-serving behavior. "Interestingly," notes the educator Alfie Kohn, "the characteristics we explain away in this fashion are almost always unsavory; an act of generosity is rarely dismissed on the grounds that it is 'just human nature.'"[1] There is a tendency in this culture, whether with approval or dismay, to see people as inherently aggressive, acquisitive, and ruggedly individualistic. We might cherish kindness, charity, and community-mindedness— our "better natures," so to speak—but these are often spoken of wistfully, as exceptions to a hardwired rule.

Not every culture accepts this as the quintessence of humanness. The anthropologist Marshall Sahlins, who studied societies across the Pacific basin, wrote: "For the greater part of humanity, self-interest as we know it is unnatural . . . it is considered madness . . . Rather than expressing human nature, such avarice is taken for a loss of humanity."[2] Some peoples even give such madness a name. The Cree word *wétiko* (with variants in other Native languages such as Ojibwa and Powhatan) refers to a creature, spirit, or mindset of greed and domination that cannibalizes people and drives them to exploit and terrorize others. (Strikingly, in the Quechua language of the Peruvian Andes, a similar entity—associated with the gold-craving and ruthless Spanish colonizers—is called *pishtako*.) Far from embodying our nature, such a relentless pursuit of narrowly defined self-interest is seen as its opposite: "a very contagious and rapidly spreading disease," according to the Native American scholar Jack Forbes.[3]

I find discussions of a fixed human nature unhelpful and even misleading. A cursory look at our history confirms that we are not one way: Jesus was a human being and so was Hitler. We can be noble and narcissistic, generous and genocidal, brilliant in our ingenuity and buffoonish in our stupidity. We are, it seems, all of the above. So where to begin?

Rather than trying to adjudicate between the many competing visions of what a human being is, we could instead see our nature as a range of possible outcomes. I very much like this formulation by Robert Sapolsky, professor of neurology and biology at Stanford University:[†] "The nature of our nature is *not to be particularly constrained by our nature.*" If we're constrained by anything, maybe it's that very open-endedness; strange as it may sound, our miraculous talent for adaptation could also be a liability. Because our nature is so influenceable, different conditions evoke different versions of us, from benign to disastrous. When we reify—set in stone, mentally speaking—the particular way human behavior shows up in a certain place and time, we commit the fallacy of conflating how we're being with who we are. This error can keep us from considering other possibilities, even if our current way of operating isn't good for us. We then replicate conditions that are unfit for our well-being, and the sad saga continues. This is why, in seeking a vision of a healthier world, we had best disabuse ourselves of any fixed, limiting beliefs about what we're all about, and instead ask, What circumstances evoke which sorts of outcomes?

Encoded in our biology are some basic needs and potentials. How our nature unfolds depends on how well these needs are met, how these potentials are encouraged or frustrated. This is true throughout the lifespan, but at no time is it more consequential than during the process of development. Chronologically we can trace development's arc from conception through adolescence, although of course in many ways we never stop growing, changing, adapting, and developing—if we're lucky, for the healthier and wiser.

More than any other factor, it is the environment—the *conditions* under which development takes place, which either do or don't meet our multiple needs—that determines which

---

†   And author, most recently, of *Behave: The Biology of Humans at Our Best and Our Worst.*

potentials will or will not manifest. This is as true for us as for any other life-form. Consider the acorn. It is in the nature of an acorn, we might say, to become an oak tree—but only if the climate and soil are right, and provided no enterprising squirrel squirrels it away for winter sustenance. Even if it roots and sprouts successfully, the size and healthy branching of the oak tree born of that acorn would depend on what nourishment the ground can provide, climatic conditions, sunlight and irrigation, its spacing from or proximity to its fellow flora, and so on.

We, too, have needs the environment must satisfy if we are to flourish. Before exploring this dynamic, we need to once again dispense with the prevalent myth that genetic traits account for human behavior. They do not. While we have a certain biological makeup, we are not genetically programmed to feel or believe or act in any particular manner. As Robert Sapolsky put it when we spoke, "We are freer from genetics than any other species on earth." Owing to our adaptability and capacity for invention, we can inhabit a much broader range of environments, for example, than any other large mammal. Further, as we have seen in our discussion of epigenetics, the expression of genes, in themselves inert, depends on the environment. Experience, therefore, is the decisive influence on how our biology manifests in our lives. "When all is said and done, the individual [is] genetically determined *not to be genetically determined*," in the apt phrase of two French scientists, restating Sapolsky's bon mot about "the nature of our nature" in biological terms.[4]

While it is in our nature to adjust to and survive in an almost infinite array of environments—certainly many more than oak trees can—we are not necessarily at our best or our healthiest in all of them. Some of these, whether physical, emotional, or social, will make wellness an uphill battle or a luxury for the lucky, rather than a widely available norm.

The needs that set the table for human health are far from arbitrary. They emerged over millions of years with the hominid and hominin† progenitors that preceded our own relatively late advent as a species, at most two hundred thousand years ago. Insofar as it is possible to speak coherently about human needs, we have to consider how they developed for eons before oral or written history. What we call civilization encompasses little more than 5 percent of our existence as a species; for the entire span of the human genus, it represents less than 1 percent. The evolutionary crucible that formed who we are and what we need was subject to very different conditions than our own. Thus, while civilization expresses aspects of our potential, it cannot by itself be used as a reliable gauge.

In *The Continuum Concept: In Search of Happiness Lost*, Jean Liedloff proposed that all life develops as "an *expectation* for its environment." Lungs can be seen as an expectation for oxygen, our cells for water and nutrients, ears for the vibration of sound waves. This is the essence of evolution: the long-term programming of creatures and all their constituent parts to arrive at life road-ready for a certain kind of setting. The same is true for all life, from organs to organisms to species. *"If one wants to know what is correct for any species, one must know the inherent expectations of that species,"* Liedloff added (italics in the original).[5] An inherent expectation is a wired-in need, something that if denied interferes with our physical and psychological equilibrium, leading to poorer health outcomes—physically, mentally, and socially.

Here's an inherent expectation in action: You walk into a corner store and select a candy bar. You smile as you greet the person behind the counter and say hello. The cashier is having a bad

---

† "Hominid": all the great apes, including humans, along with gorillas, bonobos, and chimpanzees; "hominin": species considered to be human or directly ancestral to humans.

day—perhaps nursing a toothache, a family crisis, or a crushing last-minute playoff loss by his favorite team. He looks at you sullenly (if he looks at you at all), takes your money with a monosyllabic grunt, and brusquely hands you the change. Your physiology alters: you feel tension as your body tightens, your heart rate goes up, and your breathing becomes shallower. You are irritated. Depending on your own state of mind, you might feel angry, perhaps even imagining bad things happening to the fellow.

Why? According to the neuroscientist and seminal researcher Stephen Porges, one of our inherent needs is reciprocity, to be attuned with—"well met," as the archaic greeting goes. It is what he calls a neural expectancy. Our brain may process the lack of welcoming response as an assault, a threat to safety.

Our nervous system's inherent expectation for reciprocity and connection makes sense when we consider how we developed as a species. For most of our evolutionary past, until about ten thousand to fifteen thousand years ago, human beings lived in small-band hunter-gatherer groups.[6] Indeed, if human existence were measured in the time span of one hour on a clock, we have inhabited newer environments only for the past six minutes or so. Liedloff described these forebears of ours as "people whose good relations are more important than their bargains." Her direct observations of Aboriginal people in their jungle habitat conform with the vast body of research on hunter-gatherers as collated, for example, by the psychologist Darcia Narvaez, professor emerita at Notre Dame. We have learned that such groups held values emphasizing hospitality, sharing, generosity, and reciprocal exchange for the purpose not of personal enrichment but of connection. These values were intelligent, time-tested guidelines for mutual survival. And the traditions they generated, passed down from parent to child, generation to generation, characterized human life throughout most of our existence. Yes, there was violence and bad behavior and all the rest; we have never been "perfect." But we knew something about setting the collective context for our humanness to flourish fruitfully; arguably, we knew nothing else.

Such guidelines, and the traditions that inscribed them into cultural behavior, survived for a long time even as societies became settled (i.e., not nomadic), as Westerners in contact with Indigenous peoples have found for many hundreds of years. "The community is there for them, and they are there for the community," wrote Frans de Waal about the Bushmen of the Kalahari, also known as the San people, a group widely thought to represent ways of life reaching back far into prehistory. "Bushmen devote much time and attention to the exchange of small gifts that cover many miles and multiple generations."[7]

No hominin species could have survived long enough to evolve had its members seen themselves as atomized individuals, pitted by Nature against their fellow beings. Contrary to our present ways of operating, a traditional view of self-interest would be *enhancing one's connection and membership in the community, to everyone's benefit.* Authentic self-interest need not be conflated with a suspicious and competitive stance toward others.

Hence my working assumption that our nature, all else being equal, *expects* or even *prefers* as its baseline state a condition of caring, relative harmony, and equilibrium, of the kind that obtains when interconnectedness rules the day. It is not that our nature *is* to be those ways, but that it *wants* them to be present. When they are, we thrive; when denied, we suffer.

What to make, then, of the modern received wisdom that we are fundamentally aggressive, selfish? Where does such an idea come from?

Under a capitalist system notions and expressions of human nature will both mirror the individualized, competitive ideal and justify it as being the inevitable status quo. It makes sense: if what's normal is assumed to be natural, the norm will endure; on the other hand, when suspicions emerge that the way things are may not be how they're meant to be . . . well, the quo may not be status for long. Thus do materialistic cultures generate notions—myths, in effect—of selfish, aggressive striving and dominance as behavioral baselines, encouraging characteristics that place a lesser value on connectedness to others and to Nature itself. In our present capitalist society, Darcia Narvaez suggested to me, we have become "species-atypical," a sobering idea when you think about it: no other species has ever had the ability to be untrue to itself, to forsake its own needs, never mind to convince itself that such is the way things ought to be.

As the following chapters will explore, today's culture hastens human development along unhealthy lines from conception onward, leading to a "normal" that, from the perspective of the needs and evolutionary history of our species, is utterly aberrant. And that, to state the obvious, is a life-size health hazard.

Chapter 9

A Sturdy or Fragile Foundation: Children's Irreducible Needs

We are born not knowing who we are, we don't know how to think. We only know how to feel. It is through our feelings that how we are raised creates the trajectory for our future lives.

—Natasha Khazanov[†]

Raffi Cavoukian woke suddenly at six o'clock one morning in 1997. "I bolted upright in bed," he tells me, "jaw dropped, eyes wide open, and the words 'child honoring' were playing right in front of my eyes, as a phrase and as the name of a philosophy." For the next decade, the internationally cherished children's troubadour took time away from the concert stage and recording studio to dedicate himself to envisioning, networking, and advocating for a world that honors children. He has maintained that commitment.[1] As he speaks of it, he sparkles with the playful enthusiasm and deep respect for young people that infuse his music—the same qualities that inspired my son Aaron as a toddler to dress up as his musical hero for Halloween, complete with ukulele and face-painted beard. "At its core, child honoring is respect for personhood," Raffi says. "Children are here to learn their own song."

The question of children's developmental needs is neither

---

†   Personal communication. Dr. Khazanov is a neuropsychologist based in San Francisco.

abstract nor sentimental; it is of urgent practical importance. Although we often refer to childhood as "the formative years," our societal norms speak dismally to our appreciation of how formative these years really are, of just how much is being "formed." The individual and collective stakes are far higher than we tend to imagine.

"We discover who we are from the inside," Raffi says. "What's forming is no less than how it feels to be human. And I'm using my words carefully here: how it *feels* to be human." Our culture too often subordinates felt knowledge to the intellect. This inverted ranking system upends how we raise our children—which, in turn, serves to reinforce the error culturewide. Above all, the singer asserts, "we are feeling creatures."

He has science on his side. The neuroscientist Antonio Damasio explores the primacy of feeling in his authoritative volume *Descartes' Error: Emotion, Reason and the Human Brain.* "Nature seems to have built the apparatus of rationality not just on top of the apparatus of biological regulation, but also *from* it and *with* it," he wrote (italics his).[2] *Biological regulation* means the workings of the homeostatic† and emotional structures of our brains and bodies, which, before and after birth, are many months ahead of the thinking cortex in the developmental queue—as, in the bigger picture, they long preceded it over the course of our species' evolution.

These areas of the nervous system form the unconscious scaffolding for our thoughts and conscious feelings and, therefore, for our actions. "The earliest established components of an infant's psychobiological makeup are those most formative of his lifelong outlook," notes Jean Liedloff. "What he feels before

---

† *Homeostasis* refers to the processes by which the body maintains the stability and constancy needed for all its subsystems to function properly, including temperature regulation, pH levels, and so much more.

he can think is *a powerful determinant of what kind of things he thinks when thought becomes possible.*"[3] In fact, the impacts go well beyond the content of thoughts: research has shown beyond any doubt that early experience molds behaviors, emotional patterns, unconscious beliefs, learning styles, relational dynamics, and the ability to handle stress and regulate ourselves.

The new knowledge is summed up nicely in two brief paragraphs from an article published in *Pediatrics*, the official journal of the American Academy of Pediatrics; the authors are affiliated with perhaps the world's leading institute on childhood, Harvard University's Center on the Developing Child:

> The architecture of the brain is constructed through an ongoing process that *begins before birth,* continues into adulthood, and establishes either a sturdy or a fragile foundation for *all* the health, learning, and behavior that follow.
>
> The interaction of genes and experiences literally shapes the circuitry of the developing brain, and is critically influenced by the *mutual responsiveness of adult-child relationships,* particularly in the early childhood years.[4]

In other words, early development sets the ground—whether strong or shaky—for all the learning, behavior, and health (or lack of it) that will come later. The researchers' words, if taken to heart, would call our attention to much in our current culture that cries out for immediate renovation.

If emotion is the ground of cognition, then relationships are the tectonic plates that shape that ground. Of these, a child's early emotional interactions with their nurturing caregiver(s) exert the primary influence on how the brain is programmed—again, the unconscious comes first, followed later by things like intellect.[5] In the words of the renowned developmental psychiatrist

Stanley Greenspan and colleagues, "Emotional rather than intellectual interaction serves as the mind's primary architect."[6]

Given this order of operations, children's sense of security, trust in the world, interrelationships with others, and, above all, connection to their authentic emotions hinge on the consistent availability of *attuned*, *non-stressed*, and *emotionally reliable* caregivers. The more stressed or distracted the latter, the shakier the emotional architecture of the child's mind will be.

If that sounds like an indictment of parents, that's the farthest from my intention. At the risk of being overly repetitious, let me state again that parent-blaming isn't only cruel and unfair; it's nonsensical. Suffice it for now to say that the quality of early caregiving is heavily, even decisively, determined by the societal context in which it takes place. As we will see, children are increasingly set upon by an accumulation of potent influences—social, economic, and cultural—that overwhelm and, in many ways, subjugate their internal emotional apparatus to imperatives that have nothing to do with well-being; that are, in fact, inimical to the healthy growth of the mind. "Such growth is becoming seriously endangered by modern institutions and social patterns," according to Dr. Greenspan. "There exists a growing disregard for the importance of mind-building emotional experiences in almost every aspect of daily life including childcare, education, and family life." We see the result in the growing numbers of children, adolescents, and youths suffering so-called mental illnesses[†] such as ADHD, depression, and anxiety, or engaging in aggressive or self-harming behaviors in person or on social media.

As Dr. Gordon Neufeld told a session of the European Parliament in Brussels, "The unfolding of human potential is

---

† My reasons for using the "so-called" qualifier will be taken up in chapters 17 and 18.

spontaneous but not inevitable . . . We all grow older, but we don't all grow up. *To truly 'raise' a child, then, would be to bring that child to his or her full potential as a human being.*"7 So why, in our modern culture, do we chronically miss that goal? The problem begins with the failure to grasp the needs of the developing child.

Neufeld sums up eloquently what all young ones, whatever their temperament, need first and foremost: "Children must feel an invitation to exist in our presence, exactly the way they are." With that need in mind, the parents' primary task, beyond providing for the child's survival requirements, is to emanate a simple message to the child in word, deed, and (most of all) energetic presence, that he or she is precisely the person they love, welcome, and want. The child doesn't have to do anything, or be any different, to win that love—in fact, *cannot* do anything, because this abiding embrace cannot be earned, nor can it be revoked. It doesn't depend on the child's behavior or personality; it is just there, whether the child is showing up as "good" or "bad," "naughty" or "nice."

Do we then ignore dangerous or unacceptable behavior? No, that wouldn't be the loving thing to do either, since children's needs also include guidance and orientation, which include setting boundaries. Rather, we do our best to monitor and curtail undesirable actions *from an unconditionally loving place*: a way of being wherein children understand that nothing they might do can threaten the relationship, even if it elicits momentary anger or requires correction. Operating from this attitude may even allow us to see the child's "misbehavior" in a broader, more forgiving frame—perhaps it expresses a need frustrated, a communication unheard, an emotion unprocessed. We understand and respond to the needs and emotions the child is "acting out," rather than simply punishing the behavior and banishing the feeling.

Neufeld's point about maturation being "spontaneous but not inevitable" is crucial here. The same evolution that has over many millennia honed us to be social and empathic creatures also assumes—or, to hearken back to chapter 8, "expects"—a particular kind of developmental environment. "We are indeed born for love," assert the science writer Maia Szalavitz and the child psychiatrist and neuroscientist Bruce Perry, "[but] the gifts of our biology are a potential, not a guarantee."[8] Certain kinds of experiences water the seeds of love and empathy that Nature has planted in us; absent that consistent nourishment, growth is compromised.

The essence of those experiences can be expressed in one word: security.

My eldest son, Daniel, co-writer of this book, pinpoints the lack of security as a central feature of his own early memories. "I didn't know up from down," he says, "because up could become down at any moment, depending on what mood the two of you were in, or the state of your relationship on a particular day. I had recurring nightmares as a kid where the ground kept opening up under me, and I'd fall through into another dimension, only for it to happen again. The dreams aren't hard to decipher: in the world of my childhood, *the floor was not the floor*." Indeed, without a "floor" of secure attachment, a young person is hard-pressed to feel any stable ground on which life can be experienced.

Despite all our love for our three children, Rae and I did not know how to provide the stable milieu they required, having lacked some essential aspects of nurturing in our own early years. Nor did the setup of our late-twentieth-century lives help us create the needed environment, what with our relationship tensions and my driven, workaholic tendencies, entrenched and amplified by the exigencies of medical training and practice. We were far from unique in these limitations.

Where does a sense of security come from? Once again, warm, attuned interactions with caregivers are the key ingredient. A 2010 study from Duke University reported that "early nurturing and warmth have long-lasting positive effects on mental health well into adulthood." The scientists examined nearly five hundred mother-infant pairs, noting how affectionate the moms were with their eight-month-old babies and assigning them categories such as "warm" or "occasionally negative" or "caressing" or "extravagant" in doting and tenderness. Most moms were rated as "warm," and about 1.5 percent as "extravagant." Over three decades later the grown children underwent a battery of mental health tests assessing their level of emotional distress and anxiety. Adults who had received the highest levels of maternal affection in infancy were shown to have the lowest levels of distress.[9] The lead researcher ventured that "maybe you can't be too affectionate . . . From the policy perspective, it definitely adds to that body of research that we should be able to protect time for mothers and fathers to be affectionate to kids." I consider it a sign of cultural lunacy that something so elemental, so essential, should be under such threat that we even have to exhort policymakers to "protect" it.

For a long time, it was assumed that infants are impelled to bond with caregivers only out of their helpless dependency on food, warmth, and shelter. We now know that social and emotional needs are just as much encoded in our neural circuitry by evolution, and that our optimal development requires that they be met. The neuroscientist Jaak Panksepp termed the cerebral apparatus governing these needs the "PANIC/GRIEF" system because, like a car alarm, these are the emotions that become activated in the *absence* of secure attachment. The message: we are wired to attach, to connect with one another, which we are able to do by dint of our early bonding with our caregivers. Not only that, but the wiring goes both ways: infants are "born to cry," in

Dr. Panksepp's words, precisely to activate the nurturing brain structures and affectionate behaviors of the parents—what he called the CARE system.[†]

Pondering this information sent me back to my mother's diary. Nothing to do with war or Nazis this time—just a woman of twenty-four trying to love her baby within the constraints of cultural norms, including medical advice that ran counter to her parenting instincts. According to accepted practice of the time, the doctor prescribed that I be fed on a strict schedule. Being a physician's dutiful daughter, my mom feared to disobey. Still in the hospital, with me a couple of weeks old, my mother writes:

> Now you are really giving me what for. For a change, you howled from half past midnight until 2:00 A.M. when the nurse came in and suggested I suckle you at least a little, so you finally slept. My greedy son, I definitely must warn you that we cannot make this a habit. In fact, soon we'll have to give up the 7:00 A.M. feeding. Believe me, my precious little son, my heart is rent in two as I hear you whimper your bitter complaints, but you are old enough of a fellow by now to realize that, pardon me, nighttime is for sleeping, not for eating.

There was my mom, following doctor's orders and so, for ninety long minutes, enduring my desperate vocalizations and her own emotional distress, coping as best she could via the dry wit that would be her signature until her death in 2001.

Revisiting this material now, versed in the neurobiology of parent-child attachment, I see a young woman in whose brain

[†] The world-renowned Dr. Panksepp distinguished seven such major brain systems responsible for our core emotional patterns. He rendered the names of each in capital letters. Along with CARE and PANIC/GRIEF, FEAR, RAGE, SEEKING, LUST, and PLAY are the others.

the instinctual CARE system described by Panksepp is at odds with the cultural mindset. Succumbing to the unnatural dictates of medical authority, her mother's heart aches.

And what of the infant in these now yellowed pages? What does he experience? Some three decades later, in 1975, Jean Liedloff warned her readers in *The Continuum Concept* about "the current fashion to let the baby cry until its heart is broken and it gives up, goes numb, and becomes a 'good baby.' " And indeed, I became a very good baby. Even as a four- or five-year-old I would lie in my bed before dawn, stoically enduring the stabbing pain of a middle-ear infection, whimpering quietly to myself so as not to disturb my sleeping parents.

Though it no doubt runs diametrically counter to most parents' intentions, a child whose cries are not responded to, who is not fed, not held close to a parent's warm body when in distress, learns a clear if wordless lesson: that his needs will not be met, that he must constantly strive to find rest and peace, that he is not lovable as he is. By taxing my brain's PANIC/GRIEF system, my poor mother's non-responsiveness also helped wire my brain for those chronic tendencies of mine that express the overactivation of that system: anxiety and depression. "When our brains are undercared for," writes Darcia Narvaez, "they become more stress-reactive and subject to dominance by our survival systems—fear, panic, rage." Don't I know it.

"The question," Gordon Neufeld said to me, "becomes, What are the irreducible needs of the child?" By "irreducible" he means a need that the child cannot do without if she is to reach her Nature-endowed potential; one that, if not met, will incur negative consequences. As he told the European Parliament, "It is true maturation, *not* schooling, learning or genetics that is key to becoming fully human and humane." We cannot *teach* maturity; nor can we cajole, entice, or coerce a child into it. What is required of us is to ensure the developmental conditions that satisfy the child's nonnegotiable needs; from there, Nature more or less takes care of the rest. There are four irreducible needs for human maturation, in Dr. Neufeld's astute formulation. These four needs are both simultaneous and build one on the other, in pyramidal fashion. I invite you, the reader, to consider how well our culture satisfies them for our children, or fails to.[†]

1. The attachment relationship: children's deep sense of contact and connection with those responsible for them.
Observe how my own neural expectation for such contact, instilled in infant me by eons of evolution, was frustrated within the first days and weeks of my life. Keep in mind that what matters is the child's *sense* of attachment; it has nothing to do with whether or how much the parents love the child or feel connected to her. Many young and well-meaning parents, myself and my wife included, have made the error of gauging the relationship by how *they* are feeling, how much attachment *they* are experiencing. Yet what makes the biggest difference is not what is *sent* so much as what is *received* by the child. It takes relatively mature and/or well-supported parents to be able to tune into the child's emotional needs as distinct from their own.

2. A sense of attachment security that allows the child to rest from the work of earning his right to be who he is and as he is.
Once foundational security is established, the young one can relax comfortably. This is the condition Dr. Neufeld identifies as "rest," one in which the child does not have to strive for attachment with the parent nor work to maintain the right equilibrium of contact. This state is the soil in which the roots of healthy

---

[†]   Dr. Neufeld's formulation happens to mirror precisely the basic requirements offered by the parenting practices of small-band hunter-gatherer groups, according to the research gathered by Dr. Darcia Narvaez. See chapter 12.

development can firmly take hold. From there we can reliably expect emotional, social, and intellectual growth to follow.

Despite my mother's love for me, I was essentially put to work from the moment I was born—no rest for the innocent. Contrary to her anxious half-joke that, before I was three weeks of age, I ought to be "old enough of a fellow by now to realize that . . . nighttime is for sleeping, not for eating," I was *years* away from being physiologically able to "realize" anything—much less that my needs were up for barter.

3. Permission to feel one's emotions, especially grief, anger, sadness, and pain—in other words, the safety to remain vulnerable. "Since emotion is the engine of maturation, when children lose their tender feelings, they become stuck in their immaturity," Neufeld explains. For the emotions to remain accessible, the environment must allow them to be safely experienced—meaning the child's expression of feelings *cannot threaten the attachment relationship* with the parents.

For reasons we have already begun to glimpse, many children in our culture are shut off from their authentic feelings.‡ And how would they not be, given the conformist expectations of society, amplified through parenting advice liberally dispensed by behaviorist "experts"? Consider the prescription of psychologist and mega-bestselling author Jordan Peterson: "An angry child should sit by himself until he calms down. Then he should be allowed to return to normal life. That means the child wins—instead of his anger. The rule is 'Come be with us as soon as you can behave properly.' This is a very good deal for child, parent and society."[10]

Is it, though? Notice the assumption: anger in a young child is neither normal nor acceptable. Contra her inborn need for unconditional warmth, any positive response to the child is to

---

‡   Chapter 7.

be distinctly *conditional*. She is not to be accepted for who she is, only for *how* she is. Here's the problem: even if the parent wins the behavior-modification game, the child loses. We have instilled in her the anxiety of being rejected if her emotional self were to surface. This exacts a heavy toll on both physical and mental health. While the expression of an emotion can be inhibited, or even its conscious experience blocked, the emotion itself is energy that cannot be obliterated. By banishing feelings from awareness, we merely send them underground, a locked cellar of emotions that will continue to haunt many lives.

I know for myself that the early hardening of my heart to my own pain shielded me not only from grief but also from joy. Rediscovering joy—or better yet, discovering it newly—remains part of my life's journey to this day.

4. The experience of free play in order to mature.
Rather than a frivolous activity to "grow out of," play is a requirement for the healthy development of all mammalian species. Jaak Panksepp coined a name for the neural system governing true recreation, to go with PANIC/GRIEF and CARE. "The PLAY system," he wrote, "may be especially important in the epigenetic development and maturation of the neocortex." A lack of secure infant bonding and a lack of early play, he asserted, can be contributory factors in the genesis of conditions such as ADHD, as well as of adult irritability and aggression.[11] Authentic play—agenda-free, interactive, engaging joy and imagination, and, rarer than ever these days, person-to-person—is easily compromised when children are under conditions of stress or deprivation. (Nor is it compatible with being distracted and mesmerized by digital technology, a vexing issue we will revisit in chapter 13.)

If the overall goal of development is to foster in children a felt sense of being alive in a nurturing world—"how it feels to be human," in Raffi's wonderful phrase—then we have utterly lost the plot. It takes a culture in good running order, with societal structures that take their cue from Nature's dictates, to support parents in ensuring the child's irreducible needs. How and why so many of our children's needs are going unmet will be the subject of our next chapters.

Chapter 10

Trouble at the Threshold: Before We Come into the World

My Tristram's misfortunes began nine months before
he ever came into the world.

—Walter Shandy, in *The Life and Opinions of Tristram Shandy,*
Gentleman (1759), by Laurence Sterne

Dear little son/daughter, I feel you kicking inside me. I am terribly sad and discouraged and frightened now but I love you and will protect and nourish you with all the love in the world. This adrenaline you feel is not meant for you nor flows because of you. One day I'll tell you about your gestation and I hope that if you carry with you ambivalent or painful memories, when I tell you the truth you will be able to heal. Dear little child: your Daddy will love you, too, when he gets to know you. He can't feel you moving inside him as I do inside me.

So wrote my wife when we were expecting our unexpected third child. It was a difficult period for us, and especially for Rae. She was stressed, unhappy, and anxious; what should have been a period of joy and mutual preparation felt like a lonely slog. I, the Daddy in the story, was in my mid-forties, outwardly a successful physician and columnist. Yet who was I within myself and within the four-walled world of our home? A depressed, anxious,

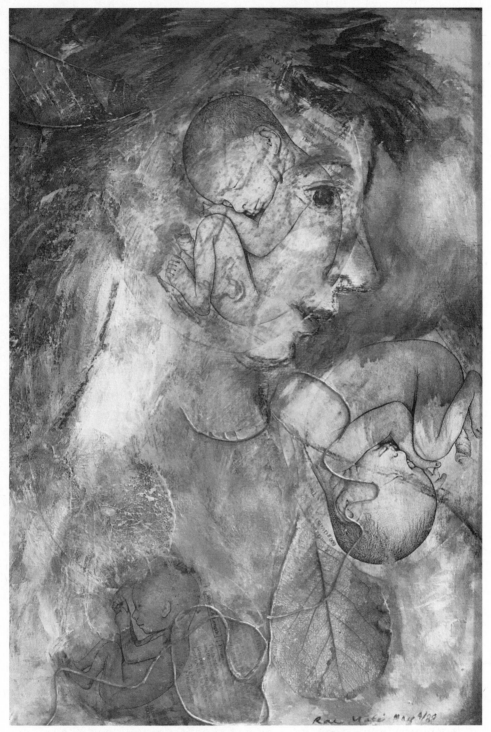

Gestation Self-Portrait, Rae Maté, 1988, mixed media. Rae created this painting during the first half of the pregnancy depicted in this chapter.

psychologically underdeveloped man, years away from addressing his core wounds; a man whose family bore the burden of his dysfunctional, erratic, and emotionally hostile behaviors; a man whose workaholism took the form at home of physical and emotional absence, even negligence; a man addicted to his own internal drama, not knowing how to be responsible for his actions and mind states or their impacts on his family, least of all his child-to-be.

Rae's diarized correspondence with the baby growing inside her showed how much she intuitively understood, long before I did, about human development and about the dynamics that so often distort its natural course in this culture. In our chapter on trauma, I pointed out that prior to becoming creators of our environment, we are its *creations*. Before we develop the capacity to take part in constructing our universe, the world fashions us. By what medium? At the beginning, through the bodies and minds and circumstances of our parents, who themselves are molded by the state of the world around them and by the histories of preceding generations. In this way, our own bodyminds are products of the larger culture from the start, a life course that begins with conception.

Before proceeding further, a necessary caution. Many readers will feel some alarm at the phrase "begins with conception," which has been heavily politicized in the ongoing cultural/religious debate over abortion rights. It is easy to see how a science-based recognition of the needs of the unborn can become political fodder for an anti-choice/"pro-life" view. All the more reason that I be extremely clear about what I do and don't mean. As a physician, I am well aware of the suffering imposed when women's right to choose is denied. There is no argument in this chapter, or anywhere in this book, for denying the right of autonomy when it comes to making such life decisions.

It has never been more vital that we speak about human development and its womb-to-tomb trajectory. It is also a highly delicate matter. For one thing, looking squarely at anything involving harm to children is difficult, often painful. Worse, when these topics arise, mothers and fathers might get the impression they are being judged, castigated, or impugned, which is doubly unfortunate: first, because in this culture too many parents—and I speak as one myself, three times over—already shoulder crippling guilt, already feel defensive; second, because blame is neither helpful nor remotely justified. We are all doing our best. My contention—really, the thrust of this whole book—is that our best *deserves to be better*, and *can* be if we incorporate the growing body of knowledge now available to us. I aim only to shed light on dynamics our entire culture needs to understand. This and the next chapter begin at our very beginnings, tracing our culture's failure to follow the developmental templates of gestation and birth as laid down by evolution.

The child's "ambivalent or painful memories" that Rae foresaw in her pregnancy journal are no poetic invention. Intrauterine experiences may not be accessible to conscious recall, but they can live on as a different kind of memory: emotional and neurological imprints embedded in the cells and nervous system of the human organism. The psychiatrist Thomas Verny calls this process *"bodywide memory."* A pioneer in recognizing the long-term influence of the intrauterine period on emotional health, Verny published his groundbreaking *The Secret Life of the Unborn Child* in 1982. In his sequel to that book, he wrote, "Before the event of birth, before we have even had a glimmer of sight or sound in the womb, we record the experience and history of our lives in our cells."[1]

In recent decades, a deluge of fresh information has underscored the crucial importance of women's physical environment, health, and emotional balance during pregnancy to the optimal development of the infant. Meanwhile, our era has also brought substantial increases in the number of children, adolescents, and young people facing depression and anxiety and other mental health challenges. Genetics on their own cannot begin to account for such abrupt shifts. If we are serious about reversing trends like these, it is critical that we connect the dots by looking to *the environment*. "Environment does not begin at birth; environment begins as soon as you have an environment," the neuroscientist Robert Sapolsky has said. "As soon as you're a fetus, you are subject to whatever information is coming through Mom's circulation, hormone levels, and nutrients."[2]

A very early factor is the stresses pregnant women are under—emotional, economic, personal, professional, and social. As the physician and psychoanalyst Ursula Volz-Boers points out, "Intrauterine life is not a paradise as some people try to make us believe. We are the receiver of all the happiness and of all the anxieties and difficulties of our parents."[3] But of course, even the earliest factor has its own earlier factors: namely, the intolerable pressures contemporary society places on the rearing milieu, the family, and on the developing young—and, as epigenetics teaches us, on the very activation of DNA itself. We need to consider to what extent our culture, including employment and the health care and insurance systems, supports or undermines women's capacity to hold their unborn infants' needs as a high social priority.

How many women are asked during prenatal checkups about their mental and emotional states, what stresses at home or on the job they may be experiencing? How many future physicians are even taught to pose such questions? How many spouses are helped to understand their responsibility to protect their expectant partners from undue stress and travail? How many businesses make provisions for their pregnant employees' relief? That last question has an especially dismal answer: women frequently report a pregnancy-hostile work milieu, especially in lower-paid jobs. But even in supportive workplaces, women are often burdened by the pressure they have absorbed and put on themselves to perform, advance, even excel in a competence-mad society. Work rarely "stays at work."

As Rae intuited, the baby feels the mother's stress directly. "By listening intently to movements and heartbeats, researchers are finding that the fetuses of mothers who are stressed or depressed respond differently from those of emotionally healthy women," the *New York Times* reported as far back as 2004. "After birth, studies indicate, these infants have a significantly increased risk of developing learning and behavioral problems and may themselves be more vulnerable to depression or anxiety as they age." Essential neurotransmitters such as serotonin and dopamine that later play key roles in mood regulation, impulse control, attention, motivation, and the modulation of aggression—and are implicated in the very learning, behavioral, and mood difficulties the article mentions—are affected by prenatal stress on the mother. Babies of moms stressed in pregnancy have lower levels of these brain chemicals and higher levels of the stress hormone cortisol. Not surprisingly, the same study showed that these newborns also had less developed learning skills, they were less responsive to social stimulation, and they were less able to calm themselves when agitated.[4]

Beyond brain substance levels, there is evidence suggesting that maternal mind states during pregnancy and postpartum shape *the very structure* of the infant's developing brain. In one study, nursing professor Dr. Nicole Letourneau, Canada research chair in parent-infant mental health at the University of Calgary, and her colleagues found that the child's gray matter, the cerebral cortex, was thinner on MRI scanning of the brains of preschool children whose mothers had suffered depression in the middle three months of pregnancy. As they point out, their brain-scan findings may presage later problems such as depression, anxiety, impaired impulse control, and attention difficulties in the child.[5] Postpartum depression had similar effects, indicating that there are certain critical periods in development, both before birth and after, during which the young human is particularly vulnerable to the environment. Such findings align with those of multiple other studies, which point to maternal-stress impacts on such brain structures as, for instance, the fear- and emotion-processing amygdala[6] and on neurological conditions such as autism.[7]

Other findings suggest strongly that many adult health challenges—everything from mental health disorders to hypertension, heart disease to diabetes, immune dysfunction to inflammation, and poor glucose metabolism to hormonal imbalance—are made more likely by intrauterine stress.[8] Among researchers there is a "universal consensus," to cite a major review paper, that what are called the developmental origins of adult disease begin in the womb.[9]

Remember telomeres, the chromosomal markers of health and aging? These structures were shown to be shorter—that is, more prematurely aged—in twenty-five-year-old adults whose mothers had undergone major stress during pregnancy.[10] We also know from our section on epigenetics that a mom's high stress levels during gestation can negatively influence the genetic functioning of the offspring, potentially impairing his lifelong stress-response capacities. Such effects have been shown to last well into midlife.[11]

Maternal stress during pregnancy has even been correlated with a poor makeup of the infant's gut microbial flora—a less healthy mix of bacteria—based on fecal samples taken from newborns days and even months after birth, with a higher incidence of intestinal problems and allergies among these babies.[12] (A deficit in infant gut microbial flora is also seen after many C-sections, when the infant does not travel through the maternal birth canal.)

Though a mother's emotional stress exerts a direct influence on the child's development and future health, it is not an isolated factor: interpersonal biology holds sway once again. As was the case with Rae and me, there is a complex interplay between a woman's psychological states and those of the father. A large Swedish survey recently showed that *paternal* depression in the year from preconception to the end of the second trimester elevated the risk of extreme prematurity (coming between weeks twenty-two and thirty-one of gestation) by nearly 40 percent. This effect was *greater*, in fact, than that of depression in the mother herself, which raised the risk only of moderate preterm birth (thirty-two weeks or after).[13] "Paternal depression is also known to affect sperm quality, have epigenetic effects on the DNA of the baby, and can also affect placenta function," one of the researchers pointed out.

At first blush, the father's melancholy posing a greater risk than the mother's seems an anomaly. As always, context is everything. The social context for procreation in our world assigns women untenably stressful roles in every facet of life, including intimate relationships. Besides being the bearers of children, they've generally been expected to assuage the psycho-emotional stresses of the men in their lives. Mothering a child may be a mandate from Nature, but mothering a grown man is both unnatural and impossible. No wonder the father's stress gets outsourced to the mother, at a cost to children and even to the gestating infant.

There is a predictable socioeconomic link, too: in a recent

Wayne State University study that examined a low-resource, high-stress U.S. urban setting, abnormalities in brain connectivity were identified in scans of yet-unborn infants of mothers who reported elevated levels of depression, anxiety, worry, and stress during the last three months.[14] Needless to say, physical factors such as nutrition and air quality interact with socioeconomic status, predisposing children to such problems as depression, anxiety, and ADHD.[15] "Poor people have more exposure to these things on all counts, whether the bad air, or psychosocial stress and other things," Dr. Shanna Swan, reproductive endocrinologist and vice chair of preventive medicine at Mount Sinai Medical Center in New York, pointed out. "That's a societal problem and the changes are not going to be on an individual level. They're going to be on a societal level."[16] Thus does inequality of opportunity, even in the basic biological sense, begin in the womb.[17]

Long before we had brain scans, blood tests, ultrasounds, and fetal heart monitors, ancient peoples intuitively understood the sanctity of the intrauterine environment. I spoke once about addiction to a First Nations group here in British Columbia, quoting studies on prenatal development such as cited above. A young man came up to me afterward. "You know," he said, "in our clan, tradition was that if you were angry or upset, you weren't even allowed to go near a pregnant woman. We didn't want you to inflict your troubles on her baby." In some African tribal societies, infants were greeted by rituals while still in the mother's belly, including with songs that would later welcome them into the world.[18] Imagine hearing your own melody and lyrics, already familiar to you, as you are ceremonially ushered into your new home, the outside world.

Such collective traditions have mostly been lost to colonialism and atomization, but we can still learn from them and apply their lessons.

"We know prenatal depression and stress and anxiety can predict behavior problems in the child," Professor Letourneau told me. "We can try to fix those behaviors in the kid years later, or we can medicate the child, or we can give pregnant women the support they need in the first place."

Support. If we want to build a world that provides it, we could start by asking its would-be recipients what the word means to them. I recently asked Rae—if I could do it over again, I would have done so long before now—what would have supported her back then. I can't improve upon the wisdom, nor the accuracy, of her answer:

"It would have helped if I had had a community in place. If there existed a larger consensus in our culture of what is required to gestate a baby. It would have helped if I had had a doctor or a social worker or family member who could have stood up for me. If the doctor had asked me, even once, how I was faring emotionally . . . If anyone had phoned my husband: 'Are you aware you are hurting your baby? Whatever problems you have with your wife, your role now is to be protective of her and of the infant she is carrying.' We all need to realize that entering a pregnancy should be like entering a shrine, a sacred place and time: a baby is being built.

"Mental health needs to be on the curriculum as soon as a woman gets pregnant—just as there are prenatal classes for the physical birth, so there should be for the emotional birth. The woman's focus must be on the baby, and not on the husband or even the job; the husband's focus—everyone's focus—must be on supporting the woman. Parents need to know that their job is mutual, that while the wife is pregnant, the husband is also pregnant. Society needs to protect pregnant women because everybody is creating this child. It takes a world to make a baby."

Chapter 11

What Choice Do I Have? Childbirth in a Medicalized Culture

At the beginning of the twenty-first century, we have to rehumanize birth, realizing there are limits to our domination of Nature.

—Michel Odent[†]

Over my decades as a family physician, I attended nearly a thousand deliveries. Standard operating procedure was to perform an episiotomy on every woman giving birth, just as I'd learned in medical school. "Time to make a little cut now," I would announce as the infant's head reached the perineum, ready to exit the birth canal. Having injected local anesthetic near the vaginal opening, I would make an incision a few inches long, "catch" the baby, and hand it to the nurse. I then set about repairing the wound I had inflicted. I knew no other way.

Years later I happened to learn from some midwives—who, in the Dark Ages of the 1980s, were still working illicitly here in British Columbia—that episiotomies are completely unnecessary in most labors. There was an organic process trying to happen, they kindly explained, which allowed a child to be born without my surgical intervention: Who knew? More surprises

---

[†]   Personal communication from the famed French obstetrician and author of *Childbirth and the Evolution of Homo sapiens*, among other books.

followed. Women can, it turns out, deliver babies without their feet in stirrups and even without reclining on a narrow metal contraption. "Try taking a shit while lying down and your legs in the air," a midwife suggested when I questioned her wisdom. Other startling news was that, barring complications, the newborn is best handed to the mother for skin-to-skin contact, rather than being poked and prodded under bright lights and having plastic suction tubes shoved in its mouth. Nor does the cord have to be cut immediately: it can be allowed to complete its pulsations, delivering more oxygen-carrying red blood cells to the infant.[1] It's almost as if Nature knows what it's doing.

These once-heretical practices have since been validated by solid medical research. At long last, doctors now have—more accurately, ought to have—permission to support in good conscience what human beings, with or without any "professionals" assisting, have been doing for hundreds of thousands of years. As the American journalist Anne Fadiman describes in her illuminating work on the clash of medical cultures besetting Hmong immigrants to the United States, these Asian women stubbornly resisted some of our "best practices" in favor of their own ways, including "squatting during delivery and refusing permission for episiotomy incisions to enlarge the vaginal opening . . . Many Hmong women were used to being held from behind by their husbands, who massaged their bellies with saliva and hummed loudly just before the baby emerged."[2] In short, they had tradition, intuition, innate body sense, Nature, and—no doubt unbeknownst to them—the most up-to-date science on their side.[3] Not to mention their husbands, who literally had their backs.

The advent of modern obstetrics has brought much to be grateful for, sparing many women and infants from avoidable suffering, illness, and death. The problem is that, along with its triumphs, and in line with the mechanistic approach of Western medicine in general, obstetrical practice ignores the genuine and natural needs of mothers and babies—in fact, it often runs roughshod over them. Bringing infants into the world is not simply a question of pushing and pulling and cutting and catching. It is a major threshold in human development, and how it is crossed has potentially lifelong consequences. By pathologizing the birth process, present-day medical practice contradicts the wisdom of Nature and of the human body. More damningly, it frequently violates even its own commitments to align itself with science and to, first, "do no harm." We need not abandon the great achievements of medical work to honor traditional wisdom, rooted in age-old experience. We can embrace both.

I will not be advocating for any particular type of birth, "natural" or otherwise, or railing against any other, much less judging any woman's individual choices around this vastly significant event. My interest, in keeping with this book's overall focus, is the cultural context in which, these days, such choices are made—which includes *by whom* and *in what manner* they are made. As the poet Adrienne Rich put it in her book *Of Woman Born*: "In order for all women to have real choices all along the line, we need fully to understand the power and powerlessness embodied in motherhood in patriarchal culture." Reducing women to passive recipients of medical care during perhaps the most momentous passage of their lives is dehumanizing, and not only figuratively: it disrupts physiological, hormonal, and psychological processes that have evolved in our species over millions of years to ensure the necessary bonding of mother and baby and the healthy development of our young.

A few years ago I spoke with Dr. Michel Odent, world renowned for his embrace of and advocacy for demedicalized birth practices. "We have to deindustrialize childbirth, to stop disturbing the first contact between mother and baby," he said in a charming French accent. "Imagine," he said with a laugh, "the mother gorilla giving birth and you try to pick up her newborn baby. And then you will understand what a maternal protective aggressive instinct is. In our civilization we have suppressed that instinct for a long time." Suppression of innate knowledge is one of medicine's unfortunate tendencies.

Medical intervention, which in a sane system would be deployed only when necessary to reduce risk, maximize health, and ensure survival, has become the default approach. A clear example is the steeply rising rate of the cesarean section: a lifesaving intervention when needed, a potentially noxious interference when not. According to the best estimates, about 10 to 15 percent of deliveries ought to end with C-sections to ensure healthy outcomes. Here in my home province of British Columbia that rate now approaches *40 percent*, as it does in many other parts of the world, with some countries exceeding that mark; worldwide, the number of these surgical deliveries doubled between 2000 and 2015. "Markedly high CS use was observed among low obstetric risk births, especially among more educated women in, for example, Brazil and China," noted a detailed, near-global survey by the *Lancet* in 2018.[4]

That would be acceptable if there were some demonstrable "value added" from such procedures being widespread, but there isn't. "Cesarean section use has increased over the past 30 years in excess of the 10–15% of births considered optimal, *and without significant maternal or perinatal benefits*," noted the *Lancet* report.[5] Even the American College of Obstetricians and Gynecologists raised, in 2014, "significant concern that cesarean delivery is overused."[6]

"If we want to find safe alternatives to obstetrics, we must rediscover midwifery," Odent told a birthing conference in 1986, when the medical profession in North America was still fighting a tooth-and-nail battle to keep midwives from fulfilling their traditional role. In many jurisdictions that struggle is far from over, while in many others there reigns a grudgingly observed truce, at best. "To rediscover midwifery is the same as giving back childbirth to women," Odent added. "Imagine the future if surgical teams were at the service of the midwives and the women instead of controlling them."[7] In effect, he was suggesting that medicine be Nature's attendant, not its ruler—a radical reinterpretation of the phrase "attending physician."

The issue is autonomy, an indispensable human need. Birthing practices express the hidden or overt values of a culture in terms of who wields power and how much genuine control people are able to exercise over their own bodies. Modern research finds that maternity-care interventions may disturb hormonal processes, reduce their benefits, and create new challenges.[8] What then, I asked Sarah Buckley—a New Zealand–based physician, advocate, and author of a highly regarded overview of the normal physiology of childbearing—explains the rapidly growing rates of medicalized interference? I expected an answer based purely on medical concerns. In fact, her response was sharply perceptive as to how acculturation into the much broader myth of normal takes place. "Doctors," Dr. Buckley said, "are the agents of our society's expectations that we imprint on mothers, when they are very open and vulnerable, that technology is superior to the body and that women's bodies are intrinsically bound to fail. It really is obvious that the culture wants to impress upon women this view of their bodies as inherently defective and needing high-level technological care." And that will carry on, she added, "*into how she brings up the child to be in accord with the demands of the culture.*"

Though systemic sexism tilts the playing field against women in particular, there is also a broader cause of unnecessary medical interference, one foundational to the Western medical view: a distrust of natural processes and fear of what can, may, or will go wrong.[†] Michael Klein, former head of the family practice department at BC Women's Hospital in Vancouver, has done extensive research on medical birthing. "You learn in a very biased environment that sees childbirth as scary and dangerous," he told me. The paradigm that dominates medical training "sees birth as nothing more than an accident waiting to happen, an opportunity for your pelvic floor to be bent out of shape. The women are unexploded bombs that need defusing." Throughout my medical schooling and internship, I was trained to anticipate the problems, complications, and dangers of birth. All good, as far as it went. The problem was, nothing in my training encouraged me *to align with Nature*. It was left to my patients and my midwife colleagues to teach birth to me as something more than a mechanical procedure of extracting a baby from the mother's body—something with ingrained, evolutionarily derived purposes, both physiological and emotional.

Sherri Dolman, a California woman I've come to know, had to wage an intense and protracted struggle for autonomy around her pregnancies. Despite a triumphant ending, her tale is a medical horror story. "I tried to conceive that child for three years," she told me. "But when I became pregnant, I was no longer able to make decisions for my child or for myself. I will never shake that for the rest of my life." Dolman was coerced into a cesarean section she did not want and, as she subsequently proved, never needed. "My doctor did not respect my decisions," she said, "and I don't think he respected me as an autonomous human being. I believe he thought he knew better than me. I can't think of one

---

[†] And in the litigious U.S. system, the terror of lawsuits and high insurance premiums.

single instance where a man is told what he can and can't do with his body, but women are told this every day."

At age thirty-four Dolman was already the mother of a seventeen-year-old son, born when she herself was a scared teenager. Because her labor had progressed slowly, likely owing to her stressed state of mind, she'd had a C-section. She was intent on a vaginal birth next time. After three years of trying, she and her partner got pregnant with a daughter. "From the first moment I vowed that I would not have a cesarean section this time around. I would deliver my daughter the way that Nature intended me to. I would trust my body, I would get the proper support I needed to do this." She did her due diligence, interviewing as many doctors as she could. "They all said, 'Once a cesarean, always a cesarean.' They weren't even willing to speak with me about it. 'I'll take you as a patient,' they told me, 'but we're going to be scheduling your cesarean.'"

Medically speaking, the doctors were completely off base. By the time of her daughter's conception, the safety of vaginal birth after cesarean section (VBAC) had long been documented, with the supposed risk—the uterus tearing under the pressure of labor contractions—shown to be negligible, posing no impediment to an unmedicated delivery. Indeed, a high-risk perinatal specialist who had evaluated Dolman's uterus with a detailed scan affirmed that her chance of such a mishap was no greater than if she had never been pregnant. In a sign of how deep the indoctrination runs, the obstetrician still balked at the vaginal option. The one doctor who had finally agreed to support Dolman's preference for natural labor got cold feet at the last possible moment.

Following a routine fetal-monitoring session, which showed no abnormality, Dolman was physically barred from leaving the hospital, threatened with arrest, and browbeaten into accepting the surgical delivery of her daughter. After this harrowing experience, she suffered what she calls "a version of PTSD . . . I was unable to function in my daily life. I felt like a failure as a mother, unable to comfort or touch my daughter in her first moments of life. I felt like I had nothing to do with her even being here. I felt disconnected from her. She cried if she needed me, but I didn't feel that I was enough. Throughout the first year of her life, I cried myself to sleep every night."

Dolman's subsequent two births were her redemption, the reclaiming of full agency.

Under the care of a midwife, she succeeded in a joyful vaginal birth at the completion of her third pregnancy. Though she described it as "very, very painful," she counts it among "the most amazing and exhilarating experiences" of her life. As is the case for so many women, Dolman's license to make her own choices was key to getting to the other side of the suffering. "No matter how painful it got, I had support and I was in control of my own body. That was very empowering to me no matter what came my way—being in charge of my own body was what it came down to." Ten years later, the telling of it still brought tears to her eyes. "Tears of joy," she quickly assured me. "My daughter asks me all the time: 'Tell me the story about how I was born.' She finds it hilarious that while I had the skin-to-skin contact with her, she pooped all over me, and she laughs every time I tell the story. That in itself was a bonding experience, just even sharing that with her. It's part of life." In 2011 Dolman brought forth another child, a healthy nine-pound, three-ounce boy. That birth, too, was vaginal, also in hospital under the care of a midwife, five years after she had been sternly admonished by ten board-certified obstetricians not to attempt such a delivery.

The triumphs don't all look the same, nor should they. "I know from my medical experience that you don't want to hold too fast to anything," said Danielle, a resident in anesthesiology.

"Still, I had beliefs and ideas about how I saw things going . . . I intended originally to have a home birth in water, at a cottage here that we had rented in the forest." It didn't turn out that way. After prolonged labor with little progress at home, the midwife recommended hospitalization and an epidural to allow Danielle some relaxation. The birth hormone oxytocin was given to promote progress, to no avail. After thirty-six hours of intense labor, Danielle accepted the necessity of surgical delivery. To this day, she is elated about her experience.

Although Danielle's process took a different form than Sherri's, the two births resembled each other in one core aspect: the mother felt herself to be in charge. "I was listened to. Everyone made time to hear what I was concerned about. Even the assistant to the surgeon came in to see me, a woman in family practice here. She met me, and she looked me in the eyes, and she was fully present. I just felt safe with everyone in there." In those words we hear the second factor determining the quality of women's experience: safety and support.

A health care system that honors women's strengths and their vulnerabilities gives them the best chance at a childbirth experience they can cherish. This view runs through a little gem of a pregnancy primer, *A Is for Advice (The Reassuring Kind)*, by the Brooklyn-born, B.C.-based midwife Ilana Stanger-Ross. "The women who report the most positive birth experiences," she observes, "are those who feel they understood all the decisions made and had a say in the decision-making process. That holds even for complicated births among women who had been hoping for 'natural' deliveries—births that require multiple interventions, births that end in surgery."[9]

To learn about the physiology of childbearing is to marvel at the innate wisdom of Nature and its highest evolutionary achievement, the human body. The biological bottom line is this:

Mammalian labor is more than a process of expelling an infant from a womb. It is preparation for life. Labor, as Nature designed it, promotes the release of hormones such as estrogen, oxytocin, and prolactin that activate a host of neural systems governing the emotions and behaviors, ensuring the baby's well-being in the short and long terms: warmth, nurturing, bonding, protection, and so on. In other words, birth prepares the template for the mother-infant relationship, which itself is the central locus of the child's early development.[10]

Having been out of the baby-catching game for some decades, I was caught off guard by a phrase Stanger-Ross used when we spoke: "obstetrical trauma." "That has become a term," she said. "Unfortunately, a lot of women feel that their birthing experience was one of trauma, which, of course, is going to have impacts on the parent-child relationship. If the birth was traumatizing, then how does that translate when now you have a newborn in your arms?"

Right on cue, I was given a textbook illustration of this alarming trend via a conversation I had the day I finished this chapter. I was being interviewed over video conference by a New York journalist reporting on the COVID-19 pandemic, which at the time was engulfing her city. At one point, Courtney, as I'll call her, proudly showed off her three-month-old cherub. When she learned what I was working on, she poured out the awful story of her recent experience at Mount Sinai Hospital at the hands of one of New York's most prominent and well-regarded obstetricians. It is as clear a tale of normalized obstetrical trauma as can be imagined.

Thirty-seven years old and healthy, Courtney was expecting an uneventful delivery. At thirty weeks the physician phoned her to announce, as if by decree, that, given her age, labor would be induced at thirty-nine weeks. This, the doctor said, was "the office protocol here" for anyone older than thirty-five. "She had known my age from the beginning, since I walked into her office last May," Courtney said. "I was so shocked that I hung up the phone—I barely said a word. I had to have half a glass of wine. I was so upset, I didn't sleep all that night." It went downhill from there. Courtney recalled with pain "the sudden disappearance of flexibility and the imposition of a tyrannical dictate. It was not the kind of care I expected. I'm not used to being bullied by doctors or talked down to. The tone became so toxic . . . and then she also kept saying, 'The baby is *huuuge*. He's going to be *huuuge*.' I said to her, 'Wait, I heard that growth scans are notoriously bad at predicting weight.' She responded, 'Not at Sinai. He's going to be nine pounds at least.' " (The baby's actual birth weight: less than eight pounds.)

Courtney considered looking for a new physician, but this late in pregnancy and still in awe of the specialist's credentials, she stayed put. "By week thirty-eight, she was saying, every week, 'This is really not looking good for vaginal, it's really not. I don't know what to tell you.' I just kept saying, 'I really don't want a C-section.' And this was our dynamic week after week. I was in a terrible state of mind for the last three or four weeks of the pregnancy: sobbing, nervous breakdown . . . At the appointed time, we show up at Mount Sinai, and it's a horrible scene. We're in this waiting room for three hours, a million different things going on, and I kept saying to my partner, 'Why the fuck am I here? We are totally within our rights to go back to Brooklyn and go into labor naturally.' " Feeling disempowered, having her intuition invalidated at this most vulnerable time of her life, being intimidated by a highly extolled medical specialist, and having been raised in a culture where "expert" authority trumps one's own, Courtney lacked the wherewithal to assert herself. She finally acceded to the induction and, after fifteen hours of fruit-less labor, the inevitable surgery.

"I was so weak. I'd been throwing up. Everything about this was like the biggest nightmare. I said, 'Fuck it—let's just do the C-section. Like, what choice do I have at this point?' So we roll into the OR, and I'm throwing up on the table, and I'm a basket case, sobbing. Scared out of my mind, shaking. They start the surgery; it takes forever. She then says to me, 'Oh, I didn't realize your abdominal muscles were this strong.' They were, because I've done Pilates for twenty years. I'm thinking, 'Why didn't you realize it? You've been examining me regularly for nine months and anticipating this surgery for weeks.' And the following morning she said to me—can you even make this up?—'I'm going to call the Mount Sinai scanning department and complain about how inaccurate your growth scans were!' All that week in the hospital I would just lie awake at night, sobbing at how violated I was."

I asked Courtney whether she had thought of working with a midwife. "I'm not that left-wing," she said. "I'm not that far-out. I completely bought into the system."

Now consider that this galling story took place in a privileged, white, middle-class context. For poor women, especially women of color, treatment of mothers in labor can be considerably more brutal, with consequences that range all the way to fatal. According to a 2019 World Health Organization report, "42% of the women [in a global survey] said they experienced physical or verbal abuse or discrimination during childbirth in health centers, with some of the women being punched, slapped, shouted at, mocked, or forcibly held down."[11] Nor is this limited to the so-called third world. In my own country, a cell phone video emerged recently of hospital staff in a Quebec facility taunting and verbally abusing an Indigenous woman in labor. Nurses "are heard calling her stupid and saying she's only good for sex and would be better off dead." Minutes later, she was.[12]

"For me, the ideal birth situation is a woman alone in a silent room, lights dimmed, with a midwife calmly sitting with her and knitting," Michel Odent told me—a wry but astute comment on the harmful effect of bright lights, noisy machines, and bustling, hectoring medical personnel on the labor process.

This brings us back to the discussion of "inherent expectation" in our chapter on human nature. We, like all organisms, arrive on the scene with the anticipation that life will unfold within certain parameters. Being the adaptable creatures we are, we can endure less than the best—at a cost. "The baby's experiences during a birth without trauma have got to be those, and only those, which correspond to his and his mother's ancient expectations," writes Jean Liedloff in her study of an Aboriginal forest society. Whereas other mammals seek dark, quiet, solitary places for birth, she points out, we invite birth trauma with "the use of steel instruments, bright lights, rubber gloves, the smells of antiseptic and anesthetic, loud voices or the sounds of machinery."[13]

Mothers feel it, even if no one else sees anything out of the ordinary. I still remember my wife whispering to me during our first birth, regarding the nurse who kept haranguing her to "Push, girl, push," to "Please tell that woman to shut up."[†] A person's body seizes up in the absence of safety and emotional connection, especially under the effect of sensitizing hormones. Oblivious to the woman's needs for silence, safety, and attunement,

---

†   That earnest nurse and I became very friendly colleagues years later at the labor and delivery suite of B.C. Women's Hospital.

hospitals create a self-perpetuating cycle, instigating many of the labor complications they then must intervene to resolve.

Ilana Stanger-Ross summed up traditional wisdom and modern science in words that, in a saner system, wouldn't even need to be said: "We need to approach someone in labor as a full person who is experiencing a sacred life passage," she told me. "They're not a sick patient. They are a person in labor—*which is a very normal thing to be.*"

Chapter 12

Horticulture on the Moon: Parenting, Undermined

We've all lost our children . . . Just look at them, for God's
sake—violent in the streets, comatose in the malls, narcotized
in front of the TV. In my lifetime something terrible
happened that took our children away from us.

—Russell Banks, *The Sweet Hereafter*

Modern society is awash in parenting expertise. Peruse any bookstore and you will behold shelves upon shelves of volumes devoted to helping moms and dads navigate this rocky terrain, from conception through college drop-off. Parenting blogs, social media groups, and online lectures abound. A playlist on the TED Talks website offers "Stories from the Front Lines of Parenting." Even if tongue-in-cheek, the war-zone language resonates for many; the struggle to be "good parents" can seem like a protracted battle against time, against ourselves, even against our kids. We arrive at the bookshelf already lost, seeking direction. We want to do right by our children; we just don't know *how*. If only we had some internal compass to guide us.

The good news is, we do: all of us, by virtue of being human, are endowed with a natural drive and talent for child-rearing. The bad news is that our society's guiding assumptions and prevailing prejudices serve to alienate us from that innate knowledge, so inherent to our species that it cannot be taught, only activated or disabled.

In this chapter we'll look at two ways modern Western culture's idea of normal undermines parenting: the erosion of our instinct for the enterprise, and the creation of isolating or stressful conditions inimical to raising healthy children. If it takes a world to raise a child, it takes a toxic culture to make us forget how to.

Suppressing Instinct, by the Book

Recently a parenting manual by an economist with no background in developmental psychology, beyond being a mother herself, became a bestseller. Having crunched the numbers, Emily Oster presents *Cribsheet: A Data-Driven Guide to Better, More Relaxed Parenting, from Birth to Preschool*. It devalues, among other things, such ancient practices as breastfeeding and co-sleeping with one's newborn. As a sympathetic *New Yorker* profile expressed it, "A major refrain of [this] book is that a parent's preferences are important. What do *you* want?" The plaudit is telling: the governing principle is what the parent *prefers*, not what the child *needs*. Here's the problem: any cultural context is bound to shape the preferences of its members in its own image. What we adults "prefer" in unnatural circumstances may well clash with what our nature would have us opt for. It so happens that parents today take their cues from a culture that has lost touch with both the child's developmental needs *and* what parents require to be able to meet those needs.

Oster's intentions are no doubt good. Around the time her book was published, the *New York Times* ran an op-ed by her with the online title "The Data All Guilt-Ridden Parents Need."[1] Freeing fellow parents from shame is a laudable objective. But quite aside from the fact that even the most carefully selected data are a poor antidote for guilt, what if the issue is more complicated? What if the angst parents feel speaks not to a lack of information or figures but to a long-brewing, culturally induced alienation from their own deepest instincts? Quite like the genes in which they are coded, instincts do not assert themselves in an automatic or autonomous way. Rather, they have to be evoked by the proper environment, or else we are liable to lose touch with them. This is as true for human beings as it is for other animals forced to live in unnatural circumstances. We might consider that the proliferation of "parenting experts" in our time is a sign of this disconnect and not its solution.

Of course, early twenty-first-century culture isn't exactly unique in this respect. Just as with theories of human nature, child-rearing attitudes, approaches, and doctrines throughout Western civilization have reflected—and reinforced—their particular time and place. It is a mostly dismal trajectory that includes infanticide, terror, and abuse: all, of course, normalized in their day. Around the fourteenth century, as the psychohistorian Lloyd deMause writes, "there was no image more popular than that of the physical molding of children, who were seen as soft wax, plaster, or clay to be beaten into shape."[2] The intent was to break the child's independent spirit, from birth onward. It was also around this time, he points out, that parenting manuals began to multiply in earnest.

In the mid-nineteenth century arrived what deMause terms the *socializing mode*, the goal of which is the fostering of a socially functional personality, one that "plays well with others"—that is, conforms to society's expectations. This approach became "the source of all twentieth-century psychological models." Among them is one popularized by the iconic Dr. Benjamin Spock, parenting pundit for millions. In *Baby and Child Care*, his bestseller that influenced generations, the good doctor proposed a cure for what he called "chronic resistance to sleep in infancy." The way to ensure that the infant doesn't "get away with such tyranny," he wrote, was to "say good night affectionately but firmly, walk out of the room, and don't go back." That's right: the "tyranny" of a baby who is physiologically and emotionally programmed to crave physical closeness with the parent, as do all mammalian young.

Today the socialization mode still dominates much of the advice parents continue to receive from "experts" and peers. Recently Jordan Peterson weighed in on how to raise "sophisticated denizens of the world outside the family." In his mega-selling *12 Rules for Life: An Antidote to Chaos*, Peterson cautions parents: "You love your kids, after all. If their actions make you dislike them, think what an effect they will have on other people, who care much less about them than you. Those other people will punish them . . . Don't allow that to happen. Better to let your little monsters know what is desirable and what is not."[3] To achieve this goal, Peterson recommends gestural and physical intimidation.

"Socialization" may be a kinder approach than treating kids as inanimate putty, yet it still centers something other than their needs: namely, the dictates of the society for which the parents act as the well-meaning but unwitting agents. To see what else might be possible, it is instructive to look at cultures more time-tested and Nature-informed than our own. Such cultures needed no "parenting experts" because the wisdom was passed down generationally, whether by instruction or simple emulation. Contrast Dr. Spock's counsel with what an elderly Cree woman once told me: "In our clan, children weren't even allowed to touch the ground until they were two years old. They were in our arms all the time." Or compare Peterson's tips for managing "little monsters" with the anthropologist Ashley Montagu's description of traditional parenting practices among Netsilik Inuit in Canada's Northwest Territories: "The Netsilik mother, even though she lives under the most difficult of conditions, is an unruffled personality who bestows warmth and loving care upon her children. She never chides her infant or interferes with it in any way, except to respond to its need."[4] Somehow, it seems, these children managed to grow into productive and yes, socialized, members of their communities—even without Dr. Peterson's stern admonishments.

It turns out that our innate parenting instinct is perfectly calibrated to ensure the provision of the thing many "experts" would have us ignore: the child's developmental needs.

And here's a plot twist: we are not talking *only* about children's needs. In a real sense, we cannot even speak about the infant's needs without considering those of the mother. "There is no such thing as a baby," the British pediatrician D. W. Winnicott once said, explaining, "If you show me a baby, you certainly show me someone else who is caring for the baby . . . One sees a 'nursing couple' . . . The unit is not the individual, the unit is the individual-environment set-up."[5] Or, in Ashley Montagu's words, "When a baby is born, a mother is born. There is considerable evidence that at this time, and for months thereafter, her needs for contact exceed those of the infant."[6] Good thing, too: Were there not built-in physiological and emotional incentives for the ones doing the caregiving, parenthood would be even more of a slog than it already is. Fewer babies would have their survival needs met if fulfilling those needs were not rewarding for parents. With its usual brilliance, our interpersonal-biological makeup dictates that our requirements be mutual. (One of the unfortunate impacts of our culture's way of doing things is that stress tends to whittle down these innate rewards, making parenting more frustrating and daunting than it rightly ought to be.)

The poet Adrienne Rich expressed the profound joys of this reciprocal design: "I recall the times when, suckling each of my children, I saw his eyes open full to mine, and realized each of us was fastened to the other, not only by mouth and breast, but through our mutual gaze: the depth, calm, passion, of that dark blue, maturely focused look. I recall the physical pleasure of having my full breast suckled at a time when I had no other physical pleasure in the world except the guilt-ridden pleasure of addictive eating."[7] Neurobiologically, Rich was right on target. On imaging studies, a baby's smile will light up the same reward areas in the mom's brain activated by junk foods or addictive drugs, releasing the same pleasure chemicals and triggering the same high.[8] Nature, that unscrupulous drug-pusher.[†]

Like all complex brain structures, mammalian bonding systems—whether of whales or chimps or rats or humans—are experience-dependent for their development and activation. For the brain circuits of nurturing to function—to "come on line," as it were—the environment must evoke and then sustain them. Both men and women have latent child-nurturing circuits in their brains, "waiting for the right environment to amplify their potentials," in the words of neuroscientist Jaak Panksepp—he of the PANIC/GRIEF, PLAY, and CARE nomenclature. Dr. Panksepp identified and mapped the specific brain centers, circuits, connections, and associated neurochemicals that choreograph what he called "the enchanting ballet of emotions between a mother and her infant." These include chemical messengers such as vasopressin, oxytocin, and endorphins—the body's natural opiates—all of which awaken in parents nurturing habits that are essential to the survival of the young. Recall,

---

†   I kid, but also not. The connection between the impaired supply of these feel-good chemicals early in life and later patterns of addiction, whether to drugs or compulsive behavior patterns, is a central theme of my previous book *In the Realm of Hungry Ghosts: Close Encounters with Addiction*, and will be revisited here in chapters 15 and 16.

these are the chemicals that, blended, form a "love cocktail" released by natural labor. Skin-to-skin contact and suckling also elicit their flow in the mother. The physiology of infant and parent is thus co-regulated by their interactions, and the effect of these interactions—or their absence—can be imprinted in the young human for a lifetime. Likewise, in the dearth of such interactions, parenting instincts may become muted, with long-term consequences for the parent-child relationship.[9] In this, as in other crucial ways, our culture has become contact-starved.

Let's remind ourselves that civilization, beginning with the Neolithic revolution and the advent of agriculture, is but a blip in the course of our species' existence, no more than twelve thousand years out of the millions that hominins have trod the earth and the estimated two hundred thousand years or less since our own species arrived on the scene. Until then, and in many places until much more recently—even up to today, in a few isolated locations—people lived in small-band hunter-gatherer groups. "The common early experiences of our ancestors (and cousins, the small-band hunter-gatherers) provided *a social commons for the development of human nature*—the essence of being human," writes Dr. Darcia Narvaez. (Italics hers.) The research she has surveyed identified seven early child-rearing practices shared by hunter-gatherer groups, practices that constitute what she calls the "evolved nest." As you read this list, I invite you to compare the experiences it includes with those of the average baby or toddler of our own time.

Amid the stresses generated by our culture, even educated middle-class parents are challenged to provide these needs—if they are even aware of them:

- Soothing perinatal experience
- Prompt responsiveness to the needs of the infant and prevention of distress

- Extensive touch and constant physical presence, including touch with movement (carrying and holding)
- Frequent, infant-initiated breastfeeding for two to five years, with four as the average weaning age
- A community of multiple, warm, responsive adult caregivers
- A climate of positive social support (for mother and infant)
- Creative free play in Nature with multi-aged mates.[10]

"The nest," Dr. Narvaez told me, "includes the mother relaxed and not stressed during pregnancy, gentle birth processes, soothing perinatal experiences, no separation of mom and baby, no infant circumcision,[†] no painful procedures, breastfeeding, and then affectionate touch constantly in the first year and throughout childhood and life, really." Recall that it was Narvaez whose contention about human beings being *species-atypical* I quoted in chapter 8—the only beings on Earth who routinely thwart their own species' inbuilt needs for healthy growth. "In our culture," she said, "we have pretty much unnested our children. We are missing most of the components of what helps a baby grow into their full potential, their systems to develop properly. That's the unnestedness."

Among the Indigenous people who hosted her in the South American jungle, Jean Liedloff once observed an exception to tribal practices that proved a cardinal rule regarding parental discipline of children: "I saw a young father lose patience one day with his year-old son. He shouted and made some violent motion as I watched and may even have struck him. The baby screamed with deafening, unmistakable horror. The father stood

---

[†] I flinched when she mentioned circumcision—I used to perform this procedure myself, one that in the North American context has no health benefit and has been shown to cause suffering to the child, especially in the medical form I was trained in.

chastened by the dreadful sound he had caused; it was clear that he had committed an offense against nature. I saw the family often, as I lived next door to them, but I never saw the man lose respect for his son's dignity again."[11]

The word "dignity" stands out: how many of us think of babies this way? And yet that omission may only underscore our blind spots when it comes to children. Think about it: even if you've never called an infant "dignified," odds are you've met quite a few *indignant* ones. The word is not figurative, either. Even babies— perhaps they especially—know when their physical and emotional integrity is being ignored or violated. Liedloff's anecdote comports with Dr. Narvaez's findings about small-band hunter-gatherers and what has been generally observed about Indigenous cultures: by and large, these did not normalize hitting their kids, and still don't. Landing on the shores of the "New World," the European Christians steeped, or so they believed, in the gentle spirit of Jesus, found it appalling to witness that the "savages" of North America avoided the corporal punishment of children.[12] By contrast, the Puritan ethic was to "engage rod and reproof," in the words of one seventeenth-century Massachusetts minister.[13]

This ethos may have fallen from favor since then, but not entirely. "To hold the *no excuse for physical punishment* theory," writes Jordan Peterson (italics his), assumes "that the word *no* can be effectively uttered to another person in the absence of the threat of punishment."[14] The good professor's "another person" is, in this case, a two-year-old, whom elsewhere he charmingly calls "the determined varmint." For Peterson, steeped in behaviorist ideology, discipline is often a matter of intimidating children, something we can accomplish, he writes, because we are "larger, stronger and more capable than the child" and can, therefore, back up our threats. He proudly boasts, "[When] my daughter was little, I could paralyze her into immobility with an evil glance." In Britain, two headlines in the *Telegraph* from 2011 and 2012, respectively, signaled that such attitudes are far from isolated: "The Rod Has Been Spared for Far Too Long: Allowing Teachers Even the Lightest Touch of Physical Force Will Improve Discipline" and "School Discipline: Sparing the Rod Has Spoiled the Children—What Can Be Done to Reverse the Collapse of Discipline Since the Banning of the Cane?"

Back in the world of science, the American Academy of Pediatrics, having reviewed nearly one hundred studies, issued a statement in 2018 that aligns with ancestral wisdom. It called for the end of spanking and of harsh verbal punishment of children and adolescents. Such treatment, the organization of sixty-seven thousand pediatric specialists pointed out, only increases aggression in the long term and undermines the development of self-control and responsibility. By elevating stress hormone levels, it may cause harm to healthy brain development and lead to mental health problems.[15] More recently, a Harvard study showed that the damage wrought by spanking to the child's nervous system and psyche may be as severe as that caused by more intense violence.[16] The good news is that the tide is turning, with young parents less and less likely to employ corporal disciplining—a welcome instance, perhaps, of the future leading us back to the past.

For another example of the modern disconnection from instinct and body, take breastfeeding. According to massive surveys in North America and internationally, the practice confers physical health benefits on both the child and, in the long term, the mother.[17] As Dr. Lori Feldman-Winter, chair of the American Academy of Pediatrics, told the *New Yorker*, the economist Emily Oster, in devaluing the practice, simply gets the science wrong. "It's basically as bad as the anti-vaxxers," the physician said.[†]

---

†   To clarify, Feldman-Winter's comment regarding anti-vaxxers preceded COVID-19 days.

Elsewhere, Oster writes that "motherhood can be lonely and isolating." Too true—but those attributes pertain not to motherhood itself but to motherhood in an alienating culture. Horticulture on the moon would doubtless be a maddening endeavor, but that tells us nothing about gardening, only that certain conditions must be in place if we hope to succeed. At one point, Oster recounts an experience of attending her brother's wedding, "trying to nurse my screaming daughter in a 100-degree closet." It is hard to conceive of a more apt metaphor for the abnormally stressful conditions our culture imposes on infants and mothers than that closet: shamed or shunned into isolation, hidden away, claustrophobic, cramped, sweltering. Given how interpersonal neurobiology works, is it any wonder the infant is screaming? In a stressed environment, as I often witnessed in family practice, breastfeeding itself can become an onerous and frustrating chore, a source of maternal misery and infant distress.

The same goes for some forms of "sleep training." The assumption that infants need to be trained to sleep is based on a cultural view that the child should adjust to the parents' schedule and agenda—which, for working parents or for stressed parents lacking support, may be a legitimate, even unavoidable longing. But we should be clear on what is being lost. As the psychologist Gordon Neufeld points out, being in physical touch is the infant's only way of connecting with the parent. Her "resistance" to being put down and having the parent follow the Spockian counsel to "say good night affectionately but firmly, walk out of the room, and don't go back" is simply an expression of her essential need. Shutting down our response to a baby's distress may also weaken our own parenting instincts, with consequences that long outlast the child's infancy.

In 2006 I wrote a newspaper article titled "Why I No Longer Believe Babies Should Cry Themselves to Sleep," pointing out that leaving small infants alone stresses their brains, with potential negative effects. It also hurts a mother's heart. I quoted my late mother-in-law, Monica, who had a painful memory of being a young mom in the late 1940s and early '50s and following medical counsel to ignore her infants' cries. "It was torture for me to do it," she told me. "It went against all my motherly emotions." Some years later the paper's website republished the piece, which was quickly shared over eighty thousand times, drawing many responses. One of them was priceless: "This article is nothing more than prefrontal lobe BS. There is no way an infant's brain patterns are permanently psychologically damaged at such a young age. There is no way that your prefrontal cortex will permanently adopt patterns that will translate into adulthood. No way. If that would be the case, then the last 3 generations to rule this earth (boomers, pre-boomers, Generation X) would have all been emotionally unstable and plagued with psychological issues." "Well, then," I thought to myself, "I rest my case."

Why Parental Stress Matters

Especially in infancy, but throughout childhood, the young human uses the emotional and nervous systems of the caring adults to regulate her own internal states. The interpersonal-biological math is elementary: the more stressed the adult, the more stressed the child.

Extensive research has demonstrated that when stressed, parents are less patient and more punishing and harsher with their young children. Stress impairs their capacity to be calm, responsive, and attuned. As a recent review by leading researchers pointed out, "In more stressful environments for parents, children not only experience less protection from environmental stressors but also are more likely to have stress-inducing relationships with caregivers."[18] Another study showed that, while elevated stress induced more punitive attitudes in mothers, increased levels of support favorably diminished them. Contemporary science affirms ancient wisdom once more.

Parental stress expresses itself in less overt ways, too, such as distraction and emotional absence. Many parents, though loving, are frequently preoccupied by genuine concerns about relationship issues or economic troubles or personal problems and, as a result, just aren't as attentive or "present." This affects development as surely as does parental rage or coldness. "Primate experiments show that infants can undergo severe separation reactions even though their mothers are visually, but not psychologically available," reports the renowned researcher, psychologist, and theorist Allan Schore.[19] Dr. Schore calls such noncontact "proximate separation"—so close, but yet so far. It's a dynamic that many children in our society experience, owing to the stresses parents habitually endure. The message the child gets is "You are not worthy of my attention. You must work to earn it." Whether or not we explicitly recall such experiences, their imprints survive in our unconscious and in our nervous systems.

Making matters more stressful is the alienation imposed by financial hardship. "The relentlessness of modern-day parenting has a powerful motivation: economic anxiety," the *New York Times* reported in 2018. "For the first time, it's as likely as not that American children will be less prosperous than their parents. For parents, giving children the best start in life has come to mean doing everything they can to ensure that their children can climb to a higher class, or at least not fall out of the one they were born into."[20] The unintended impact of such fearful, status-driven child-rearing is that the child's irreducible emotional needs fall secondary to the desperation of parents striving to ensure the academic and financial success of their offspring. Recently I was told, by a close eyewitness, of a middle-class mother yelling at her five-year-old son who balked at doing his homework: "You're not thinking of your academic future!" the poor mom shouted at the preschooler. If only the youngster could have retorted, "Yeah? Well, you're not thinking of my psycho-emotional future!"

For some two-parent families of a certain social class, having both parents working may be a choice. "I love my kids! They are amazing," writes Oster. "But I wouldn't be happy staying home with them. It isn't that I like my job better—if I had to pick, the kids would win every time. But the 'marginal value' of time with them declines fast . . . The first hour with my kids is great, but by the fourth, I'm ready for some time with my research. My job doesn't have this nose-dive in marginal value—the highs are not as high, but the hour-to-hour satisfaction declines much more slowly."[21] Oster is wise to value the quality of the hours she spends parenting over their mere number, and has every right to claim her choice, as we all do. For far too long women's self-expression and validation through the fulfillment of meaningful work apart from homemaking were squelched and frustrated.

And of course, neither the opportunity to return to meaningful employment nor the pressure to resume working, no matter what the cost to parenting, is equally distributed among women: class, as always, is a hugely significant variable. Many parents are compelled to enter the workforce from dire economic necessity, or to rejoin it far too prematurely. How can they think of their children's future when they can barely provide for the present? This is particularly the case in the United States, where fewer than 20 percent of new mothers have access to paid leave. The problem is even worse for families of color, Myra Jones-Taylor, chief policy officer at the child development nonprofit Zero to Three, told the *Guardian*. "Parents," she said, "just can't afford to stay home with their babies."[22] There are much more civilized policies in place in some countries, particularly in northern Europe, where even fathers are offered paternity leave.

One in four American women returns to work within two weeks of giving birth, a mere third of the length of postpartum maternal leave suggested by the American College of Obstetricians and Gynecologists. Even that paltry recommendation by the ACOG seems intended only to allow the maternal body to heal and recover from the travails of labor—given especially how many births these days involve surgical intervention. Such a brief postpartum absence from work leaves the needs of the child entirely out of consideration. For healthy child development, according to the child's neurobiological requirements, a much longer period with the mother is necessary—ideally for a *minimum* of nine months until the infant reaches a stage of relative biological maturity. The sudden loss of maternal contact is, for the infant, a shock—as we know from animal studies, even creatures whose period of dependence is much shorter than ours.[†]

All the Lonely Parents

The British anthropologist Colin Turnbull spent three years living with Pygmies in what was then known as Belgian Congo, in Central Africa. Until recently these tribal people followed ways of life dating back, likely with little alteration, for thousands of years. He related his observations in his classic work *The Forest People*. "The infant," he writes, ". . . knows his real mother and father, of course, and has a special affection for them and they for him, but from an early age he learns that he is the child of them all, for they are all children of the forest."[23] In the small-band hunter-gatherer milieu, the extended family and clan formed an indispensable network of warm, responsive support. Far from being

---

† For example, rats weaned just one week earlier than their Nature-appointed times are more likely to get habituated to alcohol as adults.

a two-person show (much less a solo performance), parenting originally functioned within a broad circle of attachments, the multigenerational clan, where consistent affection was modeled, encouraged, and shared.

It was also *supplemented,* in a manner both merciful and utterly commonsense, by a select group of other caregivers that Narvaez terms *allomothers,* the Greek-derived prefix *allo-* denoting "something other than the usual." Allomothers "take the baby when mom needs a break . . . They carry, rock and play with the child. They take care of mundane tasks . . . They are the buffer for the mother-child, father-child relationship." We know from many studies that the more support parents receive, the more responsive they can be to their children. "It used to be the tradition in most every society," Narvaez writes, "to have a 'lying in' period for mom and new baby where women of the community wait on the mother, giving her nutritious teas and foods that promote breastfeeding and healing. They took care of everything in the household so she could stay in her bed and give her full attention to bonding with and breastfeeding her baby."[24] In effect, these cultures had a socialized "Child Care for All" policy, to their great benefit.

As I worked on this chapter, in mid-May 2020, a horrific terrorist assault on a hospital in Kabul, Afghanistan, killed twenty-four people, including some nursing mothers. In one of the most moving news videos I have seen, women arrived to nurture and nourish these orphaned infants. "I have come here today to breastfeed these babies," one young local woman said through her COVID-19 face mask, "because they lost their mothers in this bloody attack. I have a four-month-old baby . . . and came here to give them a mother's love by breastfeeding them."[25] It may be that the allomothering instinct is as natural as that of mothering itself.

Bottom line: It was never Nature's agenda, if we can speak of it as such, that a distressed and confused young mother such as Emily Oster should have to struggle in closeted isolation, or to compromise on her instincts and desires to bond calmly with her child. It's not the job description of parenting that imposes these stresses on mothers and fathers; the problem lies with, so to speak, the sociocultural job site.

To say we have drifted afield from a community-parenting model would be an understatement. Today's insulated nuclear family unit is a distant cry from our "evolved evolutionary niche," traces of which grow fainter with each new decade, with every fresh turn of the wheel of economic or technological "progress." With evolutionary precedents shattered, we are made to endure serial breakages of our instinctual inheritance.

Consider what has happened to local communities within just a very few generations. I and many others in my age cohort can still remember growing up in neighborhoods where nearly everyone knew one another, where children played throughout the day in the streets, and where every adult, known to us all, was a surrogate parent, keeping an eye on us or ready to call us to order when out of line. Families shopped in neighborhood stores; the grocer, the baker, the hardware dealer, and the car mechanic offered their goods and services within walking distance. (A personal note: During my childhood in Budapest, the sidewalk outside our building was almost as wide as a playground, and served as such for the dozens of children from the neighboring apartment houses. I visited my old neighborhood on a recent speaking trip to Hungary, to find the sidewalk now narrow, a multilane freeway coursing along it and, on the other side, a drive-through McDonald's and a gas station.)

How quaint such memories seem now, almost like something out of *Sesame Street*. Local stores are an endangered species.

Notwithstanding thriving communal settings in some localities, in general more and more of us drive, often by ourselves, to work or to shop at some soulless and/or windowless facility far away. In place of people we know, we encounter strangers purveying mass-manufactured products. Economic interactions once informed by personal relationships, whether at the bank, gas station, or large-store checkout counter, have been increasingly replaced by emotionally sterile and ever more mechanized transactions. Suburban sidewalks, largely vacant, are no longer enlivened by the raucous play of children of mixed ages: for the most part, kids attend schools segregated into same-age groupings. The need to make a living impels many people to move far away from their extended families.

Church attendance and other vectors of socially minded participation are on the wane. "Without at first noticing, we have been pulled apart from one another and from our communities over the last third of the century," Harvard professor of public policy Robert D. Putnam wrote in 2000.[26]

Social creatures by natural design, we have become fish out of water.

Mothers, whose need for connection is an especially high-stakes matter, are among the hardest hit by these shifts. Adrienne Rich notes that during the relative affluence of the mid-twentieth century, "the move to the suburbs, to the smaller, then the larger, private house, the isolation of 'the home' from other homes . . . The working-class mothers in their new flats and the academic wives in their new affluence all lost something: they became, to a more extreme degree, house-bound, isolated women."[27] Such tendencies are exerting themselves internationally and with growing force under the sway of globalized capitalism.

While there is no sense in pining for some idealized once-upon-a-time, a decline in cohesion and community support is discernible, and lamentable. "In earlier decades, the social ties were in place," James Garbarino, a lifelong student of child development and a professor of humanistic psychology at Chicago's Loyola University, told me in an interview. "Even though the value of individualism was there, the social structures that bound people together were more evident. Many of those have atrophied or people have chosen to opt out of them, not realizing how important they were for their well-being in the past. These structures—people didn't consciously know how important they were, and so they felt they could get rid of them with no cost." Joni Mitchell was right: we truly don't know what we've got till it's gone.

A culture where Nature has become the exception is a culture in trouble. To do the job evolution has tasked us with, and to access and trust our natural instincts designed for that job, we need each other, and we need communal and social support—just as surely as our children need us. Isolated parenting is stressed parenting, as is trying to keep up with the latest counter-instinctual "expert" advice from the (apologies to Dwight Eisenhower) parenting-industrial complex.[†] Troubled parenting, in turn, is a breeding ground for personal and societal malaise.

[†]   Near the end of his presidency, "Ike" famously warned about the "military-industrial complex."

Chapter 13

Forcing the Brain in the Wrong Direction: The Sabotage of Childhood

There can be no keener revelation of a society's soul than the way it treats its children.

—Nelson Mandela[‡]

"Do you ever get accused of mother-blaming?" I asked the Harvard-based pediatrician and researcher Jack Shonkoff. "I worry about that a lot," he said. "If we talk about how influential the environment of relationships is, you can end up on a slippery slope, with people saying, 'Parents are doing a bad job—it's their fault.'" Dr. Shonkoff, whose work has illuminated much of the science of early development, then summed up the core dilemma faced by anyone who tries to engage with these issues honestly: "You can't say that parents are incredibly important in the lives of their children, yet if there's a problem it has nothing to do with the parents. But the truth is, parents don't raise their children in isolation from society."

A wiser view requires a wider lens. Yes, parents are responsible for their children; no, they did not create the world in which they must parent them.

---

‡   Address by the South African president at the launch of the Nelson Mandela Children's Fund, Pretoria, May 8, 1995.

Our cultural ecology does not support attuned, present, responsive, connected parenting. As we have seen, the destabilization begins with stress transmitted to infants still in the womb, with the mechanization of birth, the attenuation of the parenting instinct, and the denial of the child's developmental needs. It continues with the increasingly intolerable economic and social pressures on parents these days and the erosion of community ties, and magnifies with the disinformation parents receive on how to rear their young. Reinforced by educational systems that too often stress students with pressures to compete, the process culminates in the exploitation of children and youth for the glory of the consumer market.

Parents do their loving best; I know I did. I also know full well how my "best" was constrained by what I didn't yet know about myself, nor about child-rearing. However noble our intentions, our ability to carry them out is heavily influenced by our own early experiences and unresolved traumas, by the social expectations we are charged with transmitting to our children, and by the stresses of life. Does that knowledge liberate me from feelings of guilt, especially when I see the marks left on my kids by my limitations as a younger man? No, not automatically. But at least I'm aware that guilt and blame are unhelpful and beside the point, especially when we understand the context. As James Garbarino urged in 1995, "We need to put aside blaming parents and take a good hard look at the challenge of raising children in a socially toxic environment."[1]

Garbarino, at that time codirector of the Family Life Development Center and professor of human development at Cornell University, noted that among the many facets of the socially hazardous environment for child-raising were "violence, poverty and other economic pressures on parents and their children, disruption of relationships, nastiness, despair, depression, paranoia, alienation—all the things that demoralize families and communities." He also wrote of "many, many others that are subtle yet equally serious. High on the list is *the departure of adults from the lives of kids*."[2] This radical disruption of evolutionary norms is taken for granted, to the point where we barely even notice it. Worse, we mistake it for the natural state of things.

An automatic consequence of the weakening of communal and family ties is that our kids must seek their attachment needs elsewhere. Children, like the young of many species, must attach to *someone* in their lives: their neurophysiology demands it. Absent a reliable attachment figure, they experience fear and disorientation. Their brain wiring will go, well, haywire. In effect, essential brain circuits having to do with capacities such as learning, healthy social interaction, or emotional regulation will not develop appropriately.

Nothing in a child's brain tells her *to whom* she should attach. Nature's assumption, if we can put it that way, is that the parents will be consistently present. Children are born with this expectation coded into their bodies and nervous systems. The immature brain cannot abide what Gordon Neufeld calls an "attachment void"—a situation in which no attachment figure is there to connect with. Inevitably, just as a newborn duckling, in the absence of its mother, will trustingly follow the first creature it sees—the nearest goose, squirrel, park ranger, or even a robotic toy car— the vacuum must and will be filled by whoever is around.

For our young today, "whoever is around" from an early age onward is most often the peer group. Unmoored by the decline of the multigenerational adult-led community, children and adolescents have to seek acceptance from one another. This is, developmentally speaking, a fool's errand.

To be clear, the desire, even the need, to form close connections with one's own age group is natural and healthy. Such friendships can be among the richest bonds forged in a life-time. But from the perspective of emotional development, *peer orientation*—the displacement of adults as the *primary* source and locus of attachment for the child, in favor of her own age cohort—is disastrous.[†] The proverbial blind can do a better job of leading the blind than immature creatures can successfully guide one another to psychological maturity. Aaron, the younger of my two sons, now forty-three, sees in hindsight how this dynamic has limited him. "As a teenager I was consumed by what my friends thought of me, how much they liked me, what it took to fit in with their expectations," he recalled recently. "That kept me immature into my adulthood." Of course, his peer orientation was not about his peers per se: it was a natural outcome of his parents' lack of availability as emotionally attuned adults in his early years.

As we've discussed, emotional safety, formed in secure connections with a baseline of unconditional worth, is a prerequisite condition for maturation. Generally, once kids are absorbed into the peer world, they lose the safety of the primary connection with adults.[‡]

In cultures with their priorities in order, young friendships blossom in a community setting, overseen by nurturing adults. In our society, peer interactions occur not in the context of protective adult relationships but away from them.

When children spend much of their waking time away from caring adults, their brains are compelled to choose between competing attachments: the natural call of parental connection or the siren song of the peer world. If parents lose the contest,

---

[†] The phenomenon of peer orientation is documented extensively in Gordon Neufeld's book, which I co-wrote, *Hold On to Your Kids: Why Parents Need to Matter More Than Peers*.

[‡] Assuming, of course, that the adults themselves are emotionally stable, supportive, and available to provide safety. For abused children, the peer group, inadequate as it is, may be a lifeline in some cases.

children must, by default, look to one another. Which means that they, too, lose. All this is exacerbated by the blandishments of a pop culture that holds up immature adolescent celebrities as idols to be "followed"—a telling word—on social media by multiple millions of children and teens. In a previous age, these young people would have seen mature adult figures as the ones to emulate.

Some parents reading this may protest, "But *my* kid's friends seem lovely, accepting, and open-minded!" Real and worth celebrating as those qualities may be, a child finding her *primary* succor and comfort in her peer group is more a sign of "cope" than a cause for hope, especially at younger ages. The noblest of peers are hard-pressed to supply the abiding connection that developmental safety demands. Among other shortcomings, children cannot count on each other to remain internally consistent: many of us can recall an unhappy first day of school when we were shocked to realize that our erstwhile friends had morphed over the summer into something far less friendly. Nor can they offer one another the unconditional positive regard that nourishes healthy growth, a quality even well-meaning adults often find challenging to provide. As a rule, immature peers are constitutionally incapable of accepting each other "as is"; or holding space for the vulnerable experience of emotion, let alone its open expression; or relieving one another's stressed states; or celebrating or even tolerating temperamental differences. Left to its own callow devices, the peer group can offer only acceptance that is highly conditional and thus insecure, often demanding self-suppression and conformity in place of true individuality.

In more dire cases, peer orientation exposes children to the threat of rejection, ostracization, and bullying. According to a 2001 article by Natalie Angier in the *New York Times*, "The news bristles with reports that bullies abound. In one of the largest studies ever of child development, researchers at the [U.S.] National Institutes of Health reported that about a quarter of all middle-school children were either perpetrators or victims (or in some cases, both) of serious and chronic bullying, behavior that included threats, ridicule, name calling, punching, slapping, jeering and sneering."[3] Similar patterns have been reported in Europe.[4] From Spain to Germany, England to the Czech Republic, public officials and school administrators have had to confront the issue. The World Health Organization estimated in 2012 that one-third of children report having been bullied by their peers.[5] These days we hear too many accounts of children or teens manifesting or, at least, feigning indifference at real-life suffering, even finding "kicks" in it. We read frequent reports about bullying or of sexual assaults being shared on social media by adolescents as if they were amusing bits of life, even though the pain caused has also led to suicides and self-harming.

The 2019 overdose death of a troubled adolescent in a Vancouver suburb shocked the world. As the *National Post* reported, "On August 7, Carson Crimeni, a 14-year-old boy described in news reports as lonely and desperate to fit in, took drugs with a group of older teens at a skate park in Langley, B.C. As he grew increasingly incoherent, the older kids filmed him. They mocked him and laughed. They uploaded the clips online and spread them around. '12-year-old tweaking on Molly,'[†] one wrote over a video of a sweaty Carson. He looks tiny in the clip, in his gray hoodie and black pants. He's '15 caps deep,' someone wrote over another clip, according to *Global News*. In later videos, his eyes pop and spin. He sweats through his sweater. He swipes at his nose." Hours later, the boy was found near death, too far gone to be resuscitated. Even at that dire moment, reported the CBC,

---

† Slang for the psychoactive drug MDMA.

"another teen posted a picture of the ambulance on social media with the jocular caption, 'Carson almost died LOL.'"[6] Very soon after, there was no "almost" about it.

Carson Crimeni's tragedy may have been an extreme case, but many children these days live under the shadow of peer rejection, mockery, or bullying—or may themselves become bullies. In such an atmosphere, a child's protective response is to shut down her vulnerable emotions. That flight from vulnerability—whether instigated by stressful situations at home or in the context of the peer group—inhibits maturation, the emergence of a truly independent self.

"There are indications that children today are losing their tender feelings," Gordon Neufeld said in his penetrating European Parliament address.[7] "Many children have lost their sadness and disappointment . . . their feelings of alarm . . . their feelings of shame and embarrassment. Interestingly enough, research reveals when children lose their blush, they also lose their empathy. It turns out that caring too is a vulnerable feeling as it sets us up for disappointment. We know that the most wounding of all experiences is facing separation . . . Unfortunately, today's children are subjected to more [parental] separation and more peer interaction than ever before." The result, he concludes, is "a significant loss of feeling," as the young brain's defensive apparatus becomes stuck in an effort to "defend . . . against a sense of vulnerability that is too overwhelming." Again, we see the child's emotional apparatus being weakened, their felt sense of being human impoverished.

But why should our children remain open to their own vulnerability? Are we supposed to *want* them to be woundable? Gordon and I addressed the subject in the book we co-wrote:

> Our emotions are not a luxury but an essential aspect of our
> makeup. We have them not just for the pleasure of feeling

but because they have crucial survival value. They orient us, interpret the world for us, give us vital information without which we cannot thrive. They tell us what is dangerous and what is benign, what threatens our existence and what will nurture our growth. Imagine how disabled we would be if we could not see or hear or taste or sense heat or cold or physical pain. To shut down emotions is to lose an indispensable part of our sensory apparatus and, beyond that, an indispensable part of who we are. Emotions are what make life worthwhile, exciting, challenging, and meaningful. They drive our explorations of the world, motivate our discoveries, and fuel our growth. Down to the very cellular level, human beings are either in defensive mode or in growth mode, but they cannot be in both at the same time. When children become invulnerable, they cease to relate to life as infinite possibility, to themselves as boundless potential, and to the world as a welcoming and nurturing arena for their self-expression. The invulnerability imposed by peer orientation imprisons children in their limitations and fears. No wonder so many of them these days are being treated for depression, anxiety, and other disorders.

The love, attention, and security only adults can offer liberates children from the need to make themselves invulnerable and restores to them that potential for life and adventure that can never come from risky activities, extreme sports, or drugs. Without that safety our children are forced to sacrifice their capacity to grow and mature psychologically, to enter into meaningful relationships, and to pursue their deepest and most powerful urges for self-expression. In the final analysis, the flight from vulnerability is a flight from the self. If we do not hold our children close to us, the ultimate cost is the loss of their ability to hold on to their own truest selves.

Why does the flight from vulnerability inhibit maturation? Nothing in Nature "becomes itself" without being vulnerable: the mightiest tree's growth requires soft and supple shoots, just as the hardest-shelled crustacean must first molt and become soft. The same goes for us: no emotional vulnerability, no growth. Even our "tougher" qualities like resilience, determination, confidence, and bravery, if authentic and not mere bluster, have that softer state as a necessary precursor.

Apart from impeding maturation, the shutdown of vulnerable feeling reinforces the sense of emptiness. It fosters boredom, impairs genuine intimacy, undermines curiosity and learning, fuels the demand for distraction from the present moment, and drives a compulsion for overstimulation through competitive games, unrelenting background noise, hazardous social situations and behaviors, the hunger for products, and the pursuit of escape through substances.

The profit imperative animating materialistic society is superbly adept in exploiting these culturally generated pseudo-needs of children and youths. "We should be gravely concerned about our society's soul," the University of British Columbia law professor Joel Bakan writes in *Childhood Under Siege*.[8] As meticulously documented as it is shocking, Bakan's book depicts the multiple ways corporations deploy a sophisticated and sinister understanding of children's emotional needs to generate profit. Here the manipulation has been, and continues to be, very conscious indeed. In 1983 corporations spent $100 million in direct advertising to children. Less than three decades later, that figure had shot up to $15 billion.[†]

Even as parental stress and peer orientation weaken children's connections with nurturing adults, the corporate siege of

† Although these are U.S. figures, given the hyper-contagious influence of U.S. culture internationally, the impact is global.

immature minds has exploited and exacerbated the void created by the loss of connection. They act symbiotically to drain childhood of the emotional richness our development thrives on. A decade ago Bakan warned, "The average child in the United States watches 30,000 television advertisements a year—most of which pitch products directly to them . . . and all conveying a series of subtle, and corrosive, messages: that they will find happiness through their relationships with products—with things, not people; that to be cool and accepted by peers, they need to buy certain products; that fast food and toy companies, not parents and teachers, know what is best for them; that corporate brands are the true bases of their social worth and identities."[9] These trends have only accelerated since then with the further spread of social media and digital advertising.

Bakan has interviewed some of the world's leading children's marketers. One of them, Denmark's Martin Lindstrom, expressed serious qualms about the results of his work. According to Lindstrom, Bakan writes, "children's constant and deepening exposures to marketing is leading to a 'disaster in terms of kids and their futures . . . very unhealthy, and it's just the beginning we are seeing now.'" Lindstrom predicted that his industry would continue to erode children's imaginations and creative capacities. For all that, he stayed on the job. "These marketers are smart, insightful, and quite evil," Bakan told me, "because they understand what they're doing. [Lindstrom,] when you talk to him, he has his own kids, and he's quite critical of it all and thinks it's all going in a horrible direction."

Lindstrom's understanding of the child's mind, as summarized by Bakan, is alarmingly on point: "Emotions drive everything for children . . . and marketers, to be successful, must engage the most fundamental emotions at the deepest level. *Love*, which connotes nurturing, affection, and romance, is one of these fundamental emotions . . . *Fear*—as in violence, terror, horror, cruelty, and war—is another. Then there is *mastery*, kids' aspiration to gain independence from adults." (Italics in original.) This deft analysis is not intended to help the child's mind develop toward health, dignity, genuine mastery, and authentic independence, but the polar opposite: to deliberately turn that mind into prey and a lifelong captive of profit-driven market forces. It aims at the direct sabotage of childhood: the period of growth in which the young human is designed by Nature to move toward her full capacities, mature emotionally, deepen in empathy and self-understanding, learn how to connect with others in mutually beneficial ways, begin to realize her creative potentials, and acquire the template for nurturing the next generation.

Everything the corporate juggernaut foists upon children— prefabricated play options, video games, mass-manufactured toys, gadgets, peer-centric online platforms, and saccharine and superficial television programs targeted at toddlers and preschoolers, along with the mainstreaming of glossy, soulless, porn-inflected depictions of sexuality available to teens and, increasingly, even younger kids—has detrimental effects. "We are forcing the brain in the wrong direction," Lindstrom confessed to Bakan. Psychologically and neurobiologically, the marketing whiz was 100 percent correct. That Facebook (recently rebranded as "Meta"), through its Instagram brand, has knowingly marketed programs that harm the mental health of teenage girls is only the latest revelation of the corporate assault on children's minds.[10]

Although the threat posed to children's brains and minds by the ubiquitous, compulsive, commercialized world of digital devices and media raised profound alarm from the start among those who were observing the impacts, it continues to burgeon and metastasize. I refer here both to the use of digital devices by young children *and* to their compulsive use by adults in their presence.

I spoke with Dr. Shimi Kang, a Harvard-educated psychiatrist, specialist in adolescent addiction, and author, most recently of *The Tech Solution: Creating Healthy Habits for Kids Growing Up in a Digital World*. "Right now we have mothers who are on their phones while they're nursing, or giving an infant a phone during a diaper change," she said. "The diaper change used to be this whole dynamic experience between the caregiver and infant. You'd have to find a way to get them to sit still, and now you just give the child a phone and they lie quietly. You can go to any restaurant and see that many, many, many children are being fed in front of an iPad or a computer. You see it all over the place. The phone is so attractive to that young brain." What gets displaced is the neurobiology of attachment, the release of bonding and mood-regulating brain chemicals like oxytocin, serotonin, and endorphins, present in the cerebral circuits of both parent and baby when they lock eyes in attuned, responsive connection—chemicals, Dr. Kang points out, that are known to be "the key to long-term happiness and success." The unintended but wounding message to the child is, again, "You don't matter."

Although it doesn't take a brain scientist to see what makes these devices "so attractive to that young brain," brain science certainly factors into their design. "Video games, social media, gadgets, and apps are engineered to keep young brains glued to their screens by finding ways to reward them with hits of dopamine," Dr. Kang writes.[11] Dopamine, as we will see, is the essential chemical in the addiction process, whether to substances or behaviors. It is one of the brain's "feel good" chemicals, inducing a state of excitement, motivation, aliveness, and gratification. When Kang asserts that digital apps and gadgets are "engineered" to hit children's brains with bursts of dopamine, she is being very precise. "The phone," she told me, "has been designed by the world's top neuroscientists and psychologists, who have taken all of our most sophisticated brain research and understanding of human motivation and reward cycles and have embedded it into devices." She cited as an example a company with a name and mission so on the nose that one would think it came out of a satirical film or novel: Dopamine Labs. "It was started," she said, "by a neuroscientist and software developers whose entire business platform is to consult companies to help them engage and release dopamine . . . It's called *persuasive design*." Addiction, of course, is the whole point. Viewed from a corporation's bottom line, one could not imagine a more desirable consumer profile than those who can't get enough of what they don't need but feel they must have.

A 2019 study published in the prestigious journal *JAMA Pediatrics* was among the first to investigate the neurobiological effects of screen watching on children. "In a single generation," the authors wrote, "through what has been described as a vast 'uncontrolled experiment,' the landscape of childhood has been digitalized, affecting how children play, learn and form relationships . . . Use begins in infancy and increases with age, and it was recently estimated at more than 2 hours per day in children younger than 9 years, aside from use during childcare and school . . . [The] risks include language delay, poor sleep, impaired executive function and general cognition, and decreased parent-child engagement, including reading together." The study, conducted with preschoolers by means of advanced brain imaging, found increased screen time associated with poorer white-brain-matter functioning "in major fiber tracts supporting core language and emergent literary skills."[12]

Mari Swingle treats many youths with troubled behavior, attention issues, and addictive patterns. A neuropsychologist, she is the author of perhaps the most comprehensive book on the brain and the digital culture, *i-Minds: How and Why Constant*

Connectivity Is Rewiring Our Brains and What to Do About It. "We're seeing autistic-like characteristics in children without autism," she told me. "Lack of smile response, delayed verbal skills, what I used to affectionately call 'busy children': now these are just kids that are kind of running around aimlessly or conversely zombified when they're not on the tech . . . You have kids—for that matter, adults now—that are used to being on the tech for extensive periods of time. A walk won't do it, canoeing won't do it, even speed skateboarding—a lot of things—skiing, even those are now challenged." Dr. Swingle, too, is very concerned about the impacts of relentless screen exposure on brain development: "Less ability to focus on the normal, the baseline, including states of observation, contemplation, and transitions from which ideas spark—what many under the age of twenty now consider a void, proclaiming boredom . . . On a biological as well as a cultural level, such brain state changes affect learning, socialization, recreation, partnering, parenting, and creativity—in essence all factors that make a society and a culture. The neurophysiological processes that regulate mood and behavior are deregulating."[13]

She understands digital media's appeal to well-meaning parents, namely that it acts "as a stress and fatigue mediator." Engaging with it requires little or no pre-planning—it "is instantly available, and provides parents, caretakers, and even educators with much-needed moments of respite and solace." Here we have a case of the solution to one dilemma fueling another. These forms of relief, understandable as they are in these wickedly stressful times, have a cost—and it is our children who pay the lion's share.

As in marketing, the people who invent and propagate these technologies are conscious of the problematic nature of their wares, and even take it to heart—when it comes to their own children, that is. A 2019 *Business Insider* article details how many major Silicon Valley executives—including founders and CEOs of Apple, Google, and even the explicitly kid-targeted Snapchat app (!)—go to concerted lengths to limit their own kids' screen time at home.[†14] Tellingly, the late Apple CEO Steve Jobs forbade his young children to play with the then newly launched iPad.

Is it all bad news? Of course not; nothing is that simple. Ellen Friedrichs, a Brooklyn-based health educator who works with a diverse array of young people, notes that for some of her students, "the internet has been a lifeline. For that queer kid living in some small town, in a religious community where they have to sit through a homophobic sermon every Sunday . . . you can go online and find 'your people' in a way that you never could." Nor is the "lifeline" solely for marginalized youths. As I write this, for the past year and counting, my primary contact with family, friends, and students worldwide has been via a computer screen. Most of us living through the COVID-19 crisis have newfound appreciation for how technology can promote community and, for many, ease otherwise intolerable isolation. However, we should not be lulled into false optimism or complacency by these upsides. The pleasures and boons of online connectivity can neither keep pace with the burgeoning crises of disconnection nor allay concerns about what the digital world is encoding into our kids' cognitive and emotional operating systems.

––––––––––––

When schools in the Canadian province of Quebec reopened after the COVID-19 lockdown in May 2020, omitted from the curriculum were the supposed nonessentials of music, drama, art, and physical education. The assumption was that academic subjects were more important—raising the question,

†   Similar sentiments are heard from Silicon Valley execs throughout the hit 2020 Netflix documentary *The Social Dilemma*.

More important for what? Prioritizing "job readiness" is a far cry from foregrounding healthy development, which ought to be the primary agenda of the educational system, as of child-rearing in general. Even on narrow "skill building" grounds, our prevailing educational ideologies miss the boat, since cognitive skills in fact depend on firm emotional architecture, of which play is an indispensable builder.

"We used to think that schools built brains," Gordon Neufeld said in Brussels. "Now we know that it is play that builds the brains that school can then use . . . It's where growth most happens."

Those subjects deemed superfluous by Quebec school authorities tap into essential cerebral circuitry. All young mammals play, and for critical reasons. As the neuroscientist Jaak Panksepp identified, we have a designated "PLAY" system in our brains in common with other mammals. Play is a primary engine of brain development and is also essential to the emotional maturation process. "As a species, we have evolved culturally in a large part because of our playfulness and all that it produces by way of intelligence and productivity," James Garbarino writes.[15] And true play, Gordon Neufeld insists, is not outcome-based: the fun is in the activity, not the end result. Free play is one of the "irreducible needs" of childhood, and it's being sacrificed to both consumerism and the digital culture. "The culture is not respecting normal developmental tasks," the neuroscientist Stephen Porges told me. "Normal developmental tasks are to play with another person, not with an Xbox. Not to talk on a cell phone or text, but to make face-to-face interactions. All these things are neural exercises that provide resilience, creating an ability for an individual to regulate their internal emotional states."

To be up front: I think the influence of the digital/screen problem is almost unfathomably pernicious. In 2016 it was reported that British children ages five to fifteen years were spending three hours a day on the internet, and over two hours watching TV. By contrast, the time spent reading books for pleasure declined from an hour a day (as recently as 2012) to just over half an hour four years later.[16] The vast majority of "gaming" these days takes place alone in front of a screen, with pixelated avatars and disembodied voices standing in for actual playmates. Just what time does all that leave for free, creative, emergent, interactive, individual, or collective play? What kind of brains are we creating?

The same question might be asked about the educational system. In 2016, an American professor and Fulbright scholar named William Doyle, just returned from a semester-long appointment at the University of Eastern Finland, wrote in the *Los Angeles Times* that for those five months, his family "experienced a stunningly stress-free, and stunningly good, school system." His seven-year-old son was placed in the youngest class—not because of some developmental delay, but because children younger than seven "don't receive formal academic training . . . Many are in day care and learn through play, songs, games and conversation." Once in school, children get a mandated fifteen-minute outdoor recess break for every forty-five minutes of in-class instruction. The educational mantras Doyle remembers hearing the most while there: " 'Let children be children,' 'The work of a child is to play,' and 'Children learn best through play.' " And as far as outcomes go? Finland consistently ranks at or near the top of educational test score results in the Western world and has been ranked the most literate nation on Earth.[17]

"The message that competition is appropriate, desirable, required, and even unavoidable is drummed into us from nursery school to graduate school; it is the subtext of every lesson," writes educational consultant Alfie Kohn in his excellent book *No Contest: The Case Against Competition: Why We Lose in Our*

Race to Win, which documents the negative impact of competition on genuine learning, and how competition, praise, grades, rewards, and sanctions imposed on recalcitrant children destroy intrinsic motivation and undermine emotional security.[18] "Does praise motivate kids? Sure it does," Kohn sarcastically remarks. "It motivates kids to get praise."

"And?" you might ask. "What's wrong with well-deserved kudos?" It turns out that there's praise, and then there's praise. Developmental psychologists agree that praising a child's *effort* is helpful and promotes self-esteem, while valuing the *achievement* only programs kids to keep seeking external approval—not for who they are but for what they do, for what others demand of them. It's yet another barrier to the emergence of a healthy self.

For all our love and dedication as parents and educators, the world in which we must rear children these days undercuts our best efforts in a multitude of ways, all masquerading as "just the way it is." There is no "just" about it: the consequences are massive. The present, as it presently is, beggars the future.

Chapter 14

A Template for Distress:
How Culture Builds Our Character

"And that," put in the Director sententiously, "that is
the secret of happiness and virtue—liking what you've got
to do. All conditioning aims at making people like
their inescapable social destiny."

—Aldous Huxley, *Brave New World*

Recall Bessel van der Kolk's crisp remark that "our culture teaches us to focus on our personal uniqueness, but at a deeper level we barely exist as individual organisms." I don't know whether the comparison will discomfit or comfort (perhaps both?), but we humans are, in our lack of an independently self-determined self, not altogether different from our fellow social creature, the ant.

In an ant colony, all larvae are hatched with virtually the same set of genes: the queen, the workers, the warriors are created equal. Which creature becomes what, including what biological features they manifest, depends entirely on the needs of the clan. The oncologist and author Siddhartha Mukherjee described this phenomenon in a fascinating article in the *New Yorker*: "Ants have a powerful caste system. A colony typically contains ants that carry out radically different roles and have markedly different body structures and behaviors." Genetically identical siblings will become differentiated into biologically variable adults based purely on signals from the physical and social environment.

When a queen is removed from a jumping ant hive, for example, the worker ants "launch a vicious, fight-to-the-death campaign against one another—stinging, biting, sparring, lopping off limbs and heads"—until a few workers win and become, well, monarchical. Without any alteration in DNA structure, the physiology of a new queen changes; "she" now becomes fecund and dominant and will live longer than she would have in her previous worker incarnation.[1] Psychiatrist Michael Kerr, formerly of Georgetown University, noted this same dynamic in his book on human family systems. "What each larva becomes is dictated by a colony level process. In this sense, a young larva is born into a functioning position in the colony and his development is determined by that position."[2]

For all our attachment to our individual self-concept, we are rather antlike in this respect. "There is far less autonomy for a human being than we would like to think," Dr. Kerr told me in an interview. "How we function as individuals cannot be understood outside of our relationship to the larger group." In other words, our character and personalities reflect the needs of the milieu in which we develop. The roles we are assigned or denied, how we fit into society or are excluded from it, and what the culture induces us to believe about ourselves, determine much about the health we enjoy or the diseases that plague us. In this, and in many other ways, illness and health are manifestations of the social macrocosm.

If the modern nuclear family forms the primary container for childhood development, that container is itself held within a larger context, formed by entities such as community, neighborhood, city, economy, country, and so on. In our times, the context of all contexts is hypermaterialist, consumerist capitalism and its globalized expressions worldwide. Its fundamental—and, it turns out, quite distorted—assumptions about who and what we are show up in the bodies and minds of those living them out. Given the myriad links between biography and biology, cultural norms can also make themselves known in our physiology.

We see here the attachment/authenticity tug-of-war writ large. Just as we are conditioned to fit into the family, even if that means a departure from our true selves, so we are prepped—one might even say groomed—to fulfill our expected social roles and take on the characteristics necessary to do so, no matter the cumulative cost to our well-being.

I first met Ulf Caap about fourteen years ago. Then vice president of human resources for IKEA North America, Ulf seemed to have everything going for him. And yet this internationally respected business leader had sought me out as part of a personal journey born of deep existential dissatisfaction. He had been visited by a most uncomfortable realization: his well-compensated life—a runaway success by our society's "normal" gauges—and the everyday way of being it demanded of him, amounted, as he recalled, to "a sham, an illusion, a fake . . . There was virtually none of *me* in it." Another wildly successful person by societal standards, the writer-actor Lena Dunham, of *Girls*[†] fame, said something similar in our interview. In a rehab program for substance addiction, she had been assigned the exercise of writing down her own values. "I realized," she said, "that I could not think of a single value that did not belong to somebody else."

Ulf has since become a friend and sometime collaborator: we have codesigned and led workshops for high-level executives who share that same sense of their authentic selves and their work personas being at diametric odds. I don't mean merely that they leave their true thoughts, feelings, desires, and needs at the office door,

---

[†] The acclaimed HBO series of which Dunham was both creator and star.

only to retrieve them at day's end as one would a parked car. For the "sham" to be sustainable, these authentic parts of the self must be placed in long-term storage and the key misplaced. "I would negate my personal values to make a success," Ulf admitted. Now in his mid-seventies and the very picture of health, he is convinced his self-suppression and disconnect were draining his life energy: "I recognized that my steps going to work were not so light as they used to be. I was being drawn toward illness."

Ulf has had the good sense—and, he would agree, the privilege—to explore and transcend his alienation. "I spent forty years in insanity," he said, looking back. "My focus was ninety-nine percent on what success looked like in society and in the corporation I worked for. I had no focus whatsoever on what I needed. If I did what the corporation required, I would be successful." He could not have provided a more precise illustration of the insight that the young Trappist monk Thomas Merton, the most influential American Catholic writer of the twentieth century, articulated in his autobiography, *The Seven Storey Mountain*: "The logic of worldly success rests on a fallacy: the strange error that our perfection depends on the thoughts and opinions and applause of other men! A weird life it is, indeed, to be living always in somebody else's imagination, as if that were the only place in which one could at last become real!"[3]

Identity crises such as Ulf experienced are not consciously self-authored—they are the outcome of how we develop in our assorted contexts, from the family outward. "The success I had was one hundred percent external," Ulf said to me. "Totally external—and based on a mental construct I built as a five-year-old and a fifteen-year-old of what it takes to be accepted." In this sense, as the social psychologist Erich Fromm pointed out, the family acts, unwittingly, as the "psychic agent" for society to form what he called the *social character*.

The social character is, in Fromm's words, "the core character common to most members of a culture." This is different from the *individual* character we each possess and display to the world. The social character, to the extent it defines and governs us, assures that we will fit the "normal" mold in our particular culture. Fromm's concept strikes me as a potent rendering of how we function in society—antlike.

I speak here not only of the "we" in an individual sense. The collective "we" is far more blind and dangerous. For example, none of us like to see people sleeping in the streets, but as a society we countenance growing levels of homelessness. Nobody wants life on Earth imperiled, yet the march of climate change seems inexorable. Something in us normalizes such calamities, whether the result is that we actively enable them, deny them, or merely look on in passive resignation. All my life, no doubt spurred by the horrors that shaped my childhood, I have wondered how it is that so many good people can be hypnotized into compliance with the indefensible. There has to be some mechanism to acculturate us to accept as normal what is inimical to ourselves and to the world we inhabit; it is certainly not an inborn inclination. Somehow the system's values and expectations get under the skin, to the point where we confuse them with ourselves.

As Fromm put it, often people's behavior is not a matter of conscious decision to follow the social pattern, but of "wanting to act as they have to act."[4] In this way a culture creates members who will serve its purposes. It is instructive to juxtapose reality with fiction. In Aldous Huxley's *Brave New World,* individuals are "so conditioned that they practically can't help behaving as they ought to behave."[5]

Thus, what is considered normal and natural are established not by what is *good* for people, but by what is expected of them, which traits and attitudes serve the maintenance of the culture. These are then enshrined as "human nature," while deviations from them are seen as abnormal. For the most part, absent an awakening—often of the rude variety—of the authenticity drive, people will develop and behave in ways that seem to confirm the dominant ideas.

What are some of the features of the social character imbued in our culture?

The First "Character" Trait: Separation from Self

I have said that acquired personality traits such as excessive identification with socially imposed duty, role, and responsibility at the expense of one's own needs can jeopardize health. This and other conditioned characteristics are the result of a child's developmental needs being denied, of Nature being thwarted. Culture cements them through reinforcement and reward, encouraging people to perform tasks even if chronically stressful, under circumstances they might naturally want to avoid. My own workaholism as a physician earned me much respect, gratitude, remuneration, and status in the world, even as it undermined my mental health and my family's emotional balance. And why was I a workaholic? Because, stemming from my early experiences, I needed to be needed, wanted, and admired as a substitute for love. I never consciously decided to be driven that way, and yet it "worked" all too well for me in the social and professional realms.

Mechanisms for estranging people from themselves abound. They begin acting on us from the earliest moments of our existence with stresses in the parenting environment and socially sanctioned child-rearing practices that negate the child's needs. The flight from self is powerfully compounded by overt trauma, of course. But even in the absence of personal wounding it can be impelled by a conformist and competition-centered educational system, by social expectations to "fit in," the drive for peer acceptance, and a socially induced, pervasive anxiety about one's status.

In an image-mad culture that sustains itself in large part by making people feel inadequate about themselves—or, more insidiously, capitalizing (pun half intended) on these preexisting feelings—the media holds out ideals of physical perfection against which young and old measure themselves and which lead people to be ashamed of their very bodies. My friend Peter Levine wrote an article some years ago on the cosmetic procedure of injecting people with botulinum toxin; the substance relaxes muscles, temporarily, so as to remove the natural wrinkles from aging. But it also renders the face unnaturally less responsive. "There are nursing mothers taking Botox," Peter told me. "They are not able to communicate their emotions with their babies, or even pick up the babies' emotions. They lose that kind of contact." In many other spheres, including social media, we too often present an artificial, "Botoxed" version of ourselves: an image not of who we are but of how we would like to be perceived by others. "What we have with the internet is sort of a Botox for the masses," Peter said. "We have just lost this capacity to be real, which is fundamentally what makes us human, and what makes us feel connected to each other."

The Second "Character" Trait: Consumption Hunger

Among the great achievements of mass-consumption culture has been to convince us that what we have been conditioned to fervently want is also what we need. In the words of the French-Bulgarian psychoanalyst Julia Kristeva, "Desires are manufactured as surely as are the commodities meant to fulfill them. We consume our needs, unaware that what we take to be a 'need' has been artificially produced."[6] I'm reminded of a response a young Bob Dylan gave on a 1965 tour of England to two desperate autograph seekers. "We need your autograph," one of them begged through the rear-door window of the singer-songwriter's limo. Dylan demurred. "No, you don't *need* it," he said drily. "If you needed it, I would give it to you." And that's just the point: the social character hatched by our consumerist society confuses desire with need, to the point that the nervous system becomes riled when the objects desired are withheld. Supply, meet demand.

As Thomas Merton noted dolefully in 1948, "We live in a society whose whole policy is to excite every nerve in the human body and keep it at the highest pitch of artificial tension, to strain every human desire to the limit and create as many new desires and synthetic passions as possible, in order to cater to them with the products of our factories and printing presses and movie studios and all the rest."[7]

Constantly living at that "highest pitch of artificial tension" leaves many people dissatisfied, on edge, anxious—utterly captured by an addictive process that alienates them from real needs, real emotions, real concerns, real life.

If unable to achieve what we desire, we experience this as a personal failure—even if social conditions are arrayed against us so that success is out of reach. "I remember when I was a kid, I used to love to look at Tide soap commercials," the American actor, director, and political activist Danny Glover told me. "When I look at it now, it was not because I had this affinity to anything about Tide. I would look at it from the vantage point of that I wished my kitchen was like that, I wished my washing machine looked like that, I wished all the things . . . We're put in this situation where we're surrounded by all these things that ninety-nine percent of the time we'll never have, and that creates a sense of valuelessness, because you are not able to have those things." Glover's words track perfectly with social critic Neil Postman's observation as far back as 1985 in his seminal cultural critique, *Amusing Ourselves to Death*. Commercials full of happy-looking people "tell nothing about the products being sold. But they tell everything about the fears, fancies, and dreams of those who might buy them. *What the advertiser needs to know is not what is right about the product but what is wrong about the buyer.*"[8]

Driven by a culturally fueled conviction of insufficiency, we become addicted to consumption. "Consumption is a way in which you mute the pain," Glover said to me. "I know people who have plenty of resources to divert the pain by buying unnecessarily . . . The structure of capitalism creates a situation where people's value relies on their capacity to consume. I don't care if it's consuming from Walmart or from Saks Fifth Avenue. When we talk about addiction, whether it be to drugs or whether it be to other forms of behavior, they all symbolize the sense of being devalued as a human being within a system. That's basically it: feeling alienated within the system."

The Third "Character" Trait: Hypnotic Passivity

Unlike the denizens of Huxley's dystopian fantasy future, we are not automatons, engineered in test tubes to be a certain way and programmed to carry out only certain preordained functions. As citizens in ostensibly democratic countries, we have free will, up to a point—but in practice that freedom rarely strays beyond the frontier of what is socially acceptable. Not daring to rock the boat, we risk sinking with it.

Self-abandonment programmed into the social character makes us passive even in the face of threats to our existence as a species. Healthy people connected to their real emotions and authentic requirements would not be susceptible to blandishments inciting artificial needs and the products to satisfy them, no matter how cleverly packaged. Nor would they accept the unacceptable, except perhaps under threat of force—and even then, they would not be inclined to internalize it as the way things ought to be.

"Children," the great public intellectual Noam Chomsky has remarked, "are constantly asking *why*—they want explanations, they want to understand things." But soon, he says, "you go to school, you're regimented. You're taught this is the way you're supposed to behave, not other ways. The institutions of the society are constructed, so as to reduce, modify, limit the efforts and control of one's own destiny."[9]

The problem originates in how children are raised in the bosom of the modern family, itself a microcosmic representative of the culture. "The family," Erich Fromm pointed out, "has the function of transmitting the requirements of society to the growing child." It does so in all the ways we examined in our chapters on child development. The social character is seeded when children are deprived of breastfeeding; when their Nature-imbued expectations for being held are frustrated; when they are left alone to "cry it out"; when they are compelled to repress their feelings; when they are programmed to fit in with the expectations of others; when they are denied spontaneous free play; when they are "disciplined" by punitive measures such as "time-out" techniques that threaten them with the loss of what they most crave—unconditional positive acceptance; when they are denied a connection with Nature. These all contribute to the inner emptiness, the void that addictions and covetous compulsions will later attempt to fill, even as our independent spirit is subjugated to the demands of an imbalanced, materialist culture.

How lovely it would be if the democratic ideal of "we, the people" creating the society in which we wish to live were true. It's certainly a dream worth pursuing. But believing in it is not nearly enough. It will not and cannot come to pass until we reckon squarely with how things are today: it is *we* who are made in the image of our distorted, disordered, denatured world—the better to keep it running, even as it runs us into the ground.

Part III

Rethinking Abnormal: Afflictions as Adaptations

Much Madness is divinest Sense—
To a discerning Eye—
Much Sense—the starkest Madness—
'Tis the Majority
In this, as all, prevail—
Assent—and you are sane—
Demur—you're straightway dangerous—
And handled with a Chain—

—Emily Dickinson

Chapter 15

Just Not to Be You: Debunking the Myths About Addiction

*I have absolutely no pleasure in the stimulants in which I
sometimes so madly indulge. It has not been in the pursuit of
pleasure that I have periled life and reputation and reason. It has
been in the desperate attempt to escape from torturing memories.*

—Edgar Allan Poe

Bruce, a vascular surgeon in Oregon, was donning his surgical
gown when the police barged in. "I was hauled out of the hospital in handcuffs," he recalled of that sunny day seven years ago.
"It was beyond humiliating. I was practicing in a small town, so
everybody knew. I was on the front page of the local paper multiple times. It became quite a fall from grace." This trusted local
figure had been writing prescriptions in his patients' names,
only to retrieve them himself to feed his addiction. "I was using
enough, writing enough prescriptions," he recounts, "that the
initial suspicion by the police department was that I was running
some sort of drug ring." In a few short months, the jig was up.

What could bring a highly trained, accomplished physician
like Bruce, married, father of adolescents, to such depths of self-deception, dishonesty, and professional malfeasance? Surely
he understood he was jeopardizing his health, family, and livelihood. Why, for that matter, would anyone indulge—if that is the
right word—in such self-destructive behaviors?

That question has confronted me almost daily throughout my career but most insistently in my twelve years working in Vancouver's Downtown Eastside, a neighborhood notorious as North America's most concentrated area of drug use. Within its few square blocks dwell thousands of people living lives of desperate dependence on substances of all kinds, inhaling or ingesting or injecting alcohol, opiates, nicotine, cannabis, cocaine, crystal meth, glue, rubbing alcohol. Even visitors from New York or Detroit or Bristol are routinely shocked by what they see there.

"If the success of a doctor is measured by how long his patients live," I would often say, "then I'm a failure, because many of my patients die young." They died from complications of HIV, or from hepatitis C, or infections of their heart valves, brains, spines, bloodstreams. They fell victim to suicide, overdose, or violence, or to vehicles that struck them while they stumbled in a drugged-out haze onto busy streets. Unlike "high-bottom" addicts such as Bruce, now rehabilitated and back on the job, my patients had lost everything—their health, looks, teeth; their families, work, homes. Some had squandered lives of middle-class comfort, and a handful had gone, surprisingly, from riches to rags. All along, they knew full well they were facing the ultimate forfeit: their lives. And still, having struck bottoms lower than most of us could conceive of, they persisted in their habits, as I depicted in my 2009 book on addiction, *In the Realm of Hungry Ghosts*.

Prevailing views about addiction have progressed somewhat in the past decade, in the direction of more compassion, science, and sense. For all that, deceptive and dangerous myths about addiction's provenance and its very nature still reign in many circles, from medical treatment to criminal justice and policy. Even the well-meaning world of rehabilitation and recovery has its blind spots. Given the evident shortcomings and even ruinous harm wrought by our standard approaches, many voices are finally calling for a fresh view.

As a prelude to considering this, let's deal directly with the two leading misconceptions: that addiction is either the product of "bad choices" or else a "disease." Both fail to explain this unrelenting societal plague, just as they hobble our efforts toward remedying it.

The *bad choices* view should by now barely warrant mention, given the scientific advances in understanding, except that it still has a vise grip on many people's thinking and underlies the legal system's assault on drug users. It is so wrongheaded as to be laughable—and it would be, if its consequences were not so tragic. It was expressed succinctly in 2017 by then U.S. attorney general Jeff Sessions, hearkening back to the bad old days of the 1980s drug war: "We need to say, as Nancy Reagan said, 'Just say no,'" he told a Virginia audience. "Educating people and telling them the terrible truth about drugs and addiction will result in better choices by more people."

The precise success of all the war on drugs campaigns, which have had a half century to make good on their stated goals, can be seen in one sordid fact: even as Sessions spoke, his country was losing as many lives to overdoses every three weeks as had been claimed by the 9/11 terrorist attacks. That year, more than 70,000 Americans would die of a drug overdose.[1] Four years later, in 2021, that figure exceeded 100,000.[2] In the same year, my home province of British Columbia saw over 1,700 such deaths, nearly double the number killed by COVID-19 in the province as of this writing.

The "bad choices" view of addiction—which, if we're honest, amounts to little more than "It's Your Own Damn Fault"—is not only disastrously ineffective; it is utterly blind. I have never met anyone who, in any meaningful sense of the word, ever "chose" to become addicted, least of all my Downtown Eastside patients whose lives slowly ebbed away or were rapidly extinguished in the streets, hotel rooms, and back alleys of Vancouver's drug ghetto.

If a socially conservative dissenter were to protest, "Didn't they choose to *stay* hooked?" I would offer this quote by Dr. Nora Volkow, head of the U.S. National Institute on Drug Abuse: "[Recent] studies have shown that repeated drug use leads to long-lasting changes in the brain *that undermine voluntary control.*"[3] Translation: when it comes to addiction, "free will" is in many ways a neurobiological non sequitur.

In fact, I would take it much further: most addicted people had little choice even *before* their habits took hold. Their brains arrived on the scene *already* impaired by life experience, especially susceptible to the effects of their drug "of choice" (another dubious expression). Actually, that's true whether the target is a substance or a behavior. In short, the choice model ignores the question of what would drive a person toward addiction in the first place.

Though the *disease* paradigm still embraced by most addiction specialists and treatment programs is more compassionate, it, too, misses the human element. It separates mind from body—or, in this case, brain from mind, seeing the brain in purely biochemical terms. The fact is, personal and social life events, filtered through the mind, shape the brain throughout the lifetime. You cannot, scientifically, cleave biology from biography, especially when it comes to a process as psychologically layered as addiction.

Not that there's no value in considering addiction's neurochemical side. The brilliant work of Dr. Volkow and others has demonstrated that substances of dependence do, over time, change the brain so that essential functions, such as impulse regulation—which would aid someone in resisting addiction's pull—become significantly compromised, even as the circuits of reward and motivation become trained on the desired drugs. In this sense, the brain *does* become an impaired organ, with diminished capacity to make rational choices, obsessively intent instead on satisfying the addictive drives.

We err, however, when we focus on drugs alone: *it does not take a substance addiction to bring about changes in brain chemistry.* Scans have shown similar deleterious changes in the brains of nonsubstance addicts as well, such as inveterate internet gamers.[4] The compulsive intake of foods that trigger the brain's reward apparatus can also produce such effects.[5]

For all that, the equation of addiction with a largely genetically programmed, treatable disease[†6] is, as mentioned, scientifically and humanely a step forward from the shaming "bad choices" model. Just as we wouldn't think of blaming the owner of a diseased kidney, it makes no sense to reproach someone for having a "sick" brain, especially if that "sickness" was inherited.[‡] The problem is that, in typical medical fashion, the disease paradigm turns a process into pathology. Note, too, that "treatable" is a far cry from "healable"—which says less about the nature of addiction than about the medical system's failure to understand it.

The word "disease" also crops up frequently in the world of twelve-step recovery. People in programs like Alcoholics Anonymous or Narcotics Anonymous will speak about "my disease," as in "My disease wants me dead" or "My disease made me hurt the people I love." No doubt such programs have helped millions, and the language used is a big part of helping people think and act

---

†   The American Society of Addiction Medicine defines "addiction" as "a treatable, chronic medical *disease* involving complex interactions among brain circuits, genetics, the environment, and an individual's life experiences. People with addictions use substances or engage in behaviors that become compulsive and often continue despite harmful consequences" (2019).

‡   According to the American Society of Addiction Medicine and the U.S. surgeon general's 2016 report on substance use, up to 50 percent of the "disease" is due to genetic factors. I'll have more to say about the flaws in that view later in this chapter.

in new ways. I will only suggest that "disease" is more therapeutically useful as a metaphor rather than a literal fact. As with most chronic conditions, viewing addiction as a dynamic process to be engaged with rather than a demonic force to be feared or battled can ultimately expand the possibilities for healing.

For a more grounded take on addiction, we need to consider not just people's genes or brain circuitry, but also their real encounters with their world. We need to look closely at people's life experiences.[†] Addictions of any kind are not abnormal ailments, willfully self-inflicted maladies, brain disorders, or genetic short straws. Properly understood, they are not even that puzzling. As with other ostensibly mysterious conditions named in this book, they are rooted in coping mechanisms. To be sure, they may take on some *features* of disease: a dysfunctional organ, tissue damage particularly with extensive drug use, physical symptoms, impairment of certain brain circuits, cycles of remission and relapse, even death. But to call them "diseases" is to miss both the point and the opportunity to deal with them intelligently. Addictions represent, in their onset, the defenses of an organism against suffering it does not know how to endure. In other words, we are looking at a natural response to unnatural circumstances, an attempt to soothe the pain of injuries incurred in childhood and stresses sustained in adulthood.

Two Essential Questions

Over my decades of medical practice and thousands of conversations, I have learned that the first question to ask is not what is wrong with an addiction, but what is "right" about it. What benefit is the person deriving from their habit? What does it do for them? What are they getting that they otherwise can't access?

---

†   The American Society of Addiction Medicine's disease-oriented definition, cited earlier, does point to life experiences without naming or exploring them in detail; we need to go further and get more specific.

This inquiry is key to understanding any addiction, whether to substances like alcohol, opiates, cocaine, crystal meth, sniffed glue, or junk food, or to behaviors such as gambling, compulsive sexual roving, pornography, or binge eating and purging. Or to power and profit, for that matter—here, of course, we begin to shade toward addictions that go well beyond individual habits into the realm of collective fixations.

Just as I have never met anyone who chose to become addicted, neither have I met anyone whose addictions did not, at their onset at least, provide for some essential human need. Over and over again, for example, I've heard that people's addictions lubricate the gears of social connection. The Canadian Métis‡ writer, professor, and former inmate Jesse Thistle, author of the memoir *From the Ashes*, told me his substance use gave him "access to friends. And it gave me power, confidence. And it worked for a while—it worked for about the first three years. I became almost, like, bulletproof." For her part, the multitalented television artist Lena Dunham recalled, "It made me more social. It made me more relaxed. It made it easier for me to communicate." In her case, "it" was a dependence on, among other things, tranquilizers: highly addictive medications too freely dispensed by physicians. The boost extended to her creative self-expression: the drugs, she told me, "made me write like a demon because I just completely lost my inhibitions."

"Warmth" is an oft-heard descriptor for the feeling of being high—it captures a felt sense that addicts know well. The actor and children's author Jamie Lee Curtis spoke to me of "this warm bath: the way it feels when you're cold and you step into a warm, not hot, but a warm, really warm bath where that feeling of ease rises as you lower into the warmth. It was a very familiar feeling

‡   Métis are people of mixed Indigenous and European ancestry, mostly in the Western Canadian context.

to me, and it was one that I loved. I chased that feeling for ten years in and out of everything from stealing opiates to manipulating doctors for opiates."

Curtis's words reminded me of what I often heard from my hypermarginalized Downtown Eastside (DTES) patients. "What does the heroin do for you?" I once asked a patient just admitted to Onsite, the detox venue above Insite—then North America's only supervised injection site, where I was staff physician. In his late thirties, with weightlifter arms, a shaved head, and a large brass ring piercing his right earlobe, this fierce-looking man looked right at me and said, "Doc, I don't know how to tell you this, exactly. It's like when you're three years old, sick, shivering with fever, and your mother puts you on her lap, wraps you in a warm blanket, and gives you warm chicken soup—that's what heroin feels like." His fellow DTES resident, the poet Bud Osborn, also spoke of the soothing thaw heroin allowed him to experience. "I felt this warmth in the pit of my gut, which had always been really cold."

The rock guitarist[†] and reality-TV star Dave Navarro told me that he found in his addictions "a kind of love and acceptance," another running theme among users. His fellow podcaster and author, the British comedian Russell Brand, also spoke of love. "The first time I took heroin, it felt so sacred and spiritual and warm and maternal," he said. "I felt like I was held . . . I felt like nothing mattered, and I felt safe." His use of the word "maternal" is more than metaphorical: it speaks directly to the neurobiology of opiate addiction.

Others find in their compulsive habits a kind of experience that people spend years pursuing in caves, monasteries, and high-priced retreat centers. "Alcohol," the comedian and former

---

†   Jane's Addiction, Red Hot Chili Peppers.

Saturday Night Live mainstay Darrell Hammond said when we spoke, "gives you three or four hours of peace. Just peace. The talk in the head stops, the negative thinking. It's precious." Peace and quiet are not qualities most of us associate with the life of an addict, but these "precious" states are often what is sought—and, for a while, found.

Lena Dunham's tranquilizer dependence provided the temporary illusion of normalcy—an illusion reinforced by the fact that, in our society, her drugs of choice are often acquired via "legitimate" means—a doctor's prescribing pad. "Pharmaceuticals hold this magical promise of making you function normally, or better than normally," she says. "Alcohol, you smell it on someone; crack . . . you end up under a bridge. Klonopin,‡ you can go for a pretty long time thinking, 'Wow, I found the cure to not being able to function in the way that I think people should be able to function in the world.' "

It's worth asking: Who has ever heard of a "disease" that makes you "feel normal"? Or, when's the last time getting sick made you "function better than normally"?

In light of these testimonials, how much more absurd Jeff Sessions's insistence on "better choices" sounds. Shall we do Nancy Reagan one better by erecting more truthful highway billboards and school cafeteria signs: "Just Say No to Pain Relief"? Or "Just Say No to a Warm, Nurturing Feeling in the Belly"? To inner peace; to calmness, empowerment, a sense of self-worth; to community and friendship; to unfettered self-expression; to an elusive sense of comfortable normality; and to love? "I did notice," Navarro told me, "that whenever I started using substances again, I got a sense of *what a human being is supposed to feel like*." Try saying no to that.

---

‡   Klonopin is a trade name for clonazepam, a tranquilizer of the benzodiazepine class, to which also belong such chemical relatives as Valium (diazepam) and Ativan (lorazepam).

When it comes down to it, all addiction's incentives can be summed up as an escape from the confines of the self, by which I mean the mundane, lived-in experience of being uncomfortable and isolated in one's own skin. Underneath however many surface layers of "normal" functioning, that alienated discomfort can be disturbing to the point of torment: a persistent sense of being abnormal, unworthy, and deficient. Keith Richards of the Rolling Stones, perhaps the world's best-known former heroin addict, crystallizes this escape strategy in his autobiography, *Life*: "It was a search for oblivion, I suppose . . . the convolutions you go through just not to be you for a few hours."[7]

Why would the self need to be escaped? We long for escape when we are imprisoned, when we are suffering. Addiction calls to us when waking life amounts to being trapped in inner turmoil, doubt, loss of meaning, isolation, unworthiness; feeling cold in our belly, devoid of hope; lacking faith in the possibility of liberation, missing succor; unable to endure external challenges or the inner chaos or emptiness; incapable of regulating our distressing mind conditions, finding our emotions unendurable; and most of all, desperate to soothe the pain all these states represent. Pain, then, is the central theme. No wonder people so often speak about the benign numbing effect of their addictions: only a person in pain craves anesthesia.

As a quest for self-escape, the internal logic of addiction is inescapable. *Where I am is intolerable. Get me out of here.*

Here we arrive at the second cornerstone query regarding addiction, one that has become something of a mantra with me: *Ask not why the addiction, but why the pain.* This is the question neither the prevailing disease-based medical paradigm nor popular prejudice can possibly answer or would even think to raise. Yet without it, we can have no clue as to why this affliction of mind, body, and spirit is so rampant.

To map the hard and inhospitable terrain from which addiction springs, it's worth asking the people who have traversed it. Listening to their lived experiences leaves one with no confusion about what needs to be soothed, and why. We lack the space to chronicle all the tragic origin stories of the many individuals I interviewed for this book, from the well known to the unknown; what follows is a brief and representative sample.

- When the Canadian hockey legend Theoren Fleury was fourteen, his coach began sexually abusing him. "He started a routine whenever I was over—masturbate on my feet, then give a blowjob, then let me sleep." And that was far from all, he told me. In his chaotic family of origin, with an alcoholic father, he had no one to turn to. On the contrary, he was desperate to make his economically downtrodden and emotionally dysfunctional parents happy. Years later, earning millions of dollars a year as a scrappy offensive star for the New York Rangers, he was hopelessly addicted to alcohol and cocaine.
- The opiate-dependent surgical specialist Bruce also lived through a childhood bereft of nurturing. "My father was not present," he said. "I did not have a father in my life, growing up. He walked out when I was quite young, four years old. And my mother was too young to assume the duties I needed from her. My mother had me when she was sixteen, and she just was a child herself, essentially. I lived my formative years really not having any support. I lived with a lot of pain."
- The world-renowned photographer Nan Goldin, who says she did drugs "most of my life," was eleven when her older sister died by suicide at eighteen. "That was a huge defining trauma for me," Goldin says. Defining, but

not primary. "I grew up in a very neurotic family," she recalls, understating things by some magnitude. "There was constant turmoil around my older sister . . . Some of my earliest memories were of her throwing things at everyone except me. They put her in mental hospitals, and even sent her to an orphanage. There was a lot of violence, a lot of chaos, a lot of screaming."

- When the late Downtown Eastside street poet Bud Osborn was three years old, his father hanged himself in jail, where the Toledo police had taken him after he tried to throw himself out of a window. "As a child Osborn regarded one person as a refuge: his grandmother," the Vancouver journalist Travis Lupick writes in *Fighting for Space*, his book on the drug policy reform movement, of which Osborn became a prominent leader. "She was shot and killed by his aunt, who then turned the gun on herself." As a five-year-old, Bud witnessed his mother being beaten and raped. A year later he hurled himself off the porch in an attempt to take his own life.

- Former *Saturday Night Live* star Darrell Hammond was physically and emotionally brutalized by his mother, as anyone will know who has watched the painful and self-revealing autobiographic documentary *Cracked Up*.

- Lena Dunham suffered sexual abuse at a young age, along with a factor that ensures such experiences will leave lasting traumatic effects: emotional isolation. In a recent therapy session under the influence of the medication ketamine, she experienced "witnessing this overwhelming grief about being alone in my childhood."

While each life history is particular, and while trauma has many faces, some generalization is both possible and necessary, particularly where abuse and neglect meet the lower strata of racial and class status. During my dozen years in Vancouver's Downtown Eastside, I came to learn that every one of my female patients—many of whom were Indigenous, many caught up in the sex trade—had been sexually abused in childhood or adolescence, one marker of the multigenerational legacy born of Canada's brutal colonial past. Multiple large-scale studies attest to the dynamic of childhood trauma, including sexual abuse, potentiating later addiction. According to one survey published in 1997, looking at more than one hundred thousand students, adolescents who had experienced either physical or sexual abuse were two to four times as likely to be using drugs as those who reported no such molestation.[8] The ones who suffered both physical and sexual abuse were at least twice as likely to be using drugs as others who had been subjected to either abuse by itself. Alcohol consumption has shown a similar pattern: in a national sample of ten thousand adolescents, those with histories of sexual abuse were three times more likely to begin drinking in adolescence.[9]

Now that we have cleared away the thicket of mistaken beliefs about addiction, gotten a sense of what it does for people under its sway, and begun to consider what sorts of life experiences would make those "perks" so palpable and attractive, I propose to pull back the curtain even further in the next chapter. It is yet another myth—at once convenient and highly damaging—that in our world there is a category we can label "addicts," designating some identifiable group of poor, unfortunate souls, and then, neatly segregated from "those people," there are the rest of us "normal" folks.

To twist a line from the great George Carlin, it's a big club—and we're all in it.

Chapter 16

Show of Hands:
A New View of Addiction

We are long overdue for a new perspective—both because
our understanding of the neuroscience underlying
addiction has changed and because so many
existing treatments simply don't work.

—Maia Szalavitz[†]

Having delineated what addiction is and isn't, and recognizing
its impetus and function in people's lives, I'd like to offer a new
working definition, one I believe is truer and more powerful
than its antecedents. In eschewing genetic determinism, it entails the possibility of healing. I should issue a caution, though.
While more precise and more hopeful, my definition is also
more ecumenical—it makes addiction's "big tent" even bigger.
You might just find yourself under it.

Addiction is a complex psychological, emotional, physiological, neurobiological, social, and spiritual process. It
manifests through any behavior in which a person finds
temporary relief or pleasure and therefore craves, but that
in the long term causes them or others negative conse-

[†]   From an article in the *New York Times* by this prolific journalist and author, herself in long-
term recovery ("Can You Get Over an Addiction?," June 25, 2016).

quences, and yet the person refuses or is unable to give it up. Accordingly, the three main hallmarks of addiction are

- short-term relief or pleasure and therefore craving;
- long-term suffering for oneself or others; and
- an inability to stop.

Two things to note right away: First, my definition omits disease—which is not to say that it must exclude it. As I articulated in chapter 6, most illnesses are best understood as complex processes manifesting a person's entire life, rather than discrete "things" in themselves. In the end, as with many conditions, calling addiction a disease may capture relevant aspects of it without coming close to explaining the phenomenon, let alone granting us a workable pathway to healing it at its source.

Second, this definition is not restricted to drugs. The same drive that often devotes itself to substances can activate any number of behaviors, from compulsive sexual roving to pornography; from inveterate shopping to the internet (both of which habits I know well); from gaming to gambling; from any sort of binge eating or drinking to purging; from work to extreme sports; from relentless exercising to compulsive relationship-seeking; from psychedelics to meditation. The issue is never the external target but one's internal relationship to it. Are you craving and partaking of something that affords you temporary relief or pleasure, inviting or incurring negative consequences but not giving it up? Welcome to the meeting. Free coffee in the back.

If you've seen me speak on this topic, whether in person or on YouTube, you'll probably know what I'm about to ask next. I usually pause here to invite a show of hands: "Who, by the definition just given, is now or ever has been addicted?" No matter the audience size, virtually no one's hand ever stays lowered— except, I like to jest, for the occasional liar's. That is how down-right normal addictions are in our culture today. I invite you, fearless reader, to put yourself to the same test, with or without the hand-raising.

Of course, not all addictions are created equal, except in the broadest of broad strokes. My HIV- and hepatitis-C-ridden pa-tients in the Downtown Eastside surely stand apart from most of us in the degrees of suffering that hurled them into their hab-its, in the extent to which their dependencies dominate their lives, and, too, in the dire consequences their habits visit upon them. This is to say nothing about the diminished inner or outer resources available to them, often for socioeconomic and racial-ized reasons not of their creation. They differ also in the degrees of ostracization and punishment society has inflicted and contin-ues to inflict on them.

These acute differences of degree do matter, and we should not flatten or erase them. But they do not change the fact that the addiction process has certain intrinsic features known to all who live it. It spares no one, not even people at the top. That includes those whose destructive habits, in our culture's topsy-turvy value system, are spun as "success." Nor do these differences obviate the fact that most of us "normal" citizens bear far more resem-blance than we'd be inclined to admit with those we deride or pity for their more severe or glaring dependencies. It's not even a fine line that separates "us," the upstanding, from "them," the downtrodden: it's a made-up one.

Here it helps to remember the severity spectrum when it comes to trauma. All kinds of suffering, from the less obvious de-velopmental wounds we have called small-*t* to the more overt big-*T* traumas, can cry out for addictive pain relief. Again, trauma/injury is about what happens *inside* us, and how those effects persist, not what happens *to* us. An inquiry into "Why the pain?" has to leave space for the kinds of emotional injuries that may elude conscious recall or, much more often, seem unremarkable to the person doing the remembering.

It is not uncommon for people to tell themselves they enjoyed a "happy childhood." As long as life is going reasonably well, we may lack any reason to question this narrative. When addiction is present in oneself or a loved one, some inquiry is definitely in order.[†] Looking inward with compassion, most people will be able to locate themselves somewhere on the trauma/psychological-injury spectrum. Genuine happy memories do not rule out emotional suffering, but the usual bias is to recall the former and to suppress awareness of the latter. It has been my experience that even people with the most insistent "happy childhood" narrative will, if asked the right questions, very quickly come to realize that their autobiography has been riddled with blind spots.

In 2015, the writer and theater artist Stephanie Wittels Wachs lost her younger brother, Harris, to an overdose. She herself is a self-acknowledged workaholic, to the detriment of her family life. Until she invited me onto her *Last Day* podcast, she was convinced—adamant, in fact—that she and Harris had grown up in a normal, happy home. Her remembered evidence for that normalcy and happiness included their mother's involvement in many school activities—field trip chaperone, president of the PTA, and so on—and a home life where the spousal roles were stable in the traditional sense: working dad, housewife mom. The sense of security inspired by all these arrangements may well have been real; it certainly sounds like Wittels Wachs

---

[†] This inquiry, of course, need not be exclusive to uncovering the sources of addiction: anyone manifesting any of the signs of developmental injury covered in this book, from mild to severe, mental or physical, stands to benefit from a compassionate self-investigation into their own histories of distress.

grew up with a mother and father who loved their children as best they could and provided for their physical and social needs. Yet embedded in that "normalcy" were experiences of profound emotional hurt she had completely discounted, until they were conjured up from the depths by my questions. "This whole exchange caught me off guard," she confessed to her listeners afterward. "He is absolutely fucking correct. My talking points on my happy childhood are incomplete."

David Sheff was likewise "caught off guard" by a similar realization. His book, *Beautiful Boy: A Father's Journey Through His Son's Addiction,* which depicts his son Nick's nearly fatal stimulant habit, was a bestseller and, more recently, the subject of a poignant film starring Steve Carell and Timothée Chalamet. There had been no big-*T* trauma in this family, no child abuse or dire adversity. Perplexed, Sheff was forced to ask himself uncomfortable questions to understand what had impelled his talented, vivacious, highly sensitive eldest child into a life-threatening addiction. Looking back, Sheff saw that Nick's pain must have originated early on, in the crucible of a dysfunctional parental relationship. "We shouldn't have been together," he told me. "We had terrible, terrible problems in our marriage." Self-delusion played a major role: even while engaging in an extramarital affair with a family friend, Sheff harbored "this fantasy in my mind that, you know, if I was happy and she was happy, the kids would be together and then we'd have this happy family and we'd be sort of freeing them from these two traumatic families . . . I actually believed that I was doing this in some ways for Nick. I was justifying it, trying to make it okay." It is to Sheff's credit that he has been willing to look back with open eyes at how it actually was. I don't know the details, but Sheff did say that he and his son are now having candid and mutually compassionate conversations about those days, with the shared understanding that the pain of Nick's childhood was a major driver of his later difficulties.

As I have, Dr. Dan Sumrok has met the occasional trauma skeptic. With a long, graying beard hanging mid-chest and a passionate oratory style, this friend and colleague of mine in addiction medicine seems the very vision of a biblical prophet. But if Dan is an evangelist for anything, it's sanity. Over his career as a family physician, first at the University of Tennessee medical school in Memphis, then in Nashville, and more recently in a rural area, he has treated nearly twenty-five thousand people with opiate addiction. He, too, sees past the medical view of addiction as disease, genetic or otherwise; in his experience, too, trauma is the foundational factor. "I began writing about this in 1980 when I was just discharged from the military. I was a first-year medical student, and my life was flying apart. I would say my best friends were George, Jack, and Jim—the whiskey brothers."† "Some people," Dan relates, "the real militant Twelve-Steppers, will say to me, and some of the treatment programs have said, 'You know, it's not all about trauma, Dr. Sumrok.' I do want to reassure them, so I say, 'I promise you, I'm keeping an open mind. I'm waiting to see the first person for whom it's not all about trauma.'" One would have to wait a long time.

Whatever the degree of injury, all addiction is a kind of refugee story: from intolerable feelings incurred through adversity and never processed, and into a state of temporary freedom, even if illusory. Again, try saying no to that.

———————

It may surprise many to learn that no drug is in itself addictive, not even the most notorious "high risk" ones like crack or methamphetamine. Most people who try drugs, any drug, even repeatedly, never become addicted. The reasons why throw further light on the nature of addiction.

---

† The Tennessee whiskey brands George Dickel, Jack Daniel's, and Jim Beam.

I often ask audiences, "Is alcohol addictive: yes or no? Is food addictive: yes or no? Or work: yes or no? Or sex: yes or no? Or pornography, or shopping: yes or no?" The right answer, embedded in the question, is "yes or no," depending on the degree of pain one needs to soothe.

San Diego internal medicine specialist Dr. Vincent Felitti was one of the lead investigators of the now famous (though not famous enough) Adverse Childhood Experiences (ACE) Study. The study emerged after Felitti decided to listen to the life histories of patients at an obesity clinic who all reported childhood traumas. Carried out in the 1990s in California's Kaiser Permanente health care network, the research showed that among a cohort of over seventeen thousand mostly Caucasian, middle-class persons, the more adversity a child had been exposed to, the greater the risk of addictions, mental health issues, and other medical problems they faced in adulthood.[1] Adversity was categorized under three general headings: abuse (psychological, physical, sexual); neglect (physical, emotional); household dysfunction (alcoholism or drug use in the home, divorce or loss of a biological parent, depression or mental illness in the home, mother treated violently, imprisoned household member). The impacts of such experiences did not merely add up; they multiplied each other. An adult reporting an ACE score of 6 had a risk of intravenous drug use forty-six-fold greater than a child with none of the adversities named.

"It is commonly believed," Felitti said, discussing his research, "that repeated use of many street drugs will in itself produce addiction. Our findings challenge those views . . . Addiction has relatively little to do with the supposed addictive properties of certain substances, other than their all providing a desirable psychoactive relief . . . In other words, this is an understandable attempt at self-treatment with something that *almost* works, thus creating a drive for further doses."[2]

Felitti's childhood adversity findings lay further waste to the myth of genetic determinism that I began debunking in the chapter on epigenetics. No single addiction gene has ever been found—nor ever will be. There may exist some collection of genes that predisposes people to susceptibility, but a predisposition is not the same as a predetermination. What's true of physical illness is just as true of addiction: genes are turned on and off by the environment, and we now know that early adversity affects genetic activity in ways that create a template for future dysfunction. Human and animal studies have both confirmed that any genetic risks for substance abuse can be offset by being reared in a nurturing environment.[3]

One of the happiest email acknowledgments I ever received was from the grateful mother of a four-year-old. Her husband, a former alcoholic, refused to have children, so afraid had he been of passing the "alcoholism gene" to his offspring. Having read my book on addiction, he recognized the traumatic sources of his alcohol habit and gave up his fear of this nonexistent gene. And just in time—his wife had been nearly past the child-bearing age. I couldn't suppress a self-satisfied chortle. I'd been thanked before for "saving" the lives of people I had never met, but never for having been the cause of one at long distance.

The way childhood adversity engenders the neurobiology of addiction has to do with the interpersonal-biological science we have already examined. Experiences of stress in the womb can predispose to addiction, for example, by altering the brain's ability to respond to stress in functional ways. They can also have long-term influence on the parts of the brain that modulate the incentive-motivation system impaired in all addictions, whether to drugs or behaviors.[†] As the psychiatric practitioner, neuroscientist, author, and leading trauma researcher Dr. Bruce Perry told me, "We've done work, and a lot of other people have done work, showing that essentially the number and density of dopamine receptors in these [brain] areas is determined in utero."[4]

Whoever coined the slang term "dope" for drugs was onto something, because all addictions, whether to drugs or behaviors, involve *dopamine*. Dopamine is the essential neurotransmitter in the motivation system, without which all mammals are inert, inactive, and lacking all incentive. A hungry laboratory mouse whose brain is artificially denuded of its dopamine apparatus will starve himself while standing in front of a plate of food. In fact, every addict is a dopamine fiend, outsourcing the hunt for the homegrown chemical hit that makes the present moment exciting and vibrant. For virtually every "positive" feeling or quality people derive from their substances or behavior of choice, there are endogenous—naturally occurring—brain chemicals implicated. Addiction begins as an attempt to induce feelings that we were biologically programmed to generate innately, and would have—if unhealthy development hadn't got in the way.

Sex addiction, for example, has nothing to do with a "high sex drive" and everything to do with dopamine. New York social worker and former Fordham and Rutgers Universities adjunct professor Zachary Alti specializes in sex therapy and behavioral addictions, particularly addiction to porn. "Studies are suggesting," he told me, "that when viewing a pornographic image, we get a dopamine spike in our brain. When viewing images after images, we get spike after spike after spike. Whereas with substance addictions you typically get one or a few spikes just before use, with behavioral addictions dopamine itself is the substance,

---

†   Or what Dr. Jaak Panksepp identified as the brain's SEEKING apparatus.

the primary component. Especially in pornography addiction, these dopamine spikes happen over and over and over again." As with smartphone and app companies, pornographers are well aware that their profits rest on the hijacking of their consumers' brains. The sociologist Gail Dines, author of the bracing 2010 book *Pornland: How Porn Has Hijacked Our Sexuality*, reports on an article in the trade publication *Adult Video News*, in which an industry insider trumpets a Stanford University study on cyber-sex addiction showing that 20 percent of porn users are hooked. "In a true capitalist approach," she notes, the article is cheerfully headed "Exploiting the Data."[5]

What about the feelings of love that people find in addictions, particularly with opiates—the warmth Jamie Lee Curtis and others spoke of? That is, in large part, a function of the brain's internal opiate apparatus in which endorphins, our own natural, endogenous opiates, are the neurotransmitters. Dr. Jaak Panksepp suggested twenty years ago that opiate addiction is rooted in the evolutionary brain mechanisms that promote social bonding: nurturing, emotional closeness, and social affiliation. "We would anticipate," he wrote, "that individuals who experience especially intense social distress and insecurities would be especially vulnerable to opiate abuse, and this prediction has been affirmed by some clinical research. Indeed, the same dynamic may help explain why opiate addictions are especially prevalent among the socially disenfranchised."[6] The current opioid overdose crisis in the United States, and to lesser degrees in Canada and the U.K., has tragically borne out the acuity of this observation.

The endorphin system, too, is dependent on supportive, attuned relationships early in life for its development. "Face-to-face interactions activate the child's sympathetic nervous system," writes Louis Cozolino, a clinical psychologist, neuroscientist, and professor of psychology at Pepperdine University. "These higher levels of activation correlate with increased production of oxytocin, prolactin, endorphins, and dopamine; some of the same biochemical systems involved in addiction."[7] A child's closeness with the attuned, emotionally available parent promotes the optimal growth of brain systems; the lack of it inhibits healthy development.

Work has been the main, but not only, addiction of singer-songwriter Alanis Morissette. In endorphin-friendly terms, she now speaks of it as a compensation. "There's an attachment-craving in being famous," she said when we spoke. "If you think about it, eyeballs are on you. Everyone's hyper-responsive. Everyone's paying attention to you . . . You keep chasing that sense of being loved and adored and stared at." Morissette was seeking to attain through her fame that state of infant bliss so many miss out on or experience all too briefly.

When Robert Palmer sang about being addicted to love, he might have been speaking to all of us with our hands raised—all the drug addicts, all the workaholics, all the compulsive gamblers and shoppers and eaters, all those hopelessly chasing the next exciting high or soothing low. Except it's not really love we get hooked on but our desperate attempts to cope with its lack, by any means necessary.

Sobering stuff, I know. But we might as well face it.

Chapter 17

An Inaccurate Map of Our Pain: What We Get Wrong About Mental Illness

We don't understand any major mental disorder biologically.

—Professor Anne Harrington[†]

At age nineteen, a freshman journalism student at the University of Florida, Darrell Hammond was plunged into his first experience of searing mental distress. "I was in unspeakable terror," the comedian recalled. "That level of fear—I don't even know how I survived it. The doctors were treating me for depression and paranoia, and for psychosis because I told them that I had seen someone talking, and the words didn't come out at the same time their mouth was moving." He was prescribed an antidepressant, amitriptyline, as well as the antipsychotic thioridazine. Over the subsequent decades, Hammond estimated that he was evaluated by up to forty psychiatrists and labeled with multiple diagnoses, including depression, bipolar disorder, and complex PTSD, and he didn't recall what else. The assumption that guided his treatment was the same one that dominates much of medical thinking: that such torments are caused by a biological disease of the brain. Accordingly, he was treated with an ever-changing cocktail of medications. Throughout

†   Historian of science at Harvard University and author of *Mind Fixers: Psychiatry's Troubled Search for the Biology of Mental Illness*. CBC Radio interview, October 2019.

years of professional success, including an unprecedented fourteen-year run on *Saturday Night Live*—his range expressed in roles from Bill Clinton to, perhaps most belovedly, a jocularly vulgar Sean Connery—he continued to feel lost, irritable, isolated, and despondent. The only recourses he could find to interrupt his misery were self-medicating with alcohol and overt self-harm: his body still bears the scars of over fifty self-inflicted cuts.

Thirty-five years into his psychiatric odyssey, Hammond met a clinician, Dr. Nabil Kotbi at New York City's Weill Cornell Medical College, who changed his life with two short sentences: "I don't want you to call what you have a mental illness. You have been injured." The insight that his symptoms were not the manifestations of some mysterious medical condition, Hammond told me, "was a 'Hallelujah Chorus' moment . . . What [Dr. Kotbi] seemed to be saying to me was that mental illness comes from somewhere very specific. It has a story, and in that story, you're the only one that has no power." In the decades between his first encounter with the mental health system and his meeting this particular psychiatrist, no one had asked Hammond about traumatic childhood experiences. "I can't describe what it was like to go into a doctor's office, in acute pain, and have them look at me and go, 'You shouldn't be feeling this way.' No one at the time was saying, 'Hey, you're probably a victim of child abuse.' At that time, if you felt bad for no apparent reason, they called you bipolar. That's all they knew. 'He has unexplainable highs and lows,' you know. They treated me with [the mood stabilizers] lithium and then Depakote. Neither of those were successful. *Nothing* was really successful until the truth about my life was acknowledged." The truth of Hammond's life included a cavalcade of abuse at the hands of his mother.[†]

[†]   The hit Netflix documentary *Cracked Up!,* directed by Michelle Esrick, catalogs the real-life horror show Hammond endured as a child. Dr. Kotbi is interviewed in the film.

While mental ailments certainly exhibit some features of illness—the brain seeming to function like a disordered organ—mainstream psychiatry takes the biological emphasis too far, reducing everything mostly to an imbalance of DNA-dictated brain chemicals. Psychiatrist Kay Redfield Jamison, one of today's most eloquent authors on manic-depressive illness, also known as bipolar disorder, wrote the memoir *An Unquiet Mind*. This book is essential reading for anyone wanting to appreciate the experience of an exquisite consciousness oscillating from episodes of hyper-elation to immobilizing despair. And yet, embedded in Dr. Jamison's gorgeously rendered recollections are faulty assumptions that exemplify the simplistic genetic narrative to which psychiatry still clings. Here she recalls a manic episode: "My mind was flying high that day, *courtesy of whatever witches' brew of neurotransmitters God had programmed into my genes*." In truth, neither God nor genes have much to do with it.

In her *Touched with Fire*, an equally poignant book, Jamison puts it more explicitly, asserting that "the genetic basis for manic-depressive illness is especially compelling, indeed almost incontrovertible."[1] Twenty-five years on, we know that the hard, scientific evidence is not only not compelling; it is nearly nonexistent. The "almost incontrovertible" proof Dr. Jamison relied on is the literature on family histories, adoption, and twin studies, all of which are riddled with false assumptions.[‡] The proof she alludes to for

---

‡   Traits can be passed on from one generation to the next without any DNA sequences being involved; and in identical twins, one cannot separate genetic effects from environmental ones, given identical siblings were gestated in the same uterus and most were brought up in the same family. If adopted to different families, they had still shared the same uterine environment and the same trauma of separation from their birth mother. I won't fatigue the reader here with a further critique of adoption studies, a subject I covered extensively in two of my previous books, on ADHD and addiction, respectively. See especially *In the Realm of Hungry Ghosts: Close Encounters with Addiction*, Appendix I: "Adoption and Twin Study Fallacies." In brief, for all the attention they have received, twin and adoption studies prove very little, if anything. For an exhaustive refutation of twin-study "findings," see *The Trouble with Twin Studies*, by the psychologist Jay Joseph.

genetic causes is only "compelling" if one is already a believer: on the evidence itself, it is pure science fiction.[2] It is also inelegant: in my work with mental distress and addictions—including my own—I've always found more than enough in people's personal histories to account for their psychic suffering, without superimposing a narrative dominated by genetic predetermination.

The term "mental illness," even as it describes real phenomena, focuses our attention centrally on brain physiology, analogous to how, say, anginal pain connotes a restriction of oxygen supply to the heart muscle, owing to narrowed cardiac arteries. It also implies that the problem necessarily falls within the domain of medicine. Despite whatever partial truths they contain, these assumptions are highly questionable and limit our understanding. Worse, they generate harm, both in the sense that they leave many people subjected to inappropriate treatments and in that they displace perspectives that could be far more complete, humane, and helpful. The biological determinism that governed Darrell Hammond's physicians also placed his condition beyond his own agency to heal, thereby reinforcing the "You are the only one that has no power" story he spoke of. Such a view threatens to keep the sufferer largely in the position of passively receiving treatment, his symptoms ameliorated by medications to be ingested, in many cases, for a lifetime.

In its predominantly biological approach, psychiatry commits the same error as other medical specialties: it takes complex processes intricately bound with life experience and emotional development, slaps the "disease" label on them, and calls it a day.

Little in the training of doctors prepares them to wonder about their patients' lived experience, much less to seek the sources of their malaises therein. Simplistic explanations, which require little time or emotional energy, are an attractive fallback position. Many doctors are intensely uncomfortable facing their own hidden sorrows and wounds—what Carl Jung called our shadow side. And not only doctors: as a well-known colleague told me, "Patients play into this as well. They don't want to look at their lives, either. It would involve getting into recovery, changing something. It's enormous work to recover from our childhoods. It's incredibly worthwhile, but it's a lot of work." The gospel of genetic causation shields us from having to confront our hurts, leaving us all the more at their mercy.

If anything, this limitation is especially calamitous in the realm of mental suffering, and even less justified. After all, unlike in cancer or rheumatoid arthritis, no physical findings, blood tests, biopsies, radiographs, or scans can either support or rule out psychiatric diagnoses. That statement may surprise many readers, so it bears repeating. There are *no measurable physical markers* of mental illness other than the subjective (a person's description of their own mood, say) and the behavioral (sleep patterns, appetite, etc.).

Like all concepts, mental illness is a *construct*—a particular frame we have developed to understand a phenomenon and explain what we observe. It may be valid in some respects and erroneous in others; it most definitely isn't objective. Unchecked, it becomes an all-encompassing lens through which we perceive and interpret. Such a way of seeing can say as much about the biases and values of the culture that gives rise to it as about the phenomenon being seen, whether a religious concept like "sinful" or a biomedical one like "mentally ill."[3] In some cultures, for example, people with visions may become prophets or shamans. In ours, most likely they would be deemed insane. One wonders how a Joan of Arc or the medieval saint and composer of sacred music Hildegard of Bingen would fare at the hands of the contemporary mental health system. I once speculated out loud, in front of an audience of hundreds, what would happen if I strode up to the prime minister of Canada and pronounced, Joan-like, that I have seen the future in which he leads the global fight against climate change, beginning with giving up his reliance on campaign funding from the fossil fuel industry.

Other than modern culture's typical, left-brain materialist bent, how did we arrive at this view of mental illness as an essentially biologically rooted phenomenon? In part, it seems to be a holdover from a once tantalizing aspiration in medical science, a mission unaccomplished. "Psychiatry today stands on the threshold of becoming an exact science, as precise and quantifiable as molecular genetics," wrote the journalist Jon Franklin in a Pulitzer Prize–winning series in 1984.[4] As with the ultimately unfulfilled promise of the genomic revolution to explain health and illness, the initial enthusiasm for the prospect of a science-based psychiatry was virtually unbounded. Nearly forty years later we are no closer to crossing this imagined threshold; if anything, we are further away. When the fifth edition of the *Diagnostic and Statistical Manual of Mental Disorders (DSM-5)* was published by the American Psychiatric Association in 2013, Dr. David Kupfer, head of the task force responsible for it, acknowledged as much. "In the future," he stated in a press release, "we hope to be able to identify disorders using biological and genetic markers that provide precise diagnoses that can be delivered with complete reliability and validity. Yet this promise, which we have anticipated since the 1970s, remains disappointingly distant. We've been telling patients for several decades that we are waiting for biomarkers. We're still waiting."[5]

The journalist and author Robert Whitaker, formerly the director of publications for Harvard Medical School, was a firm believer in the chemical-imbalance theory of mental illness—until he wasn't. "When I first started writing about psychiatry, I believed that to be true," he told me. "I mean, why wouldn't I?" His disillusionment arose from research he uncovered while reporting for the *Boston Globe*. "I said to people, 'Can you just tell me where you found that depression is due to serotonin or where you actually found that schizophrenia is due to too much dopamine?' I asked to read the source materials and, I swear to God, they said, 'Well, we didn't really find that. It's a metaphor.' The most amazing thing was, when you trace it in their own research, you find they didn't find it! The divergence from what you're being told from what is in their own scientific literature— that's the key—it was just stunning to me." These conspicuous non-findings are documented in Whitaker's book *Anatomy of an Epidemic* and have been corroborated in other literature.[6]

Contrary to what I, too, used to believe, a diagnosis like ADHD or depression or bipolar illness explains nothing. *No diagnosis ever does.* Diagnoses are abstractions, or summaries: sometimes helpful, always incomplete. They are professional shorthand for describing constellations of symptoms a person may report, or of other people's observations of someone's behavior patterns, thoughts, and emotions. For the individual in question, a diagnosis may seem to account for and validate a lifetime of experiences previously too diffuse or nebulous to put one's finger on. That can be a first and positive step toward healing. I know this from firsthand experience.

The dead end comes when we assume or believe that the diagnosis equals an explanation—an especially futile view when it comes to illnesses of something as inherently abstract as the mind. As the British psychologist Lucy Johnstone said to me, "In physical illness you have, in principle, a way of checking it out. You can say, 'Let's look at the blood test or the enzyme levels.' And you could, in most cases, confirm or disconfirm it. But in psychiatry, it's simply a circular argument, isn't it? Why does this person have mood swings? Because they have bipolar disorder. How do you know they have bipolar disorder? Because they have mood swings." My mind goes to A. A. Milne's Pooh and Piglet walking in the snow in an unwitting circle, shuddering as they come across yet more "Heffalump" tracks at every turn.

An oft-heard objection to mental health diagnoses, particularly with regard to children, is that they "pathologize" or "stigmatize" ordinary, healthy feelings or behaviors. Aren't kids supposed to get bored or antsy, angry or sad? My answer would be yes—and it's not that simple. While overdiagnosis is certainly a risk, I don't see the spike in, say, ADHD cases over the past decades as being due solely to gullible parents, hapless teachers, overzealous school shrinks, and unscrupulous drug companies. As I discussed in earlier chapters, the world into which kids are being born these days might as well have been designed to promote disruptions of cognitive function and emotional self-regulation. Everything I have seen tells me we *are* witnessing a sea change in children's mental well-being.

Why, then, do I persist in my critique of the diagnostic model? Because diagnoses reveal nothing about *the underlying events and dynamics that animate the perceptions and experiences in question.* They keep our gaze trained on effects and not their myriad causes. There could be multiple reasons why a child may have trouble paying attention or be restless, disengaged, and fidgety: anxiety, stresses at home, boredom with material she finds uninteresting, resistance to the constraints of sitting in a classroom, fear of bullying, an authoritarian teacher, trauma—even birth month, believe it or not. A University of British Columbia study looked at the prescription records of almost one million B.C. schoolchildren over an eleven-year period and found that kids born in December were 39 percent more likely to be diagnosed with ADHD than classmates born the previous January. The reason? December kids entered the same grade nearly a year younger than their January counterparts—they were eleven

months behind in brain development. They were being medicated not for a "genetic brain disorder" but for naturally delayed
maturation of the brain circuits of attention and self-regulation.[7]

Or consider the *DSM-5* diagnosis of oppositional defiant disorder (ODD), often tacked on to ADHD and other "diseases."
"If your child or teenager has a frequent and persistent pattern of
anger, irritability, arguing, defiance or vindictiveness toward you
and other authority figures, he or she may have oppositional defiant disorder," advises the Mayo Clinic.[8] The clue is in the word
"toward": oppositionality, by definition, can arise only in the
context of a relationship. I can suffer symptoms of a cold in isolation, or break my ankle on my own. I cannot oppose anyone or
be angry or irritable with anyone unless that "anyone" is in some
relationship with me. "If you don't believe me," I sometimes tell
audiences of therapists, parents, teachers, or medical professionals, "just lock yourself in your room tonight, make sure you
are absolutely alone, and oppose somebody. If you succeed, put
it on YouTube—it'll go viral in no time."

Given that a child develops in the context of relationships,
her behavior will be intelligible to us only if we look at the relational environment. Seen this way, these so-called ODD kids
turn out to be ones who lack sufficient connection with nurturing adults and have a natural resistance to being controlled by
people they do not fully trust or feel close enough to. This aversion, furthermore, is only magnified by all attempts to shame or
cajole it into submission. To call this "disordered" says nothing
about the child's inner experience; it reflects only the perspective of the ones who find his recalcitrance inconvenient. It is also
completely obtuse about how emotional power dynamics work:
there is nothing disordered in resisting authority figures that, for
whatever reason, we do not feel confident in and safe with.

If we are today seeing more youngsters in automatic resistance mode, the question we must return to is, How does this culture disrupt healthy adult-child relationships? Why are we diagnosing children with a disorder, instead of "diagnosing"—and treating—their families, communities, schools, and society?

The psychiatrist, author, and leading trauma researcher Bruce Perry[†] has come to disdain diagnoses almost completely. This is no knee-jerk prejudice: his dim view of the norms and practices of his field follows decades spent assessing tens of thousands of troubled children, and extensive contributions to the vast literature on adversity and what we define as "disorders." "When I got into psychiatry," Dr. Perry told me, "it became clear really quickly that the diagnoses were not connected to the physiology, that they were just descriptive, and that there were hundreds of physiological routes to somebody having an attention problem, for example. And yet the profession acted as if these descriptive labels were *really a thing* . . . I knew that if we were doing 'research,' if we were using these hollow descriptors which we call 'diagnoses' and then study interventions and outcomes, we would just get garbage. And that's what we've done."

These days Dr. Perry is adamant that "even playing the *DSM* game is completely wrong." When invited to contribute to one of the manual's editions, he refused. "I said, 'Listen, in twenty-five years they are going to look back and won't believe that we thought about people that way.' It's not a valid way to think about the complexities of human beings." He practices what he preaches in the clinic he helps run. "We haven't used diagnoses for fifteen, twenty years," he said, "and it really has not interfered with our ability to do good clinical work. In fact, we're able to do better clinical work without using those labels."

[†] Currently senior fellow of the Child Trauma Academy in Houston, Texas, and an adjunct professor of psychiatry and behavioral sciences at the Feinberg School of Medicine in Chicago, and, most recently, coauthor, with Oprah Winfrey, of the bestselling *What Happened to You?*

Based on my observations in family practice and my under-standing of human development, I have followed the same lines. When I work with any mental health condition, say depression or anxiety or ADHD or addiction, I'm not so interested in the formal diagnosis as such. My "diagnostic" focus goes to the spe-cific challenges the person is facing in their life and the traumas animating those challenges. As for "prescriptions," I am primar-ily interested in what will promote the healing of the psychic wounds the ongoing traumatic patterns represent.

Now, here's a perhaps surprising assertion: I'm not anti-pharmacology. No one who's felt or witnessed the beneficial effects of psychiatric drugs can deny that neurobiology must, indeed, play a role in the dynamics and potential easing of men-tal distress, just as it does in all our experiences. Sometimes the healing of which I just spoke can be helped along—not made to happen, certainly, but assisted—by the intelligent use of these medications. That is not just my professional opinion but my personal experience as well.

In my mid-forties, I decided to go on the serotonin-enhancing drug Prozac. (Among the brain's principal neurotransmitters, or chemical messengers, serotonin is believed to be active in such functions as mood regulation and the dampening of aggression.) The skepticism I harbored about this growing trend to medicate millions was eclipsed by my hunger for respite from the daily se-verities of my state of mind, as summed up grimly in a diary entry from that time: "*I have no energy for life. I have spent every week-end for the past two months—every free weekend—in an enervated, passive, demoralized state, depressed and depressing to be with.*"

I was soon a different person. Within days, my wife noted with relief the softening of my facial features. I now greeted morn-ings with vim instead of venom, lost my irritability around my fam-ily, smiled and laughed a lot more, and could feel and express tenderness where before I'd been cold and brittle. It was as if someone had bandaged my aching heart so that it no longer hurt or bruised at the slightest touch. I found myself marveling to my sister-in-law: "You mean people can feel like this normally? I had no idea!" My experience was similar to what, some years later, the writer Elizabeth Wurtzel would depict in her 1994 personal account *Prozac Nation*. "One morning I woke up and really did want to live," she wrote. "It was as if the miasma of depression had lifted off me, in the same way that the fog in San Francisco rises as the day wears on. Was it the Prozac? No doubt."

As happens with many new converts, my initial reticence quickly gave way to a period of outsize enthusiasm. In my medical practice I became something of a Prozac booster, succumbing to the error of looking for pathology where there was only everyday unhappiness. "You have a chemical imbalance in your brain—you are lacking serotonin," I would earnestly explain to patients in whom I detected symptoms of depression, prescription pad at the ready. Little did I know that I was uttering scientific nonfacts. Yes, the medication was helping me, at least in the short term. And yes, I have witnessed other cases where psychiatric drugs were life-enhancing and even lifesaving. But we have to avoid the fallacy of inferring from medication's (in some cases) observable benefits that the proven *origin* of mental illness rests in the biochemistry of the brain, let alone that physiological disturbances are genetically caused.

That a medication has a certain positive effect reveals nothing about the genesis of a symptom. If aspirin eases a headache, can the headache be explained by an inherited brain deficiency of acetylsalicylic acid, the pill's active ingredient? If a shot of bourbon relaxes you, is your tense nervous system suffering from a DNA-dictated whiskey shortage? There are fifty or more neurotransmitters in the brain whose complex interactions we are only now beginning to explore, not to mention the almost infinite possibilities inherent in the lifelong intersection of experience with the biology of body and brain. Once again, the physiology of the brain is a manifestation and a product of life in motion and in context.

Further, as Bruce Perry writes, "The brain is a historical organ. It stores our personal narrative." Since it does so in the form of its chemistry and its neural networks, it is no wonder that difficult experiences may result in disturbed neurobiology. Even when brain scans show certain abnormalities—as they do, for example, in many traumatized people—these do not prove that the "disorder" has a neurochemical *source*. A recently published thirty-year study followed people from early life to age twenty-nine. Poor quality of care in infancy was, nearly three decades later, associated with a higher volume of the emotionally key brain structure, the hippocampus, as well as with an elevated risk for "borderline personality" features and suicidality. In other words, the brain's genetics did not "cause" either the "illness" or the neurophysiological differences: all were the result of life experience.[9]

The British author Johann Hari has explored addictions and depression from both the personal and journalistic points of view. In his bestselling work *Lost Connections*, he relates his own experience of devastatingly low moods, followed by his initial elation at the depression diagnosis that, at last, "explained" his disturbing mind states. "This will sound odd," he writes, "but what I experienced at that moment was a happy jolt—like unexpectedly finding a pile of money down the back of your sofa. There is a term for feeling like this! It is a medical condition, like diabetes or irritable bowel syndrome."

Like mine, Hari's first experience of medications was positive.

"It was only years later," he relates in *Lost Connections*, "that somebody pointed out to me all the questions the doctor didn't ask that day. Like: Is there any reason you might feel distressed? What's been happening in your life? Is there anything hurting you we might want to change?" The answers would have been yeses all around: Hari was carrying both past trauma and present stress that he took to be part of his "normal." Over time, he came to recognize that the narrow medical model that had helped him manage his symptoms was also leaving him far short of healing. He is not entirely jaded about the biological approach, he told me, but he also noted with sorrow that "it has crowded out the much more common-sense insights that people have about why they become distressed and how to resolve their distress. Really—how do I put it—it's given us an inaccurate map of our own pain."

It is known beyond controversy that the greater the degree of childhood adversity, the higher the risk of mental disturbances, including psychosis. One study found that people who had suffered five types of maltreatment in childhood were multiple times more likely to be diagnosed with psychosis than those who had not experienced such traumatic events.[10] A major review in 2018 in the *Schizophrenia Bulletin* concluded that the severity of childhood traumas was correlated with the intensity of delusions and hallucinations.[11] Richard Bentall, a clinical psychologist, academic, and Fellow of the British Academy, summed up the science a few years ago: "The evidence of a link between childhood misfortune and future psychiatric disorder is about as strong statistically as the link between smoking and lung cancer," he wrote. "There is also now strong evidence that these kinds of experiences affect brain structure, explaining many of the abnormal neuro-imaging findings that have been reported for psychiatric patients."[12] This mirrored a Harvard study that concluded,

"These brain changes may be best understood as *adaptive responses to facilitate survival and reproduction in the face of adversity*. Their relationship to psychopathology is complex."[13]

There is something scientists reviewing research papers will not say, although it is manifestly evident to many clinicians working with mental distress: overt maltreatment is not necessary to exert negative impacts on the neurobiology of the brain or the functioning of the mind. Neurobiology is a continuum, as are "mental illness" and health. Emotional injury during development can have physiological consequences, even *without* abuse or neglect. As Bruce Perry explains, adverse childhood experiences—of the big-ticket kind that merit the official ACE designation—are of consequence, but "not as determinative as your history in relationships . . . The most powerful predictor of your functioning in the present is your current relational connectedness and then the second most powerful component that we see is your history of connectedness."

"Don't be so sensitive," people are often told. In other words, "Don't be so yourself." Genetic vulnerabilities do not code for illness, but they may confer sensitivity for a person being more impacted by life's vicissitudes than someone else with a hardier predisposition—a far from trivial effect. Sensitive people feel more, feel deeply, and are more easily overwhelmed by stress, not just subjectively but physiologically. Both monkeys and humans, for example, can inherit genes involved in the production of certain brain chemicals such as serotonin that can make them more susceptible to negative experiences—or, on the other hand, more amenable to the effect of positive ones. (And, of course, sensitivity, too, is a continuum.)

"Genes affect how sensitive one is to environment, and environment affects how relevant one's genetic differences may be," the leading geneticist R. C. Lewontin has said. "When an environment changes, all bets are off."[14] Some people will feel more pain and will therefore have greater need to escape into the adaptations that mental illness, or addiction, represent. They will have more need to tune out, to dissociate, to split into parts, to develop fantasies to account for realities they are unable to endure. But that's a far cry from saying that they have a heritable neurobiological disease. These are the children that Tom Boyce, a professor of pediatrics and psychiatry at the University of California, San Francisco, describes as *orchids*, "exquisitely sensitive to their environment, making them especially vulnerable under conditions of adversity but unusually vital, creative, and successful within supportive, nurturing environments."[15] The same "sensitivity" genes that in a stressed environment can help potentiate mental suffering may, under positive circumstances, help promote stronger mental resilience and therefore happiness.[16] Sensitive people have the potential to be more aware, insightful, inventive, artistic, and empathic, if their sensitivity is not crushed by maltreatment or disdain. The most sensitive of our kind have made some of the most lasting cultural contributions; many of these have also suffered the most intense pains during their lives. Sensitivity can be the quintessential combo package: gift and curse, all in one.

Many of the people I've met with mental illness exhibit this quality, sometimes to astounding degrees. I'll never forget a conversation I had as a medical student with a psychotic young man about my age. Tall and disheveled, he gazed at me with piercing eyes as I lobbed him some questions related to a meaningless research project for which I was getting paid. Inwardly, I was awed by his insights into life, society, the secrets of existence, into human beings. I was wishing as I listened that I could have access to such awareness. "It's not true what you're thinking," he abruptly interjected. "It's not true I'm more intelligent than you are."

Despite the genetic hoopla in the popular media and all the lavishly funded DNA-hunting in the scientific world, no one has ever identified any gene that causes mental illness, nor any group of genes that code for specific mental health conditions or are required for the presence of mental disorder. Professor Jehannine Austin, an academic and researcher, leads a genetic counseling clinic for mental health in Vancouver.[†] "Everybody has some genes that predispose to mental illness," she told me, but these are "a very, very long way away from causing anything . . . Literally what separates those of us who do suffer from those of us that don't is *what happens to us during our lives*."

I believe there is more than meets the eye when it comes to the persistent appetite for genetic causes. There are the factors I've already covered: reticence to face trauma on the one hand, and the neglect of developmental science on the other. There is also the standard-issue preference for a simple and quickly understood explanation, along with our tendency to look for one-to-one causations for almost everything. Life in its wondrous complexity does not conform to such easy reductions.

Other psychological and sociological dynamics add to the adhesive appeal of genetic theories. The first shouldn't come as any news: we all hate feeling culpable. Whether as individuals for our own actions, as parents for our children's hurts, or as a society for our many failings, we have our ten-foot poles at the ready when accountability comes to call. Genetics—that neutral, impersonal

---

[†] Full credentials: Ph.D., FCAHS, CGC; professor and Canada research chair, UBC Departments of Psychiatry and Medical Genetics; executive director, BC Mental Health and Substance Use Services Research Institute.

handmaiden of Nature—seems to absolve us of responsibility and of its ominous shadow, guilt. If genes truly rule our fate like capricious, microscopic gods, then we are off the hook.

The genetic argument is used to justify social inequalities and injustices that are otherwise hard to defend. Much like junk sciences of the past—phrenology, eugenics, and so on—it serves a deeply conservative function: if phenomena like addiction or mental distress are determined mostly by biological heredity, we are spared from having to look at how our social environment supports, or does not support, the parents of young children, and at how social attitudes, prejudices, and policies burden, stress, and exclude certain segments of the population, thereby increasing their propensity for suffering. The writer Louis Menand said it well in a *New Yorker* article: " 'It's all in the genes': an explanation for the way things are *that does not threaten the way things are*. Why should someone feel unhappy or engage in antisocial behavior when that person is living in the freest and most prosperous nation on earth? It can't be the system! There must be a flaw in the wiring somewhere."[17]

There is a stark paradox in all this. To the extent that we cling to genetic fundamentalism to avoid the discomforts of personal responsibility or societal reckoning, we radically—and unnecessarily—disempower ourselves from dealing either actively or proactively with suffering of all kinds. It is entirely possible to embrace responsibility without taking on the useless baggage of guilt or blame. Even more regrettably, we miss the excellent news that if our mental health is not dictated by our genes, then we are not their victims. On the contrary, there is much we can do, each and all.

Chapter 18

The Mind Can Do Some Amazing Things: From Madness to Meaning

Perhaps the line between sanity and madness must be drawn relative to the place where we stand. Perhaps it is possible to be, at the same time, mad when viewed from one perspective and sane when viewed from another.
—Richard Bentall, *Madness Explained: Psychosis and Human Nature*

If we are not to see mental distress solely as illness, then what is it? The view I have come to favor is of a piece with how I approach many other conditions under the "illness" umbrella: rather than seeing it as an intruder from the outside, consider what it might be expressing about the life in which it arises. This framework is, if anything, all the more intuitive when it comes to afflictions that take up unwanted residence in the mind, in a person's emotional world, in the personality.

Let's begin with something rather simple, now on the rise: depression, a state I know intimately. The word's literal meaning is quite telling. To *depress* something means to push it down, as one might a beach ball in a swimming pool. I like that analogy especially because one can easily feel how much concerted force it takes to keep the ball submerged, and the way it "wants" to find a way back up to the surface. Keeping it down takes a toll.

What is pushed down when a person is depressed is easily identified by its absence: emotion, the continual flow of feelings that remind us we're alive. Unlike the wrangler of the beach ball, a depressed person doesn't choose this submersion of life energy—it imposes itself, turning a once-vibrant emotional landscape into arid desert. The only "feeling" that remains, typically, is more sensation than emotion, a thrumming, indistinct pain that threatens to consume everything, and sometimes does. If we label this depression of feeling a disease, we risk not recognizing its original adaptive function: to distance oneself from emotions that are unbearable at a time in life when to experience them is to court greater calamity. Recall what I called the tragic tension between authenticity and attachment. When experiencing and expressing what we feel threatens our closest relationships, we suppress. More accurately, *we* don't: our mind does that automatically and unconsciously on our behalf.

The origin story of my own depression is easy to trace. It is documented in the trove of family photographs, from infancy onward, in which there is hardly ever even a hint of a smile on my face. Gazing at you from these pictures is a child who, at best, is serious beyond his age, when not morose. Under the conditions of war and genocide, I absorbed the feelings of my grief-stricken and terrorized mother; in my earliest photos I see my little self almost mirroring them. "The child can . . . feel the tension, rigidity and pain in the body of the mother or of anyone else he is with," writes the psychological thinker and spiritual teacher A. H. Almaas. "If the mother is suffering, the baby suffers too. The pain never gets discharged."[1] I could not have endured such emotional torment if I had felt it fully—no infant could. Nor was there room for my own sorrow and rage at the separation from my mother at less than one year of age.

As I have noted before, such extreme circumstances as beset my infancy and childhood are not required to induce a splitting from self. The riskiest emotions, and thus the most frequently exiled, are acute grief and healthy anger, two feelings that often get tarred as "negative."† Of course, a child may also have cause to banish her joy, enthusiasm, or pride if these arouse disapproval, envy, or just blank incomprehension on the part of parents too stressed, distracted, or depressed themselves. Either way, repressing the rejected emotion is the surest way of escaping overwhelming levels of vulnerability, of avoiding a too-painful rift between oneself and the ambient world. There is a catch, however: we cannot select which emotions to force below consciousness, nor willfully reverse the mechanism even after it has outlived its usefulness. "Everybody knows there is no finesse or accuracy of suppression," wrote the American novelist Saul Bellow in *The Adventures of Augie March*; "if you hold down one thing, you hold down the adjoining." Thus the repression of emotion, while adaptive in one circumstance, can become a state of chronic disconnect, a withdrawal from life. It becomes programmed into the brain, embedded in the personality.

The neuroscientist Jaak Panksepp, who studied the biology of the brain's emotional systems as thoroughly as anyone, had scathing words for the physiological disease model. "Popular depictions of depression as a 'chemical imbalance' are trivial . . . [All] problems in living, including death, are accompanied by 'chemical imbalances,' " he pointed out. He, too, saw depression as an adaptation of the brain to the loss of connection, as a physiological "shutdown mechanism" to terminate distress, "which, if sustained, would be dangerous for infant mammals."[2] In other

---

† By contrast, recall that we are born with evolution-programmed RAGE and GRIEF circuits in our brains.

words, far from expressing inherited pathology, depression appears as a coping mechanism to alleviate grief and rage and to inhibit behaviors that would invite danger. It is not that neurotransmitters are not involved in depression—only that their abnormalities *reflect* experiences, rather than being the primary *cause* of them. Brain disturbances manifest the stresses of existence during formative periods and, once established, become a source of further stress. Hence follow, Dr. Panksepp concluded, "the diverse symptoms and variants of depressive illness."

It has been transformative for me to realize that my own mental health issues carry genuine meanings that arose from my life within my family of origin in a particular historical context. I have found the same to be true universally, no matter where I look, whose mental "illness" I consider, or indeed how extreme the condition happens to be. If anything, the more flagrant ones are easier to decode. When examined, the manifestations of all the various mental health diagnoses have meaning, from depression through what is called schizophrenia to attention deficit hyperactivity disorder, from troubled eating patterns to self-cutting.

———————

"Before becoming a clinical psychologist, I was considered by some to be a seriously mentally ill patient," New York therapist Noël Hunter recalls in her book *Trauma and Madness in Mental Health Services*. Prior to seeking help in early adulthood, she had been living with intense distress and a sense of "being controlled." "I was just all over the place," she told me, "and was very scared of being hospitalized. I saw about six or seven different psychologists, social workers, psychiatrists at that time, and accrued about eight different diagnoses throughout all of that as well." She was placed on five medications, which she was assured she would have to rely on for the rest of her life. "I feared having my own children one day lest I pass on my genetic faults," she writes. "The fact that there was unfathomable abuse throughout my entire family, that coldness and greed superseded nurturance and love, and that emotional neglect was balanced only by an intrusive lack of boundaries all seemed irrelevant."[3] The meaning, once sought, was crystal clear and had nothing of the insane in it: Hunter's "paranoia" was a faithful, unerring emotional imprint of childhood. Without getting into the details, there had been a time in her life when, young and helpless, she *was* controlled by powerful, hostile figures in ways she found hurtful and scary, ways that violated her neural expectations and distorted her sense of reality.

The mind is a meaning-making machine. It will generate stories that "make sense" of the emotions that, at a vulnerable time, it could not contain and perhaps still cannot. Yet in the individual's unspoken history, the emotions were real, and therefore still are. They can surface in a number of different ways, such as Dr. Hunter's belief in being "controlled" as a young adult. To other minds, such narratives appear as madness itself. "It comes out as somewhat fantastical, so we say, 'That's totally non-understandable,'" Hunter remarked. In my experience, the story underneath diagnostic labels like hers is always perfectly coherent if one seeks the truth in the emotional texture and the biographical record rather than in the *content* of the paranoid fantasy. Coming to see this coherence and integrate it into her sense of self has enabled Hunter to understand and regulate herself differently. Today she is long off her "lifetime" pharmacological agents. I have witnessed many such examples and know of many more.

Forty-year-old Leslie, a recently certified therapist who is now pursuing an MA in psychology, made over a dozen suicide attempts or serious suicidal gestures from age seventeen to her mid-thirties. Leslie was plagued by chronic insomnia, cried uncontrollably, and could not maintain relationships. Her medical chart was a smorgasbord of *DSM* nomenclature: chronic depression, borderline personality disorder, dysthymia, panic disorder, ADHD, and, briefly, bipolar disorder. She had also been diagnosed with chronic cystitis and fibromyalgia. At one point she was on five different psychiatric medications, including two antidepressants, an antipsychotic, and a benzodiazepine tranquilizer, and was prescribed a third antidepressant intended to soothe her physical pain, along with an anti-inflammatory.

Leslie's healing journey—she, too, is no longer on any medications—has centered on finding the meaning in her multifaceted sufferings. Her crushing belief in her unworthiness revealed itself to be a self-protective strategy gone awry. Odd as it may sound, it was the best worst option. A suffering child, as Leslie was—again, the details matter less than the contours— has two possible options when it comes to processing her experience. She can conclude either that the people she relies on for love are incompetent, malicious, or otherwise ill-suited to the task, and she is all alone in this scary world; or that she herself is to blame for, well, everything. As painful as the latter explanation is, it is far preferable to the other one, which paints a life-threatening picture for a young being with zero power or recourse. The first option is not an option at all. Better to believe "It's my fault; I'm bad," which lets you believe there's the chance that "if I work hard and be good, I will be lovable." Thus, even the debilitating belief in one's unworthiness, nearly universal among people with mental health diagnoses and addictions, begins as a coping mechanism, a topic we will revisit in chapter 30.

What of Leslie's chronic state of panic? Her supposed "brain disorder" was, in fact, the expression of a mind alarmed by early hurt. It is adaptive for the brain of a child in her situation to be in a state of hyperalert fear, even when no immediate danger is present. These adaptations to adversity, once habitual, cannot discern between major and minor threats—or no threat at all. The capacity to recognize safety or threat will evolve in a healthy way under conditions of safety but be disrupted by prolonged early insecurity. Possible outcomes include feeling besieged when there is no threat, or conversely, remaining oblivious to danger when it is present.[4]

Leslie has even learned to have compassion for her self-hurting compulsions. "They were actually trying to protect me from the deep pain that I was in or trying not to feel," she said. These included hitting herself with a leather belt, as her mother had done when Leslie was a child. When I asked her what that did for her, she answered: "It would kind of calm me down a bit. I would be *less dysregulated*." Surprising but true: the very mental patterns and behaviors that seem to throw our lives into such chaos originate as an attempt, a temporarily and partially effective one, to *regulate* our nervous systems, to bring our bodies and minds to equilibrium.

The incidence of self-cutting is rising, particularly among young people. If we resist the default to "mental illness" as an explanation for such acts, we might ask instead: Why do people harm themselves? As in Leslie's case, these behaviors play the role, paradoxically enough, of self-soothing. They bring short-term relief. That more and more people are resorting to self-harm is a marker of the growing prevalence of stress and trauma. The comedian Darrell Hammond told me that cutting himself afforded him "a crisis that's more manageable than the terror inside you, the one that's going on in your head . . . You look at a cutter's arms; those aren't suicide cuts. Those aren't death cuts. Those are either 'I want someone to know I'm in distress,' or 'When I start patching this arm up, running and finding the Band-Aid, and cleaning myself up, I have a crisis, but it's manageable, and the one in my head was not.'" The Canadian Indigenous writer Helen Knott depicts the same process with scorching eloquence: "Those brief moments of the sharp blade dragging across skin provided me with a relief from the hate that I felt for myself. It was as if the moment the skin opened up, it became a vent that poured out all of my fucked-up whirling emotions . . . I didn't want to die at that time—that's not what cutting was about. I was doing it so I could put up with living."[5]

Thus, many actions and beliefs that look like pure insanity from one perspective make sense from another—and *always made sense at the start.* It is our task, if healing is the goal, to make sense of them newly, now, with the benefit of adult discernment and compassion.

We can derive this same lesson from the tragic life of the great comic actor Robin Williams. On August 10, 2014, the night before he died by suicide, Williams attended a soiree in his posh San Francisco Bay Area neighborhood. The others at the party would have seen the effervescent, people-loving persona for which he was so well known. Underneath that mask, he was in despair.

Williams was in the throes of Lewy body disease, a neurodegenerative brain disorder characterized by Parkinsonian symptoms and advancing dementia. Unlike depression or anxiety, this ailment does have distinct physiological markings, even if they can be identified only in an autopsy. "Robin was losing his mind and he was aware of it," his wife revealed after his death. "He kept saying, 'I just want to reboot my brain.'" The thought of suicide, however, was not new to him; in a 2010 interview he recriminated himself for "not having the balls to do it."

In addition to the madcap, on-the-fly brilliance of his work as a comic, he had a sweetness and vulnerability that touched many hearts, a love that poured out into the world but that he could never extend to himself.

The founts of the comedian's anguish can be located in his

childhood. The author Anne Lamott grew up near Williams in Illinois. In a much-circulated Facebook post, she wrote that, as children, "we were in the same boat—scared, shy, with terrible self-esteem and grandiosity." His lifelong dilemma, she said, would remain "how to stay one step ahead of the abyss."

In the same post, Lamott alluded to heredity as a likely cause of her friend's sufferings. Yet I hear in Williams's own words more than enough information to account for his mental-emotional woes without resorting to genetic superstitions. "My only companions, my only friends as a child were my imagination," he once said, an admission of profound loneliness.[6] He initially honed his extraordinary capacity to generate strange and hilarious imaginary characters as a way of breaking his isolation, in a family with an emotionally distant mother and a father he recalled as "frightening." As many sensitive kids are in the peer culture, he was bullied at school. He found some freedom in fantasy, as his characters "could say and do things I was afraid to do myself." His comic skills had the original function of gaining him some closeness with his mother. "You get this weird desire to connect with her through comedy and entertainment," he told the podcaster Marc Maron in 2010. His wording was unkind to himself: there is nothing weird about a child seeking attachment with his parent. What is abnormal is that any child should have to do so. Hence the same coping mechanisms that potentiated his greatest gifts ended up becoming the bars of his prison—the double bind of the hypersensitive child, once again. Underneath his brilliantly turbulent comic persona, he learned to suppress his real feelings. He was past master at that, until his death.

Cocaine, he once implied, gave him respite from his super-charged energy, just as a hyperactive child may be given the stimulant Ritalin to settle him. He had the addict's lifelong discomfort with the self, the need to flee from his consciousness of himself:

"sleepwalking with activity," he called it. In an episode of the hit 1970s television series *Mork & Mindy*, he played both the outer space arrival Mork and his real self. "You know, if you learned to say no, you'd probably have a lot more time to yourself," Mindy tells the comedian. "Maybe that's the last thing I want," Robin replies, with an ineffably sad expression on his face.

It wasn't for lack of self-awareness that the abyss got the better of Williams in the end. Long before he developed a degenerative disorder, he suffered from what he called "please-love-me syndrome," a self-diagnosis far more penetrating than anything a *DSM*-toting psychiatrist could come up with. I find myself wishing someone had guided him to connect the dots, to see that "syndrome" as the emotional endoskeleton of his manic-depressive swings, addictions, and suicidality, and very likely his terminal brain condition as well.[†] From there, he could have traced the links back even further to the scared, isolated child he once had been. He might have found the meaning that could have saved him.

What, then, of conditions widely believed to be brain diseases, largely rooted in genetics, such as the group of diverse behaviors and thought patterns called schizophrenia, marked often by psychoses, delusions, and hallucinations? The science is clear and, again, belies popular prejudice. No "schizophrenia gene" has ever been found—or, more accurately, claims of its discovery have had to be serially retracted. Broad surveys have found that at most only about 4 percent of the risk can be attributed to a wide variety of genes—none of them specific to this condition, as they are also seen in cases of ADHD or autism.[8] Again, what

---

†   A scientific aside to Williams's story is that research has now linked the onset of Parkinson's—a close relative of Lewy body disease—with chronic depression and stress. See endnote 7 to this chapter.

is being transmitted, if anything, is sensitivity and not disease. Even the nomenclature should give us pause: the Greek origin of "schizophrenia" means "split mind." The question follows naturally: Why would a mind need to split itself?

Self-fragmentation is one of the defenses evoked when the experience of how things are cannot be endured. Only those who know real life to be an insufferable bane are impelled to check out from it. No fixed genetic destiny here, but a survival need composed of constitutional vulnerability and overwhelming life experience. One way for an organism to escape that agony, whatever its source, is to disconnect whenever the distressing emotions are triggered. In the face of trauma, splitting from the present is a form of instantaneous self-defense.[9] From that perspective, it is a miraculous dynamic allowing vulnerable creatures to survive the unendurable.

In psychoses there occurs a prime feature of severe mental illness, disintegration. In such extreme states, with normally related mental processes utterly separated, the person may be completely detached from the here and now. Such is the case in schizophrenia, but absenting oneself from reality can show up in a range of forms from mild to severe, depending on the degree of hurt and the genetic sensitivity of the individual.

A milder flight from reality is dissociation. Helen Knott, subjected to sexual exploitation when very young, describes it well: "My feelings left my body. My spirit sat outside of me like an unacknowledged apparition. I didn't know whose life I was living, whose body I inhabited. This wasn't my story, my life, my reality . . . I was scared that if I tried to lean into my feelings, I would fall off the emotional edge and I didn't know what I would do to myself."[10] What we call a disorder is revealed to be an ingenious means for an assaulted psyche to absent itself from agony.

Such is also the recollection of the former National Hockey League star Theoren Fleury, who was sexually assaulted by his coach as a teenager and went on to become an advocate for child-hood victims of sexual abuse. "The first few times he got at me weren't so bad because I was gone. I would open my eyes and he would be standing over me, cleaning himself up. I knew something had happened, but I was not sure what. The mind can do some amazing things. Even years later in therapy, when telling the counselor about it, I would check out—leave my body. She'd have to literally shake me to bring me back."[11] Horrific though the inciting circumstances were, I hear in Fleury's use of the word "amazing" an appreciation for the parts of himself that mobilized way back when to protect him from pain—an attitude I heartily recommend to anyone making similar discoveries.

A chronic, reflexive tuning out is one of the hallmarks of atten-tion deficit hyperactivity disorder (ADHD),[†] now being diag-nosed worldwide with increasing and alarming frequency. This is not dissociation-level "out of body"–ness, but it does disconnect one from oneself, from one's activities, and from other people in ways that disrupt functioning and are, as I personally attest, often highly frustrating. ADHD's features include poor attention span, distractibility and low boredom threshold, poor impulse control, and (mostly in males) difficulty being still. Millions of children are receiving stimulants as a result, and hundreds of thousands are even being treated with antipsychotic medications—not for psychosis, but simply to calm them, to make them more pliable. This amounts to a vast and uncontrolled social experiment in the chemical control of children's behavior, since we don't know the

---

†   Also known as ADD, to denote that the hyperactivity may not always be present. In practice, and confusingly, the two acronyms are often used interchangeably.

long-term effects of such drugs on the developing brain. What we do know from adult research should give us pause. It has been understood since at least 2010 that prolonged use of antipsychotics is associated with shrinkage of brain volume in adult subjects.[12] In children we are already witnessing some short-term systemic harm. Here in Vancouver, British Columbia Children's Hospital has had to establish a special clinic just to deal with the metabolic consequences of such drugs, which include obesity, diabetes, and threats to cardiovascular health.

ADHD is sometimes said to be the "most heritable" mental illness, which in my view is a bit like calling quartz the most chewable crystal. Some experts estimate—I should say misestimate—the heritability of ADHD traits to be in the range of 30 to 50 percent.[13] The genetic thesis never made sense to me, even though two of my children and I myself have been diagnosed with this "brain disease." Tuning out is dissociation's less extreme cousin, part of the same family of escapist adaptations. It is invoked by the organism when the circumstances are stressful and there is no other recourse for relief, when one can neither change the situation nor escape it. Such was the imperative in my own infancy. Such, too, was the situation for my three sensitive children—a trait they may well have inherited, as discussed in the last chapter—in an emotionally chaotic home characterized, amid plenty of love, by parental anxiety, depression, and conflict. This adaptation then becomes wired into the brain, without the brain itself being the original source of the problem.

It's true that we are seeing more troubled children these days, but blaming a child's behavior on her brain makes no sense—nor does blaming the parents. As we have seen with other conditions, when a syndrome rises sharply in frequency over a short period of time, genetics cannot possibly be the cause. Jaak Panksepp suggested that ADHD is not a brain disease but a problem stemming partly from the thwarted development, in modern societal conditions, of what he called the innate PLAY system. His proposed solution: more play opportunities for children, to encourage the "construction of the social brain."[14]

Just as depression is "explained" by the biologically minded as resulting from a lack of the neurotransmitter serotonin, ADHD is chalked up to an insufficiency of dopamine, the brain's incentive-motivation molecule. So we prescribe dopamine-enhancing stimulants, such as Ritalin or Adderall. While dopamine certainly seems to be implicated, here, too, medical practice ignores the interaction of physiology and environment. Today, voluminous research has linked the symptoms of ADHD to trauma or early stress, and has shown that both can impact the dopamine circuits of the brain and that adversity can interfere with a child's subsequent capacity to focus and to organize tasks.[15, 16] Such trauma or early stresses can include maternal depression or more overt disturbances in the family milieu. One study reviewed data involving sixty-five thousand children aged six through seventeen years. The parents of those diagnosed with ADHD reported much higher prevalence of adverse events.[17]

The time has come to address the swiftly changing and ever more stressful environments our children are growing up in, before we interfere chemically with children's brain physiology. When I saw children who met the criteria for this condition, my approach was to consider the family milieu and to help parents understand the stresses they were unwittingly transmitting to their offspring. These children were in every case the proverbial canaries in the coal mine. Sensitive to the nth degree, their "symptoms" expressed the unresolved travails of the entire family system, itself often overwhelmed by the pressures exerted by a culture increasingly unfriendly to development. If we saw the condition and its associated traits as manifestations of biopsychosocial underdevelopment rather than as symptoms of a disease, we would ask ourselves how to provide the right conditions for healthy brain plasticity and psychological growth. We—physicians, parents, educators—would honor the neurobiology of relationship above all.[†]

We might well learn from our canine friends. A veterinary publication in 2017 reported that some "problem dogs"—more hyper, more distractible, and less obedient than others—can be treated with stimulant medications to abate the "symptoms," rendering them more trainable. "Of more interest is the fact that certain environmental and social conditions affect the appearance of ADHD symptoms," reported *Psychology Today*. "Dogs which have lots of social contacts with other dogs and many interactions with people seem to show fewer symptoms [typical] of ADHD. The more that you physically connect with and play with the dog, the fewer the problems. Dogs that are left alone for extended periods of time are also more likely to show hyperactive symptoms on your return. Another interesting association the researchers found is that dogs who sleep alone (isolated from their owner or other dogs) have more problems."[18] If only psychologists, physicians, and educators had as much insight and empathic imagination as these veterinarians, perhaps fewer children would be medicated.

Meaning, when sought, readily shows up as well in bipolar illness, also known as manic-depressive disorder. "I got sick for the first time when I was twenty-one," Caterina recalled. "It turned into a full-blown psychotic episode. I thought I was the epitome

---

[†] Though I am not categorically against the use of medications in ADHD, I decry the automatic, extensive, long-term, and almost exclusive reliance on them. For more, see my book *Scattered Minds: The Origins and Healing of Attention Deficit Disorder*.

of evil. I felt I was this horrible thing that doesn't deserve to exist. I would go into catatonic states and hear voices, all telling me about my unworthiness, my evil nature."

This interview was unique in that it took place in the presence of Caterina's parents, instead of the usual one-on-one. They had intuited that their daughter's problems arose from something beyond her brain chemistry and requested my input.

Caterina's manic episode ensued after a hostile argument with her mother. "I felt hurt and angry at something she said," Caterina reported. "I thought I had ruined my family and that we were all going to fall apart. At first it was scary . . . but then it started feeling really good, and it progressed and progressed until I felt like I was very powerful—I could save the world. I wasn't a force of destruction anymore; I could put all the art back in the world." (Now twenty-six, she studies art in Toronto.) Typically for the manic state, Caterina felt hyperenergized and did not sleep for a week until she was admitted to a psychiatric hospital. The medications she was prescribed eased her symptoms, but she was not guided to ponder the source of her delusions of malevolent or magnificently benign power. "Do you think that is something we have to look at?" she asked me. "My psychiatrists thought that delusions are just like having a fever." I replied with a question of my own. "What if your delusions are perfectly accurate? Not accurate in a concrete sense, but accurate to your emotional reality?" I pointed out that both fantasies—"I had ruined my family" and "I could save the world"—have something in common. Caterina was quick to catch the similarity: "In both, I have a sense of control! I'm very powerful."

The source of that sense of overweening power soon began to surface. "My parents went through a really hard time when I was eleven," Caterina recalled. "They would have horrible fights at night . . . and they would scream at each other. My dad would cry to me . . . *understandably,* because he was going through a lot, and we were really close." That "closeness," really an unhealthy lack of boundaries that psychologists call "fusion," had persisted throughout Caterina's formative years. Harmful as the dynamic was, in Caterina's mind it was her moral duty to protect her parents: she wore her inability to hold her family together like a badge of shame, proof of her unworthiness. Absorbing a parent's sorrow is not the Nature-given responsibility of a child. "The reversal of roles between child, or adolescent, and parent, unless very temporary, is almost always not only a sign of pathology in the parent but *a cause of it in the child,*" wrote the great pioneer of attachment research and personality development, the British psychiatrist John Bowlby.[19]

Caterina's psychotic phase can be seen as a kind of inner haunting wherein all the intense emotions she'd had to stuff away as a child in order to carry out her "understandable" role came to take over her adult mind. Her parents, who had themselves been traumatized in their families of origin and by political tragedies in their home countries, were unable to handle their own emotions, never mind their young daughter's. All in all, her self-accusations of ungodly wickedness and her delusions of near-divine potency were two poles of a "power" she never should have been burdened with.

A study in 2013 looked at nearly six hundred French and Norwegian subjects with a bipolar diagnosis. "Our results demonstrate consistent associations between childhood trauma and more severe clinical characteristics in bipolar disorder," the researchers reported. "Further, they show the importance of including emotional abuse as well as the more frequently investigated sexual abuse when targeting clinical characteristics of bipolar disorder."[20] Once again, let's note that the subtler forms of emotional injury, such as those Caterina sustained as a child, while more difficult to study, are no less harmful to the sensitive youngster.

"So, do you think people should focus on the emotional content of delusions and try to understand them?" Caterina asked me as we wrapped up. "Do you think that's a way of healing, rather than medicating them?" "It's not necessarily a question of *rather than*," I suggested. "If you weren't on medication, you'd not be able to have this conversation right now. My problem with the usual approach is not that doctors give medication; only, too often, that's all they do."

I advised the family to pursue therapy to sort out their individual traumas and mutual enmeshment.

Extensive scientific literature now links disordered relationships to food, as well, with early trauma and family stress. Recall that the seminal Adverse Childhood Experiences (ACE) Study began after the lead investigator, Dr. Vincent Felitti, began to pay heed to the life histories of patients at the obesity clinic where he served as medical director. "We could help them lose weight," Dr. Felitti told me, "but not to keep it off. I kept wondering why, until I finally got the message. 'Don't you get it?' they said. 'We're stuffing down our pain.'"

As with other people with "genetic" mental health problems, which anorexia is often considered to be, the personal histories of individuals always reveal meaning. A medical colleague who suffered from anorexia as a teenager, for example, is a self-described perfectionist, a trait that nobody is born with. Rather, it arises as an adaptation to fit in with an environment where one perceives no welcome for being just who one is, with all one's "imperfections."

Much as with addictions or self-harming behaviors, or conditions like obsessive-compulsive disorder, there is always a "pay-off" with disordered eating patterns. At age seventeen, Andrea, now twenty-seven, became "super, super meticulous" about what she would eat. "I would cook for other people, and I would never eat it. But everything that I would eat for myself was always weighed out, measured out. When I was in university, I remember eating Greek yogurt and granola or muesli for breakfast, and I would measure out absolutely everything in measuring cups. Everything would go into a tracker so I knew what I was eating. It was the ultimate form of control." At five feet seven, Andrea went down to 106 pounds.† She did not menstruate for seven years.

When asked what she "got" from her self-denial, she said: "It's that sense of control, and also self-acceptance. It made me feel better about myself, because I had control of what I was doing, essentially." Although she recalled a "not bad" childhood, her mother, Cathy—who participated in our interview—was able to correct the record. She and her husband divorced when Andrea was six, after years of intense marital stress. A child in such circumstances is prone to lack self-acceptance and yearn for agency in an emotionally unstable environment.

This desperate drive to seize some command at least of their own body amid turmoil is almost universal among people with anorexia or bulimia that I have interviewed. The psychologist Julie T. Anné, who specializes in treating eating disorders, nails it: with her clients, she says, "three lacks" are typical—lack of control, identity, and self-worth—along with a need to numb pain. "In a relational world . . . the human psyche devises a brilliant means to emotionally survive," she told me. "In our culture, this becomes the pursuit of perfection vis-à-vis the body and self. Also known as anorexia." And yet these deeply wounded individuals, like the

---

† 170 cm and 48 kg, respectively.

bearers of every mental-emotional burden we have touched on, are all too rarely asked the key questions: *Where did this come from?* and *What valid problem is it trying to fix?*

One of Robin Williams's most beloved performances, for which he won an Academy Award, is in *Good Will Hunting*, where he appears in the role of a kindly psychologist tasked with helping an angry Boston janitor after the latter assaults a cop. Played by Matt Damon, this gifted man—he turns out to be an intellectual diamond in the rough—has stuffed his vulnerability underneath a layer of ossified rage and defiance. The most iconic scene from the movie features Williams's therapist getting right in Damon's face and repeating a simple but powerful statement, "It's not your fault," until the latter finally collapses, sobbing, into his embrace. That message, "It's not your fault," conveys not just undaunted compassion, for which Damon's character was starving inside, but wisdom, too. From behavioral problems to full-blown mental illness, it's not *anyone's* fault—nor, as we've seen, the fault of their brains or their genes. It is an expression of untended wounds, *and it is meaningful.*

The meaning extends beyond people's individual lives, their families of origin, and their childhoods. If we are going to address the myriad afflictions to which this book has devoted its attention so far, we need to look through a wider lens at the bigger story. If I could distill my message and insert it into that beautiful cinematic moment, I would have Robin Williams look all of us in the eye—including himself—and say with assurance: "It's not your fault . . . *and it's not personal.*" It's about our hurting world, manifesting the illusions and myths of a culture alienated from our essence.

We turn to that bigger picture next.

Part IV

The Toxicities of Our Culture

Making an injury visible and public is often the first step in remedying it, and political change often follows culture, as what was tolerated is seen to be intolerable, or what was overlooked becomes obvious.

—Rebecca Solnit, *Hope in the Dark*

Chapter 19

From Society to Cell: Uncertainty, Conflict, and Loss of Control

The history of the world is the history of a ten-thousand-year
war of brains between the rich and the poor . . . The poor
win a few battles . . . but of course the rich have won the
war for ten thousand years.

—Aravind Adiga, *The White Tiger*

We know that chronic stress, whatever its source, puts the nervous system on edge, distorts the hormonal apparatus, impairs immunity, promotes inflammation, and undermines physical and mental well-being. I see it on a daily basis, and I agree with János Selye, the father of stress research, who "without hesitation" asserted "that for man the most important stressors are emotional."[1] At this stage in our exploration of trauma, illness, and healing I would only add that the main determinants of human emotional stress extend from the personal to the cultural. We are, in effect, biopsycho*societal* beings.

To review what we've seen about stress so far: First, its physiology and consequences include the acute or chronic activation, potential overactivation, and even exhaustion of the hypothalamic-pituitary-adrenal (HPA) axis that connects our brain's emotional centers and the body's entire physiological apparatus.[†] Then there's what Bruce McEwen has called "allostatic load": the wear and tear on the body of having to maintain its internal equilibrium in the face of changing and challenging circumstances, trauma salient among them. In this culture many people are fated to be bearers of heavy allostatic loads, to the detriment of their mental and physical health, as demonstrated, if more proof were needed, by a recent Yale study showing the cumulative impact of stress on accelerated biological aging. "Our society is experiencing more stress than ever before, leading to both negative psychiatric and physical outcomes," the researchers noted.[2]

Of course, there is no "equality of opportunity" in stress, any more than there is in economic life. The structure of a society based on power and wealth, with built-in disparities along racial and gender lines, leaves some people far more physiologically burdened than others. It is true that in a culture that recruits individuals and groups into a fearful competition against others, the psychological triggers for stress spare no social tier, but the fact remains that their effects are unevenly distributed. And while the *personal* stresses of a disconnect from the self and the loss of authenticity may cut across class lines, the allostatic strain imposed by imbalances of power falls most onerously on the politically disempowered and economically disenfranchised.

What, in our society, are the most widespread emotional triggers for stress? My own observations of self and others have led me to endorse fully what a review of the stress literature concluded, namely that "psychological factors such as *uncertainty, conflict, lack of control, and lack of information* are considered the most stressful stimuli and strongly activate the HPA axis."[3] A society that breeds these conditions, as capitalism inevitably does, is a superpowered generator of stressors that tax human health.

---

†   Chapters 2 and 3.

Capitalism is "far more than just an economic doctrine," Yuval Noah Harari observes in his influential bestseller *Sapiens*. "It now encompasses an ethic—a set of teachings about how people should behave, educate their children, and even think. Its principal tenet is that economic growth is the supreme good, or at least a proxy for the supreme good, because justice, freedom, and even happiness all depend on economic growth."[4] Capitalism's influence today runs so deep and wide that its values, assumptions, and expectations potently infuse not only culture, politics, and law but also such subsystems as academia, education, science, news, sports, medicine, child-rearing, and popular entertainment. The hegemony of materialist culture is now total, its discontents universal. We explore how it affects our very health in this and the following chapters.

In medical school I was trained to think of life and health in purely individualistic terms. That we have a hard time *not* seeing things this way is, itself, a quintessential feature of the "normal" worldview engendered by capitalism.

In this, as in much else, the medical system mirrors and reinforces the prevailing ethic. In an atomized, materialistic culture people are induced to take everything personally, to see their own mental and physical distress as misfortunes or even failures belonging to them alone. Take the picture painted by the former British prime minister Tony Blair, to this day a sought-after, well-remunerated spokesperson for the desocializing ethic—that is, for bleaching the "social" out of society. Many health problems, he said, are "not, strictly speaking, public health problems at all. They are questions of lifestyle: obesity, smoking, alcohol abuse, diabetes, sexually transmitted diseases . . . These are not epidemics in the epidemiological sense—they are the result of millions of *individual decisions*, at millions of points in time."[5] This perspective denotes a blithe unawareness of the many studies linking all these "millions of decisions" to trauma and stress, including the stresses imposed by low socioeconomic or occupational status, and poverty—a festering sore in British society since the dismantling of the "welfare state" and communal institutions, along with the disempowering of labor unions. That underlying such "individual decisions" is the social milieu fostered by late-stage capitalism seems not to have occurred to Mr. Blair, despite considerable evidence. This is no surprise: a refusal to recognize broad economic and political conditions as relevant to individual health and happiness is a core feature of materialistic ideology. No one inclined to connect those dots would ever be entrusted with the keys to the kingdom.

Culture acts on our well-being via all manner of biopsychosocial pathways, including epigenetic causes; stress-induced inflammation; impairment of telomeres and premature aging; how and what we eat; toxins we ingest or inhale. It exerts its influences through many other outside-in mechanisms, too: through effects passed on from parents to children; from one person to another; from social, political, and economic conditions to individual bodies—"from society to cell," in the words of the molecular scientist and researcher Michael Kobor. Contra the Blairite view, it also powerfully influences and constrains nearly all the "individual decisions" most of us make with regard to our well-being.

All stressors represent the absence or threatened loss of something an organism perceives as necessary for survival. An impending loss of food supply, for example, is a major stressor for any creature. So is, for our species, the absence or threatened loss of love, or work, or dignity, or self-esteem, or meaning.

In 2020, a few weeks before the novel coronavirus metastasized to devastate the world economy, no less a figure than Kristalina

Georgieva—head of the International Monetary Fund, that executive planning committee of international capital—was already warning that the global economy risked returning to the woeful conditions of the Great Depression, owing to inequality and financial-sector instability. "If I had to identify a theme at the outset of the new decade," she said, "it would be increasing uncertainty."[6] The majority of the population in my own country, for one, did not require this alarming forecast to know that things were not looking up. Just a month before the IMF head issued her prediction, nearly 90 percent of Canadians expressed the concern that food prices were rising faster than their incomes. About one in eight Canadian households experienced food insecurity in the previous year.[7] In my home province of British Columbia in 2017, 52 percent of women reported "extreme emotional stress" regarding their financial situation.[8] Such trends are international and have been growing for decades.

The burgeoning of chronic mental and physical health conditions across many countries in the past decades, from depression to diabetes, can be no coincidence. "Neoliberalism[†] has made the world of work far less secure and consequently more stressful and health damaging," write two British health academics, ". . . resulting in a myriad of chronic diseases including musculoskeletal pain and cardiovascular disease."[9] I find that unsurprising, living as we do under a system that habitually foments the stress of mass uncertainty. Globalization, with its ruinous policies dictated to so-called developing countries by bodies like the International Monetary Fund and the World Bank—such as cutting back social supports, suppressing workers' rights, and

---

[†]   Although the term "neoliberalism" is mostly employed nowadays by critics of the erosion of social programs, the increasing power of the corporations, their laissez-faire ideology, and their sway over governments under late-stage capitalism, it was originally coined in the 1930s by prominent advocates of just such policies. My use of it is in itself neither critical nor laudatory: it refers to an objective reality whose health impacts we are investigating.

encouraging privatization—has also permeated the industrialized nations. It's what the Canadian political philosopher John Ralston Saul called "the crucifixion theory of economics: you had to be killed economically and socially in order to be reborn clean and healthy."[10]

The health impacts of our economic system are neither hard to understand nor difficult to track. A 2013 study comparing the health and stress status of young Swedes to young Greeks during the financial catastrophe then engulfing Greece found the Athens students to be at a marked disadvantage. They reported higher levels of stress, harbored "lower hope for the future," and suffered "significantly more widespread symptoms of depression and anxiety," as well as, ominously, *lower* cortisol levels.[11] The latter is a marker of long-term stress: a sign that people's healthy, protective stress-response mechanism was burning out. It often augurs future disease.[†] "One can suspect that the social crisis in Greece is beginning to have biological effects on the residents of the country," the study warned. Similarly, in Canada it was found that when women are under economic pressure, their children's stress-hormone levels rise markedly by age six, elevating the risk of illness later in life.[12]

Many people exist at the mercy of forces completely beyond their power to affect, let alone control. Who knows when the next cyclic recession will strike or when yet another megabusiness will downsize, merge, or relocate so that livelihoods are jeopardized with barely a day's notice. Even prior to COVID-19's economic ravages, one had become almost inured to news that yet another corporation was declaring masses of employees redundant. "High Street Crisis Deepens as 3,150 Staff Lose Jobs in a Week" was a headline in the *Guardian* in January 2020, a few

---

†   To clarify, both chronically elevated *and* lowered cortisol levels signal overburdening of the body's stress apparatus: the former its excessive activation, the latter its debilitation.

weeks before the pandemic arrived in Britain. Only months earlier, the *New York Times* had reported on the deepening insecurity of American families: "The costs of housing, health care and education are consuming ever larger shares of household budgets and have risen faster than incomes. Today's middle-class families are working longer, managing new kinds of stress and shouldering greater financial risks than previous generations did."[13] As the famed anthropologist, researcher, and author Wade Davis remarked recently in a broadly circulated *Rolling Stone* piece, "Though living in a nation that celebrates itself as the wealthiest in history, most Americans live on a high wire, with no safety net to brace a fall."[14] A better blueprint for allostatic overload could not be imagined.

Although the world's most advanced capitalist country evinces the rawest individualistic ethic, leaving the majority of its people mired in insecurity, we are not speaking of a uniquely American trend. Such is the overweening economic and cultural influence of the U.S. throughout the world that, as Morris Berman has argued, "If the twentieth century was the 'American century' the twenty-first will be the 'Americanized century.' "[15] The Organisation for Economic Co-operation and Development reported that pressures on the middle class around the world have increased since the 1980s.[16] Thus on the very terrain in which capitalism stakes its greatest claims to success—economic achievement—we find many people in a state of chronic uncertainty and loss of control, subject to stress-inducing fears that translate into disturbances of the hormonal apparatus, of the immune system, and of the entire organism.

No wonder, then, that insecurity about work or the loss of it can instigate disease. Studies in the United States showed that the risk of stroke and heart attacks in people fifty-one to sixty-one years of age more than doubles in the aftermath of prolonged job loss.[17] The results hold even after the expected increase in stress-related behaviors such as smoking, drinking, and eating are taken into account. In fact, multiple job losses have been shown to raise the risk of heart attacks as much as cigarettes, alcohol, and hypertension.[18] Even the *fear* of losing one's job is just as strong a predictor of an older person's health as it actually happening. In the decade and a half between the late 1970s and the mid-1990s, the proportion of American employees of major corporations who professed themselves "frequently concerned about being laid off" nearly doubled, from 24 to 46 percent.[19] Jobs with time pressure, fast pace, and high workload, coupled with decreased control over such factors, are also associated with increased stress and ill health.[20]

A signature marker of stress is inflammation. I've encountered the links between the two in many of the patients under my care. Inflammation is implicated in an extensive range of pathologies, from autoimmune conditions to vascular disease of heart and brain, from cancer to depression. One of my most penetrating interviews for this book was with the scientist Dr. Steven Cole. "A theme that comes up over and over again," Cole said, "is this increase in inflammatory gene activity in people confronting a sense of threat or insecurity for more than a short period of time. We can detect these same in mice, in monkeys. As far down as in fish, you can see that the more stress or threat or uncertainty you're exposed to, the more the body turns on this defensive program that involves more inflammation."

———————

While most people experience loss of control and waning security, others enjoy a surfeit of these. For this stratum of society, even conflict is not such a source of stress—in any struggle, the greater the power, the less the threat. It used to be that only people accused of Marxist tendencies would speak of "class war." In recent years, though, the actuality of elite dominance and the assault on the middle and lower classes has struck home across ideological lines. No less an authority than the multibillionaire investment tycoon Warren Buffett has seen the writing on the wall. "There's class warfare, all right," he told the *New York Times* in 2006, "but it's my class, the rich class, that's making war, and we're winning."[21] The ice-cream magnate Ben Cohen, a wealthy man with a social conscience, put it even more frankly, telling the same paper in 2020: "What we have in America is a democracy that's run for the benefit of corporations. That's a disaster. We're looking at it, we're living it and it continues to get worse."[22] In our globalized world, America's way of doing things is the template for many countries.

Even Nobel Prize–winning economists like Joseph E. Stiglitz have joined the chorus. Stiglitz is as credentialed an expert as they come: apart from his Nobel laurels, he was chief economist for the World Bank and chairman of President Bill Clinton's Council of Economic Advisers. As such, he used to formulate many of the policies whose effects he has now come to rue. Currently a professor at Columbia University, he has documented and decried the social, political, and health impacts of rising inequality throughout the elite-ruled globalized world. He laments what he calls a shift "from social cohesion to class warfare."

"The political system seems to be failing as much as the economic system," Stiglitz writes in his 2012 book, *The Price of Inequality*. In the eyes of many, he continues, "capitalism is failing to produce what was promised, but is delivering on what was not promised—inequality, pollution, unemployment, and *most important of all*, the degradation of values to the point where everything is acceptable and no one is accountable."[23] (Italics in original.)

Here the analysis by Stiglitz and other latter-day critics of capitalism reveals its limitations. What if, I would put to them, the system is not failing at all but succeeding magnificently? To suppose that its demonstrated harms represent a "failure" is to ignore that for some people—who also happen to be the class gaining most of the wealth and wielding the most power—the system is functioning smoothly indeed. The Swiss bank UBS reported in October 2020 that during the COVID-19-induced market turmoil the international billionaire stratum had grown their fortunes to over ten trillion dollars between April and July of that year. The world's then richest individual, Amazon founder Jeff Bezos, had increased his wealth by over $74 billion; Tesla owner Elon Musk by up to $103 billion.[24] "Canada's top 20 billionaires collectively have become $37 billion richer," the *Toronto Star* reported. "That's in the midst of an economic crisis that has left millions of Canadians unemployed or working reduced hours and struggling with bills, and our governments are borrowing to fund emergency financial aid for individuals and businesses to stave off even greater hardship."[25]

The notion that capitalism is *meant* to provide equality and opportunity for all must be taken on faith, since history and material reality provide no evidence for it.

In the realm of political decision-making, a widely circulated U.S. study showed that the views of ordinary people make no difference to public policy: a lack of control on a mass scale.[†] "When a majority of citizens disagree with economic elites or with organized interests, they generally lose," the authors concluded, adding that "even when fairly large majorities favor policy change, they generally do not get it."[26]

"Why do the rich have so much power?" asks a *New York Times* piece by Stiglitz's fellow Nobel laureate in economics Paul

---

†   Reported extensively, for example, in the *New York Times*, the *New Yorker,* and in many other publications, not to mention the academic literature.

Krugman—another erstwhile advocate, since reformed, of the globalizing impetus fueling the dominance of multinational corporations over governments and the public. Because, he answers his own question, "America is less of a democracy and more of an oligarchy."[27] In this light, I find little reason to question the astute assertion of consumer advocate and social crusader Ralph Nader that the two leading political parties in the United States are, in practice, "one corporate party wearing two heads and different makeup." In many other countries, too, behind the democratic facade real power is wielded by the moneyed few.

Where does that leave the rest of us? When he was installed as rector at Glasgow University in 1972, the spirited Scottish labor leader Jimmy Reid gave an address that the *New York Times* called "the greatest speech since President Lincoln's Gettysburg Address."[‡] Reid may not have studied the psychology or neurobiology of stress, but he understood everything about uncertainty, loss of control, and conflict in the lives of the people he represented. "Alienation is the precise and correctly applied word for describing the major social problem in Britain today," he declared. "People feel alienated by society . . . Let me right at the outset define what I mean by alienation. It is the cry of men who feel themselves the victims of blind economic forces beyond their control. It's the frustration of ordinary people excluded from the processes of decision-making. The feeling of despair and hopelessness that pervades people who feel with justification that they have no real say in shaping or determining their own destinies."[28]

Keep in mind, Reid's speech was given at the tail end of a brief postwar era of relatively enlightened social programs, at a time the system he excoriated was exhibiting its most benevolent face. What might he say today?

[‡] A Scottish friend of mine opined that the *Times* thereby flattered the American president.

Chapter 20

Robbing the Human Spirit:
Disconnection and Its Discontents

*Whereas individual people can become dislocated by
misfortunes in any society, only a free-market society
produces mass dislocation as part of its normal functioning,
even during periods of prosperity.*

—Bruce Alexander, *The Globalization of Addiction*

As a speaker on stress and trauma I'm often asked what lessons we may derive from the COVID-19 pandemic. Chief among them, surely, is the indispensability of connection—a quality globalized materialism has increasingly drained from modern culture, long before the isolation imposed by the virus reminded us of life's spiritual impoverishment without it. The health impacts are immeasurable.

It is now de rigueur for observers of all political hues and philosophical persuasions to bewail the glaring, growing absence of social feeling. "That basic sense of peoplehood, of belonging to a common enterprise with a shared destiny, is exactly what's lacking today," the oft-insightful conservative columnist David Brooks wrote recently in the *New York Times*.[1] Lacking, we might say, by design: qualities like love, trust, caring, social conscience, and engagement are inevitable casualties—"sunk costs," in capitalist argot—of a culture that prizes acquisition above all else.

A society that fails to value communality—our need to belong, to care for one another, and to feel caring energy flowing toward us—is a society facing away from the essence of what it means to be human. Pathology cannot but ensue. To say so is not a moral assertion but an objective assessment. "When people start to lose a sense of meaning and get disconnected, that's where disease comes from, that's where breakdown in our health—mental, physical, social health—occurs," the psychiatrist and neuroscientist Bruce Perry told me. If a gene or virus were found that caused the same impacts on the population's well-being as disconnection does, news of it would bellow from front-page headlines. Because it transpires on so many levels and so pervasively, we almost take it for granted; it is the water we swim in. We are steeped in the normalized myth that we are, each of us, mere individuals striving to attain private goals. The more we define ourselves that way, the more estranged we become from vital aspects of who we are and what we need to be healthy.

Among psychologists there is wide-ranging consensus about what our core needs consist of, some of which we have already explored. These have been variously listed as:

- *belonging, relatedness,* or *connectedness*;
- *autonomy*: a sense of control in one's life;
- *mastery* or *competence*;
- *genuine self-esteem*, not dependent on achievement, attainment, acquisition, or valuation by others;
- *trust*: a sense of having the personal and social resources needed to sustain one through life; and
- *purpose, meaning, transcendence*: knowing oneself as part of something larger than isolated, self-centered concerns, whether that something is overtly spiritual or simply universal/humanistic, or, given our evolutionary

origins, Nature. "The statement that the physical and mental life of man, and nature, are interdependent means simply that nature is interdependent with itself, for man is a part of nature." So wrote a twenty-six-year-old Karl Marx in 1844.[2]

None of this tells you anything you don't already know or intuit. You can check your own experience: What's it like when each of the above needs is met? What happens in your mind and body when it's lacking, denied, or withdrawn?

Bruce Alexander is the author of the essential volume *The Globalization of Addiction: A Study in Poverty of the Spirit* and a professor emeritus of psychology at Simon Fraser University. We both worked with the socially ostracized drug-user community in Vancouver's Downtown Eastside in the early 2000s. To hear Bruce tell it, such a choice of career path would have confounded his younger self, enthralled as he was by the ideology of materialist selfishness. "As I saw it then," he said, "it doesn't matter if a few people are going to die around the edges, but us strong guys, we're going to make it good for ourselves and for everybody. Now I've converted. Those ideas are incredibly toxic. They simply do not allow people to be people."

Just as I have named authenticity and attachment as two basic needs, so Bruce has identified people's "vital need for social belonging with their equally vital needs for individual autonomy and achievement" and calls the marriage of the two *psychosocial integration*.[3] A sane culture, Bruce and I agree, would have psychosocial integration as both an aim and a norm. Authenticity and attachment would cease to be in conflict: there would be no fundamental tension between belonging and being oneself.

Dislocation, in Bruce's formulation, describes a loss of connection to self, to others, and to a sense of meaning and purpose—all of which appear on the roster of essential needs above. Lest the word "dislocation" conjure something hazy like "being lost," he is quick with a graphic metaphor. "Think of a dislocated shoulder," he said, "a shoulder disarticulated, out of joint. You didn't cut off the arm, but it's just hanging there and not working anymore. Useless. That's how dislocated people experience themselves. It's excruciatingly painful." More than an individual experience, the same intense pain often occurs at the social level when large groups of people find themselves cut off from autonomy, relatedness, trust, and meaning. This is *social dislocation,* which, along with personal trauma, is a potent source of mental dysfunction, despair, addictions, and physical illness.[†] Abnormal from the perspective of human needs, such dislocation is now an entrenched facet of "normality" in our culture. Extreme examples include the physical and psychic dislocation forced upon North America's Indigenous populations by colonialism and, more recently, the globalization-induced economic hollowing out of entire regions in the United States, from the Rust Belt to the mining towns of the Appalachians—which has resulted in a vast increase in suicides and overdose deaths among the working class. The latter have been called "deaths of despair" by the Princeton economists Anne Case and Angus Deaton, her Nobel laureate spouse.[‡]

Dislocation spares no class of people, even if it shows up differently in different strata of society. Societal privilege may insulate some of us from being outwardly wrecked by dislocation's

---

[†]   Alexander acknowledges the Hungarian American economist Karl Polanyi as the originator of the concept of social dislocation, in the latter's 1944 work, *The Great Transformation.*

[‡]   As in their much-lauded 2020 book, *Deaths of Despair and the Future of Capitalism.*

gale-force winds, but it cannot exempt us from the inner impacts of having our needs for interconnection, purpose, and genuine self-esteem denied. Neither achievements nor attributes nor external evaluations of our worth can possibly compensate us for such a lack.

Recall that the Scottish labor leader Jimmy Reid defined "alienation" as the estrangement of people from a society that bars them from shaping or determining their own destinies. The word has other meanings as well, including estrangement from our essence, from ourselves, and from others. Already in the mid-nineteenth century Karl Marx recognized all these and added one more: disconnection from our labor as a meaningful activity over which we have agency and control. In this, Marx was prescient. Work encompasses several of the core needs noted above, including competence, mastery, and a sense of purpose. Just 30 percent of employees in the U.S. feel engaged at work, according to a 2013 report by Gallup; across 142 countries, the proportion of employees who feel engaged at work is only 13 percent. "For most of us," wrote two leading economic consultants in the *New York Times*, "work is a depleting, dispiriting experience, and in some obvious ways, it's getting worse."[4]

Alienation is inevitable when our inner sense of value becomes status-driven, hinging on externally imposed standards of competitive achievement and acquisition, and a highly conditional acceptance—I should say "acceptability"—in others' eyes. With the erosion of the middle class in recent decades, people who judged themselves in terms of worldly success have sustained a perceived loss of worth. The promise of the middle-class dream has largely evaporated, to the distress and deep anger of many. But even people perched atop the economic pyramid can experience a devaluation of self, for the simple reason that materialistic values run counter to the need for meaning, for purpose beyond self-serving endeavors.

There are no moral fingers to wag here. Objectively, it is the case that centering on the self's evanescent desires to the exclusion of communal needs results in a diminished connection to our deepest selves, which is to say the parts of us that generate and sustain true well-being. Whatever "wins" our personality can rack up, whatever momentary sense of security we gain through our various identities, however much we burnish our image or self-image with material gains—these are a flimsy replacement for the rewards (and challenges) of being alive to one's humanity. An investor dabbling daily in millions told Pulitzer Prize–winning journalist Charles Duhigg, "I feel like I'm wasting my life. When I die, is anyone going to care that I earned an extra percentage point on my return? My work feels totally meaningless." That loss of meaning, Duhigg says, afflicts "even professionals given to lofty self-images, like those in medicine and law." Why would this be? the author wondered. The answer: "Oppressive hours, political infighting, increased competition sparked by globalization, an 'always-on culture' bred by the internet—but also something that's hard for these professionals to put their finger on, an underlying sense that their work isn't worth the grueling effort they're putting into it."[5] It's simple economics, really: artificial inflation (of self-concept, of identity, of material ambition) is bound to lead to a downturn or even a crash when the bubble inevitably bursts.

Like our other needs, meaning is an inherent expectation. Its denial has dire consequences. Far from a purely psychological need, our hormones and nervous systems clock its presence or absence. As a medical study in 2020 found, the "presence [of] and search for meaning in life are important for health and well-being."[6] Simply put, the more meaningful you find your life, the better your measures of mental and physical health are likely to be. It is itself a sign of the times that we even need such studies to confirm what our experience of life teaches. When do you feel happier, more fulfilled, more viscerally at ease: when you extend yourself to help and connect with others, or when you are focused on burnishing the importance of your little egoic self? We all know the answer, and yet somehow what we know doesn't always carry the day.

Corporations are ingenious at exploiting people's needs without actually meeting them. Naomi Klein, in her book *No Logo*, made vividly clear how big business began in the 1980s to home in on people's natural desire to belong to something larger than themselves. Brand-aware companies such as Nike, Lululemon, and the Body Shop are marketing much more than products: they sell meaning, identification, and an almost religious sense of belonging through association with their brand. "That presupposes a kind of emptiness and yearning in people," I suggested when I interviewed the prolific author and activist. "Yes," Klein replied. "They tap into a longing and a need for belonging, and they do it by exploiting the insight that just selling running shoes isn't enough. We humans want to be part of a transcendent project."

Whatever one might say about the corporate, social, or ecological ethics of firms like Ford or General Motors, the unionized jobs they provided did keep generations of families employed gainfully and, for many, even meaningfully. The rapid deindustrialization of the working class in North America has led to a loss not only of income security but also of meaning, exacerbating the dislocation epidemic. The proliferation of service jobs and Amazon warehouse gigs hasn't replaced the sense of belonging these company jobs fostered in many communities. The eviscerating effect of these trends on people's sense of purpose and connection was expressed with heartbreaking candor by the dockworker character Frank Sobotka on HBO's *The Wire* two decades ago, who wistfully lamented to a lobbyist friend: "You know what the trouble is, Brucey? We used to *make* shit in this country, *build* shit. Now we just put our hand in the next guy's pocket."

———————

Not only does our individual and societal sanity depend on connection; so does our physical health. Because we are biopsychosocial creatures, the rising loneliness epidemic in Western culture is much more than just a psychological phenomenon: it is a public health crisis.

A preeminent scholar of loneliness, the late neuroscientist John Cacioppo and his colleague and spouse, Stephanie Cacioppo, published a letter in the *Lancet* only a month before his death in 2018. "Imagine," they wrote, "a condition that makes a person irritable, depressed, and self-centered, and is associated with a 26% increase in the risk of premature mortality. Imagine too that in industrialized countries around a third of people are affected by this condition, with one person in 12 affected severely, and that these proportions are increasing. Income, education, sex, and ethnicity are not protective, and the condition is contagious. The effects of the condition are not attributable to some peculiarity of the character of a subset of individuals, *they are a result of the condition affecting ordinary people*. Such a condition exists—loneliness."[7]

We now know without doubt that chronic loneliness is associated with an elevated risk of illness and early death. It has been shown to increase mortality from cancer and other diseases and has been compared to the harm of smoking fifteen cigarettes a day. According to research presented at the American Psychological

Association's annual convention in 2015, the loneliness epidemic is a public health risk at least as great as the burgeoning rates of obesity.[8] Loneliness, the researcher Steven Cole told me, can impair genetic functioning. And no wonder: even in parrots isolation impairs DNA repair by shortening chromosome-protecting telomeres.[9] Social isolation inhibits the immune system, promotes inflammation, agitates the stress apparatus, and increases the risk of death from heart disease and strokes.[10] Here I am referring to social isolation in the pre-COVID-19 sense, though the pandemic has grievously exacerbated the problem, at great cost to the well-being of many.

The rise of loneliness as a health hazard tracks with the entrenchment of values and practices that supersede any notion of "individual choices." The dynamics include reduced social programs, less available "common" spaces such as public libraries, cuts in services for the vulnerable and the elderly, stress, poverty, and the inexorable monopolization of economic life that shreds local communities. By way of illustration, let's take a familiar scenario: Walmart or some other megastore decides to open one of its facilities in a municipality. Developers are happy, politicians welcome the new investment, and consumers are pleased at finding a wide variety of goods at lower prices. But what are the social impacts? Locally owned and operated small businesses cannot compete with the marketing behemoth and must close. People lose their jobs or must find new work for lower pay. Neighborhoods are stripped of the familiar hardware store, pharmacy, butcher, baker, candlestick maker. People no longer walk to their local establishment, where they meet and greet one another and familiar merchants they have known, but drive, each isolated in their car, to a windowless, aesthetically bereft warehouse, miles away from home. They might not even leave home at all—why bother, when you can order online?

No wonder international surveys show a rise in loneliness. The percentage of Americans identifying themselves as lonely has doubled from 20 to 40 percent since the 1980s, the *New York Times* reported in 2016.[†][11] Alarmed by the health ravages, Britain has even found it necessary to appoint a minister of loneliness.

Describing the systemic founts of loneliness, the U.S. surgeon general Vivek Murthy wrote: "Our twenty-first-century world demands that we focus on pursuits that seem to be in constant competition for our time, attention, energy, and commitment. Many of these pursuits are themselves competitions. We compete for jobs and status. We compete over possessions, money, and reputations. We strive to stay afloat and to get ahead. Meanwhile, the relationships we prize often get neglected in the chase."[12]

It is easy to miss the point that what Dr. Murthy calls "our twenty-first-century world" is no abstract entity, but the concrete manifestation of a particular socioeconomic system, a distinct worldview, and a way of life.

———

Is it possible nevertheless that our consumer culture does make good on its promises, or could do so? Might these, if fulfilled, lead to a more satisfying life?

When I put the question to renowned psychologist Tim Kasser, professor emeritus of psychology at Knox College, his response was unequivocal. "Research consistently shows," he told me, "that the more people value materialistic aspirations as goals, the lower their happiness and life satisfaction and the fewer pleasant emotions they experience day to day. Depression, anxiety, and substance abuse also tend to be higher among people who value the aims encouraged by consumer society." He points to four central principles of what he calls ACC—American corporate capitalism: it "fosters and encourages a set of values based on *self-interest*, a strong desire for *financial success*, high levels of *consumption*, and interpersonal styles based on *competition*."[13]

There is a seesaw oscillation, Tim found, between materialistic concerns on the one hand and prosocial values like empathy, generosity, and cooperation on the other: the more the former are elevated, the lower the latter descend. For example, when people strongly endorse money, image, and status as prime concerns, they are less likely to engage in ecologically beneficial activities and the emptier and more insecure they will experience themselves to be. They will have also lower-quality interpersonal relationships. In turn, the more insecure people feel, the more they focus on material things. As materialism promises satisfaction but, instead, yields hollow dissatisfaction, it creates more craving. This massive and self-perpetuating addictive spiral is one of the mechanisms by which consumer society preserves itself by exploiting the very insecurities it generates.

Disconnection in all its guises—*alienation, loneliness, loss of meaning*, and *dislocation*—is becoming our culture's most plentiful product. No wonder we are more addicted, chronically ill, and mentally disordered than ever before, enfeebled as we are by such malnourishment of mind, body, and soul.

Chapter 21

They Just Don't Care If It Kills You: Sociopathy as Strategy

Not all psychopaths are in prison. Some are in the boardroom.

—R. D. Hare, Ph.D.[†]

Rob Lustig asserts that endocrinologists are the unhappiest of doctors, the most prone to suffer burnout. He would know, being one himself. Endocrinologists specialize in metabolic diseases, those of the hormone-producing glands such as the adrenals, the thyroid, the pituitary, and the pancreas. I asked him why gloom is such an occupational hazard for him and his colleagues. "Increasingly, we look after people who don't get better," Dr. Lustig replied. "It's like we're ladling water out of the proverbial leaky boat with a teaspoon while it keeps pouring in through a gaping hole at the bottom." He is all the more saddened by such futility since his subspecialty is working with children, among whom rates of obesity, diabetes, and related conditions have been escalating over the past several decades. Increasing numbers of children are showing markers of cardiovascular disease previously found only in adults.[‡]

The tide that keeps flooding the ship, Dr. Lustig says, stems from a culture in which many major corporations, unregulated

---

[†]   Professor emeritus, University of British Columbia, and a world-renowned expert on psychopathy.

[‡]   As Dr. Lustig documents in his book *The Hacking of the American Mind: The Science Behind the Corporate Takeover of Our Bodies and Brains.*

by governments, have deliberately and with the utmost ingenuity targeted the brain circuits of pleasure and reward to foster addictive compulsions. "That's why they hire neuroscientists and use fMRI machines," he told me. Neuroscience, originally meant to unlock the mysteries of consciousness and the brain, has become another handmaiden of the profit motive. There is actually a field called—and I'm not making this up—*neuromarketing*. "Their aim is to market happiness in a bottle," Lustig added. Or in a hamburger, or in a new smartphone or one of its many apps. In short, these corporations are acting as unscrupulous pushers in the open-air, perfectly legal market of mass addiction.

What the system sells as happiness is actually pleasure, a philosophical and economic distinction that makes all the difference between profit or loss. Pleasure, Rob Lustig pointed out, is "This feels good. I want more." Happiness, on the other hand, is "This feels good. I am contented. I am complete." This tracks perfectly with my understanding of addictions and brain chemistry. While similar in some ways, pleasure and happiness run on different neurochemical fuels: pleasure employs dopamine and opiates, both of which operate in short-term bursts, while contentment is based on the more steady, slow-release serotonin apparatus. It is very hard to get addicted to serotoninergic substances or behaviors. *All* addictions, however, commandeer the dopamine (incentive/motivation) and/or opiate (pleasure/reward) systems of the brain. Pleasure in the absence of contentment, and especially when sought in instant gratification, may be addictive, hence profitable. Contentment sells no products—except when evanescent, in which case it is no contentment at all, rather the bogus kind of "happiness" meant by *Mad Men's*[†] fictional ad whiz Don Draper when he

---

[†]   The critically acclaimed cable TV series about the mid-twentieth-century advertising business.

muses, "What is happiness? It's a moment before you need more happiness." True happiness, being a non-commodity, does not make itself obsolete.

Neuromarketing is a strategic invasion of human consciousness, consciously aimed at the hyperactivation and constant agitation of the dopamine/endorphin functions of the brain. This endeavor was abundantly cataloged, for example, in Michael Moss's 2013 work of investigative journalism on the food industry, *Salt Sugar Fat: How the Food Giants Hooked Us*, one of the most widely read books of the year. He, too, documented a deliberate corporate conspiracy to hook people on addictive junk foods, with no regard for health consequences. Painstaking work combining the expertise of scientists and marketing wizards was undertaken to find the "bliss spot," that perfect blend of sugar, salt, and fat‡ that would most excite the brain's pleasure centers. This mind-hacking—in today's parlance—to induce mass addictions directly undermines free will, and I mean that neurochemically. By design, the power of the prefrontal cortex to override cravings is dampened, and the capacity of the lower emotional circuits to subvert rational thought ratcheted up. It's an appalling example of how rampant free-enterprise materialism has hijacked the science of neurophysiology to deregulate the brain, just as it "deregulates" the financial markets.

To call such activities a "conspiracy" is no hyperbole, even if the word has lost some of its meaning through overuse, particularly in post-9/11 and COVID-19 times. Yet if nonsensical conspiracy theories take hold too readily among the credulous and the enraged, the underlying fear of being manipulated is downright sensible. The history of corporate wrongdoing, including

---

‡ Or, as the case may be, other addictive substances such as caffeine: for example, the dopamine-boosting drink Red Bull, which, if advertising were honest, would add a qualifier to its label, billing itself as a *"non-renewable* energy drink."

direct assaults on health, is a compendium of well-documented schemes to deceive the public for profit. Each one is secret until it's not. Far from aberrations, they are all rigorously faithful to the system's acquisitive logic. Life-impairing but lucrative deceptions have been repeatedly exposed in virtually every industry and in the most prestigious firms, from pharmaceuticals to the extraction of raw materials, from air travel to car manufacturing to food production. We need not belabor the point here, except to remind ourselves that the folks in control are powerful and "respectable" people, even philanthropists, in whose minds the denial of prosocial values has become acceptable, more virtue than sin, and either way, a requirement.

It no longer surprises me that even when exposed, such manipulations do not create any significant long-term pushback from a public too desensitized to protest, or too resigned to imagine meaningful alternatives. Popular outrage, even when it bursts into flame temporarily, does not translate into structural change. Massive public assaults on human health and humane ethics are, for lack of a better word, entirely normalized. "The greatest conspiracies are open and notorious," the whistleblower Edward Snowden told British comedian and podcaster Russell Brand in 2021. "They are not theories but practices: practices expressed through law and policy and systems of government, technology, finance . . . We become inured to it. This leaves us unable to relate *the banality of the methods of their conspiracy to the rapacity of their ambitions.*"[1] This is conspiracy realism, not conspiracy theory. That widespread chicanery in the top rungs of society is ignored or, at best, tolerated by much of the population speaks to the effectiveness of elite control and to the passivity of the social character inculcated by our culture.[†]

---

†   Social character was the topic of chapter 14.

Rob Lustig calls the United States "the drug capital of the world," and he isn't talking about cocaine, heroin, or methamphetamine, nor even mass-marketed opioids like OxyContin. He is referring to sugar, a substance that, in 2013, the chief health officer of the Netherlands declared to be "addictive and the most dangerous drug of all times." "Addictive" is not too strong a term. A Harvard Medical School study found that people ingesting foods with a high glycemic index—meaning, in practice, junk foods that rapidly elevate blood sugar levels—got hungrier faster. On fMRI scans, they showed activation of the same brain regions stimulated by drugs such as cocaine or heroin.[2] Never missing a profitable beat, multinational corporations vigorously market sugar-laden concoctions to children, and prey on people who, owing to trauma, penury, and grinding oppression, are especially vulnerable to addictive substances. The latter include poor Black people in the United States and the denizens of Brazil's makeshift villages, the *favelas*. In many "developing" countries—a term that manages to be both condescending and euphemistic—troops of impoverished women are recruited to go door-to-door, selling such junk products to already undernourished compatriots.

The costs in health and longevity are far greater than even the worst projections for the COVID-19 pandemic. A report published in the *Lancet* found that eleven million deaths worldwide in 2017 could be attributed to diets deficient in vegetables, seeds, and nuts but laden with salt, fat, and sugar.[3] According to another study presented to the American Heart Association, sugary drinks alone may be responsible for up to 180,000 deaths around the world.[4] Coca-colonization, this has been called.

As a result of the corporatization of agriculture, a built-in outcome of the North American Free Trade Agreement, Mexico now vies with the United States for world leadership in obesity and its related diseases. "About 73% of the Mexican population is overweight, compared to one-fifth of the population in 1996, according to a study by the Organisation for Economic Co-operation and Development," the BBC reported in August 2020.[5] "Childhood obesity tripled in a decade and about a third of teenagers are [overweight] as well," according to CBS News. "Experts say four of every five of those heavy kids will remain so their entire lives."[6] More than four hundred thousand cases of diabetes are diagnosed in Mexico every year, with the numbers dying exceeding those killed in that country's appalling drug wars.[†]

Canada is swiftly catching up, with Australia, New Zealand, and Asia also in the race. In China, the adult obesity rate doubled in the two decades between 1991 and 2011, from 20.5 to 42.3 percent. There, too, Coca-Cola has wielded major influence in shaping government policy to enhance its profits.[7]

British prime minister Boris Johnson, formerly a man of notorious girth, became a weight-loss evangelist in the wake of his close encounter with the novel coronavirus, which, for a few days in 2020, had him in intensive care. "I'm not normally a believer in nannying, or bossing type of politics," said the PM after his recovery. "But the reality is that obesity is one of the real co-morbidity factors. Losing weight is, frankly, one of the ways you can reduce your own risks from COVID." He instituted government policies advocating healthier eating habits and regulating the advertisement and marketing of junk food. Spot-on, one might say. Yet, had he chosen to be scientific, Johnson might have listed poverty and being BAME—Black, Asian, or minority ethnic—as major risk factors for coronavirus morbidity and death. He might also have

---

[†]   In a desperate and probably futile attempt to reduce high obesity and diabetes rates, the Mexican state of Oaxaca has banned the sale of junk food and sugary drinks to children.

recognized obesity itself to be a socially engendered condition, dramatically on the rise internationally since the advent of the austerity and laissez-faire policies his party has championed for almost a half century now. Nearly two-thirds of adults in his country are obese or overweight, as are a third of children six years of age. According to the National Health Service, in the statistical year 2018–2019 there were 876,000 hospital admissions in Britain in which obesity was a factor, an increase of nearly 25 percent over the preceding twelve months.[8]

Not all food- or tobacco-related ill health can be ascribed directly to the commercialized "hacking" of the public mind, any more than the epidemic of prescription drug deaths is due exclusively to corporate manipulation. It is truer to say that the manipulation is made possible by the very stresses, disconnections, and dislocations of life entrenched by globalized capitalism. Ted Schrecker and Clare Bambra—professors of public health policy and of public health geography, respectively, at Durham University—have studied the health impacts of recent economic trends. "The countries which are currently the most neoliberal and experienced the greatest increases in neoliberalism during 1980–2008 . . . had correspondingly higher rates of obesity and overweight," they note. "This shows that the timing and international spread of the obesity epidemic mirror the rise and diffusion of neoliberalism."[9] That's the issue Boris Johnson was not about to confront in his weight-loss promotion campaign.

The worldwide obesity epidemic is a marker of the international stress epidemic discussed in our previous chapters, and of the attendant lifestyle challenges endemic to our modern era: lack of time, lack of exercise, growing insecurity, lack of family connection, loss of community, and erosion of the social network. There are many aspects of life that drive people to follow unhealthy diets and engage in self-harming habits, the main culprits being emotional pain, stress, and social dislocation. And as we have seen, compulsive overeating—like all addictions—is itself a response to stress and a way of soothing the impacts of trauma. "It's not what you are eating," someone cleverly said, "it's what's eating you." Stress induces people to "choose" unhealthy foods and to put on weight in the wrong places, promoting disease. It also depletes the serotonin/contentment circuits, shifting the brain's functioning toward the short-term, dopamine-fueled pleasure mechanisms.

The corporate elite, served by their amply compensated minions in the fields of science and psychology, well know how to profit off the stress generated by the system that gives them power. They wouldn't be doing their jobs if they didn't.

Big Food is no outlier when it comes to hoodwinking the public. The pharmaceutical industry "systematically manipulated the entire country for 25 years," wrote Nicholas Kristof in the *New York Times* in 2017, "and its executives are responsible for many of the 64,000 deaths of Americans last year from drugs—more than the number of Americans who died in the Vietnam and Iraq wars combined. The opioid crisis unfolded because greedy people—Latin drug lords and American pharma executives—lost their humanity when they saw the astounding profits that could be made." And the government response? In Kristof's words, "Our policy was: 'You get 15 people hooked on opioids, and you're a thug who deserves to rot in hell; you get 150,000 people hooked, and you're a marketing genius who deserves a huge bonus.' "[10] It has been broadly established that Big Pharma, such as Purdue, the company controlled by the Sacklers, promoted opiates like

OxyContin to doctors as relatively safe analgesics. They did so in full awareness of their drugs' addictive potential. Over the years, hundreds of thousands of people have died.

All the while, the Sacklers garbed themselves in the cloak of virtuous public benefactors: an established phenomenon in the world of major-league philanthropy. The drug-profiteering family bestowed their largesse—and their names, beautifully embossed—on hospitals, medical schools, and museums around the world, from North America to Europe to Israel.

Kristof's point about differential consequences was all too close to my own experience. If any patient of mine in the Downtown Eastside was arrested selling a couple of ounces of cocaine—as many were, in their desperation to fund their arbitrarily illegalized habits—they were subject to imprisonment. Meanwhile, this week as I write, a court settlement was announced that infuriated many: at the cost of a paltry $4.5 billion fine, the Sacklers get to keep their wealth and face no criminal charges. Free as birds—vultures, perhaps—holding billions in their beaks.[†]

To be fair, the drug companies were only following their tobacco-industry exemplars who for decades, and with equally casual disregard for human life, denied and actively concealed the health hazards of their product, and who continue to resist efforts at regulation.[11] Tobacco kills about forty-five thousand Canadians annually, ten times as many as die from opioid overdoses—not to mention the hundreds of thousands who suffer smoking-related illness and debility. The worldwide death toll due to tobacco use exceeds seven million each year.[12] For every person who dies, thirty live with chronic illness.

---

†   This settlement has since been overturned on appeal and, as this book goes to edits, the court saga continues. More on the Sacklers in chapter 33.

Like the skilled pushers they are, the tobacco corporations miss no angle, targeting the most vulnerable. "For decades, menthol cigarettes have been marketed aggressively to Black people in the United States," reported the *New York Times*. "About 85 percent of Black smokers use menthol brands, including Newport and Kool, according to the Food and Drug Administration. Research shows menthol cigarettes are easier to become addicted to and harder to quit than plain tobacco products."[13] (As of this writing, the Biden administration has indicated plans to ban the sale of menthol cigarettes.) Now restricted, though far from curtailed, in hawking their products in the wealthier countries, the multinational merchants of tobacco, alcohol, sugary drinks, and junk food have cast their gaze on the so-called developing world, where rules are more lax and governments even more pliant. Millions will fall ill, millions will die—not "will," are dying.

What kind of people would knowingly cause the illness and deaths of countless millions? Law professor Joel Bakan,[†] whose book *The Corporation: The Pathological Pursuit of Profit and Power* became the basis of the award-winning documentary of the same name, set out to assess corporations in the light of standard mental health measures we would apply to people. The appraisal is entirely fair, given that U.S. law has, since the late 1800s, regarded corporations as "persons." "Viewed from such a vantage," he told me, "many corporations meet the criteria of 'sociopaths,' acting without a conscience: not caring about what happens to other people as a consequence of their actions, having no compulsion to comply with social or legal norms, not feeling guilt or remorse." It's an airtight case—from a mental health perspective, how else to regard nonaccountable "persons" with limitless power, quite willing to obscure truths and broadcast lies, sowing illness and death?

---

† See chapter 13.

If anyone requires a second opinion, the New York psychoanalyst Steven Reisner is ready with one.[‡] "Narcissism and sociopathy describe corporate America," he told me. "But it's flat-out wrong to think in twenty-first-century America that narcissism and sociopathy are illnesses. In today's America, narcissism and sociopathy are *strategies*. And they're very successful strategies, especially in business and politics and entertainment." Call it the myth of abnormal, this notion that somehow these antisocial traits go against the grain; truer to say they are the grain.

Why would such strategies be pursued? That patron saint of unbridled free-market ideology, the Nobel Prize–winning economist Milton Friedman, put no fine point—nor any ethical handbrake—on it. "Well, first of all, tell me," he once remarked in an interview, "is there some society you know that doesn't run on greed? You think Russia doesn't run on greed? You think China doesn't run on greed? . . . The world runs on individuals pursuing their separate interests."[14] Friedman also laid down as an ironclad rule that "there is one and only one social responsibility of business—to use its resources and engage in activities designed to increase its profits."[15] Note the use of the phrase "social responsibility": Friedman believed to his bones that self-interested, minimally regulated corporate capitalism is *what's best for everyone*. Thus spoke not a mustache-twirling movie villain self-aware of his perfidy, bound to get his comeuppance by film's end, but a theorist whose still-eminent standing in "normal" political-economic circles speaks volumes about what sort of society we are.

Bakan told me that he originally imagined corporations as unhealthy life-forms plaguing "a basically healthy, democratic society." He no longer believes that. "The pathology has metastasized—the pathogen has infected the host," he said.

---

‡   Reisner hosts *Madness: The Podcast,* an engaging look at "where psychology and capitalism collide."

Humanity faces no challenge of more gravity and consequence than the climate crisis that, as of this writing, is devastating many areas of the world and threatens planetary life itself. To my mind, no issue illustrates more vividly the sociopathic behavior of those in corporate and government spheres who had plenty of advance warning but for decades minimized or denied the menace for the sake of profit or power.

It was in the year 1800 that the great German naturalist and geographer Alexander von Humboldt first sounded the alarm about the impact of human activity on the climate, having seen the environmental damage wreaked by colonial plantations in Venezuela. He prophesized that our interference with the ecology could have "unforeseeable impact on future generations."[16] Over two centuries later, more than eleven thousand leading scientists from 153 nations found it necessary to endorse an urgent warning. "We declare clearly and unequivocally that planet Earth is facing a climate emergency," they wrote. "To secure a sustainable future, we must change how we live. [This] entails major transformations in the ways our global society functions and interacts with natural ecosystems."[17] Four decades earlier the first international climate conference had been held in Geneva, and largely ignored. Ever since then, alarms have been sounded again and again by scientists, activists, and health professionals around the world. In 1992, long before the climate advocate Greta Thunberg called out the world's politicians on their failure to protect the climate—indeed, well before Thunberg was born—the Canadian activist Severn Cullis-Suzuki, aged twelve, addressed leaders gathered at the first U.N. Earth conference in Rio de Janeiro. "Coming up here today, I have no hidden agenda," she said. "I am fighting for my future. Losing my future is not like losing an election, or a few points on the stock market. I am here to speak for all generations to come." We know what has been done—or, more accurately, *not* done—in the face of a looming catastrophe that is now affecting people's well-being around the world and threatens the very basis of our existence.

"Health is inextricably tied to climate change," warned the *Journal of the American Medical Association* back in 2014. The health impacts are well documented. Four years later, the *Lancet* reported: "Vulnerability to extremes of heat has steadily risen since 1990 in every region, with 157 million more people exposed to heatwave events in 2017, as compared with 2000."[18] Yet more recently, in what the *Wall Street Journal* called "an unprecedented plea," editors of two hundred health journals internationally, including the *Lancet*, the *British Medical Journal*, and the *New England Journal of Medicine*, called the failure of political leaders to confront the climate crisis "the greatest threat to global public health."[19] The harms of climate change include acute and chronic physical illness such as cardiovascular disease and susceptibility to infections, along with mental health challenges. Especially at risk are people with heart or kidney conditions, diabetes, and respiratory ailments. I need hardly mention food and water insecurity, major stressors already affecting millions.

Underlying the active and callous disregard of our Earth's health is the sociopathology of the most powerful entities, whose planetary poison-pushing removes any hint of metaphor from this book's subtitular phrase "toxic culture." "The oil companies pumped billions of dollars into thwarting government action. They funded think tanks and paid retired scientists and fake grassroots organizations to pour doubt and scorn on climate science. They sponsored politicians, particularly in the U.S. Congress, to block international attempts to curtail greenhouse gas emissions. They invested heavily in greenwashing their public image." So reported the *Guardian* in 2019, a scenario also amply chronicled by the *New York Times* and many other publications. Nor are we talking only about the past: in 2020 the top one hundred or more American corporations channeled their political donations largely to lawmakers with a record of stalling climate legislation. No doubt, such openhanded generosity owed much to the certainty that these same politicians would also avidly support the interests of big business. Compared with financial gain the climate is, well, small change.

From a medical perspective Joel Bakan's comment about the pathology metastasizing could not be more apt. If in the body a cell begins to multiply at the expense of the entire organism, destroying tissues nearby and spreading to other organs, robbing the host of energy, disabling its defenses, and eventually threatening its very life, we call that unchecked growth a cancer. Such abnormal and malignant transformation is now besetting our world, run by a system that seems rigged against life. The abnormal has become the norm; the unnatural has become the inescapable.

In the logic of profit, greed is creed, and health nothing but collateral damage. "It's not that they want you to die," the endocrinologist Rob Lustig told me in a tone of mock reassurance. "They only want your money. They just don't care if it kills you."

Chapter 22

The Assaulted Sense of Self: How Race and Class Get Under the Skin

My brother raised his hand when Dad told us we were
Indians, and through the tears in his eyes he asked our father,
"But we're still part human, right?"
—Helen Knott, *In My Own Moccasins*

As a child in postwar Hungary, in the aftermath of the genocide that had claimed the lives of most of my extended family and community, I was often insulted for my ethnic identity. I'll never forget how a friend came to my defense once: "Leave him alone," he chided the bullies. "It's not his fault he's Jewish." I carried the corrosive shame of that blameless "fault" for a long time, having absorbed other people's view of me.

Despite such firsthand experience of having been "othered" early in life, my status since adolescence as a privileged member of a dominant culture—a white-presenting middle-class male in North America—has also seeped into how I see the world. I am still prone to having blind spots around what people from other backgrounds are carrying, what trials they must endure. It's all too easy for the privileged among us to assume we walk the same streets as everyone else. Though a satellite view of Earth may suggest we do, that's not how it plays out at ground level. Do

Indigenous people in Canada or Black people in America tread the same ground as their Caucasian counterparts, face the same daily obstacles, navigate the same sorts of adversity? Surely not.

Early in his posthumously published autobiography, the revolutionary Black leader Malcolm X recalls his self-abasement when he tried to remake himself according to the standards of a society that rejected who he was. As a young man he was "conking," searing his scalp to obliterate his hair's natural curliness. "This was my first really big step toward self-degradation," he writes, "literally burning my flesh to have it look like a white man's hair."[1] Many years later, as a leader in the Nation of Islam, Malcolm challenged his audience to confront their own self-loathing. "Who taught you to hate the texture of your hair?" he asked. "Who taught you to hate the color of your skin to such an extent that you bleach to get like the white man? Who taught you to hate the shape of your nose and lips? Who taught you to hate yourself from the top of your head to the soles of your feet?" I winced in recognition when I read those words, having been all too conscious of my own easily identifiable "ethnic" appearance in Eastern Europe.

Malcolm's withering questions probe far beyond mental or emotional self-concept. Self-rejection has powerful physiological dimensions that pertain to every aspect of well-being. From an early age it is one of racism's sharpest and most intimate harms.

Canadian physician Dr. Clyde Hertzman[†] minted the concept of "biological embedding," by which he meant precisely what we've been looking at in myriad ways in this book: that our social environments and experiences, in his words, "get under the skin early in life," shaping our biology and development. Hertzman

---

[†]   Until his untimely death at age fifty-nine, Dr. Hertzman was professor of the Department of Health Care and Epidemiology at the University of British Columbia and Canada research chair in population health and human development. He was internationally renowned for his explorations of the social determinants of health.

meant "under the skin" literally, referring to what life events do to skin, nervous system, and viscera. It is no outcome of genetic destiny, for example, that in Canada Indigenous people suffer more illness and die earlier than others. Racism and poverty do get under the skin, in so many ways.

This chapter is a brief, trauma-informed look at a huge subject: how two major social determinants of health—race and economic status—become biologically embedded. I'll take up a third, gender, in the next chapter. But although I'm treating them separately here, it would be a fallacy to think of them as independent operators. For many individuals they intersect in ways that make it almost impossible to tease out what is a function of which—hence the term "intersectional." It is difficult to separate, for example, the health impacts of being a woman in a patriarchal system and at the same time a person of color in a racialized climate, of being poor in a culture that worships wealth, or living as a gay or lesbian person in a society where homophobia is still endemic.

An African Canadian-British friend of mine, the public speaker, mindfulness teacher, and author Valerie (Vimalasara) Mason-John, has intimately experienced the nexus of all four of these variables.[‡] All contributed to their descent into bulimia and substance addiction, beginning with the racial torment they experienced as a young child in Britain at the Barnardo orphanage, Barkingside, Essex. "Daily I'd have this kid who would come up and say, 'Hey, woggamatter? Niggamind—go black home and eat your coon flakes, and you'll be all white in the morning.' That was relentless," Vimalasara told me. "People kept telling me my hands looked like a monkey's. By age four I was trying to bleach my skin." And now as an adult in Canada, they said, "It

---

‡   Vimalasara's preferred pronouns are "they/them." The racial pejoratives are cited above with their express permission.

is impossible to isolate my sexuality from my gender and/or my race—they can be all at play when someone is relating to me. The intersection of these determinants has impacted my whole life. Who knows which identity of mine will be oppressed when I walk out of my home in the morning. Sometimes it is all, and sometimes it's just one, but the identity that continually becomes a threat to others is my Black skin."

As the Black American writer Ta-Nehisi Coates tersely asserts, "Race is the child of racism, not the father." In other words, the very concept of race emerges from the distorted imagination of the racist. Though racism's impacts are real, in physiological or genetic terms race does not exist. Superficial differences in skin color, body morphology, or facial features do not create "races." Historically the idea of race arose from the impulse of European capitalism to enrich itself by subjugating, enslaving, and, if necessary, destroying Indigenous people on other continents, from Africa to Australia to North America. Indeed, the word "race" did not exist in any meaningful way until it was created in the late eighteenth century. Psychologically, on the individual level, the "othering" racism entails is an antidote to self-doubt: if I don't feel good about myself, at least I can feel superior to *somebody* and gain a sense of power and status by claiming privilege over them. "The anti-Semite," wrote the French philosopher Jean-Paul Sartre, "is a man who is afraid. Not of the Jews, to be sure, but of himself and his own consciousness, of his liberty, of his instincts, of his responsibilities, of solitariness, of change, of society, and of the world . . . The existence of the Jew merely permits the anti-Semite to stifle his anxieties."[2] The pernicious impact of racism flows from its very nature, which is to see and treat another, in essence no different from you, according to your self-serving, resentful, and twisted fantasy of who they are. The brilliant writer James Baldwin once said, "What white people have to do is try and find out in their own hearts why it was necessary to have a n—— in the first place. If you, the white people, invented him, then you've got to find out why."

Recalling the shame I felt as a child at being Jewish, I completely resonate with a powerful formulation by the Black American psychologist Kenneth Hardy:[†] the "assaulted sense of self." In this state, Dr. Hardy says, "the soul of one's being gets perpetually punctured . . . It's when one's definition of self is defined by someone else. It is when my sense of self is defined by what I am not, rather than by what I am." He adds, "Who I am thus becomes a response to how I am defined; it's always in response to something else."[3]

The author Helen Knott, who is of Dane-zaa, Nehiyaw, and European descent, knows well this experience of the assaulted self by virtue of being Indigenous in modern Canada. "I became 'the other' in my eighth-grade social studies class," she writes. "The outcast. The wild Indian. Merciless Indian savage."[4] The stain and the strain of being defined by outside prejudices could not but penetrate her core sense of who she was.

Knott and I met by Zoom one winter morning in 2019, shortly after I read *In My Own Moccasins*, her poetic memoir of trauma, addiction, and redemption. "Othering was socialized into me," she said. "It was present within my family and how they interacted with the outside world. With my mom, there was a lot of 'You're not brown enough, you're not white enough.' No matter where you go, you're always aware of your otherness within a room. You could be sitting somewhere and you're calculating, 'Is this a safe space for me to have the conversation that I want to have? Do I make myself less visible or more visible?' It's an almost unconscious calculation of safety, almost at all times."

---

† Kenneth V. Hardy, Ph.D., is president of the Eikenberg Academy for Social Justice and a professor of marriage and family therapy at Drexel University, Philadelphia.

Knott had been reflecting on how the women in her life hold racism's marks in their very bearing—"even," she says, "how their bodies transform in public [white-dominated] spaces." She gave me a vivid example: "When my grandma goes into a grocery store, ever since I can remember, she will suddenly . . . her shoulders will hunch in, and her head will face the ground. She doesn't make eye contact with people; she will just shuffle along. This happens in any kind of larger public space. Her whole presence changes. Outside of that, she has been our matriarch where she *holds* space. She's the one telling stories and calling people and telling people to do this or that. In her old age, because now she's seventy-nine, it changed a bit in the last few years. She's taken a few more liberties because she's like, 'I don't care anymore.'"

When asked why he "keeps bringing up race all the time," Dr. Hardy offers a response as medically apt as it is candid: "If I don't bring it up, I have all these physiological things inside." Emotional suppression and its biological harms are, indeed, among the many wounds racism inflicts. In chapter 3 we mentioned that racism shortens lives. A study that examined the chromosome-protective telomeres of Black American men found that overt experiences of racism *and* the assaulted sense of self, including the internalization of racial bias, "operate jointly to accelerate biological aging."[5]

Socially entrenched bigotry, whether in its subtle or overt forms, takes an enormous and, until very recently, mostly unspoken toll on health. This silence—not in science or data but in public discourse—was finally breached following the May 2020 murder of George Floyd and the advent of the novel coronavirus. The former, one of a string of countless such killings of unarmed Black people, brought home to millions worldwide the venomous racial injustices structurally entrenched in Western societies, most egregiously in the United States; the second demonstrated all too clearly that police brutality is but one vector of lethal racism. Latino and Black Americans have been three times more likely to be infected by COVID-19 and twice more prone to dying of it. In Britain, too, communities of color were disproportionately affected, owing to deprived housing conditions, economic disadvantage, and preexistent health problems rooted in discrimination and inequity.

Behind the studies and dismal statistics are the tormented lives of real human beings, depicted with bitter eloquence by many great authors. No research paper, for example, could possibly convey the stress-inducing experience of confinement, deprivation, fear, and suppressed outrage with more force than the words of Ta-Nehisi Coates as he recalls his youth in inner-city Baltimore: "We could not get out. The ground we walked on was trip-wired. The air we breathed was toxic. The water stunted our growth. We could not get out . . . Not being violent enough could cost me my body. Being too violent could cost me my body. We could not get out."[6]

"In America, it is traditional to destroy the black body—*it is heritage*," Coates states. While that destruction has been most blatantly evident in the lynch-mob rampages of bygone eras and in officially sanctioned violence persisting to this day, it achieves more insidious and even more widespread effects through the direct imprint of racism on the body. Importantly, these effects show up in people's physiology as if programmed there from the start. "Heart disease, diabetes, obesity, depression, substance abuse, school success, premature mortality, disability at retirement, and accelerated aging and memory loss all have social determinants in early life," Clyde Hertzman pointed out.[7] Not surprisingly, Black people in the United States suffer more diabetes, obesity, and hypertension, along with life-threatening complications such as strokes, for which their risk is doubled.

For example, a forty-five-year-old African American man re-siding in the Southeast has the stroke propensity of a fifty-five-year-old white man in the same region and a sixty-five-year-old white man residing in the Midwest. Reviewing the literature, I found it most stunning that the race differentials in blood pressure rates are measurable already in children and adolescents.[8] Why? "Hyper" means "too much," "tension" means "tension," and racial discrimination induces it. For similar reasons, Black American children are six times more likely than non-Black kids to die of asthma.[9]

This is all of a piece with what we have seen throughout this book. For young children, being subordinated in their social milieu—whether family or classroom—leads to heightened car-diovascular, nervous system, and hormonal responses to stress and higher risks of chronic medical conditions. That remains true for adults as well. The suppression of individual authen-ticity plays havoc with biology, breeding illness; even greater mayhem will ensue for bodies belonging to groups whose self-suppression has been systemically imposed, often with great violence.

James Baldwin once said that "to be a Negro in this country and to be relatively conscious, is to be in a rage almost all the time." Baldwin uttered those words in 1961. They still ring true, decades of civil rights advances and a Black president later. Bald-win also understood that rage on its own, even if come by hon-estly, could not be the end of the story. In the very next sentence, he described "the first problem" as being "how to control that rage so that it won't destroy you."[10] I am convinced such anger, and moreover its obligatory suppression in a society that fears and punishes Black rage, contributes to the elevated risk Black American men face for dying of prostate cancer and Black Ameri-can women do of succumbing to cancer of the breast.

The racial differences, independent of genetics, defy economic categories: for example, the abovementioned breast cancer risk for Black women cuts across class lines. Around birth, Black mothers are dying at three to four times the rate of non-Hispanic white mothers. And their infants are at least twice as likely to die as white babies—another trend that holds across education levels and socioeconomic status. "Put simply," warned a recent article in the magazine of Harvard's T. H. Chan School of Public Health, "for black women far more than for white women, *giving birth can amount to a death sentence.*"[11] And how not to be startled at the finding that having a non-Black doctor doubles a Black baby's risk of dying—the baby's "penalty," we might say, for the crime of being born while Black.[12] For white infants the race of the physician makes no difference. In short, it is "racism, not race itself, that threatens the lives of African American women and infants," a recent review of multiple studies concluded.[13]

We have seen how emotional stressors, among which racism ranks as a frontrunner, get "under the skin": the triggering of inflammation-promoting genes, the premature aging of chromosomes and cells, tissue damage, elevation of blood sugar, the narrowing of airways. Even *without* economic disadvantage, the stresses of racial prejudice mount over time, toxifying the body and undermining its capacity to maintain itself. That allostatic load, the wear and tear, just becomes too much. When so-called biomarkers such as blood pressure, stress hormones, blood sugar indicators, inflammatory proteins, and lipids were measured, they were significantly higher in Blacks than in whites, with Black women showing consistently higher scores than Black men. In both races poor people scored higher than their economically advantaged counterparts, but *non-poor* Blacks had a greater probability of high scores than *poor* whites. Differences were especially pronounced among non-poor Black women, compared with non-poor white women—once more illustrating the intersection of race and gender as they determine health in a racially stratified society.[14]

"When you have racism as a mechanism, there's generational trauma," the Tennessee psychotherapist Eboni Webb told me. The softness of her voice during our Zoom call could not mute the harsh realities of her family history. "All the women in my family are very fair," Webb said. "We didn't have Caucasians come into our story willingly, but forcibly. The women in my family have been subjected to brutalization through the generations. That assault itself is trauma, but the trauma is also how we have had to armor ourselves. I remember my parents telling me if something happens at school, you come home and cry. Don't cry there. Talk about emotions being traumatizing: What happens to a people that can't show the full range of their emotions? For people of color raising children, the lens is not just 'racism exists,' but 'racism can be life-threatening.' Our childhood experience is one of learning how to live out of our survival defenses, and that just hasn't changed. We don't have the luxury of raising our kids in any ideal manner." Living out of survival defenses is a formula for the lifelong activation of the body's stress apparatus, with myriad consequences.

I was thirteen in 1957 when, along with nearly thirty-eight thousand fellow Hungarians, refugees from a brutal Stalinist dictatorship, my family and I were welcomed with open arms by Canada. The North really seemed true and strong and free, in line with the words of this country's national anthem. What I didn't know and what no one was speaking of was that in the same year, even as we were adjusting to the advantages of life in British Columbia, a four-year-old First Nations child, Carlene, had a pin stuck in her tongue on her first day at a federally mandated, church-run residential school not far from where I lived. Her crime had been to speak her Native language in the classroom. For an hour this little girl could not put her tongue back in her mouth for fear of cutting her lips. Soon after, years of sexual abuse began. By age nine Carlene was an alcoholic and later became dependent on opiates to soothe her pain. We met at a healing ceremony not long ago and that was when, sobbing and trembling with emotion, she told me her story. I thought I had heard everything. I had not. Now a grandmother and years sober, she grieves to see her grandchildren suffer the throes of addiction. For her, our national anthem was a cruel hoax: there was no "true North strong and free!" Nor is there yet.

And so it is that in Canada, where looking down on Americans is something of a national indulgence, we have nothing to feel superior about. Police prejudice, including brutal violence, is notoriously inflicted on Indigenous peoples and on people of color. Nearly 30 percent of the jail population in this country is composed of Indigenous people, who make up no more than 5 percent of the general population.[†]

About the same proportion of my impoverished, addicted clients in Vancouver's Downtown Eastside were of Indigenous background, the inheritors and carriers of a toxic colonial legacy of extermination and expulsion; the genocidal destruction of communal existence; many decades of the involuntary placement of Indigenous children in state-enforced, rigidly Christian residential schools where Native languages and culture were outlawed on pain of punishment and a culture of appalling, entrenched sexual and physical abuse reigned; the period known as "the Sixties Scoop,"[‡] when the Canadian child-welfare (!)

[†]   Among women inmates, the ratio is 50 percent.

[‡]   In fact, the phenomenon lasted at least into the 1980s.

system abducted thousands of First Nations children from their homes and placed them with non-Indigenous families; atrocious living situations on reservations; ongoing multigenerational trauma; and the persisting encroachment on and pollution of Indigenous lands for economic projects that profit distant corporations. In 2021 the world was horrified at the discovery of thousands of small bodies at the former sites of residential schools across Canada. Many other thousands are known to have disappeared whose remains are yet to be found and whose deaths, deeply etched and grieved in the consciousness of their families and communities, have not until recently been formally acknowledged by the governmental and ecclesiastic institutions responsible. Nearly two thousand unmarked graves have been identified as of late 2021. Another five thousand to ten thousand such graves likely exist and await finding.

Health and living conditions among our First Nations populations are scandalous, matched only by the chronic failure of governments at all levels to remedy the social, economic, and cultural circumstances that foster them. The lifespan of Indigenous people is fifteen years shorter than that of other Canadians, infant mortality two to three times higher, and type 2 diabetes four times more widespread: this among a population that knew no diabetes a little over a century ago.[15] Elevated blood sugars are the least of it: diabetes is a leading cause of blindness, heart and kidney failure, and limb amputations. First Nations people are developing the disease in their forties, while among other sectors of the populace its onset is mostly in the eighth decade. The rates are rising. "By 2005," a 2010 study found, "almost 50% of First Nations women and more than 40% of First Nations men aged 60 or older had diabetes, [compared] with less than 25% of non–First Nations men and less than 20% of non–First Nations women aged 80 or older . . . First Nations adults are experiencing a diabetes epidemic that disproportionately affects women during their productive years."[16] Youth suicide rates in some Indigenous communities in Canada—First Nations, Inuit, Métis—were higher, according to a 1994 paper, than of any other culturally identifiable cohort in the world.[17] That continues to be the case.

Dr. Esther Tailfeathers is an Indigenous physician at the Blood Tribe Reserve in Alberta, a community that has had more than its share of severe substance dependence. She has invited me there twice to support their addiction programs, once in the wake of a three-month span when the community of 7,500 people lost 20 people to overdoses.[†] I asked Dr. Tailfeathers what it was like for her, now a successful professional, to grow up Indigenous in Canada. "At times horrific," she said. "We were one of the first Native families to move into the town of Cardston and rent a home. There was no school bus, so I had to walk a long way from the school on the other side of town. In grade one, I remember being followed by a group of children all the way home. The leader of this group picked up a big stone and threw it at me, and subsequently all the other children all threw stones. That was my first lesson on bullying and hatred." It wasn't her last. "When I was about nineteen, we had huge land-claim protests. I was beaten by the RCMP[‡] and thrown in jail.

"Sadly," she added, "you'd think things would have improved, because we know what had happened starting in residential

---

[†] By contrast, the province of British Columbia, with a population of 5 million, had 170 overdose deaths in July 2020, its highest ever. Proportionately to this Blood Tribe tragedy, B.C. would have lost over 4,000 people in one month.

[‡] RCMP: the Royal Canadian Mounted Police, the much-venerated national police organization among whose tasks, from its inception until today, has been to suppress the resistance of Indigenous people to the takeover of their lands and resources, and—during the residential school era—even their children.

schools and progressing forward. I don't think it has improved. It's gotten worse."

In 1848 a twenty-seven-year-old Berlin physician, Rudolf Virchow, was dispatched to Upper Silesia to investigate a deadly outbreak of typhus, a bacterial infestation then plaguing that impoverished, mostly Polish-speaking region of Germany. Along with his medical recommendations to counter the epidemic, Virchow caused an uproar by calling for social, political, and economic reforms. These included the introduction of Polish as an official language, separation of church and state, the creation of grassroots organizations, free education for both sexes, and, above all, *free and unlimited democracy."*

Virchow, these days honored as the father of modern pathology, disdained any separation of health from social conditions and culture. "Medicine has imperceptibly led us into the social field and placed us in a position of confronting directly the great problems of our time," he wrote. When challenged that his advice had more to do with politics than with medicine, Virchow issued his timeless retort: "Medicine is a social science, and politics nothing else but medicine on a large scale."

For all Virchow's renown, nearly two centuries later many doctors and scientists internationally are still striving in the face of political, professional, and social indifference to impart the broader lessons he derived from his investigations. When the contemporary epidemiologist Sir Michael Marmot[†] began his research into the impact of social stratification on health, he discovered that "inequality and health was completely off the agenda, bar a few trailblazers, writing about the evils of capitalism."[18] His

---

†   Sir Michael Marmot is professor of epidemiology and public health at University College London and in 2015 was president of the World Medical Association.

findings over the decades, published in numerous papers and books, have richly demonstrated the links between social and health disparities.

There's no need to repeat the science in detail. Both inequality and poverty stir the by now familiar brew of disturbed genetic function, inflammation, chromosomal and cellular aging, physiological wear and tear, hormonal disturbances, cardiovascular effects, and immune debility, all of which combine to bring illness, disability, and death. Biologically embedded in utero, in childhood, and throughout adolescence, all these are further exacerbated by adversity or threat at any stage of life. Stress hormone levels, for example, are much higher among children of low economic status—a biological hazard for future illness of many kinds.[19]

While we Canadians like to pride ourselves on our publicly funded health care system—and rightly so, especially as we peer over the 49th parallel at the law-of-the-jungle morass to our south—research shows that, at most, only about 25 percent of population health is attributable to health care. A full 50 percent is determined by social and economic environments.[20]

In my view there is plenty of reason to think that even this 50 percent is a serious underestimate. "Tell me your zip code," asserted a speaker at a 2014 Chicago health conference, "and I'll tell you how long you'll live." The life-expectancy gap between Chicago's poorest and most affluent neighborhoods is close to thirty years.[21] "Basically the difference between Iraq and Canada, within a few miles," a physician friend of mine commented. Canadians given to patriotic smugness might look at a similar study in our own country, done in 2006. In the city of Saskatoon, people in the poorest neighborhoods were two and a half times more likely to die in any one year. The infant mortality rate was triple in the city center than in its more affluent environs.[22]

In 1974 the anthropologist Ashley Montagu, cited earlier in this book, coined the phrase "sociogenic brain damage." Technologies since available to us confirm that stressed environments, including penury, do interfere with brain development. More recently, one scientist has called poverty a "neurotoxin." Brain scans of children and young people from deprived backgrounds have shown reduced surface area of the cerebral cortex, as well as smaller hippocampi and amygdalae—the subcortical regions involved in memory formation and emotional processing.[23] The brain's serotonin system in adolescents has been seen to be impaired by the stresses of poverty, increasing the risk for emotional turbulence.[24]

Toronto physician Gary Bloch, who serves an impoverished inner-city population, has been waging a campaign within the medical profession and beyond to raise awareness of how penury, race, and gender inequities intersect to promote disease. He wants doctors to recognize poverty as a risk factor for ill health, just as they would regard high blood pressure, smoking, or a poor diet. In practice, of course, these all tend to accompany one another. An affable forty-seven-year-old with an open smile and earnest demeanor, Gary—a long-time family friend of ours— writes prescriptions for diet supplements and refers people to financial aid workers to help with subsidies and tax problems: anything that could help ease their poverty. He shared a telling anecdote he heard from a social worker. "A physician says, 'Take this antibiotic three times . . . on a full stomach,' and I always laugh hysterically, and the women I know who are working poor laugh because they know that, 'Yeah, three meals, like what's he talking about three meals? A *full stomach?*' Another said, 'I had an old guy that needed diabetes medicine who lived in a shelter in Toronto . . . He was elderly and had mobility issues, and he didn't take any of his diabetic medication because the side effect it caused for him was diarrhea, and he was living in a shelter with sixty younger men and two toilets . . . He had no chance of getting to the toilet if he needed to quickly, so he wasn't going to take his pills.'"

"The missing piece I've been addressing is the link between knowing how social issues affect people's health and what to do about them," Gary told me—a Sisyphean task, given current social conditions. "Societal trauma is something I deal with all the time," he said. "I honestly cannot remember being taught that when I was in medical school. The traditional body of knowledge, medical culture, hasn't included interventions into social issues as a core part of what medicine is. Social trauma is a huge beast to come up against, and I can almost tangibly feel how strong and real an entity it is. It is daunting to try to confront it."

Were health professionals to take to heart information about social determinants, Canadian health expert Dennis Raphael mockingly suggests, they would stop issuing injunctions such as "Stop smoking," dispensing instead "Don't be poor" and related prescriptions: "Don't live in damp, low-quality housing"; "Don't work in a stressful, low-paying manual job"; "Don't live next to a busy major road or near a polluting factory"; "Be able to afford to go on a foreign holiday and sunbathe."[25] In other words, immigrate to a kinder, saner, more equitable parallel universe.

The beast of inequality has many tentacles with which to squeeze the life out of people's lives. For one thing, inequality's biological imprint doesn't affect only the very poor. In societies dominated by materialist principles, your relative position on the social ladder is a predictor of health across all strata. The linking of social rank with health is known as the *social gradient*, a slope that runs through all segments of society. It is easy to see why. Status grants people higher or lower degrees of control, the absence of which we already know to be a trigger for physiological stress and illness. This was shown in Michael Marmot's famous Whitehall studies, which found that people's rank in the British civil service correlated with their risks for heart disease, cancer, and mental health diagnoses.[26] The further down the position on the ladder, the higher the risks, independent of behavioral factors such as smoking or blood pressure. And this among a cohort of people with relative economic security and respectable, middle-class employment! "It is easier to vacate contaminated buildings than to change social structures," another leading chronicler of inequality, the British epidemiologist Richard Wilkinson, has commented. "We could speculate on how different the response would be if the slope of the social gradient in death and disease ran in the opposite direction, so that the highest-status people did the worst."[27]

Finally, amid a culture grounded in values of competition and materialism, we confront not only actual material conditions, pertinent as they are, but also how people are induced to *see* themselves. When people judge themselves or are judged by others according to financial achievement, being lower on the pyramid—even if in a relatively stable position—is itself a source of stress that undermines well-being. In the neuroscientist Robert Sapolsky's tart phrase, "Health is particularly corroded by your nose constantly being rubbed in what you do not have."[28]

Racism, poverty, inequality—in this society, people's faces are constantly rubbed in what they do not have and what the system daily reminds them they do not deserve.

Chapter 23

Society's Shock Absorbers: Why Women Have It Worse

Many of my female patients have no idea how to express their anger in healthy ways. Their suppressed anger contributes to their depression and, I believe, other medical symptoms as well.

—Julie Holland, M.D., *Moody Bitches*

This chapter aims to pierce an apparent medical mystery: Why do women suffer chronic illness of the body far more often than men, and why are they far more likely to be diagnosed with mental health conditions? I say "apparent," because from all that is known about the *bodymind* unity and our biopsychosocial nature, the answers are staring us in the face and are entirely predictable. That we don't recognize them has everything to do with our taking for granted the "normal" way of things in a culture of patriarchy, which, despite centuries of female resistance and progress, is ruled as often by subliminal male concerns as by overt power dynamics.

By "we" I'm referring not only to my profession of medicine and to society at large but to my own membership in the dominant sex class and the conditioning that such an affiliation has instilled in me. The truth is, I talk a much better gender-equality game than I sometimes play. It has taken, and continues to take, a very strong and determined woman—my wife, Rae—to keep alerting me, far more frequently than she should have to, to such realities in our own personal relationship. Looking around me, I sense that Rae and I are far from unique in manifesting how unconscious transactions between men and women play out daily in our culture, to the detriment of both sexes but especially at the cost of women's physical and emotional well-being.

The gender gap in health is real, if underappreciated. Women are more subject to chronic disease even long before old age, and they have more years of poor health and disability. "Women have it worse," a leading U.S. physician wrote recently, pointing out that women are at much higher risk of suffering chronic pain, migraines, fibromyalgia, irritable bowel syndrome, and autoimmune conditions like rheumatoid arthritis.[1] As noted in chapter 4, rheumatoid arthritis strikes women three times more often than it does men, lupus afflicts women by a disproportionate factor of nine, and the female-to-male ratio of multiple sclerosis has been rising for decades. Women also have a higher incidence of non-smoking-related malignancies. Even when it comes to lung cancer, a woman who smokes has double the chance of developing the disease.[2] Women also have double men's incidence of anxiety, depression, and PTSD.[3] "We are creating a new normal that isn't normal at all," the New York psychiatrist and author Julie Holland said when I interviewed her. "Perhaps one out of four or more American women right now are taking psychiatric medications, but if you add in things like sleeping pills and antianxiety meds, it's even higher. At any given staff meeting or PTA meeting, you've got about a quarter of the people, maybe more, who are taking daily medicines to moderate the way they feel and the way they behave." Alzheimer's dementia, too, seems to affect women disproportionately, just as it does Black people in the United States.[4]

That last fact alone ought to give us pause, containing as it does a significant clue as to the sources of such conditions. This book has, after all, been tracing the physiological impacts of developmental needs not being met, of stress and trauma. A consistent theme, beyond scientific doubt, has been that such emotional disturbances frequently trigger inflammation and other forms of physiological and mental harm. We might ask ourselves what burdens, what stresses, could women of any color and class share with Black people as a group? To me the answer is clear: they are both especially targeted by a culture that does not honor but demeans, distorts, and even impels people to suppress who they are. If that is an accurate assessment, we would expect that as these pressures intersect and compound each other, so would the incidence of disease rise. And it does, hugely.[5]

In the previous chapter we examined the biological embedding of racism and inequality and the resulting health disparities. Here we take the logical step of looking at the stresses of being female in a patriarchal society. These, too, get under the skin, playing havoc with all systems of the body, including the immune system.

A feisty thirty-eight-year-old small-town Manitoba firefighter I will call Liz told me of her health calvary when we met at a health conference in Toronto. By then she had been off the job for nearly a year with Crohn's disease, the intestinal autoimmune condition we encountered with Glenda's story in chapter 2, with such symptoms as fatigue, bloody stools, and abdominal cramping. When that condition resolved, she came down with manifestations of post-traumatic stress: debilitating fear, horrendous fantasies, insomnia. "I had shaking every day," she told me. "I was terrified of things I had no reason to be afraid of. I developed a mistrust of myself, not knowing how I would react in a lot of situations. I would cry at the drop of a hat for reasons I couldn't explain . . . when I was in public or when I was doing things. I had suicidal thoughts. And I used a lot of alcohol to manage these symptoms; I started drinking every day."

By now, it will be no surprise for the reader to learn that there was early trauma in Liz's history. She had been sexually abused at age seven, a violation that recurred throughout her childhood and adolescence. We know that sexual trauma is a risk factor for all manner of conditions of mind and body, and that girls are more likely than boys to be subjected to it. It is no longer a secret that well beyond childhood, females in this culture face the constant menace of sexual harassment in both private and professional life. While the advent of #MeToo advocacy has thrown necessary light on this scourge, it has long been thus. When my wife was sixteen, working at an ice-cream store, she heard her boss, old enough to be her grandfather, snigger to his son as they walked behind her: "I wouldn't mind getting into her pants." "I was shocked and disgusted and weirded out," Rae recalls. "I had never heard that expression before, but it felt gross. It was total objectification. Naturally, I kept silent." Or unnaturally, as it were—but either way, an experience for women and girls so regular as to be entirely "normal." And that is the case worldwide.[6] In such a sexualized and threatening climate, how can many women avoid developing that "assaulted sense of self" Dr. Kenneth Hardy identified as one of the deep imprints of racism, along with the damage it does to physiological and psychological well-being?[†]

We are hearing more and more about the hazards women face in traditionally male fiefdoms such as policing and firefighting. Along with the risk of secondary trauma faced by all first responders, an atmosphere of toxic masculinity on the job also took a toll on Liz, helping to trigger her gut inflammation and mental distress. If she showed vulnerability, upset at the tragedies she often witnessed, she was treated with derision and contempt. "It was a very macho scene," she recalled. "If you have any issues, you're a

---

†   For Dr. Hardy's concept of the assaulted sense of self, see chapter 22.

liability. Particularly if you are a woman, if you talk about it, you're considered a 'pussy.' They'll physically do stuff to you, sabotage you in some way. They threw tampons into my bed. I don't even know why. It was very much a symbol of femininity." Such bullying, too, assaults the body and the spirit. In a 2017 study of female firefighters, harassment and threats on the job were linked to suicidal ideation and more severe psychiatric symptoms,[7] findings that extend into other, less male-dominated professions as well. Not only mental but also physical health suffers.[8]

One healthy response to assault for any sentient creature is anger, a function of the evolutionary RAGE system in the brain whose purpose is to defend our boundaries, physical or emotional.[‡] My friend Dr. Julie Holland's comment in the epigraph to this chapter about women's anger being subdued to the detriment of their health tracks invariably with my observation among people with depression, autoimmune disease, and cancer. The ingrained abdication of the natural, spontaneous "no" is not restricted to women in this culture, but it is certainly imposed on them more widely and with greater force. The dynamic goes even deeper than deliberately holding in anger. As I distinguished earlier, repression (as opposed to suppression) occurs with no conscious awareness, as healthy feelings are banished beneath the level of consciousness: out of mind, out of sight. "Sugar and spice don't make space for anything that's not nice," Holland writes. "When we don't even know we're angry, we can't converse with the person responsible or otherwise tackle the problem. We cry; we eat; we soothe ourselves a thousand different ways."[9]

Early childhood mechanisms of self-suppression are reinforced by persistent, gendered social conditioning. Many women end up *self-silencing*, defined as "the tendency to silence one's thoughts

---

[‡] The neuroscientist Jaak Panksepp's identification of the brain's emotional systems CARE, PANIC/GRIEF, FEAR, PLAY, LUST, SEEKING, and RAGE was introduced in chapter 9.

and feelings to maintain safe relationships, particularly intimate relationships." This chronic negation of one's authentic experience can be fatal. In a study that followed nearly two thousand women over ten years, those "who reported that, in conflict with their spouses, they usually or always kept their feelings to themselves, had over four times the risk of dying during the follow-up compared with women who always showed their feelings."[10] As at home, so on the job. Another study showed that for women with non-supportive bosses, the squashing of anger—a natural adaptation to an environment in which to self-express would be to risk the loss of employment—increased the risk of heart disease.[11]

Recall from chapters 5 and 7 this array of self-abnegating traits that predispose to disease: a compulsive and self-sacrificing doing for others, suppression of anger, and an excessive concern about social acceptability. These personality features, found across all autoimmune conditions, are precisely the ones inculcated into women in a patriarchal culture. "I was denying myself as a person, denying my own desires, my wants," the first responder Liz said. "I was not paying attention to what I needed. Everyone else was far more important. My job was way more important than any concern that I had. I wasn't listening to myself in any regard."†

That "not listening to self" in order to prioritize others' needs is a significant source of the health-impairing roles women assume. It is among the medically overlooked but pernicious ways in which our society's "normal" imposes a major health cost on women. More on that below.

———

The sexualization of women is another source of ill health. Being valued for the use another can make of you is an assault on the self.

---

† Typically, none of the physicians treating Liz for her Crohn's ever inquired about her childhood traumas or current stresses or about her relationship to herself.

Girls and women are much more likely to be subjected to it, even sold the seductive idea that there is empowerment in it. The famed Canadian singer-songwriter Alanis Morissette spoke to me of the "headiness of the power" she recalls feeling when the male attention she received as a young pop star and TV celebrity began to take on a carnal hue. On the one hand, she recalls, "My intellect or my being-ness was diminished almost everywhere I turned, if not obliterated entirely. At the same time, all of a sudden, I have this power that I can wield in terms of being objectified or sexualized. In some ways it was enticing to feel empowered in this way, of being found attractive or straight-up statutorily raped.‡ There was an element of it that felt like power to me. It was sort of a young perspective of 'Hey, I'll take the power wherever I can get it.' " Mind you, the era Morissette is describing came decades before the emergence of online platforms like OnlyFans, where young women provide explicit "content" of all sorts to (overwhelmingly male) subscribers. A *New York Times* headline—in the Business section, no less— said it all: "Jobless, Selling Nudes Online, and Still Struggling."[12]

Young people are increasingly getting their first round of sex education from all too easily accessed online pornography. This is not Victorian erotica we are talking about, or your stepdad's *Hustler* collection. According to sociologist and *Pornland* author Gail Dines, the most popular (read profitable) kind of internet porn today is known in the industry as "gonzo," a genre characterized by "hard-core, body-punishing sex in which women are demeaned and debased."[13] These physically violent, emotionally hostile depictions of sex are being accessed by children at younger and younger ages—most sources place the average age of first exposure around eleven years old.

---

‡   "It took me years in therapy to even admit there had been any kind of victimization on my part," Morissette says in the recent documentary *Jagged.* "I would always say I was consenting, and then I'd be reminded like, 'Hey, you were fifteen—you're not consenting at fifteen.' Now I'm like, 'Oh, yeah, they're all pedophiles. It's all statutory rape."

Girls must contend with a toxic conflation of sexuality with sub-servience. Dines notes that women's and teen magazines are fea-turing ever more content aimed at helping women make the most of the cultural shift by diversifying their skills at pleasing someone else, usually a male. Girls are encouraged to be sexual not as a nat-ural or emergent self-expression, but as a means of attracting and keeping a partner, or a way of "empowering" themselves within an oppressive power structure. Where the normalization of abusive sex meets social media attention-seeking, the results can be grue-some: in summer 2020 a viral "TikTok challenge" came to light in which teenage girls share "post-coital videos of their bruised and cut limbs, in an attempt to emulate the recent Netflix kidnap-porn film, *365 Days*."[14] Meanwhile, pornography teaches many boys to associate pleasure with domination and a shutdown of tender feel-ings. The suppression of vulnerable emotions, of course, is one manifestation of male trauma, leading inexorably to a withering of compassion for others—especially when those others have some-thing we want, as in every instance of date rape or nonconsensual sexual aggression.

––––––––––––

The burdens placed on women in patriarchal cultures, and the ways these curtail and constrain women's prospects for authen-tic self-realization, have long been recognized—by women, that is. In 1792, thirty-three-year-old Mary Wollstonecraft published her astonishingly radical book *A Vindication of the Rights of Woman,* observing that women "*are made to assume an artificial character before their faculties have acquired any strength.*"[15] Almost exactly two hundred years later, the indomitable radical feminist thinker Andrea Dworkin captured the visceral dimensions of life in a female body under patriarchy: "That loss of self is a physi-cal reality, not just a psychic vampirism; and as a physical reality it is chilling and extreme, *a literal erosion of the body's integrity and its ability to function and to survive.*"[16] I'm not sure if Dworkin knew the science buttressing her claim, but her use of the word "literal" was exactly right.

Such loss of self, in Dworkin's phrase, becomes women's portion in large part because, in addition to their role in providing for their families' economic and physical needs, they are the designated emotional caregivers, at their own expense. The task of caring, in fact, falls largely to women in this culture. The contemporary phrase *emotional labor* does a great job of conveying the joblike nature of this stress-inducing, externally imposed role. Arguably to an even greater degree than housework and childbirth, this is the proverbial "woman's work" that "is never done."

Women often serve as the emotional glue—the connective tissue, if you like—that keeps nuclear and extended families and communities together. It is no coincidence they suffer far more than men do from diseases of *actual* connective tissue, among which lupus, rheumatoid arthritis, scleroderma, fibromyalgia, and their multiple relatives are variants. Thus, these conditions, as most chronic maladies do, reflect social dynamics along the lines we have been investigating throughout, not simply individual physiology gone rogue.

It is no secret that the stress of caregiving enfeebles the immune system. The caretakers of Alzheimer patients, for example—the vast majority of whom are women—have significantly diminished immune function and poorer wound healing, suffer more respiratory illness, and experience much higher rates of depression than well-matched non-caregiving peers.[17] Immunity is not the only function impaired by caregiver stress. Mothers looking after emotionally challenged children were found to have abnormal cortisol indicators, poorer metabolic functioning as measured by blood testing, and less healthy distribution of body fat.[18] As mentioned in chapter 4, they also have shorter telomeres, indicating premature aging.

The self-stifling expectation of caregiving while ignoring one's own emotions and needs has only been reinforced by the COVID-19 pandemic. "Mothers Are the 'Shock Absorbers' of Our Society," a *New York Times* headline pronounced in October 2020. A survey of married women found that childcare was a major source of stress, with women largely internalizing their frustrations. Rather than ask their spouses to step up their domestic contributions, the researchers found, "mothers blame themselves for these conflicts and feel responsible for reducing them, including by leaving the workforce, beginning use of antidepressants, or ignoring their own concerns about COVID-19."[19]

"All this extra work is affecting women's health," the British author Caroline Criado Perez stated in *Invisible Women*, her award-winning book about the implicit male-oriented bias in virtually all aspects of social, economic, cultural, academic, and even medical life. She gives a fascinating example of the asymmetrical apportioning of chores between men and women: "We have long known that women (in particular women under fifty-five) have worse outcomes than men following heart surgery. But it wasn't until a Canadian study came out in 2016 that researchers were able to isolate women's care burden as one of the factors behind this discrepancy, noticing that women who have bypass surgery tend to go right back into their caregiving roles, while men were more likely to have someone to look after them."[20]

Our society reinforces men's sense of being entitled to women's care in a way that almost escapes being put into words. I refer here to the automatic mothering women provide their male partners, the emotional sustenance that forms the invisible mortar of many heterosexual relationships: a very conventional dynamic that speaks to how tenacious gendered social constructs are, how thoroughly steeped we are in them. Some men are aware of the care they receive only in its absence and experience intense resentment when it is withdrawn; for example, when their female partner is preoccupied elsewhere, as when children are born. Many a woman has complained to me that her spouse becomes distant and punishing when she so much as catches a cold. As I observed in family practice, the children may lose out on maternal attention when the husband demands mothering energy from his partner. (It goes without saying that the father's stable attunement with his kids is also compromised when he assumes an infantile role in the partnership.) Oftentimes the mother loses vitality or develops physical or emotional symptoms signaling her body's rebellion against being overtaxed, imposing further strain on both her and her dependents.

I confess that what I "observed in family practice" mirrored the scenario played out in our own home, especially when our children were small. Nor is it a dynamic I can honestly relegate to the past. I interviewed Rae, the world's leading authority on this subject. "It's as if your tension is my responsibility, which I have neglected," she said. "You see me through a negative lens, like it must be about me somehow. I begin to question myself. I get careful around you, as if I'm walking on eggshells. I start feeling depressed, alienated, lonely. I'm left with a lot of resentment, and that's really stressful and frustrating." And then came the expert diagnosis. "I think there is a mother rage that erupts with male frustration, and it's taken out on the woman," Rae concluded. "She has to keep him happy. He does not differentiate his anger and his frustration from her—she becomes just an object to him."

When I spoke with Dr. Julie Holland, she averred that the disproportionately high rate of anxiety and depression in women stems, in large part, from their absorption of male angst and their culturally directed responsibility for soothing it. In that sense, women are ingesting the antidepressants and anxiolytics (anti-anxiety meds) for both sexes. "Girls are given all sorts of overt and covert messages that the way to get along is to go along and seek consensus, make sure everybody else is happy," she said. "You know, they see their mothers. I definitely saw my mom doing this for my father—making dinner, doing the dishes, doing the laundry. He's reading the paper after dinner . . . You take on somebody else's pain. When I was first dating my partner, Jeremy, I remember saying to him things like 'If you're in a sad or scared place, I want to lead you out into the light.'" I nodded in recognition when Julie said this. Over half a century ago, Rae took on very much the same task, or should I say "burden." "I saw your light the first time we met," she recalls, "and I saw your shadow. I was going to heal you; I was going to dispel the darkness." An unenviable assignment, to say the least.

In *Down Girl: The Logic of Misogyny*, the contemporary feminist philosopher Kate Manne, associate philosophy professor at Cornell University, gives us a handy way of conceptualizing the expectations held of women and the demands made on them: *feminine-coded goods and services*—those which are "hers to give." They include "attention, affection, admiration, sympathy, sex, and children (i.e., social, domestic, reproductive, and emotional labor); . . . safe haven, nurture, security, soothing, and comfort." These are counterposed with the *masculine-coded perks and privileges* that are "his for the taking": for example, "power, prestige . . . rank, reputation, honor . . . hierarchical status, upward mobility, and the status conferred by having a high-ranking woman's loyalty, love, devotion, etc."[21] It is not hard to intuit which of these groupings would entail and engender (no pun intended) more self-suppression, sacrifice, and stress. Bear in mind, too, that Manne is depicting here women of relative privilege. So many others, in addition to assigned gender roles, struggle under the heavy freight of poverty, single parenthood, and racial discrimination. We have seen the cost in health these intersectional misfortunes exact.

When I speak of *patriarchy*, I mean not the conscious will nor, often, even the conscious awareness of individual men, but a system of power. Although patriarchy is ancient, having arisen with the dawn of civilization, capitalism has comfortably adapted it to its needs—we see that played out in economics, in politics, in all institutions of this society, as in the home. Men pay a price, too, even as they reap the dubious "benefits" of the system that privileges them. When I reduce my wife to an object whose purpose is to keep me satisfied, what role am I casting myself in? An impotent, dependent child whose emotional welfare hinges on Mommy's willingness to comply with my perceived needs. This child, in an adult body, struts, remonstrates, sulks, and makes demands on his caregiver. He is never sated, never satisfied. Both partners, in their own ways, are powerless.

Men's suffering, too, is part of the patriarchal cycle, in the mix as both effect and cause. The taboo against vulnerability, in particular, is deeply harmful to men as well as to women. Anger may be more permissible among men, but sadness, grief, or "weakness"—which really just means acknowledging one's limits—are not. Many combat veterans have had to overcome this patriarchal bylaw as they have struggled with anguish, depression, suicidality, and other manifestations of post-traumatic stress, from which there is no healing without a free flow of vulnerable emotion. Toxified masculinity, like the suppression of the feminine, is lethal. It claims its victims through many pathways, including alcoholism and other substance addictions, workaholism, violence, and suicidality[†]—all defenses against or escapes from vulnerability, grief, and fear.

"In our culture we 'turn boys into men,' through disconnection," says the therapist Terry Real. "To learn to disconnect from your feelings, from your vulnerabilities, and from others is what we call autonomy and independence. That's a traumatic wound, a hidden one because it's culturally normative. It's almost preverbal." In his book *I Don't Want to Talk About It: Overcoming the Secret Legacy of Male Depression*, Real speaks of male fragility and the denial of men's sensitivity. "To me, the fragility has to do with both the trauma and the injunction against being human," he told me. "The essence of [toxic] masculinity is invulnerability. The more vulnerable you are, the more 'girly' you are. The more invulnerable you are, the more 'manly' you are. So the fragility of being a human, the simple human vulnerability, is suppressed. Men are trying to live up to a standard which is inhuman, and they're dogged by a sense of falling short of that standard over and over and over again." As Real spoke, I was reminded of the male firefighters who threw tampons into Liz's bed and the vulnerability they were attempting to shame in her, as they were ashamed of their own.

"The guys that I treat are all captains of industry who've done beautifully in the world and are horror stories in their personal lives," Real confided. Male domination exacts a high price in both directions, and by all indicators, it costs more than it pays.

---

† Recent research shows that over thirty thousand U.S. veterans of the post-9/11 wars in Iraq and Afghanistan have committed suicide, over four times the number killed in combat. https://coloradonewsline.com/2021/07/08/report-veteran-suicides-far-outstrip-combat-deaths-in-post-9-11-wars/.

Chapter 24

We Feel Their Pain:
Our Trauma-Infused Politics

In insider political circles, almost all politicians are seen as difficult and even damaged people, necessarily tolerated in some civics class inversion because they were elected.

—Michael Wolff, *Landslide: The Final Days of the Trump Presidency*

Having started our journey at the individual and cellular levels, we now arrive at the outermost layer of the biopsychosocial onion: the political. You may well be wondering, What does this have to do with this book's concerns—with illness and wellness, with trauma? Why does it matter? Why, as they say, "go there"?

Wherever one falls on (or off) the political spectrum, it's not hard to conclude that politics today, and the media culture around it, are more toxic than ever. It's true that current events, from village gossip to world affairs, have always been combustible fodder for conversation. These days, they are so incendiary that it often seems no conversation is possible, to the point where many people—as many as 60 percent of Americans, according to one poll—anticipate family holidays with dread.[1] The authors of a 2019 study of Americans out of the University of Nebraska–Lincoln found that "a large number of Americans believe their physical health has been harmed by their exposure to politics and even more report that politics has resulted in emotional costs and lost friendships."[2] They may be more correct than they realize. In an article titled "Stressed Out by Politics? It Could Be Making Your Body Age Faster, Too," telomere researcher Dr. Elissa Epel (see chapter 4) suggests that the allostatic wear and tear of politics may shorten those health-maintaining chromosomal structures.[3] A D.C.-area psychologist has even coined a name for this malaise of the governed: "headline stress disorder."[4]

The toxicity of political life might be of less concern if we could get even a momentary breather from it. Our phones have become handheld stress machines buzzing urgently with updates, from the banal to the grave, about matters of conflict and uncertainty—matters largely out of our control. Social media feeds "feed" us all we can eat, and more still. It never stops.

Not that we're entirely helpless: we probably all could, for example, adjust our news consumption habits to better filter out the rancor, spite, anxiety, and doom. We could practice better listening and exercise more empathy with those with whom we disagree. We could adopt a strict mindfulness regimen: five minutes of deep breathing before and after scrolling, no exceptions. These moves would all be salutary. They would also be not enough. In my view, there is something going on beyond and beneath the oft-lamented "hyperpartisanship," "polarization," and "radicalization" we're witnessing.

The closer I look at who populates the political landscape— the people at the top and we ourselves at its base (or somewhere in between, for the more privileged among us)—the more I see the wounded electing the wounded, the traumatized leading the traumatized and, inexorably, implementing policies that entrench traumatizing social conditions. Beneath all the posturing, punditry, and politicking, the pulse of unseen emotional undercurrents thumps insistently. I can't prove it, of course. Social psychology doesn't lend itself to the kind of firm conclusions achievable in the physical sciences. What I can do is point to it, offering my observations and citing examples and research where possible, and trust people to look for themselves. I do consider the issue of enormous importance—and not just because trauma adds flammable emotional fuel to already fiery family dinner-table debates.

For one thing, political culture is among the many avenues by which toxic myths become normalized truths. Politics are intimately linked with the social character as we have discussed it: the set of desired characteristics that most dispose people to function smoothly within a given system, even if those traits are literally sickening. The same holds for those who steer the ship. A society like ours demands of its leaders a certain set of dispositions and worldviews—call it the *political character*—without which their careers would never get off the ground, given the job requirements. The traits most amenable to stewarding a socioeconomic system that traumatizes populations as a matter of course will, naturally, be ones that inure their bearer to vital aspects of emotional life, if not disable the compassion circuitry outright. This always starts with the self, early in life. There may be exceptions, but I haven't seen many, especially not at the uppermost echelons of power.

When trauma manifests on the political stage, the consequences for people and the planet are massive. Politicians make policy, after all, and policy creates or cements the very cultural conditions we know are antithetical to our health. The level of trauma awareness or blindness they and we bring to the political conversation can't help playing itself out in the world we end up living in. If disease is the *individual* body's way of alerting us to something out of joint, something contrary to what our nature intends for us, then surely social maladies like addiction and global catastrophes like climate change are all signs of something amiss in the *body politic*. So, too, is the mood of resignation and cynicism that surrounds politics in general, and the sometimes ludicrous levels of suspicion and venom that infuse public discussions of everything from elections to abortion to how we should handle health pandemics.

Phantasmagorical vaccine paranoia, for example, is not the same as healthy skepticism. Nor is contemptuous, self-righteous scorn toward vaccine or lockdown dissenters equivalent to responsible citizenship. In my work on trauma, I have observed that it is not merely the ideas people hold but, even more, the emotional resonance of how they speak and act—of *who and how they are being*—that reveal their inner psychic life. When we try to address the content of their speech or their beliefs without attending to the energetic fuel, we miss the mark. The same is true in the sociopolitical sphere: if we want to understand why individuals and groups believe and behave as they do—and we should want to, if we truly care about the consequences—then we need to be willing to see the traumatic scars underneath the extreme emotional reactions. This can be difficult when we ourselves carry strong points of view about our rightness and their wrongness—which is yet more reason to take it on.

All this is more than speculative. Traumatic childhood experience has been shown to bear very directly on adult political orientations. Michael Milburn, emeritus professor of psychology at the University of Massachusetts, found that the harsher the parenting people were exposed to as young children, the more prone they become to support authoritarian or aggressive policies, such as foreign wars, punitive laws, and the death penalty. "We used physical punishment in childhood as a marker of a dysfunctional family environment," he told me. "There was significantly more opposition to abortion, and more support for capital punishment and the use of military force, particularly among males who had experienced high levels of physical punishment, *especially if they had never had psychotherapy.*" I was intrigued by that last finding. "Psychotherapy," Milburn explained, "speaks to a potential for self-examination, for self-reflection."

The confluence of politics and trauma is not a new concept. Decades ago, the great Polish Swiss psychotherapist Alice Miller pointed to how the harsh child-rearing practices long fashionable in Germany helped prepare the template for Nazi authoritarianism. She also argued persuasively that the intense suffering and oppression in childhood of the German fascist leaders, most especially monstrous psychopaths like Adolf Hitler and Hermann Göring, played a decisive role in shaping their mental-emotional lives and, necessarily, their political inclinations. "Among all the leading figures of the Third Reich," she wrote in *For Your Own Good: Hidden Cruelty in Child-Rearing and the Roots of Violence*, "I have not been able to find a single one who did not have a strict and rigid upbringing."[5] For "strict and rigid," we can substitute "traumatizing": Miller was not, after all, speaking about homes run by kindly parents with firm curfews but the sorts of environments that would imprint on a child a fear-tinged view of the world and/or require of him to go numb in the face of suffering, starting with his own.

The subliminal beliefs leaders hold about human nature, the world, and their position in it, and the unconscious impulses that motivate their actions, are of great consequence for their politics— which is to say, for our lives and our world. The worldview they developed early in life under the impact of misfortunes they did not choose and could not control imbues how they feel about, interact with, and act upon the universe and their fellow beings decades later. And yet, as the British psychotherapist Sue Gerhardt points out, "We rarely address the underlying psychological and emotional dynamics of our public figures, or our culture as a whole."[6]

Let's briefly examine two pairs of political nemeses—first in Canada, then the United States—all four of whom have convinced millions of people to entrust them with great power. What makes each of them so appealing and so appalling, depending on who's observing, owes much to personality traits forged in the crucible of early trauma.

In my own country, former prime minister Stephen Harper was much admired by conservatives for his icy, tough-on-crime, climate-science-is-irrelevant, addiction-is-a-criminal-choice views, and reviled by progressives for the same things. Harper has recalled an idyllic childhood, despite growing up under a stern "stickler" of a dad whose own father had disappeared mysteriously years earlier and was never located. I resonate completely with *Toronto Star* journalist Jim Coyle's aside that, contrary to Harper's recollections, it is "not difficult to imagine that life under such a patriarch might have been stifling."[7] This, after all, is a man characterized by his biographer as "autocratic, secretive, and cruel," and whose former chief of staff reported him to have been "suspicious, secretive, and vindictive, prone to sudden eruptions of white-hot rage over meaningless trivia." A Canadian columnist once wrote about Stephen Harper's "dead, sociopathic eyes," while another journalist described him as "chilly and inscrutable." No child is born with dead eyes: such a look bespeaks a recoiling from seeing what is dreadful to a young soul.

The man who succeeded Harper on Ottawa's Parliament Hill exudes a very different vibe, one of terminal likability. Justin Trudeau is known for speaking in warm tones and inclusive language. He has shed public tears of sorrow at more than one press conference, including when a Canadian rock music hero died of brain cancer in 2017.[8] There is nothing wrong with a politician showing their vulnerable side—would that it were more normalized—but, as many have noted, there is also something inauthentic, even unctuous, about Trudeau's nice-guy persona.

Recently, he has had to abjectly apologize for indulging in a private family excursion on a national day created to commemorate the trauma inflicted on our native peoples, a history about which he has waxed contrite in the past.[†] Such ethical and emotional obtuseness bears the imprint of a trauma-inflected childhood. Justin grew up in a home where the father—Pierre, the eminent and irascible prime minister of the 1960s and '70s—was consumed by work, status, and virility. As a boy, Justin was under the care of a mother three decades younger than her womanizing husband, with whom she was often in conflict, her gloom deepened by bipolar disorder. At times she was given to manic high spirits and embarrassingly public sexual hijinks with the likes of Mick Jagger. The current prime minister has recalled being "desperate . . . to inject a sense of magic into every moment we did have together as a family."[9] I am speculating, I'll admit—neither Trudeau nor any politician has ever sought me out for counseling—but I see it as no stretch to say that his fraught upbringing likely primed him to make cloying sweetness and shallow ingratiation his métier.

According to the popular narrative, there could have been no more diametrical opposites in American politics, whether gauged by demographic appeal, ethical values, or personality, than 2016 presidential opponents Donald J. Trump and Hillary Rodham Clinton. The differences are easy to spot, the similarities subtler but instructive. It may come as a surprise to supporters of both, for example, to read a *Scientific American* analysis published in 2016 that pointed out how many qualities that define psychopathy are routinely found in top politicians. One was "coldheartedness," a trait on which both Trump and his then opponent Clinton scored in the upper quintile.[10]

Donald Trump's cartoonishness, the havoc he wreaked

[†]   September 30, 2021: Canada's inaugural observation of National Day for Truth and Reconciliation.

on the U.S. political system, and the cultural tumult around his ascendancy can too easily obscure what a sad, thoroughly wounded person he is. It took one who knows him better than most, his psychologist niece, Mary Trump, to cut through both the hoopla and the opprobrium to the dark heart of the matter. We now know from Mary's revealing 2020 biography, *Too Much and Never Enough: How My Family Created the World's Most Dangerous Man,* that the young Donald had plenty of cause to push reality out of mind and sight; to become grandiose, narcissistic, combative, and utterly opportunistic. "Deep down I have no problem describing him as a sociopath," Mary has said of Donald's father, Fred, the paterfamilias. "He had no real human feeling, and he treated his children variously with contempt." Her own father, Fred Jr., Donald's older sibling, was driven by childhood trauma to alcoholism and an early death at age forty-one. The world has seen what Donald has been driven to. It oughtn't to have required Mary Trump's revelations to uncover the suffering behind the huckster-president's persona, but, in our trauma-blind world, it did. "He is a poster child for trauma," the psychiatrist Bessel van der Kolk told me.

The journalist Tony Schwartz got an up-close view when he ghostwrote Trump's bestselling *The Art of the Deal.* "Lying is second nature to him," Schwartz told the *New Yorker* years later. "More than anyone else I have ever met, Trump has the ability to convince himself that whatever he is saying at any given moment is true, or sort of true, or at least ought to be true."[11] "Second nature," as we noted before, is nobody's real nature. No one's original nature impels them to lie; there are plenty of *congenial* liars, but no *congenital* ones. Friedrich Nietzsche wrote somewhere that people lie their way out of reality when they have been hurt by reality, and this is eminently true of Donald Trump's origin story. Lying, automatic or deliberate, first insulated him from devastating rejection in childhood, and later served him in the realm of political power.

Hillary Clinton is still admired and pined for by many as a tenacious survivor and the rightful winner of the 2016 election. Compared with Trump, at least, she is a paragon of poise, grace, empathy, hard work, and reason. What almost never gets asked is, Where do such relentless ambition and "tenacity" come from, and at what cost? Ought we really to celebrate it, or is it in its own way also an unhealthy norm, even if not to the same degree as Trump's bloviating bluster? Such questions were completely bypassed in the hagiographic haze of Clinton's campaign, in ways I found literally incredible. One moment in particular stuck with me; it demonstrates how readily we normalize and lionize the "winning" personalities of our leaders.

On the evening of her nomination, a video celebrating Hillary's life and achievements was broadcast to an international audience, narrated by the actor Morgan Freeman. In it, the candidate quoted a life lesson imparted to her in childhood by her stern, exacting father: "Don't whine, don't complain, do what you are supposed to do, do it to the best of your ability." By all indications, this was a whitewash. As we know from biographical accounts, the father could be capricious and cruel. "He hurled biting sarcasm at his wife and his only daughter and spanked, at times excessively, his three children to keep them in line."[12] In the video Secretary Clinton also shared, "My mother wanted me to be resilient, she wanted me to be brave." She then related an instance of how this "resilience" was inculcated. "I was four, and there were lots of kids in the neighborhood. I would come out and have a bow in my hair, and the kids would all pick on me. It was my first experience of being bullied, and I was terrified. One day I ran into the house, and my mother met me and she said to me, 'There is no room for cowards in this house. You go back outside and figure out how you are going to deal with what those kids are doing.' " That isn't a call to resilience but to repression. The message a young child receives in such a circumstance is "Vulnerability is shameful in this house, there is no room for your fear. Do not feel or show your pain, suck up your feelings, you are on your own. Don't expect any empathy here." And yet no one in the arena seemed to find this blow to a small child's sensibility disturbing. No media commentator so much as registered that this handpicked example of supposedly inspiring parenting was, in fact, a public celebration of trauma. No observer suggested that a little girl seeking the safety of the parent's embrace is hardly a coward. She is a normal four-year-old.

In any case, the life lesson about pushing through the pain did its work. More than six decades later, a campaigning Clinton was ill and dehydrated with pneumonia but hid her "weakness" from everyone until she collapsed in the street. "I'm feeling great," she unconvincingly assured the public the same day. "It's a beautiful day in New York." No doubt, the same self-suppressing dynamic compelled her to tolerate her husband's philandering proclivities, described by the late writer Joan Didion as "the familiar predatory sexuality of the provincial adolescent." In stereotypical trauma-impact fashion, Hillary blamed herself for her spouse's infidelity. He was under great stress, and she had not sufficiently tended to his emotional needs, she told a friend, thus aligning with women's assigned role in the culture of patriarchy. "She thinks she was not smart enough, not sensitive enough, not free enough of her own concerns and struggles to realize the price he was paying," this close confidant summarized Hillary's views.[13]

The internalized lack of empathy showed itself during the election campaign when she carelessly—but all the more tellingly—dubbed half of Trump's base "a basket of deplorables," revealing to a wide swath of America what they already knew in their bones: that many urban elites view them with smug contempt as people whose economic, political, and moral grievances can be ignored. The deplorables' retort came that November, in the form of a stunning political upset.

"Hillary Clinton and Donald Trump," the conservative columnist David Brooks wrote discerningly in 2016, ". . . both ultimately hew to a distrustful, stark, combative, zero-sum view of life—the idea that making it in this world is an unforgiving slog and that, given other people's selfish natures, vulnerability is dangerous."[14] That sense of danger, I would only add, started long before their forays into political life. Although their respective supporters would likely shudder at the thought of them being remotely similar, Trump and Clinton were a match made in childhood suffering.

On reading the biographies of leaders from many countries across historical periods, one sees how each of them, in their own way, had emotionally starved childhoods; each "overcame" these adversities by dint of the very personality qualities that would land them in the history books as icons and change makers, no matter what great harms they perpetrated. In each case, these traits are seen by many people to this day as laudable and worthy of emulation. That's as normal as normal can get.

And that's where the rest of us come in. Abetted and amplified by the profit-driven media machine, political culture plays on our deepest longings for surety, security, and even supremacy, targeting our damaged "inner children" with force and precision. In fact, much of politics is a lot more coherent if we see how people, many millions of them at once, unconsciously look to their leaders to fulfill their own unmet childhood needs. As the cognitive scientist George Lakoff puts it, "We all think with a largely unconscious metaphor: the Nation as Family."[15]

I asked Daniel Siegel what draws people to follow leaders who exude hostility and an authoritarian streak, such as a Donald Trump. "People may actually feel excitement that someone in the public eye is expressing aggression or assertion, the opposite of impotence," the psychiatrist and mind researcher said, noting how such traits can feel empowering to those in whom a sense of real power is wanting. "It's like a child wanting to be with a parent that will protect them. There is a sense of 'I'm going to be safe and everything is going to be okay.' " What Dan describes is also a *sense memory*, an indelible and usually unexplored imprint from childhood, a longing stored in the bodymind and activated by present-day insecurities projected into the political realm.

On the liberal side, idealizing leaders as kind, supportive, caring, and inclusive can be another form of displaced longing for attuned parenting. One prominent Democratic-supporting celebrity, the song parodist known as Randy Rainbow, tweeted out a photo of a smiling Joe Biden with Kamala Harris the night she was announced as Biden's running mate. His caption read "G'night, Mom and Dad. See you in the morning."[16] People under the sway of such childlike idealizations, even in half jest, are liable to ignore discomfiting counterevidence.

———

Adjacent to politics—increasingly overlapping with it, in fact—is the vast expanse of entertainments, professional sports, fads, and obsessions that we call popular culture. Indeed, one social function of pop culture is to divert people's attention from things that really do matter; imagine if all the energy now expended on analyzing the private lives of celebrities or the detailed intricacies of sporting events were, instead, devoted to mobilizing populations to collectively tackle the great issues of our age.

The election of a former reality-TV game show host to his

country's highest office is but one example of the dissolving membrane between the two spheres. "Movie-star handsome" is one of the accolades Canada's own current prime minister was showered with as he shot to international fame. Thirty years ago Bill Clinton, then a novice presidential candidate, entered the national consciousness by playing the saxophone on *The Arsenio Hall Show*. These days, former president Barack Obama subjects himself to fawning interviews with late-night talk show hosts,[17] when he isn't trending for his celebrity-soaked shindigs on Martha's Vineyard. News is entertainment, and vice versa.

One may bemoan such fluff as a degradation of political life. Less appreciated is the way pop culture grooms us for a particular sort of passive, spectator-like engagement with politics. The hero worship and emotional projection driving modern showbiz run on superfuel distilled in large part from trauma. Think of how expected, how exceedingly *normal*, the following phenomena are: a bright young star, often among the vanguard of their craft, flames out in a blaze of addiction, mental instability, or self-harm; revelations emerge about this or that beloved mogul or star's longtime sexual predations; an athlete or entertainer reveals having endured sexual violations throughout their career, or longer; a former squeaky-clean child star turns objectified sex symbol, often with an unhappy ending.

At best, the pop culture machine treats these incidents as sobering interruptions: we briefly bow our heads in solemn silence to remember the fallen before getting back to gawking, gossiping, consuming. And what do we consume, exactly? Art, sometimes; harmless fun, often enough. But we also ingest the pain of wounded people, packaged as entertainment, to dull or perhaps validate our own distress. We venerate the "personalities" that cover up pathological suffering, then express surprise when things go awry.

For their part, many celebrities seek fame precisely because the love of a fan base is the closest they can come to filling a lifelong void of homegrown esteem. Iconic figures such as Marilyn Monroe, Elvis Presley, Kurt Cobain, and Amy Winehouse are valedictorians of a sad class of superstars felled by the collision between their early torments and the public limelight. All four rose to superstardom on a charisma born of a blend of extraordinary ability and trauma-injected desperation, their talent idolized and exploited, their wounding ignored even when acted out on the public stage.

Many others suffer secretly over the course of long and illustrious careers, as in the case of Aretha Franklin, whose sister Erma once said, "Aretha is a woman who suffers mightily but doesn't like to show it." Of course, she *did* display it to anyone with eyes to notice. The revered singer of the self-assertive anthem "Respect" had been more than disrespected in childhood and continued to suffer abuse in her adult relationships. The disconnect is achingly apparent in the stunning concert documentary *Amazing Grace,* filmed at a Los Angeles church in 1972. With thrilling command and depth of feeling, a thirty-year-old Aretha rattles the rafters and electrifies the crowd. The confident mask only slips when her preacher father takes the pulpit to praise his daughter's gifts. In the presence of this emotionally cruel patriarch, she stiffens, her face a curious mix of practiced deference and involuntary dissociation, as if she's not quite in her body— the very same body that had been channeling the divine Word and the sweet ache of longing so transcendently just minutes before. In her music this magnificent artist conjured the power and force she could not wield in her personal life. Her lot was to be legendary in a business and a culture that would rather mythologize than empathize. We avert our gaze from the pain, lest real life intrude on the magic.

I will say that I am encouraged by the fact that celebrities such as Alanis Morissette, Dave Navarro, Lena Dunham, Ashley Judd, Russell Brand, and Jamie Lee Curtis, all interviewed for this book, and others like Oprah Winfrey and the singers Jewel, Sia, and Lady Gaga have opened up recently about their trauma and its impact on their lives and careers. In the political realm, Hunter Biden, son of the current U.S. president, has spoken publicly about some of the traumas underlying his addiction history; his father, though the owner of an infamously punitive policy record when it comes to drug-related "crime," has at least made some more compassionate statements of late with his son's troubles in the news.

All in all, the system works with cyclic elegance: a culture founded on mistaken beliefs regarding who and what we are creates conditions that frustrate our basic needs, breeding a populace in pain, disconnected from self, others, and meaning. A select few—especially those with the sorts of early coping mechanisms that prime them to deny reality, block out empathy, fear vulnerability, mute their own sense of right and wrong, and abjure looking at themselves too closely—will be elevated to power. There they govern over a majority who so crave comfort and stability, who are so ground down by cynicism and alienation, that they will trade authentic instincts and collective self-assertion for the pseudo-attachment of false promises and soothing charisma. Completing the cycle, our wounded leaders with their blinkered priorities enact social policies that keep conditions how they were, or worse.

When former Ohio state senator Nina Turner campaigned for Bernie Sanders in 2020, she was fond of paraphrasing Matthew 7:16: "And ye shall know the tree by the fruit it bears."

Judged by the current harvest, the tree of our social life and our politics is infused with trauma from the root to the fruit. If there is any hope for a different yield, a hope on which the future of the planet surely hinges, many of us—as many as are able, anyway—will have to do what so many of our leaders constitutionally (pun intended) cannot: look within bravely, the better to look out and around honestly.

Part V

Pathways to Wholeness

A change of worldview can change the world viewed.

—Joseph Chilton Pearce, *The Crack in the Cosmic Egg:*
New Constructs of Mind and Reality

Chapter 25

Mind in the Lead:
The Possibility of Healing

The mind cries out, explains, demonstrates, protests;
but inside me a voice rises and shouts at it,
"Be quiet, mind, let us hear the heart!"
—Nikos Kazantzakis, *Report to Greco*

Having navigated the concentric circles of human health and illness from the cellular to the social, and having traced the inextricable and reciprocal connections between them, we now delve into the "good news": the topic of healing. The news may be encouraging, but that's not to say it's easy. How to approach healing, after all, in these troubled times? How to move toward health in the context of a socioeconomic system staunchly uninterested in remedying any of its root maladies, and in the face of a pandemic that has both highlighted and deprived us of so much we take for granted? How to keep hope alive when the odds seem so prohibitive?

And what *is* healing, anyway?

When I speak of healing, I am referring to nothing more or less than a *natural movement toward wholeness*. Notice that I do not define it as the end state of being completely whole, or "enlightened," or any similar psychospiritual ideal. It is a direction, not a destination; a line on a map, not a dot.

Nor is healing synonymous with self-improvement. Closer to the mark would be to say it is *self-retrieval*. In fact, our modern self-improvement culture—which has to a large extent been co-opted by the same consumerist forces responsible for the conditions we have been chronicling—can too easily obscure or complicate the healing journey. When we heal, we are engaged in recovering our lost parts of self, not trying to change or "better" them. As the depth psychologist and wilderness guide Bill Plotkin[†] told me, the core question is "not so much looking at what's wrong, but where is the person's wholeness not fully realized or lived out?"

Healing is also distinct from being cured: the latter means the absence of disease; the former implies coming to wholeness. "It's possible to be *healed* but not *cured*, and it's possible to be cured but not healed," my colleague Dr. Lissa Rankin[‡] points out. "Ideally, healing and curing happen together, but this isn't always the case." We will see examples of that in the chapters to follow.

I have made a similar distinction when it comes to addiction: it is possible to be *abstinent* without being *sober*. One is the absence or avoidance of something harmful—itself a worthy objective— while the other is a new, positive capacity to live in the present, free to experience life as it is. Analogously, if cure is the banishment of life-impairing symptoms or conditions, healing is the process of reuniting ourselves with the inner qualities that still live within us as inherent possibilities, as I believe they always do, and that make life worth living. We do not heal "in order to" be cured, even if that understandable wish is present. Healing is best seen as an end in itself.

What follows is not an attempt to prescribe a one-size-fits-all solution—no size does—but to point to the possibility of healing

---

[†] Plotkin's Colorado-based Animas Valley Institute offers potent retreats, workshops, and "quests" that use Nature itself as a kind of template and teacher of human wholeness.

[‡] Rankin's own story of illness and healing was touched on in chapter 5.

on individual and societal levels, even in the context of our increasingly anxious and disordered culture. I intend also, to the best of my
ability, to offer suggestions about what healing asks of us, the inner
and outer conditions that are most hospitable to its flourishing.

———————

Any movement toward wholeness begins with the acknowledgment of our own suffering, and of the suffering in the world. This
doesn't mean getting caught in a never-ending vortex of pain,
melancholy, and, especially, victimhood; a new and rigid identity
founded on "trauma"—or, for that matter, "healing"—can be its
own kind of trap. True healing simply means opening ourselves
to the truth of our lives, past and present, as plainly and objectively as we can. We acknowledge where we were wounded and,
as we are able, perform an honest audit of the impacts of those
injuries as they have touched both our own lives and those of
others around us.

This can be exceptionally difficult, for myriad understandable
reasons. No matter what degree of discomfort our illusions cover
over, the truth hurts, and we don't like hurting if we can help it—
even if we sense that something better could lie on the far side of
the pain. As Nadezhda Mandelstam wrote in her searing memoir
of life under Stalinism, *Hope Against Hope*, "It is very difficult to
look life in the face." Many of us will be ready to seek the truth
only once we have concluded that the cost of *not* doing so is too
high, or once we become sufficiently acquainted with our own
ache of longing for the real. The Greek playwright Aeschylus was
exquisitely on point when he had his chorus declare:

> *Zeus has led us on to know*
> *the Helmsman lays it down as law*
> *that we must suffer, suffer into truth.*[1]

There are exceptions, but I myself have never encountered anyone who was not spurred along their path of growth and change by some setback or loss, some illness, anguish, or alienation. Fortunately—or unfortunately, depending on how we choose to see it—life has a way of delivering the requisite suffering right to our doorstep.

"Truth" is a big little word, easily misconstrued. I am not speaking about some ultimate spiritual Truth; nor am I referring to purely intellectual verities or verifiable facts, as in "true or false." If that were all, then we could "study, study into truth" and every academic faculty would be staffed by modern-day Buddhas. Where, for all its merits, has our mighty intellectual capacity got us? Right to where we are: an unjust world, threatened self-extinction, untold and needless pain and privation in a universe of abundance, the spread of alienation and despair. In fact, our cerebral talents are all too readily recruited by the part of us that wants to *deny* how things are: there is a reason "rationality" and "rationalize" are linguistic siblings.

The truth I speak of is much more modest and down-to-earth: a clear look at how it is, how things actually happen to be at this moment. This is the kind of truth that ushers in healing. To access it, we will have to tap into something more resourceful than our smarts.

The intellect becomes a far more intelligent tool when it allows the heart to speak; when it opens itself to that within us that *resonates* with the truth, rather than trying to *reason* with it. "And now here is my secret, a very simple secret," the fox advises the Little Prince in Antoine de Saint-Exupéry's beloved tale: "It is only with the heart that one can see rightly; what is essential is invisible to the eye." The intellect can see verifiable *facts*—provided that denial doesn't obscure or distort them, as it often does to protect the wounded or pain-averse parts of us. It is possible to declaim, declare, and insist on facts, all without a scintilla of what I'm calling truth. The kind of truth that heals is known by its felt sense, not only by how much "sense" it makes.

If any of this strikes you as vague or unscientific, recall that the heart is a living, beating organ before it is an abstract concept. Dr. Stephen Porges has brilliantly shown that the neural circuitry of social engagement and love is intricately connected with the heart and its functions. More than that, the heart also has its own nervous system.[†] The verbal-thinking cerebrum has arrogated to itself the honor of being the only brain, falsely so. Actually, it shares the distinction with the gut and the heart. In other words, the heart *knows* things, just as surely as a gut feeling is also a kind of knowing. In fact, the gut's neural plexus has been appropriately called a "second brain," as has the heart. Thus we may speak of three brains, meant to function in concert, with the autonomic nervous system connecting them all. Without that heart- and gut-knowledge, we often function as "genius-level reptiles," in someone's apt phrase.[‡]

And yet we can't ignore our minds, either, since that's where so much of the action is. If the heart is our best compass on the healing path, the mind—conscious and unconscious—is the territory to be navigated. Healing brings the two into alignment and cooperation, often after a lifetime of one hiding behind or being disregarded by the other.

"Everything has mind in the lead, has mind in the forefront, is made by the mind," the Buddha said 2,500 years ago. I return to this phrase of the great teacher Gautama because it is key to understanding our relationship to what we consider real. It is also

---

[†] The study of the neural net in the pericardium, the fibrous sheath encasing the heart, and its connections with the nervous system and brain is encompassed by the discipline of neurocardiology.

[‡] Joseph Chilton Pearce in *The Heart-Mind Matrix: How the Heart Can Teach the Mind New Ways to Think*.

the bedrock of the therapeutic approach I take to my work and, when I am conscious, to my personal path. With our minds we construct the world we live in: this is the core teaching. The contribution of modern psychology and neuroscience has been to show how, before our minds can create the world, the world creates our minds. We then generate our world from the mind the world instilled in us before we had any choice in the matter. The world into which we were born, of course, was partly the product of *other people's* minds, a causal daisy chain dating back forever.

This may sound grim. Yet the Buddha's dictum offers a way out, since we remain the ones creating the world we see, the world we think is real, in every moment. And here is where healing comes in. We can do nothing about the world that created our mind, that may have instilled in us limiting, harmful, untrue beliefs about ourselves and others. However—and here's the good news I alluded to—we can learn to be responsible for the mind with which we create our world moving forward. The capacity to heal is born of the willingness to do just that, to take on that responsibility. Such willingness is not a once-and-for-all declaration but a moment-by-moment commitment, one that can be regenerated when we lose touch with it. I, for one, have to keep reminding myself to do so. Nor is it an invitation to self-imposed naïveté or blithe so-called positive thinking. It is about the willingness to reconsider our entire view.

If the wounded mind can be tyrannical, it is a tyrant secretly longing to be deposed. I have seen this in my own life numerous times, experiencing the freedom that comes with relinquishing some unhappy belief or perception my mind had clung to just seconds prior. I have also been most fortunate, through my work, to encounter case after case of astounding turnarounds. In every instance, the essential shift transpired not in people's circumstances or histories but in how they related to them. This is evident in the following stories of two people who, in the most literal sense and in ways most of us will feel lucky to never have to experience, suffered into truth. If they can do it, any of us can.

One drizzly morning in 2019 I interviewed Sue Hanisch in her cozy cottage, located in Sedgwick, a village in England's verdant Lake District, about seventy-five miles north of Liverpool. Over a cup of tea, the soft-spoken sixty-two-year-old occupational therapist and trauma worker told me the story of her trek up Mount Kilimanjaro: a momentous feat for anyone, and all the more so for her, thirteen years after a bomb planted by the Irish Republican Army at London's Victoria Station blew off her right lower leg and severely damaged her left foot. "I remember a nurse crying and another one gagging at seeing my legs," she recalled. The explosion, from a ten-pound device left in a trash bin, occurred fifty years to the day Hanisch's grandfather lost his life in the 1940 bombing of Coventry by the Luftwaffe.

Multiple surgeries and years of despondence followed. Forty were injured that day; the man next to Hanisch had been killed instantly. Her mind carried enormous guilt about survival, and equally about her depression. "That man had been between me and the bomb. It's almost like, how dare I survive, and how dare I not take full advantage of life on planet Earth when he couldn't have that choice?"

By the time Hanisch set out to climb Kilimanjaro on her right below-the-knee prosthesis and surgically repaired, nearly insensate left foot, her psychic wounds had healed significantly. This liberation has grown with the integration of her experiences into the tapestry of her life, as she has divested energy from the limiting stories she once told herself about what it all meant. "It's a mixed blessing to be on planet Earth," she said to me softly. "It's a difficult experience. But I've also been given the opportunity to find out the gold in the wound. I've had some amazing experiences because of what's happened to me." For her, those experiences invariably involve others. "I've noticed how it's the connections that I make with people that are actually the thing worth living for, and nothing else, really. It's the connections that make me feel I am here and that also make me *want* to be here. How I can reach out to other people to help them feel connected? That's the only thing of any heartfelt importance to me."

Among the profound connections Sue made was with the last people you would have expected her to bond with. Ever the adventurous sort, some years after the explosion she found herself in South Africa's KwaZulu-Natal wilderness on a peacemaking mission with, among others, several participants from Northern Ireland, veterans of the very organization whose bomb had mangled her body and altered her life forever. "The idea," she said, "was to hear the other side of the story, to see each other's struggles, and to put us in a different environment where we would need to protect one another."

At some point the expedition had to ford a river. Sue's dilemma was that she could not expose her metallic prosthesis to water, and the anticipation made her quite agitated. She needn't have worried: plans had already been made for her safe and dry passage. Two men carried her across on their shoulders, one of them a former IRA militant. "The fact that it was an IRA guy, it made me absolutely overcome with emotion. I was crying and so was Don, the IRA man. The experience of working with these fellows made me realize just how damaged they had been by what had gone on in their lives before. Don himself was the youngest of seventeen. He had his first gun when he was eight, and he grew up in a children's home. He'd been in jail, he'd been bullied, and he'd been having a really tough time himself. He was carrying the burden of having killed people and not having a clear conscience. It was good for me to be with these people whose lives I had had no insight into before. I realized I could have easily been Don, had I grown up in those circumstances."

Hanisch's ascent of Mount Kilimanjaro came a few years later. There, too, she was accompanied by a man from Northern Ireland, someone who had heard her story and wanted to reach the mountaintop with her. Reach it they did, and then the two improbable co-climbers did something even more unlikely: they danced, giving new meaning to the term "peak experience." "I have had to be invited back into life," she reflected. "And it was love that invited me back."

Another illuminating conversation with a woman who had come through a personal hell ended up supporting my own unlikely reconciliation with the past. My interlocutor was Bettina Göring, grandniece of Hermann Göring, the Nazi Reichsmarschall whose Luftwaffe had killed Sue's grandfather, and one of the pillars of the criminal regime that murdered my grandparents. We had been brought together by the director of a documentary series that featured us both; the filmmaker intuited, correctly, that we might have something to offer each other. We spoke by Skype: I from Vancouver, Bettina from Thailand, where she now lives and does healing work with others part-time. That such an exchange actually happened, and that it was so heart-to-heart, requires a word that I don't often use: "miracle." She had initiated it, writing to express appreciation of my work. The magical quality of this meeting, for me, was the fact that two people who had begun life at such different poles—one the descendant of martyrs, the other the relative of a notorious perpetrator—would each be sent on a healing journey on which they would serendipitously encounter each other and find mutual understanding.

Born eleven years after the war, Bettina had carried a dark legacy her entire life. A hypersensitive child, she bore all the family burden of multigenerational trauma and absorbed guilt for her uncle's monstrous depravity. Having been abandoned by his mother at six weeks of age, Hermann Göring was brought up under the rigid and cruel child-rearing regimens Alice Miller identified in studying the lives of all the top Nazi leaders—what she had called the "poisonous pedagogy." Morphine addiction and compulsive eating were among his attempted escapes from his dreadful inner world, the monstrosities of which he did so much to inflict on others.

Bettina recounted how she had sought healing for herself. It was at an encounter group in Australia that she realized, she said, "how guilty I felt, even though it made no sense—I mean, from my brain, my mind, I knew it didn't make sense—but I felt it." She shuddered as she told me this. "It was very painful to face that shame and to face the horror and all that had been a part of it." A woman with acute empathic ability, she decided to use that inner resource and courageously opened herself to experience her great-uncle's psyche—that is, to its resonance and vibrations within herself. She did so not to forgive Göring, but to forgive *herself*, to let go of the darkness she had always identified with. "I faced it," she told me. "It was horrible. It was like going through the darkest night of the soul. I faced the worst of the worst, the monster. Very scary. Yet coming out of it again, I felt much freer."

That's exactly how I felt after we said our goodbyes. My own past had not changed one iota; my sense of the possible, though, had. I was reminded of something my colleague, the trauma expert Bessel van der Kolk, had said to me one balmy autumn day about ten years ago, over lunch at a conference we were both speaking at in upstate New York. I no longer recall what in the conversation or my demeanor prompted his comment, but suddenly from across the table Bessel peered over the rims of his glasses and said, "Gabor, you don't need to drag Auschwitz around with you everywhere you go." In that instant Bessel saw me. Despite all my positive engagements with life, despite the love and joy and immense good fortune that have also been my portion, that self-directed hopelessness was an ever-lurking shadow, ready to obliterate the light whenever I experienced a setback or a discouragement, and even in innocent, unguarded moments.

The mental prison camp Bessel identified was built and fenced in by *the meaning* my infant mind had forged from events that were painful and frightening and far beyond my control—*not just by the events themselves*. That meaning, the never-ending story whose moral is "I am a damaged being, beyond all hope of healing," has frequently colored my subjective experience of life, regardless of external factors and regardless of all I've witnessed and learned to the contrary, even in defiance of my core values and convictions about humanity. I have always believed—and "believed" is not a strong enough word here, because I'm speaking of a conviction more powerful than belief—that within everyone there is the potential for development and growth, no matter what they have experienced, believed, or done. And then there was me, the lone exception! Such is the power of the mind: it can rigidly maintain its convictions for a long time even when such views are self-defeating, contrary to experience, and even dissonant with other, neighboring beliefs.

The most inspiring journeys toward wholeness are the most improbable because they belie the notion that some traumas are beyond the pale. When writing this chapter, I had the pleasure of speaking with Dr. Edith Eger, a fellow Hungarian Jew, internationally beloved psychotherapist, and author, now in her nineties. The same filmmakers who had connected me with Bettina also introduced me to Edith.

Edith was sixteen years old in June 1944 when, five months after I was born, she and her family were transported to Auschwitz from Košice, the same Slovakian town where my mother grew up and from where my grandparents were deported. Very likely they traveled on the same train as the Egers. Her parents, along with my grandmother and grandfather, were sent to the gas chambers immediately on arrival. Edith's survival and, far beyond that, her transcendence of the horrors she endured are depicted in her book *The Choice*. What choice could she mean? Certainly not the choice of when and where she was born, or what befell those closest to her. Rather, she found a way to exercise the only agency she had, which lay in her own point of view and emotional attitude toward the unchangeable past. Here she explains how, decades later, she forgave Hitler himself. This happened at Berghof in the Bavarian Alps, the location of the Führer's residence from 1933 onward. "It is too easy to make a prison out of our pain, out of our past," she writes. "So I stood on the site of Hitler's former home and forgave him. This had nothing to do with Hitler. It was something I did for me. I was letting go, releasing that part of myself that had spent most of my life exerting mental and emotional energy to keep Hitler in chains. As long as I was holding on to that rage, I was in chains with him, locked in the damaging past, locked in my grief. To forgive is to grieve—for what happened, for what didn't happen—and to give up the need for a different past. To accept life as it was and as it is."[2] We could say that she came to "choose" her past, not in the sense of liking or condoning it, but by simply letting it be. "I do not of course mean," Edith adds, "that it was acceptable for Hitler to murder six million people. Just that it happened, and I do not want that fact to destroy the life that I had clung to and fought for against all odds."

When Bessel advised I could let go of Auschwitz, he meant precisely that I didn't need to keep clutching the pain and resentment of the past, nor the beliefs I developed at a time when I could not have known any better. It is a freedom worth seeking.

When I spoke with Edith Eger again in 2019, she was just completing *The Gift*, her second book of healing wisdom. I was moved, knowing I was unlikely ever again to encounter someone so intimately close to the story of my own beginnings. "Edie," I said, "I haven't got over it yet, and here I am, seventy-six years later." She laughed gently. "Gabor, perhaps you never will. You don't need to. You just need to allow yourself to be with it." Nothing needed to change, Edith was reminding me: only how I held my history in my mind.

None of us need be perfect, nor exercise saintly compassion, nor reach any emotional or spiritual benchmark before we can say we're on the healing path. All we need is readiness to participate in whatever process wants to unfold within us so that healing can happen naturally.

Anyone, no matter their history, can begin to hear wholeness beckoning, whether in a shout or whisper, and resolve to move in its direction. With the heart as a guide and the mind as a willing and curious partner, we follow whatever path most resonates with that call.

Chapter 26

Four *A*'s and Five Compassions: Some Healing Principles

Everything in nature grows and struggles in its own way,
establishing its own identity, insisting on it at all costs,
against all resistance.

—Rainer Maria Rilke, *Letters to a Young Poet*

No one can plot somebody else's course of healing, because that's not how healing works. There are no road maps for something that must find its own individual arc. We can, however, sketch out the territory, describe it, familiarize ourselves with it, prepare to meet its challenges. We can learn what natural laws seem to govern healing, specifically what attitudes and attributes it both awakens and responds to in us. Like natural childbirth, healing cannot be mandated or hastened, but it can certainly be helped along. As the poet and musician Jewel eloquently puts it, "You cannot force nature / only nurture it." That had been her personal experience of healing, she told me in an interview.

The following four *A*'s are not how-to steps or rigid injunctions. They represent healing principles that have proved useful guideposts for many people. I originally devised them while writing *When the Body Says No* and have since amended them, condensing them from seven to four. (In a later chapter I will propose two new *A*'s that harmonize individual and social healing, of which justice is a core tenet.) Each of these represents a healthy quality corresponding to a human need, often stunted or forced underground early in life by emotionally or physically inimical conditions or, in this confused and repressed culture of ours, just by environments that could not support its development. An essential aspect of healing is welcoming each of these qualities back into our life and letting it teach us its ways.

1. Authenticity

To put it bluntly, authenticity is a quality more often marketed than manifested in our culture. Even Coca-Cola is sold as "the real thing." We find ourselves surrounded by the rampant phenomenon of ersatz authenticity: someone is performing "realness" for the crowd or the camera, but it doesn't convince; maybe the words don't match the cadences, or there's too much defiance and bluster in the delivery.

Authenticity is hard to pin down. While synonyms like "genuineness," "truthfulness," "originality," and so on come to mind, authenticity itself eludes any precise definition that could fully capture its essence. Like its fellow natural state, love, authenticity is not a concept but something lived, experienced, basked in. Most of the time you know it when it's there. Have you ever tried explaining to anyone what love is in purely intellectual terms? As with love, so with authenticity.

The pursuit of authenticity is rife with pitfalls. For starters, we have the paradox that authenticity can't be pursued, only embodied. By definition, striving for some idealized self-image is incompatible with being authentically who one is. We have to begin with accepting ourselves fully, as Anita Moorjani discovered in her encounter with fatal illness.[†] "Even the slightest little resistance from the opposite person . . . like if I had displeased

---

[†]   See chapter 7.

someone even slightly—this was me *before*—I would be the one to back down," she told me. "Today, I'm not afraid of being disliked, of disappointing someone. I'm not afraid of what I used to think of as my negative qualities. I realized that they are just the other side of being who I am."

One of the most direct approaches to authenticity is noticing when it isn't there, then applying some curiosity and gentle skepticism to the limiting self-beliefs that stand in for it, or just stand in its way.

The lack of authenticity makes itself known through tension or anxiety, irritability or regret, depression or fatigue. When any of these disturbances surface, we can inquire of ourselves: Is there an inner guidance I am defying, resisting, ignoring, or avoiding? Are there truths I'm withholding from expression or even contemplation, out of fear of losing security or belonging? In a recent encounter with others, is there some way I abandoned myself, my needs, my values? What fears, rationalizations, or familiar narratives kept me from being myself? Do I even know what my own values are?

The growing capacity to admit to oneself, "Ouch, that hurts," or "You know, I didn't really mean what I just said," or "I'm really scared to be myself in this situation" is the impulse toward authenticity becoming stronger. After enough noticing, actual opportunities for choice begin to appear *before* we betray our true wants and needs. Whereas earlier, such awareness would have been clocked only after the fact, we might now find ourselves able to pause in the moment and say, "Hmm, I can tell I'm about to stuff down this feeling or thought—is that what I want to do? Is there another option?" The emergence of new choices in place of old, preprogrammed dynamics is a sure sign of our authentic selves coming back online.

2. Agency

Agency is the capacity to freely take responsibility for our existence, exercising "response ability" in all essential decisions that affect our lives, to every extent possible. Being deprived of agency is a source of stress. Such deprivation could arise from social or political conditions: poverty, injustice, marginalization, or the seeming collapse of the world around us. In the case of illness, it's often due to internal constraints.

The exercise of agency is powerfully healing. The psychologist Kelly Turner has studied many cases of so-called spontaneous remission of what had been diagnosed as terminal malignancy. "Having worked as a counselor at various hospitals and oncologists' offices," she reports, "I know firsthand that the patients who listen and follow instructions are considered 'good' patients, while the 'annoying' patients are those who ask a lot of questions, bring in their own research, or—worst of all—challenge their doctors' orders."[1] Yet these latter ones, she found, those who find ways to take control of their own healing, are the ones likely to do better in the long term. In hindsight, Dr. Turner notes, all her radical remission survivors wished they'd started much earlier to be active agents of their destinies rather than compliant patients in the hands of physicians.

As with authenticity, capitalism sells a bogus version of agency through personal-power mantras like "Be all you can be" and "Have it your way." Personal choice becomes a brand, with no attention paid to the contexts in which those choices are made. Often the freedom being advertised is the dubious freedom to choose between this or that identity-burnishing product or service that will not, cannot, satisfy us. Nor does agency mean some sort of false omnipotence or ultimate dominion over all happenings and circumstances. Life is so much bigger than us, and we do not forward our own healing by pretending to be in control where we're not.

Agency does mean having some choice around who and how we "be" in life, what parts of ourselves we identify with and act from. This often starts with renegotiating our relationship with the personality traits we have so long taken to be identical with who we really are, the ones that first arose in us to keep us safe but now keep us boxed in. There is no freedom in *having* to be "good" or the most talented or accomplished, or in the need to please or entertain or be "interesting." Nor can we wield agency when we react with automatic opposition to other people's demands: knee-jerk reactivity leaves no room for "response ability"—or what in our first chapter we called response flexibility, a capacity trauma greatly impairs.

Agency is neither attitude nor affect, neither blind acceptance nor a rejection of authority. It is a self-bestowal of the right to evaluate things freely and fully, and to choose based on authentic gut feelings, deferring to neither the world's expectations nor the dictates of ingrained personal conditioning.

3. Anger

People often ask me to define "healthy anger." Here's what it's not: blind rage, bluster, resentment, spite, venom, or bile. All of these stem from an unhealthy buildup of unexpressed or unintegrated emotions that need to be experienced and understood rather than acted out. Both anger suppressed and anger amplified out of proportion are toxic.

Anger in its natural, healthy form is a boundary defense, a dynamic activated when we perceive a threat to our lives or our physical or emotional integrity. Our brains being wired for it, we can hardly avoid it: this is the self-protective RAGE system identified by Jaak Panksepp. Its full functioning is a standard feature of our wholeness, essential for survival: think of an animal protecting its turf or its young. The movement toward wholeness often involves a reintegration of this oft-banished emotion into our repertoire of available feelings. This is not the same as stoking resentment or nurturing grievance—quite the opposite. Healthy anger is a response of the moment, not a beast we keep in the basement, feeding it with shame or self-justifying narratives. It is situational, its duration limited: flashing up when needed, it accomplishes its task of fending off the threat and then subsides. It becomes neither an experience to fear and loathe nor a chronic irritant.

The fact—and some people may need to actively remind themselves of this—is that we are talking about a valid, natural feeling that does not in itself intend anyone any harm. Anger in its pure form has no moral content, right or wrong—it just *is*, its only "desire" a noble one: to maintain integrity and equilibrium. If and when it does morph into a toxic version of itself, we can address the unhelpful stories and interpretations, the self-righteous or self-flagellating thought patterns that keep stoking it, without invalidating the emotion. We can also observe how our inability to say no fuels chronic resentment that leaves us prone to harmful combustions.

Many of us have learned to minimize our anger to the point that we don't even know what it looks like. In this case it's best not to idealize or exaggerate: picturing a bombastic eruption of ire or some righteous, curse-encrusted monologue will not help us. Like authenticity, genuine anger is not a performance. Anger's core message is a concise and potent no, said as forcefully as the moment demands. Wherever we find ourselves tolerating or explaining away situations that persistently stress us, insisting that "it's not so bad" or "I can handle it" or "I don't want to make a fuss about it," there is likely an opportunity to practice giving anger some space to emerge. Even the plainspoken admission that "I don't like this" or "I don't want this" can be a step forward.

Research suggests that anger expression could support physical health, for example in those with amyotrophic lateral sclerosis (ALS) or fibromyalgia, two conditions that baffle the conventional medical mind. We have already reported (in chapter 2) that ALS patients are perceived by their physicians as extraordinarily nice. Tellingly, in another ALS study, the most "agreeable" ones—the ones least likely to be in touch with anger, that is— also had the most rapid deterioration of their condition and of their quality of life.[2] The same is true with fibromyalgia, which many studies have linked to childhood trauma. A 2010 study in the *European Journal of Pain* concluded that "anger and a general tendency to inhibit anger predicts heightened pain in the everyday life of female patients with fibromyalgia. Psychological intervention could focus on healthy anger expression to try to mitigate the symptoms of fibromyalgia."[3]

The question for most of us is not whether to be angry but how to relate in a wholesome way to the feelings that naturally ebb and flow with life's tide, anger included.

4. Acceptance

Acceptance begins with allowing things to be as they are, however they are. It has nothing to do with complacency or resignation, though sometimes these can pose as acceptance—think of the shrugging expression "It is what it is"—just as stubborn egotism can moonlight as authenticity. Rather, acceptance is the recognition, ever accurate, that *in this moment* things cannot be other than how they are. We abstain from rejecting or condoning. Instead of resisting the truth or denying or fantasizing our way out of it, we endeavor to just *be with it*. In doing so, we foster an aligned relationship with the actual, present moment.

Acceptance also means accepting how downright difficult it can be to accept. It may seem paradoxical, but true acceptance denies or excludes no aspect of how it is, *not even our impulse to reject how it is*. Anger, sadness, trepidation, resistance, even hatred—within an accepting attitude, these all have room to say their piece. Sometimes accepting ourselves starts with facing that we don't know how we feel, or that our feelings are mixed. Rejection of *any* part of our experience is an unnatural self-rejection, one that nonetheless feels normal to many of us. You've made some serious mistakes? You find yourself filled with hatred, or resentment, or confusion? These, too, are candidates for acceptance; underneath them there is always pain. In fact, hatred, resentment, and even confusion can be the psyche's attempts *not* to feel pain or sadness. Healthy grief—the jewel so often hidden within ossified grievance—frequently waits on the other side of accepting how things are and have been. That, too, can be hard to embrace, but when we forestall the energy of mourning that wants to move through us, we only cause it to build up. As Gordon Neufeld puts it, "We shall be saved in an ocean of tears."

A distinction must be made between *accepting* and *tolerating*. Being with something and putting up with something have precious little to do with each other. Acceptance is vitalizing because it makes room for the other three *A*'s—it grants admission to *anger* if such is present, increases our sense of free *agency*, and makes room for whatever our *authentic* experience might be. Tolerating the intolerable, on the other hand, is deadening. For example, resigning oneself bleakly to conditions such as abuse or neglect involves *rejecting* crucial parts of one's self, needs, and values that deserve to be respected and integrity that needs to be safeguarded. That is far from true acceptance.

Darlene, a thirty-eight-year-old family therapist in San Jose, California, began to accept that the realities of her marriage were intolerable only when she developed an autoimmune disease. Based on her fundamentalist Christian upbringing, she had truly believed her God-given duty was to "accept"—read endure—the miseries her husband's own traumatic imprints visited upon her. "As the connection between my stress and my illness dawned on me," she related, "at one point I remember going, 'Holy shit—I've been in this kind of martyr-honoring-God position of staying in this abusive marriage, and there's just no way: this is going to kill me!'"

The same applies to injustice or oppression on the social level. To accept that whatever is currently happening is happening—the simple fact of the matter—does not mean conceding that it *should* happen. To deal with racism, poverty, or any other societal ill, we must first recognize that they are realities of life in this culture. They exist, and we must acknowledge our pain and grief that they do. Now we can ask ourselves how we might effectively work to eliminate not only their expressions but their root causes. We can move on to healthy anger, to agency, to autonomy in action.

The Five Compassions

The acclaimed neurosurgeon James Doty[†] heads Stanford University's Center for Compassion and Altruism Research and Education. "There is a subset of people who believe that compassion is soft, that it's not worthy of scientific study," he told me during a public conversation we held at the California retreat center 1440 Multiversity.[‡] "Yet, I assure you, the science we have today demonstrates these practices of mindfulness, self-compassion, and

---

[†] Author of the bestseller *Into the Magic Shop: A Neurosurgeon's Quest to Discover the Mysteries of the Brain and the Secrets of the Heart.*

[‡] A brief segment of this conversation can be viewed here: "A Neurosurgeon Talks of Vulnerability: Gabor Maté and James Doty" July 12, 2019 https://www.youtube.com /watch?v=WiAXbZmA2dU.

compassion are some of the most powerful that exist to change your physiology and to benefit you in your own health, mental and physical, and in terms of your longevity." Compassion, as both salve and salvation, is not limited to the realm of the individual. If we are to dream of a healthier, less fractured world, we will have to harness and amplify compassion's healing power.

In my work with clients and in training thousands of therapists, I have distinguished five levels of compassion that build on and reinforce one another nonhierarchically. Together, they encourage, guide, and orient us on the pathway to wholeness. As the playwright (and physician) Anton Chekhov wrote, "It is compassion that moves us beyond numbness toward healing."

1. Ordinary Human Compassion

The word "compassion" comes from the Latin, meaning "to suffer with." Whether or not we experience another's pain so vividly, entry-level compassion does mean the ability to *be with suffering*. It also means being *moved* by the awareness that someone is struggling; it does not register as a neutral fact.

Interpersonal compassion necessarily involves empathy, the ability to get and relate to the feelings of another. Our experience of it may fluctuate depending on who we are looking at and even on how we are feeling at any given moment. Certainly, it can be worn down or depleted, as anyone who has ever experienced work-related "compassion fatigue" can attest. For most of us it bounces back once we get the rest and replenishment we need. Its absence in anyone, glaring in sociopaths and psychopaths, is always a marker of a wound to the soul, or, in A. H. Almaas's words, "the suppression of hurt." When we notice such an empathy gap in ourselves, instead of self-judgment—itself a lack of compassion—we could well ask what pain *we* have not yet fully felt and metabolized. We can learn a lot about our own emotional-injury history by observing in what situations, and toward whom, our naturally open and supple hearts tend to harden and shut down.

Compassion is not the same as pity, which on some level always buys into a preexisting story about oneself or another. While compassion guides the best social policies, pity empowers no one. To take pity on you, I have to first cast us in unequal roles, looking down on your misfortune from some imagined perch. Even if there is an actual power gap between us in the world—say, one born of a racial or economic hierarchy—treating it as if it is a permanent, essential fact about us does neither one of us any favors. Self-compassion, equally necessary, also has its unhealthy analogue: "to wallow in self-pity" conveys the comfy but muddy trap of feeling perennially sorry for oneself. Self-pity takes a kind of solace in seeing oneself as an unfortunate character, beleaguered by fate. It undermines healing by reinforcing the stories that keep us ensconced in a world of hurt, and by discouraging responsibility for our own point of view. Self-compassion, by contrast, doesn't resist how things are, nor swaddle the pain in layers of narrative gauze; it just says, "I am hurting."

2. The Compassion of Curiosity and Understanding

The second compassion takes as its first principle that everything exists for a reason, and that the reason matters. We ask, without judgment, why a person or group—any person, any group—would end up being the way they are and act the way they do, even or especially when we are vexed or perplexed by it. We might also call this the compassion of context. However sincere our desire to help ourselves or someone else, we cannot do so without beholding the suffering being experienced, including knowing its source as best we can. It's not enough, for example, to feel bad for people caught in the coils of addiction without seeking to understand what pain in their lives they've been driven to escape and how that wound was sustained. Absent a clear view of the context, one is left, at best, harboring inert good wishes and engaged in well-meant but ultimately ineffective interventions. We see this limitation in the woefully inadequate addiction-treatment approaches currently in vogue.

The willingness to seek the why before leaping to the how is the compassion of curiosity and understanding in action. Though it is called for in every instance of chronic suffering, whether in the personal or social realm, it can be challenging in practice. In today's society we often default to easy explanations, quick judgments, and knee-jerk solutions. Questing with clear eyes to find the systemic roots of why things are the way they are takes patience, curiosity, and fortitude.

The Métis academic Jesse Thistle, cited in chapter 15, has authored a gripping memoir of his childhood, youth, spiral into addiction and crime, and ultimate recovery, a book suffused with precisely this kind of thoroughgoing compassion. "I wrote *From the Ashes*," Jesse told me, "mainly so that people could witness what happened to me and my brothers in our family . . . In a way, I was trying to vindicate my family and make people understand. So with my nation's history, I'm helping re-member. Not just remember, like a memory. Like re-member, reassemble this history that has been disembodied by the state and forgotten." In chronicling the events of his own life, Thistle, along with fellow writers and artists of Indigenous Canada, is reclaiming a compassionate context for his people—in both the familial and national senses of that word—to exist and be seen in the world's eyes, and their own.

3. The Compassion of Recognition

Remember Bruce from chapter 15—the Oregon vascular surgeon arrested at his hospital for forging drug prescriptions to feed his opiate habit? He views the experience, humiliating as it was, with gratitude for the life-changing awakening it sparked in him. "If it hadn't happened to me in the way it happened," he told me, "I would have gone on my merry way as the oblivious, technically proficient but emotionally retarded individual that characterizes so many of us in the surgical profession." In place of his old "self-centered" ways of relating, Bruce describes "a new attitude" characterized by seeing himself in others: "[I can say] 'I am a human being who has flaws, who struggled. You may be in that same category. Let's see how we can fix this problem together.' "

Bruce is embodying what I call *the compassion of recognition*, which allows us to perceive and appreciate that we are all in the same boat, roiled by similar tribulations and contradictions. Until we recognize our commonality, we create more woe for ourselves and others: for ourselves, because we increase our distance from our humanity and get caught up in the tense physiological states of judgment and resistance; for others, because we trigger their shame and further their isolation. If you are not sure what I mean, the next time you feel intense judgment toward anyone, check in with your body states—the sensations in your chest, belly, throat. Does it feel pleasant? Unlikely; nor is it healthy for you.

The lesson is not that you shouldn't judge, since it's not *you* that's doing it but rather your automatic mind. To judge yourself for judging is itself to keep the wheel of shame spinning. The opportunity is to inquire into your judgmental mind and body state with compassionate curiosity. Healing flows when we are able to view this hurting world as a mirror for our own pain, and to allow others to see themselves reflected in us as well—recognition paving the way for reconnection.

4. The Compassion of Truth

We may believe it an act of kindness to protect people from experiencing pain. While this is so when it comes to pain that is unnecessary and preventable, there is nothing compassionate about shielding people from the inevitable hurts, disappointments, and setbacks life doles out to all of us, from childhood onward. Such a mission is not only futile, it is counterproductive—and may even be inauthentic, the seemingly altruistic impulse arising from our discomfort with our own woundedness.

Whatever our intentions, we do no one any favors by fearing their pain or colluding in their banishment of it. As people work to heal their traumas, hurt will inevitably arise. This is why all of us go into denial, suppression, repression, rationalization, justification, hazy memory, and varying grades of dissociation in the presence of hurt. When we face all the ways we have numbed ourselves, pain will inevitably emerge—in fact, it has been waiting a long time to do so. Of course, the fear of these exiled parts is also natural. "When you have a lifetime of emotions that you have been running from," writes Helen Knott, "it seems like once they catch up they will gang-beat you and leave you crippled in an alleyway."[4] That need not happen. The compassion of truth recognizes that pain is not the enemy. In fact, pain is inherently compassionate, as it tries to alert us to what is amiss. Healing, in a sense, is about unlearning the notion that we need to protect ourselves from our own pain. In this way, compassion is a gateway to another essential quality: courage.

The compassion of truth also recognizes that truth may lead, in the short term, to further pain. Darlene, the San Jose family therapist, found this out once she left her dysfunctional marriage. "My childhood community doesn't understand me, can't see me, doesn't get it," she said. "It breaks my heart because I want to be loved and connected, but I suspect they will never be able to see me or connect with me." That some attachments may not survive the choice for authenticity is one of the most agonizing realizations one can come to; and yet, in that pain, there is freedom. It reverses and vindicates the tragic, mandatory choices we had to make in the opposite direction as we started in life. "It's a journey of ditching people-pleasing and not caring what people think," Darlene told me. "There are times when I go, 'I want that person's approval.' I can't say I've arrived, but it's an onion process: I've gotten lots of the layers off, and more and more freedom in my authenticity. I've had to find my own pockets of community where I am seen and understood. It's been a painful process, but I know it's the right thing."

Truth and compassion have to be reciprocal partners. We are not being compassionate by dumping unwelcome truths in someone's lap, perhaps justifying it on the grounds that "I'm just being honest!" "Only when compassion is present," writes A. H. Almaas, "do people allow themselves to see the truth." And without safety, the truth cannot do its healing work.

5. The Compassion of Possibility

There is more to each of us than the conditioned personalities we present to the world, the suppressed or untrammeled emotions we act out, and the behaviors we exhibit. Understanding this allows for what I call *the compassion of possibility*. I don't mean possibility in the hypothetical, future-dwelling sense, as in "maybe someday," but as a present, alive, ever-available inherent quality. Possibility is connected to many of humanity's greatest gifts: wonder, awe, mystery, and imagination—the qualities that allow us to remain connected to that which we can't necessarily prove. It's up to us to nurture this connection, because the day-to-day world will not always provide us with reassuring evidence. This deepest aspect of compassion recognizes that the seemingly impossible only *seems* so, and that whatever we most need and long for can actualize at any moment.

Staying open to possibility doesn't require instant results. It means knowing that there is more to all of us, in the most positive sense, than meets the eye. The same applies to whatever seems the most real, solid, or intractable in us or others. In a famous story, the Buddha saw the universal potential for the humane self to emerge in a notorious criminal who accosted him with murderous intent; the man became his humblest and most gentle follower.

"In order to gain possession of ourselves, we have to have some confidence, some hope of victory," wrote the Catholic mystic Thomas Merton. "And in order to keep that hope alive we must usually have some taste of victory."[5] The compassion of possibility, I would say, is a door we keep open so we can see that victory coming. If we didn't mistake ourselves or one another for whatever personality features and behavioral traits appear on the surface, "good" or "bad," if in each person we could sense the potential for wholeness that can never be lost, that would be, for us all, a victory worth savoring.

Chapter 27

A Dreadful Gift:
Disease as Teacher

Surviving breast cancer redefined who and how I am . . .
Until then, I'd spent a lifetime being a caretaker for everyone
around me. From then, I started to put myself first. I had
voices at the back of my head telling me whatever I did wasn't
good enough. Now, finally, I've silenced them.

—Sheryl Crow[†]

"I have beautiful conversations with my rheumatoid arthritis these days—it makes me want to cry," we heard forty-two-year-old Julia say in chapter 5. On its face, it's an odd and improbable statement. Wouldn't it be more natural to see a potentially crippling disease as a dire threat to be avoided, suppressed, or combated than as an intimate, life-affirming companion? And yet, as in the stories I will relate in this chapter, and as in so many others I have encountered in my work, Julia found value and meaning in her encounter with illness. Some people, more than a few, go beyond that to call their disease a cherished gift. *Blessed with a Brain Tumor* is the title of a book by a young man I interviewed, Will Pye. "This was a gift from spirit, for my soul to facilitate healing transformation and awakening," he told me. What Julia and Will had arrived at is a profound pivot away from conventional thinking: seeing disease itself as

---

†   From an interview the singer-songwriter gave the *Guardian*, July 10, 2021.

an agent of healing, or at least as an opportunity for learning and growth. Rather than merely healing *from* disease, they have somehow learned to heal *through* it.

To be clear: disease is not a "gift" I would wish on anyone. It is not a path of transformation I would direct anyone to if there were any way to avoid it. For the brave women and men whose stories follow, it was just the route their lives took. Nor do I take for granted that I, in their place, would be able to find the inner strength, courage, trust, and sagacity to approach my ailment as they have. Nonetheless, their travails can teach us much about healing, if we are willing to learn from their example.

Let's keep in mind the distinction we made in chapter 25 between healing and cure. Although I have witnessed people reversing and outliving the direst of prognoses, and have seen such cases documented elsewhere, it is not getting better but getting *whole* that we are exploring. Healing, not cure, is the blessing that disease bestowed on these people. Cure can never be guaranteed. Healing is another matter, and it is available until we draw our last breath. It is the movement toward experiencing oneself as a vital whole, whatever may be happening corporeally. Healing is not an endpoint: it is as much a process as disease is. In the following histories, illness happened to be the teacher that initiated people into their healing journey.

None of us, sick or not, need to wait for it to get that dire before we embark on our own journey.

———————

"What happens in these conversations with your rheumatoid arthritis?" I asked Julia, who, since adding therapy, meditation, and other forms of self-work to her low dose of a single drug, has experienced few flare-ups, with no progress of her disease for over a decade and significant improvement in her blood work.

"When it speaks to me," she replied, "rather than seeing it as something I've got to push through or go into a big drama about, I literally just feel it. I sit with it, get curious about what's been happening in my life, what I might be suppressing."

We saw how, in her abusive family of origin, Julia had become a hyper-responsible "nice" person who repressed her feelings to protect everyone else's. "I do my own self-inquiry," she continued. " 'What are you trying to tell me?' I wonder. This happened to me just two weeks ago, when my jaw blew up. I knew it was just there to remind me to allow some difficult feelings to arise, so I listened. I lay on my bed and breathed for an hour. I did some mindful contemplation. I didn't get upset about it, just stayed curious. Literally the next day it was gone. I didn't have to adjust my medication. I never do."

In contravention of all cultural mores, Julia expressed gratitude for her rheumatoid arthritis. "It saved me," she said. "It was my body's way of saying, 'Wake up, wake up. You're not helping yourself holding this much anger and rage deep down inside.' Anger and rage are not feelings I want to hold on to, but I do see them as guides that let me know that something in my life is out of balance. I get [rheumatoid] flare-ups maybe once a year now. When one shows up, I just accept that it's here and there is something I can do about it, something more to learn from it." This is a profound testament to the twin power of acceptance and agency—two of the core universal principles of healing we looked at in the last chapter.

I would never suggest that Julia's practice of compassionate inquiry toward herself is solely responsible for her well-being or that her medication was not beneficial. What we are witnessing is the self-transformation the disease has guided her to, along with the ensuing increase in awareness, equanimity, joy, health, and satisfaction in her life. What she learned from her condition also impelled her to grow professionally. It has revealed her true calling and fostered skills and capacities with which to support others. "It has given me so much," she said. "It led me to my doing my master's and becoming a psychologist. And now my whole field—my specialty is chronic pain in illness." That conversation took place three years ago. She recently sent me an email reporting that for the past twelve months she has "been medication-free for the first time in 16 years with zero symptoms."

To my friend the psychologist Richard Schwartz, nothing about Julia's journey is surprising. Dick is the originator of a widely practiced form of therapy called Internal Family Systems. IFS imagines the personality as an amalgam of independent "parts," each of which comes along as a response to life events. The "internal family" is a constellation of all these different aspects, some at odds with one another, some collaborating. In Julia's case, the anger and rage her childhood emotional and sexual abuse evoked would be seen as "exiled" parts: facets of herself she could not afford to experience as a child, and therefore repressed. The "nice," overachieving, hyper-responsible persona represents "protector" parts, adapted to keep the love and approval of others coming her way. Somewhere in there, and yearning to assert its leadership, is what IFS terms the Self, or what in chapter 7 I described as the "sense of self arising from one's own unique and genuine essence."

That's what the body is calling us back to, through indicators emotional or physical. Symptoms and illness are the body's way of letting us know when we have strayed from that core.

"My experience is that when parts of us can't get through to us otherwise, they don't have a lot of options, but they do have the body," Dick told me. "There are many, many different kinds of medical symptoms. As we have the client focus on the symptom itself and get curious about it, and ask questions of it, they will usually encounter the part that's using the symptom to get a message through, to try and express itself somehow, because the client has refused to listen to it otherwise. As they begin to actually listen to the part, a lot of times the symptoms go away, or they get a lot better." That was the precise finding of a study in which IFS was applied to a group of rheumatoid arthritis patients. As people listened to their "parts" and to their bodies, similarly to how Julia taught herself to do, the subjective aspects of their experience, such as pain and self-compassion, improved, as did objective physical parameters like blood markers of disease and joint inflammation.[1]

The Romanian medical doctor Bianca, also introduced in chapter 5, continues to have her own intimate conversations with her illness. As you may recall, she had flare-ups of her multiple sclerosis when stressed on the job or in her personal life—that is, when she took on too much or ignored her own needs in either realm. Her condition is stable, despite having given up the drug regimen she had been told she'd have to rely on for the rest of her life. Although her MRI findings still show signs of inflammation in her central nervous system, they have not progressed after many years and she has no symptoms, unless she neglects herself in some way. At such times, she has numbness of the skin, which she sees as a perfect metaphor for some emotion she may not be permitting herself to feel. "This is that red light," she said, "telling me, 'Okay, stop. Go back to yourself.' And that's exactly what I do. At that moment I stop, because in the last years I've learned, when I feel it, even a little bit, I stop. I relax. I meditate. I go to see how I feel, what it's telling me. And the moment I discover what it is—maybe it's some emotional pain, maybe I'm sad about something, maybe it was some trigger that took me somewhere and suddenly I'm not here—then I come back to myself. The moment I discover it, that moment the symptom disappears."

Bianca now mostly works with MS patients, most of whom suffer from post-traumatic stress and all of whom exhibit the same overcompensating tendency that used to drive her, with a focus, she said, "on overperformance and success."

In 2003 Donna Zmenak, a speech-language pathologist in Ontario, Canada, was diagnosed with cancer of the cervix. It happened in the aftermath of high stress in her life, including a bitter three-year custody battle for her three young children. The oncological gynecologist suggested that Zmenak immediately undergo a radical hysterectomy, involving removal of the uterus and some ligaments, as well as excision of multiple nodes in her pelvis and of the upper part of the vagina, all to be followed by radiation. She declined. "I told the surgeon I didn't want to live like that, my insides gutted. He said I was making a stupid decision and that he could make decisions, too. Then and there he discharged me."

That the surgeon would part with a patient unwilling to follow his professional opinion is understandable. That he should demean the patient for it is unacceptable. I was reminded of the angry outburst of the recalcitrant patient Kostoglotov in Aleksandr Solzhenitsyn's novel *Cancer Ward*: "Why do you assume you have the right to decide for someone else? Don't you agree it's a terrifying right, one that rarely leads to good? You should be careful. No one is entitled to it, not even doctors."[2]

For a year Donna did it her way, following a cleansing diet, taking supplements, and working with a medical doctor who specialized in nutrition. At the end of that period, she was devastated to be told the cancer had spread and that, without surgery, she had no more than six months to live. Once more, she declined. As I interviewed her, even in retrospect and even knowing the story's happy ending, I had trouble grasping the source of her confidence and determination. "There was just something inside of my heart saying, 'You can do this,'" she replied by way of explanation. "I thought that my inner voice had more value than the people in the world around me who were giving me their best advice. I knew they were. But I didn't feel it was the best advice for me. As a young woman, as much as I wanted to live, I did not want to live in that body. I knew enough at that point in my life that quality of life was more important to me than longevity."

Zmenak embarked on a further six-month inner and outer pilgrimage that took her to healers who taught her practices such as yoga and meditation. She also consulted former cancer patients who had forged their own paths. Along the way, she read a book, *Profound Healing* by Cheryl Canfield, another cancer survivor who had declined conventional treatment and has long outlived a prognosis of a grisly death. She met Canfield, now a hypnotherapist and wellness consultant in California, staying with her for a while and learning from her, in Zmenak's summation, the values of "acceptance, autonomy, and authenticity. She taught me all that, and she taught me how to *die well*. I went home in such a different space that I never really went back to my old ways of being."

Above all, Donna made a fundamental decision about how to live whatever lifespan remained to her: true to herself, even if her intuitions defied the opinions of doctors, family, and friends. "If I only have six months to live, my children are going to know me, the real me, who I am," she recalled telling herself. "This always makes me cry. I remember that moment. And I said, 'You know what? No more. I accept this. I'm going to be me, and I'm going to go forward being happy' . . . And I meant it. I just drew this line, and I never went back." Catching her own hyperbole, she quickly corrected herself: "I'm human, and I fall into that trap all the time. But I get out quick."

Six months into her psycho-emotional-spiritual odyssey, Zmenak heard the same prognosis from another gynecologist, stated in even more alarming terms. Without surgery, this doctor said, her death was inevitable, imminent, and would be "a smelly mess." "This time I *knew* the cancer was gone," she recalled. "I told him I don't think I have cancer anymore; as a matter of fact, I think I'd like to have another baby . . . And he looked at my partner, telling him, 'Not only will she never have a baby, but she will also never live through a baby, and she won't even live long enough to have a baby. You as her partner need to convince her to get this surgery right away, because it's not pleasant.' Then he turned back to me. 'You've got to think of the people around you. Think of your children. You've got to think of your partner.'" The irony of this doctor urging her to "think of the people around you" after years of the people-pleasing self-suppression that had helped precipitate her disease was not lost on Donna.

A short while later, repeat biopsies and scans showed no trace of cancer in Zmenak's uterus, abdomen, or lymph nodes—tests she had submitted to in full confidence she had overcome the malignancy, but also having agreed to have the surgery if she was proved wrong. She returned to see the surgeon to discuss the results. "I get into the room, and I'm sitting there on the chair, smiling, and he goes, 'Why aren't you up in the stirrups?' He was angry. I said, 'Didn't you hear the news? There's nothing there.' He said, 'You're not healed. You have cancer, you'll always have cancer. Cancer comes back, and we need to do the surgery now. You can't heal yourself. This is not possible. Don't delude yourself. You are not healed.' I just stood up and said, 'What's not coming back is me.' And that was it. I left, and I never saw him again."

From time to time since, Donna has sent this surgeon Christmas cards, including after the vaginal full-term delivery of her fifth child, now twelve years old—another feat she had been assured was impossible, given the instability of her uterine opening following the cone biopsy. "In my first Christmas card I said, 'Please don't tell anyone it can't be done. Because I'm still alive, and I'm here, and this is what I have done.' " She has never heard back.

I contacted Nancy Abrams, Zmenak's family physician, who verified every detail of the medical history. "I witnessed the whole thing. I have the records," Dr. Abrams said. "She did all that, and all of a sudden she didn't have cancer. What I really find odd is why do these oncologists not want to know how these people cure themselves? She did it. And she went on to have another child, number five, vaginally, when she had a super-big contraindication, the cone biopsy. She probably shouldn't have even had a competent cervix to carry on her pregnancy, but she did all of that and nobody says, 'Wow, how come that happened to her?' "

Such lack of curiosity is the norm. When I spoke with the oncological psychologist Kelly Turner, whose book *Radical Remission* reported on many cancer patients who recovered despite the direst of prognoses, I wondered whether the people she had studied, those whose courses eluded the grim predictions of health professionals, had found their medical caregivers open to hearing their histories of healing. "For the most part the answer is, sadly, no," Turner replied. "The vast majority of people that I researched said to me in gratitude, 'You are the first doctor . . . the first person with some kind of a health-related degree who has taken any interest in why I got well . . . I tried to tell my oncologist all the things I was doing, and the oncologist didn't want to know it.' I hear that all the time, and it really breaks my heart." The same indifference was noted by Dr. Jeffrey Rediger,[†] who, in researching his book *Cured: The Life-Changing Science of Spontaneous Healing*, documented over one hundred cases of

---

[†] An instructor in psychiatry at Harvard Medical School and medical director for the McLean SouthEast Adult Psychiatric Programs.

"spontaneous remission." "The best the doctors will say is, 'Keep it up, it's working,'" he remarked. "But they are never curious about how their patients did it."

I can understand something of these doctors' reticence. Even for someone like me, well versed in the science of mind-body unity and with a great appreciation for the power of the human spirit—the only grounds on which histories such as Donna Zmenak's make sense[‡]—it is a challenge to fathom a saga so out of line with customary medical expectation and experience. Her example is one few could emulate; indeed no one ought to without the inner resources and a genuine inclination to do so. The teaching from her trajectory is not that anyone should follow her radical choices, but that it's possible to gain the capacity to accept life as it actually is, the authenticity to search for our own truth in all situations, and the agency to choose our response to whatever occurs. Rounding out the four A's, there is healthy anger, which flashed in Donna's declaration, "What's not coming back is me." Her journey into self is not over. "I work daily at maintaining my authenticity," she says.

———

Another uniquely determined—and self-determined—person I met, Dr. Erica Harris, has undergone more medical treatments in a decade than most of us could imagine for several lifetimes, including aggressive chemotherapy, whole body radiation, a bone marrow transplant, a double lung transplant, prolonged hospitalization for a chronic infection, and repeated excisions for skin cancer—to list only the most salient ones. She would have died long ago without astute medical intervention, nor could she stay alive without it now. The potent medications that ensure her

---

[‡]   The only secular grounds, that is.

survival exact a high cost. "I've lost the vision in my right eye," she wrote to me recently, "have endless skin cancers, lost half of my lower lip, am osteoporotic, have chronic kidney damage, am on lifelong immunosuppression, have lost my monthly cycle at the age of 35 [now 44], had three strokes, require ongoing immunoglobulin infusions, blood transfusions. I have even lost my once happy marriage as a result of what cancer brought, and yet, I'm the happiest I have ever been or could ever imagine being! Truly so blessed!" For all that she has had to surrender in terms of physical health, she has given up nothing in exuberance and joie de vivre. In fact, for her those qualities have become fuller, more deeply felt, and far less conditional.

A skilled and much sought-after sports chiropractor, once a pillar of health, Dr. Harris never spared herself when it came to work. "I was passionate about my athlete clients," she told me. "I loved helping people. Let's say they had trained forever, and they endured an injury a few months before a race. My inner reward would come from seeing their joy crossing the finish line. I was a bit of a workaholic, one might say—"

"You could probably take out the 'a bit,' " I interjected.

"Yes," she concurred, "my clinic grew really, really fast. When the regular hours were fully booked, I found it really hard to leave somebody in pain. I started coming in very early and staying very, very late. People began to notice I was getting sick all the time. I had strep throat at least every month. I had a terrible disk herniation in my low back that impacted my right leg, and I would still go into the clinic. I was hobbling, trying to help others succeed through their pain, ignoring my own. I loved being busy. I loved everything about it."

If her personality loved the overwork, her body did not. At age thirty-five, on an outing with her two children, Harris got the shocking news. "There I am," she recalled, "I'm a mom of two babies, still nursing my youngest, and I'm standing at the aquarium. I had done a very routine blood test that day, and now it's the lab calling, with this tone of urgency and panic. 'Is this Erica Harris? You need to go the nearest emergency ward right now.' I ended up being diagnosed with a very aggressive form of AML, acute myeloid leukemia, a rare version of it that usually only older men get." Encouraged by the high rate of expected good results, she received two courses of chemotherapy. Neither proved effective.

In 2012 Harris was advised to enter a palliative care facility, where she was told that daily transfusions might keep her alive for no more than two months. Unwilling to yield to that grim diagnosis, she fought to stay home with her small children, going to the hospital daily to receive her transfusions. She also continued to pursue her emotional healing and spiritual path until, just before the ominous two months were up, an unlikely remission surprised both her and her physicians. "It was really hard," she told me. "I'm not sure why I'm here today, but I truly believe it was because I transformed myself from within, allowing myself to be real about everything that was going on now in the present, but also in the past. And allowing myself just the space to express it all."

Like Donna Zmenak, Harris did yoga and meditation and pursued nutritional healing. But the biggest change was that, for the first time in her life, she allowed herself to feel the entire range of her emotions, releasing a lifelong pattern of repression. She fully gave herself over to her grief and shed tears of despair. "One time during my first hospitalization, I watched my kids going home with the nanny," she recalled. "*I* wanted to be the one driving home with those babies. *I* wanted to be making them dinner. *I* wanted to be putting them to bed. I turned around from that window, and I slumped down to the floor with my back against the wall. I grabbed my knees and I wept. I wept and I wept. I didn't stop for days." As a telling sign of the reigning medical culture, the ward psychiatrist was consulted to see her. "She came in," Erica said, smiling in recounting this, "and she literally had this Hawaiian floral-print gown, and she's like, 'I'm off to Hawaii, but I can prescribe something for you to treat this depression, whatever you need. I heard you have been crying.' What I really needed was just the space to experience all of my emotions, with no pretense—no pretense, for the first time. I needed to feel the hurt of it all."

For all her recurrent health challenges, nearly ten years after her terminal prognosis of a mere sixty days' survival, Harris is vibrant, brimming with energy, raising her two children, whom she has triumphantly shepherded into adolescence, and actively inspiring and helping others on their healing path. We have plans, she and I, to work together someday. I see in her case the miracles of modern medicine joining with the power of self-transformation to achieve results neither could have achieved without the other.

The Harvard psychiatrist Dr. Jeffrey Rediger, who has explored many cases of "miraculous" recovery from terminal malignancy and other fatal diseases, told me that a transformation of identity, such as Zmenak and Harris underwent, seemed to him to be the key. "It's a nebulous concept," he conceded, "but ultimately that's where the healing is to be found. These people who get better really change their beliefs about themselves or their beliefs about the universe." This has been my observation as well, no matter with what illness: cancer, autoimmune disease, or neurological disorders like MS or ALS.[†] Some, like Donna Zmenak, refused medical treatment; others, like Will Pye and Erica Harris, wouldn't have

---

†   Even with the usually fatal diagnosis of ALS, there are dozens of medically documented and peer-reviewed published cases of partial or complete reversals in the neurological literature, or decades of survival after terminal prognoses, even after long years of people having been wheelchair-dependent and on respiratory assistance. The physicist Stephen Hawking famously outlived his two-year prognosis by over fifty years.

survived without it. In all cases, people voluntarily and with relentless courage underwent a painful but ultimately exhilarating shedding of a second skin, the blend of adaptive, self-abnegating traits I cataloged in chapter 7, on attachment versus authenticity, and grouped also under Erich Fromm's term "social character." Disease's role as teacher rests in how it leads people to question everything they had thought and felt about themselves, and to retain only what serves their wholeness.

In her own documentation of "miraculous" healing, Dr. Kelly Turner unearthed similar themes. The centrality of reorienting identity in the direction of the authentic is among her essential findings. "Everyone that I've interviewed said that they actually wouldn't trade this experience for the world," she told me. "Because the person they are now is so much more complete. They feel whole, they feel happier, they feel more grateful, that they wouldn't want to go back to who they were before that hardship. Many of them, I would dare say nearly all of them, tell me that they're a completely different person now than they were at the beginning of their journey." As I related earlier, Turner also said that many of her interviewees wished they had learned these same lessons decades before their illness. The challenge we all face is: Can we acquire that learning before life forces it upon us? Do we have to wait to "suffer into truth"?

"Every moment was precious," Erica recalled. "I needed to go deeply inward at that time and reflect on all of the layers, like I hadn't done all my life. I finally realized how my body had been screaming no all my while as a sports chiropractor, and how I had ignored it. The disease has been my greatest teacher."

———

Intrigued by her advice to Donna Zmenak, I contacted Cheryl Canfield, now decades past the uterine cancer she had been assured was terminal. I was surprised to learn that she had accepted the possibility of succumbing to the disease. "When I started writing *Profound Healing*," she told me, "the working title was 'Dying Well,' because I assumed that what the doctors were telling me was not necessarily true, but likely to be true. The probability, if not for sure the inevitability, was that I would die of this cancer. I began the book because, at forty-one years old, I had no idea how to face this totally unexpected journey that meant leaving my body early, my family, and my loved ones. I wanted to create my last project, writing something that would help me figure out how to take this path and might also help others coming along behind me. It turned out that the title had to be changed. What we need to die well is also what we need to live well. That's what the disease taught me."

I also talked with Will Pye about the experience that caused him to write *Blessed with a Brain Tumor*. This tall, athletic man had been diagnosed at age thirty-one with a malignant growth at the precise spot where, as a depressed twenty-year-old, he used to imagine pointing a gun to his head in a visual fantasy of suicide. Heeding his inner guidance and with the agreement of his neurosurgeon, he delayed surgery for two years. He pursued what medical parlance calls "watchful waiting" while engaging in intense self-healing practices, until the onset of seizures signaled an increase in the size of the malignancy. The tumor was then excised, followed by radiation. By now Pye is just beyond the outer limit of the anticipated survival period for his type of brain cancer.† For seven years he has been off his antiseizure medications, despite having been told he'd need them for the rest of his life. He cannot know how it will go for him, and yet, as the title of his

---

†   As this book goes to its final editing stage, December 2021, Will Pye reports he is now in rehab/recovery from a repeated bout of surgery this past October, owing to the recurrence of his tumor, first diagnosed in 2011. The average survival rate of his original diagnosis is five to ten years.

book asserts, he insists the disease has been a blessing. The diagnosis, he told me, served as a wake-up call.

"What did it wake you up to?" I asked.

"The finite nature of this life, for one thing. It brought the truth of my mortality into a more felt, easier-to-grasp dimension. While we all know it intellectually, psychologically we function with an avoidance or disregard for the reality of death. After the diagnosis, I'd be having conversations with people in the awareness that this might be the last conversation I ever had with that person. And that creates an extraordinary degree of shared presence, listening, care. So yes, total transformation. Day to day when I get out of bed, there is a practice of fully recognizing the gift of this moment, of this day, of this body, of this breathing happening now."

Ours is a culture wholly averse to death and even aging; think of how many products are geared toward erasing or "reversing" the signs of oncoming infirmity, the physical reminders of life's finitude. Here, then, is another sense in which healing is an upstream journey: it necessarily involves the full-hearted acceptance of the inevitability of our passing and the determination to experience all the days and moments that lead us to our earthly exit.

Some years ago, I led a retreat for people with all manner of health challenges, from mental distress such as depression through addictions to physical illness. One attendee was a sixty-four-year-old I will call Sam, with advanced ALS, that mysterious, paralyzing, and fatal degeneration of the nervous system. His form of the condition was the so-named bulbar onset type, meaning that it was not his limbs, but the muscles of speaking, chewing, and swallowing that were first affected. "I . . . came . . . here," he told the group in a voice hoarse, attenuated, and halting, "because . . . I want . . . to live." As he described himself, his pre-disease personality lined up with what I have seen in everyone with his condition: what we have earlier called superautonomous self-sufficiency, the shutdown of feelings and the almost phobic refusal to seek help or emotional support from anyone.

After a week of intense self-exploration, intimate sharing with fellow participants such as he had never been capable of, and some revelatory psychedelic sessions, Sam said he had an announcement to make. "When I first said I wanted to live," he said, his voice notably stronger and more resonant, "I meant I wanted to live longer. I don't see it that way anymore. I still want to *live*, but I now know that 'living' means not chronology but quality. I really want to be in my life every moment, experience what is ahead of me to the fullest, as I have never done before." He died a year and a half later, in keeping with his prognosis. In the months following the retreat, Sam—and after his death, his family—sent messages of gratitude and celebration for the vitality, love, and joy he was able to manifest in himself and with his close ones in the final phase of his life.

The manner of Sam's dying, measured not in numbers on a calendar but in the aspects of himself he was able to reclaim, came as close as I have ever seen to what has been called a "good death." He had not been cured of his illness, but he had healed. He had brought into harmony parts of his essence that might have remained fragmented and discordant without the unasked-for invitation his disease presented him with. He also found a way to make life-affirming meaning of what he could just as easily have viewed as cruel, destructive, or senseless—as many do view death from "untimely" illness. As his family's later communications made clear, the meaning he made has endured well beyond his bodily existence, radiating into their own lives.

"The journey," Will Pye said to me, "is to find the gift in the challenge. It impelled me to practice and cultivate the capacity to consciously choose the meaning of all that was happening."

That challenge, and the gifts of self that can ensue from engaging with it, is waiting patiently for each of us in the "what's happening" of our lives right now. The choice we have is whether to take it up now or to wait for a more urgent occasion for the learning.

Chapter 28

Before the Body Says No:
First Steps on the Return to Self

Healing has no choice but to ripple out when we are
real with ourselves and with others.

—Helen Knott, *In My Own Moccasins*

I'll say it again: disease is not the authenticity instructor I would wish for any of us. Major calamities of body and mind are only the latest and loudest summons from essential parts of ourselves we have lost touch with. To make such drastic signals less necessary, we can get better at hearing and heeding the more subtle alerts our lives unfailingly send our way, before they become a clamor. This chapter offers some simple but potent practices, distilled from my work with thousands of people, that can retrain mind and body to become more sensitive and responsive to these calls from within.

It may be helpful, in doing these exercises, to bear in mind some fundamental and by now familiar principles discussed throughout this book:

a. *Your personality is not you; you are not your personality.* The mystery of who we truly are lies somewhere beyond the veil of personality. This does not make the personality "false," any more than clothing is true or false. Unlike clothing, though, "taking off" the personality, or perhaps just some parts of it, appears to be out of the question because *it seems like who we are.* The point is not that we should (or can) suddenly strip it all away in the name of authenticity. It helps, however, to remind ourselves that it does not define us. We were not, to channel a popular song, born this way.[†]

b. *The personality is an adaptation.* What we call the personality is often a jumble of genuine traits and conditioned coping styles, including some that do not reflect our true self at all but rather the loss of it. Each personality takes shape according to how one's particular temperament reciprocally interacts with family, community, and culture. It may not express our real needs, deepest longings, and truest nature, but rather our attempt to compensate for our estrangement from them. "We suffer from a case of mistaken identity. Our culture has sold us a bill of goods about who we really are," writes marital/family therapist Dick Schwartz.[1]

The aim of healing work is not to shed the personality entirely but to free ourselves from its automatic programming, granting us access to what's underneath, to reconnect with what's essential about us. "Liberation," A. H. Almaas says, "is really nothing but the personality becoming free in the moment; the personality loses its grip, lets itself just relax."[2] Our genuine strengths remain, with more room than ever before to stretch out and make themselves known.

c. *Our bodies do keep the score.*[‡] If the authentic self can be covered by many layers of limiting self-belief and conditioned behavior, it is never obliterated. It continues to speak to us through the body. We can learn to heed the messages the body sends by learning its language.

d. *The personality, and the loss of our essential nature, is not personal.* The disconnect from self is endemic in our materialist

---

[†] Lady Gaga, "Born This Way," 2011.

[‡] A nod here to the title of Bessel van der Kolk's contemporary classic work on trauma, *The Body Keeps the Score.*

culture, encouraged and then exploited in many spheres, from economic to cultural and political. Historically speaking, of course, the search for the true self under the limiting layers of mind long predates modern society. Each of us, then, while responsible for our own healing journey, and bound to grapple with our own personality's particularities, can also take heart in knowing that we are engaging with a universal dynamic—a tale as old as time, to quote the theme song to *Beauty and the Beast*, the beloved Disney musical about unlikely transformations and recovering one's essence.

What matters in applying the practices below is not so much the letter of the law as the spirit of the endeavor. That spirit is captured in the name of a methodology I have developed: Compassionate Inquiry (CI). Compassionate Inquiry is both a professional training I have taught to thousands of therapists in over eighty countries and a practice of individual self-reflection, as outlined below. To their edification (and sometimes dismay), the professional participants in the CI course spend the first three months working on their own issues, not those of others. *Therapist, heal thyself.*

Taking the latter half of the name first, what does it mean to *inquire*? If genuine, an inquiry is an open-ended exploration. It requires, first and foremost, humility: allowing, with Socrates, that we do not already know the answer or, better yet, the very real possibility that we haven't yet happened upon the right questions. Accordingly, in what follows I recommend you do your best to suspend, at least for the moment, whatever you believe you know about yourself. In this heyday of superficial pop psychology, self-knowledge is most often a case of the personality being an expert on the subject of itself, rather than the deeper, more intimate kind of knowing that can illuminate darkened corners of our histories, the better to see our present predicaments clearly. This is what we are inquiring into here. We are out to know ourselves, not merely to know *about* ourselves.

The other piece is *compassion*. To inquire compassionately takes openness, patience, and generosity. Think of how you would treat a struggling friend or loved one in their time of need, the leeway you would grant them to be confused, perplexed, frustrated. Being compassionate to yourself is no different, except that it's often harder to practice. In compassion there is no exhortation that we should be other than the way we are, only an invitation to inquire into the what, how, and why of the beliefs and behaviors that do not serve us. I would never tell anyone that they *should* be compassionate with themselves. Compassion brooks no "should." In any case, our defended, walled-off parts do not respond positively to such demands—why would they? It is far kinder and more effective to bring attention to the *lack* of self-compassion, to notice it and be curious about how it presents in one's life. Once seen, it softens, allowing one to investigate its long-ago origins and present-day impacts.

There is nothing touchy-feely here. Compassion is distinct from conjuring up warm feelings toward anyone, including the self. It is an attitude, not a feeling. Unlike feelings, which come and go of their own accord, attitudes can be invited, generated, and nurtured in the face of *any* emotional state. The attitude here is one of inexhaustible non-judgment toward whatever one notices. When self-judgments arise—as they inevitably do—we can stay curious about their origin without believing their content.

Everything is a candidate for inquiry, even intensely negative experiences like self-loathing.† Rather than admonishing ourselves

---

†   More on the adaptive sources of self-loathing in chapter 30.

for hating ourselves, we can be curious as to why self-hatred arrived on the scene in the first place. A question posed in that spirit often illuminates. When the beauty in us can compassionately accept the beast—allow it to "be our guest," if you will—the latter may transform into a handsome and loving companion; at the very least, it can relax and stop hounding us so ravenously.

Before the Body Says No: A Self-Inquiry Exercise

Here's an exercise, to be done daily or weekly, or at whatever frequency seems right to you. It does require commitment over time—which, if I'm any example, can be hard to muster. If committing even a few minutes a day for such self-inquiry seems beyond the doable, it's worth noticing that, too, without judgment, and asking whence the reluctance.

Without judgment doesn't mean without vigilance. Our personalities are adept at throwing up roadblocks of rationalization when they sense we may be trying to unfasten or even question their hold. A commitment to healing means being hip to their tricks, as it were. The standard excuse is also the lamest: "I don't have the time." Most of us, even the busy ones, have more time than we know what to do with; what we lack is a strong sense of *intention* for its use. Default pursuits, whether noble or frivolous, quickly fill the void, and suddenly there's "no time." We don't help matters by protesting, "Oh, but I really *do* want to work on myself, it's just . . . ," and then listing all the reasons that make it impossible. If that sounds like you, ask yourself, empowered by compassionate curiosity, what discomfort it may evoke in the present to even engage in self-work. It may be that setting a strong intention opens you up to the vulnerable fact that you could be disappointed, or confronted, or pushed beyond well-worn zones of comfort. These risks are real. Whatever the case, it will not help to coerce, cajole, or shame yourself into any practice, not even ones meant to help you.

This exercise is best done in written form, in a quiet room where you can be with yourself and your experience, free from distractions. You will want to write out your answers, because doing so will engage the mind more actively and profoundly than observing your mental ideas or insights; also, because you may want a record of your progress. Writing by hand rather than typing helps create a sense of connection with yourself, while keeping the digital distractions at bay.

This exercise, I've often been told, has helped to change people's lives. The key is to do it regularly, at intervals of your choosing but at minimum once a week.

Question #1:

In my life's important areas, what am I not saying no to?
In other words, where did I, today or this week, sense a "no" within me that wanted to be expressed, but I stifled it, conveying a "yes" (or a silence) where a "no" wanted to be heard?

Get current and stay specific. Really look, and remember that we are speaking here not of occasional lapses but of chronic patterns. We all make mindful and heartfelt decisions to support others at the cost of our own convenience. Parents, necessarily, act this way all the time: most children will never know how many sleep-deprived nights a mom or a dad spent watching over them when they were ill. Or, if a friend is in serious distress, opting to meet them rather than following our desire to stay home and rest might be an authentic choice. In no way does compassionate inquiry seek to stigmatize genuine altruism. It is the *habitual, unwilled* selflessness ingrained in many people's personalities, the kind that takes a heavy toll, that we are gently bringing to the fore.

People tend to find this dynamic present in two major realms: work and personal relationships. On the job, for example, you may have accepted an additional task that you sensed would overburden you; or you took work home for the weekend, giving up time for yourself or for your family. You might not have said no to a colleague who was impinging on your personal space; or maybe someone asked your opinion, and you gave them what you thought they wanted to hear, not what was true for you.

In your personal life, you may have accepted a friend's invitation for drinks when you really needed to rest. You may have engaged in sex with a partner when physical intimacy was the last thing on your mind, or when some issue needed to be resolved before resuming erotic contact; or you may have overridden a "no" feeling that cropped up in you midway through. You may have assented when, on short notice, neighbors asked for help with moving, even though you had other pressing matters to attend to. Perhaps you needed to take space for yourself but opted against asking your partner to mind the kids for a while. Or you assumed your perennial role of family caregiver to your aging parents, rather than requesting that your siblings pitch in and lighten your load.

More generally, ask yourself: With whom and in what situations do I find it most difficult to say no? Even if I say it, do I do so reluctantly, apologetically, or with guilt? Do I beat myself up about it afterward?

There is a world of difference between a considered, conscious "yes" and a compulsive suppression of a "no." Admittedly, the realities of modern-day work can blur the distinction: we may rationally decide that holding on to a job requires saying yes to demands that tax us, demands that we would rather rebuff. All too many people find themselves in such situations for the sake of sheer economic survival. In such cases, we can ask ourselves whether the price we pay is worth the stress thereby incurred. That millions lack the freedom to even raise that question is a social problem of vast proportions. But for many among us, the absence of the "no" does not serve either our personal or economic well-being. Only you can know which denial of "no" characterizes your own situation. Even so, just getting clear that we are consciously and purposefully accepting a situation that incurs chronic stress is already a step up from doing so automatically.

Question #2:

How does my inability to say no impact my life?

You will find this impact lands in three main spheres: the physical, the emotional, and the interpersonal.

On the physical level, we are talking about bodily warning signs such as insomnia, back pain, muscle spasms, dry mouth, frequent colds, abdominal pains, digestive problems, fatigue, headaches, skin rashes, loss of appetite, or the urge to overeat.

On the emotional plane, this inquiry yields answers such as sadness, alienation, anxiety, or boredom. The impact can also manifest as emotional deficits: for example, the loss of pleasure in things that used to bring joy, a dulling of one's sense of humor, etc.

In the interpersonal realm, the most frequent impact is resentment toward the people or situations where the authentic answer was stifled. That, on close examination, is an ironic outcome. Let's say you suppress the "no" in order to maintain closeness with someone you care about. In practice, resentment drives you further away because it will contaminate your love for that person. They, too, will sense the emotional withdrawal fueled by resentment. It will show up in your facial expressions, tone, body language. You will have achieved the opposite of what you had wished for. And if you pay attention, you will know that resentment is more than an abstract emotional quality: it literally feels corrosive in your belly or chest, or tight in the muscles of your jaw, neck, or forehead. Resentment can be seen as the residue of things unsaid, feelings not honored. The word "resent" comes, after all, from the French *ressentir,* meaning "to feel again." And again, and again, and again, in our minds and bodies, until we get the memo.

For a fuller accounting, one additional place to look for impacts is slightly further out, in the material, everyday world. The question here would be "What do I miss out on in life as a result of my inability to assert myself?" Possible answers include fun, joy, spontaneity, self-respect, libido, opportunities for growth and adventure, and on and on.

Question #3:
What bodily signals have I been overlooking? What symptoms have I been ignoring that could be warning signs, were I to pay conscious attention?
The third question reverses the direction of the previous one: here we *start* with the physical impacts, trusting them to reveal where authenticity has been missing. It requires you to take an inventory of your body—a regular and deliberate scan—for the day or the week. For some people, this question is an essential backup measure, because their self-denial has become so normal that they might not be able to identify an unsaid "no"—the word doesn't even dare form itself in the mind, much less on the tongue.

The idea is to take a regular survey of ongoing symptoms— say, fatigue or a persistent headache or upset stomach or low back pain—and then ask what unsaid "no" these might be signaling. Of course, this requires pausing long enough to spot the signs. In our culture of mind-body bifurcation, many of us have become accustomed to ignoring the body's messages. The brain's reward mechanisms may even revel, in a manner very much like addiction, in the elevated levels of dopamine and endorphins that flow when others appreciate or benefit from our self-denial. There's a reason for the term "adrenaline junkies." The drive to be good to others, a genuine impulse when not compulsive, can thus overwhelm the equally authentic imperative to be good to ourselves.

Likewise, in people who are completely identified with their roles in the world, the "no" has a hard time breaking through the soundproof armor of identity to make itself heard. We confuse ourselves with our worldly job descriptions—doctor, therapist, teacher, lawyer, CEO, man of the house, supermom. Hence this third question, inviting us to proactively consider what the body has been telling us all along, how it is trying to draw our attention away from our conditioned identity and toward what we really need. This may very well prevent the body from having to shout at us more loudly or to initiate a more disastrous crash.

Question #4:
What is the hidden story behind my inability to say no?
What feeds our habitual pattern of denying our "no" is what I call *the story*. By this I mean the narrative, the explanation, the justification, the rationalization that makes these habits seem normal and even necessary. In truth they sprout from limiting core beliefs about ourselves. Most often we are not aware that they *are* stories. We think and act as if they're true.

When I pose this question in workshops, it can take people some time to identify the underlying narrative, the story beneath the story. When we get past the minutiae of the particular situation (e.g., "Well, you know how my mom is—it's just easier to say yes than to go through the hassle"), we find the deeper tale, whose internal logic determines our interpretations and reactions. This subtextual layer is always about the self, not the current circumstances.

If you have a hard time spotting the story underlying your behavior, try asking, "What must I believe about myself to deny my own needs this way?" The answer, even a speculative one, will likely be very close to the mark. Our stories, though neither objective nor accurate, are always *internally consistent* with our behavior and our experience.

Some examples of familiar stories:

- Saying no means I can't handle something. It's a sign of weakness. I have to be strong.
- I have to be "good" to deserve being loved. If I say no, I'm not lovable.
- I'm responsible for how other people feel and what they experience. I mustn't disappoint anyone.
- I'm not worthy unless I'm doing something useful.
- If people knew how I really felt, they wouldn't like me.
- If I turned down my friend/spouse/colleague/parent/neighbor, I would feel deservedly guilty.[†]
- It's selfish to say no.
- It's not loving to have anger.

Notable in these answers is the implied double standard. We usually think of double standards as differential rules of the road from which we exempt ourselves while holding others to unsparing scrutiny—as parodied in the phrase "Do as I say, not as I do." In practice, such unconscious duplicity is just as often employed *against* the self: call it reverse hypocrisy. I often ask people, "If your friend said no to some request because that's what felt true to them, would you condemn them as 'weak'?" The answer is, predictably, "Of course not." Check in with yourself: Would

---

† Befriending our compulsive guilt feelings is covered in chapter 30.

you burden anyone else with the responsibility never to disappoint others' expectations? If a neighbor had to turn down a request because they had something to attend to, would you charge them with selfishness? Would you say to your child that she is worthless unless she makes herself "useful"? I'm confident that you, like everyone to whom I put these questions, will answer in the negative.

Some people balk at saying no, out of an ingrained sense of being "the strong one" whom others respect for their uncomplaining reliability. This kind of "strength" comes at the expense of real power, a quality that involves having a say in which burdens we do or don't pick up. Most of us, given a choice, would rather live a life of conscious power and cultivated fortitude than one of unwilled strength.

Question #5:
Where did I learn these stories?
No one is imbued at birth with a sense of worthlessness. It is through our interactions with nurturing caregivers that we develop our view of ourselves. If, because of their own trauma, they treat us badly, we take it personally. If, for whatever reason, they are stressed or unhappy, we take that personally, too. Awareness of our parents' distress, which as young children we could not have alleviated, can lead us to question our own value, even if we were assured verbally that we were loved. That certainly happened to me, as came to my awareness most forcefully on a therapist's couch—an incident I will describe in chapter 30.

The intention in looking at the past is not to dwell on it but to let go of it. "The moment you know how your suffering came to be, you are already on the path of release from it," the Buddha said.[3] Hence this fifth question calls for a frank look at our childhood experiences—not as we would have liked them to be, but as they were.

Question #6:

Where have I ignored or denied the "yes" that wanted to be said?

If stifling a "no" can make us ill, so can withholding an authentic "yes." What have you wanted to do, manifest, create, or say that you have forsaken in the name of perceived duty or out of fear? What desire to play or explore have you ignored? What joys have you denied yourself out of a belief that you don't deserve them, or out of a conditioned fear that they'll be snatched away?

As with the unspoken "no," ask yourself: What is the belief keeping me from affirming my creative impulses? For me, it was the imperative to keep working at the expense of ignoring my intuition. As I wrote in *When the Body Says No*:

> For many years after becoming a doctor, I was too caught up in my workaholism to pay attention to myself or to my deepest urges. In the rare moments I permitted any stillness, I noted a small fluttering at the pit of my belly, a barely perceptible disturbance. The faint whisper of a word would sound in my head: writing. At first I could not say whether it was heartburn or inspiration. The more I listened, the louder the message became: I needed to write, to express myself through written language not only so that others might hear me but so that I could hear myself.

"Music saved my life," the Nashville songwriter and former alcoholic Mary Gauthier told me.† "The self-expression that I'm

---

†   In fact, Gauthier expressed as much in the title of her recent book, *Saved by a Song: The Art and Healing Power of Songwriting*.

able to articulate through song, and then of course the resonance when it connects with other people, has been literally a lifesaver for me. And it has kept me sober as well. It's a reason to get up in the morning that continues to move me." The creative force within, whichever way it calls us, is a powerful support to healing.

"What is in us must out; otherwise we may explode at the wrong places or become hopelessly hemmed in by frustrations," wrote that wise medical scientist János Selye in *The Stress of Life*.[4] I've learned this lesson well. Whenever something in me demanded to be uttered and I gave it no expression, I suffocated in the silence. The books I have written, including the one now in your hands, came from heeding the call of what in me needed out.

Chapter 29

Seeing Is Disbelieving:
Undoing Self-Limiting Beliefs

*Healing cannot occur if we do not accept our worthiness—that
we are worth healing, even if doing so might shake up our
view of the world and how we interact with others.*
—Mario Martinez, Psy.D., *The MindBody Code*

In a society that capitalizes on people's sense of inadequacy, the
most prevalent self-limiting story is bound to be "I am not worth
it." It underlies all the others bullet-listed in the previous chapter. Unaddressed, it sabotages our best efforts to inquire compassionately into ourselves. I felt its sting even while writing this
book. It was touchingly acknowledged by one of my friends and
mentors in the therapeutic field, Peter Levine. "I have answered
the question 'Have I *done* enough?' positively," Peter said during
a recent conversation. "I *have* done enough. But '*Am* I enough?'
I'm still wrestling with that one." I smiled in recognition.

There are many ways of working with the tall tale of unworthiness. Some teachers suggest positive affirmations. Personally, I
have found that such messages seem to evaporate precisely when
I most need them.

We should not underestimate how entrenched and insidious
this conviction of unworthiness is, or how difficult it is to dislodge with words. We were almost literally hypnotized into it. In
a neural framework, as the biologist Bruce Lipton explains, it's a

matter of brainwaves. Delta waves, the brain's lowest frequency, predominate in our first two years, then theta waves ramp up until we are about six. "A child under seven is predominantly in theta," he told me. "Theta is a hypnotic state, and it's how you absorb all this stuff for seven years. Just as under the spell of a hypnotist, you believe whatever messages you get." Only afterward does the state of conscious awareness and logical thinking associated with alpha and beta wave activity come on line. "We download our perceptions and beliefs about life years before we acquire the capacity for critical thinking," Dr. Lipton writes. "Those perceptions or misperceptions become our truths."[1] From such truths, we will henceforth generate our concepts about ourselves in the world. More precisely, from such untruths.

We strike a powerful blow for authentic autonomy when we notice where the self-deceptions reside and bring fresh perception, fueled by compassionate inquiry, to them.

———

You have pinpointed the unspoken "no" or "yes," started to identify the various impacts, looked at the stories underpinning such patterned self-denials, and inquired into their sources. Now what? While there is inherent value in knowing our stories *as* stories, what we ultimately want is to unfasten their hold on us.

The following exercise will suggest some first steps to liberating ourselves, to waking up from the hypnotic reverie of unworthiness.

For the healing section in my book on addiction, I adapted— with permission—a series of steps formulated by Jeffrey M. Schwartz, a psychiatry professor at the University of California, Los Angeles, in his book *The Mind and the Brain*.[2] Here I take the adaptation one step further, applying the method to self-limiting beliefs of all stripes.

While Dr. Schwartz originally developed these steps for healing obsessive-compulsive disorder, they readily lend themselves to reprogramming other kinds of thought loops as well. After all, negative thinking has a more-than-obsessive quality: we are compelled to it, over and over, despite deriving no pleasure from it. The idea is to retrain the brain, to strengthen through conscious effort the prefrontal cortex's capacity to break out of a past-based trance and repatriate us to the present. Any repetitively self-deprecating thought pattern can be worked with in this way.

The method is an *experiential* one, requiring commitment and mindfulness. It needs to be not only done but fully experienced. Only when attention is present can the mind rewire the brain. *"Conscious attention must be paid,"* Jeffrey Schwartz insists. "Therein lies the key. Physical changes in the brain depend for their creation on a mental state in the mind—the state called attention. Paying attention matters."

To Dr. Schwartz's original four steps, I add one more. These five steps are most effective when practiced regularly, but also whenever a self-undermining belief pulls you so strongly that you fear becoming mired in it. Find a place to sit and write, preferably a quiet place. With this exercise, too, you'll want to keep a handwritten journal.

Step 1: Relabel

The first step is to call the self-limiting thought what it is: a thought, a belief, not the truth. For example, "I *seem to believe* that I'm responsible for everyone's feelings." Or, "I'm *having the thought* that I have to be strong." Or, "I'm *acting as if I think* I'm only worthy when I'm being helpful." Bringing conscious awareness to this step in particular is vital: we are awakening the part of ourselves that can observe mental content without identifying with it—acting as our own interested but impartial observer.

The point of relabeling is not to make the self-negating thought disappear: a longtime occupant of your brain, it will resist eviction with everything it has. In fact, it is strengthened by efforts to suppress or expel it, just as surely as by giving in to it. Remember: you're not trying to debunk the story or make it wrong. Arguing with it would be like telling a two-year-old screaming, "I hate you!" over a plate of vegetables: "No, you don't. That's just a thought you're having." Nor do you try to replace it with some sort of cheerful opposite—for example, "I'm a good person," or "I am a channel of pure light." Rather, you are divesting from the *certainty* that the implicit belief is true. In doing so, you put the story in its place, gently taking it off the nonfiction shelf. It is no longer an ironclad law to be resisted or an accusation to be refuted: just a thought, painful or dysfunctional though it may be. Odds are, the thought will come back—at which point you'll relabel it again, with calm determination and mindful, vigilant awareness.

Step 2: Reattribute

In this step you learn to assign the relabeled belief to its proper source: "This is my brain sending me an old, familiar message." Rather than blaming yourself or anyone else, you are ascribing cause to its proper place: neural circuits programmed into your brain when you were a child. It represents a time, early in life, when you lacked the necessary conditions for your emotional circuitry's healthy development. You're not pushing the thought away, but you're also making clear that you didn't ask for it, nor have you ever deserved it.

Reattribution is directly linked with compassionate curiosity toward the self. The presence of a negative belief says nothing about you as a person; it is not a moral failure or a character weakness, just the effect of circumstances over which you had no control. What you do have now is some say over how you respond to the negative belief. The quality of your present-moment experience is far more tied to that choice of responses than to anything fixed or preordained by the past.

Step 3: Refocus

This one is all about buying yourself a little time. Being mind phantoms, your negative self-beliefs will pass—if you give them time. The key principle, Jeffrey Schwartz points out, is this: "It's not how you feel; it's what you do that counts." That doesn't mean you suppress your feelings or beliefs, only that you don't let them pull you under or derail your inquiry. You stay in relationship with them even as you consciously take a detour.

So here's the game plan: if you manage to catch a negative self-belief striving to seize control, *find something else to do.* This takes awareness, and it's best not to beat yourself up if you miss it at first. Sometimes these belief patterns just take over before we can swing into action.

Your initial goal is modest: buy yourself a quarter of an hour. Choose something that you enjoy and will keep you active, preferably something healthy and creative, but really anything that will please you without causing greater harm. Instead of helplessly sinking into the familiar despair of negative self-belief, go for a walk, turn on some music, do a crossword puzzle—whatever can get you through the next fifteen little minutes. "Physical activity seems to be especially helpful," Schwartz suggests. "But the important thing is that whatever activity you choose, it must be something you enjoy doing." Or, if you don't immediately have the energy for that, you might refocus on what is loving and alive in your life: on possibilities you have fulfilled or glimpsed, on what you have contributed to yourself or others, on people you have loved or who have offered you love.

The purpose of refocusing is to teach your brain that it doesn't have to succumb to the old, tired story. It can learn to choose something else, even if—to begin with—it's only for a while.

Step 4: Revalue

Here's where you take stock and get real. Up until now, the self-rejecting belief has ruled the roost, overshadowing whatever else you may consciously believe about yourself. Let's say you've told yourself, "I deserve love in my life," but all the while your mind is assigning greater value to the currency of "I'm worthless." It's that second one that tips the scales at least nine times out of ten. You can think of this step, then, as a kind of audit, an investigation into the objective costs of the beliefs your mind has invested so much time and energy in.

What has this belief actually done for me? you ask. Possible answers: *It has left me feeling ashamed and isolated. It has produced bitterness. It has stopped me from pursuing dreams, from taking risks, from experiencing intimate love. It has incurred physical illness or symptoms.* To recognize its impact, allow your answers to go beyond the conceptual. Feel your own body state as you consider the space the belief has occupied in your mind. The impacts live right there, in your physiology, as surely as they do in your actions and relationships.

Be specific: What has been the net value of the unworthiness story—or whichever identified story you are working on—in your relationship with your partner, wife, husband? Your best friend, your children, your boss, your employees, your co-workers? What happened yesterday when you allowed the belief to rule you? What happened last week? What will happen today? Pay close attention to what you feel when you recall these events and when you foresee what's predictably ahead.

A complete revaluation also takes into account any *payoffs* or *dividends* you have derived from this belief. Has it kept you safe from harm, even in the short term? Has it protected you from criticism or rejection? Include these, too: the more thorough the audit, the better.

Above all, do this exercise without judging yourself. You didn't come into life asking to be programmed in this way, and you will not be punished for what gets uncovered—on the contrary, you are trying to commute the sentence you've been living out. Remember, too, that it's not personal to you. Millions of others with similar experiences have developed the same mechanisms. What *is* personal to you is how you choose to respond to it in the present.

Step 5: Re-create

What has determined your identity up until now? You've been acting out mechanisms wired into your brain before you had a choice in the matter, and from those automatic mechanisms and long-ago programmed beliefs you have fashioned a life. It is time to re-create: to imagine a different life, one truly worth choosing.

You have values. You have passions. You have intention, talent, capability, a desire to contribute, perhaps a latent sense of purpose or calling. In your heart there is love, and you want to connect that with the love in the universe. As you relabel, reattribute, refocus, and revalue, you are releasing patterns that have held you and that you have held on to. In place of a life blighted by your compulsive obsession with acquisition, self-soothing, self-justification, admiration, oblivion, and meaningless activity, what is the life you really want? What do you choose to create? Write down your values and intentions and, once again, do so with conscious awareness. Envision yourself living with integrity, being able to look people in the eye with compassion for them—and for yourself.

The road to hell is not paved with good intentions; it is paved with lack of intention. The more you relabel, reattribute, refocus, and revalue, the freer you will be to re-create. Are you afraid you will stumble? Guess what: you will. That's called being a human being.

———————

To conclude, a word to the wise—or those who wish to be. If we remove the hyphen from "re-create," we are left with the verb form of "recreation," as in "play." An excellent reminder that we do ourselves no favors by taking ourselves, or the process of inquiry, so seriously that we lose a sense of spontaneity and vitality. These steps may not be much fun, but they still work best when infused with some lightness. I have seen more than a few people surprise themselves, mid-process, with a smile.

Chapter 30

Foes to Friends: Working with the Obstacles to Healing

My life has not been about fixing what is broken.
It has been about engaging in a loving and tender
archaeological dig back to my true self.
—Jewel, *Never Broken: Songs Are Only Half the Story*

I wish I could tell you that healing is as straightforward as apply-ing a particular mental exercise a certain number of times a week. Alas, the quest for wholeness is not reducible to any one or two (or three, or twenty, or fifty) practices, modalities, or approaches. Far from a one-and-done proposition, returning to ourselves is a road we choose, with all the twists and turns and seeming cul-de-sacs that come with following—or indeed, forging—an uncertain path. In my experience we are never as close as we hope, and never as far as we fear.

This chapter will offer a way of working with some of the most universal obstacles to healing: crippling guilt; self-loathing and its close cousins, self-rejection, self-sabotage, and self-destructive impulses; and blocks in our emotional memory, or what we may call denial of pain. Again, we're not referring here to abstract concepts. "I'm unworthy" and "I am defective" are much more than thoughts; they live in our neurophysiology and mind as "dis-crete clusters of related mental processes," in the words of Dick Schwartz. "For efficiency's sake, the brain is designed to form these clusters—connections among certain memories, emotions, ways of perceiving the world, and behaviors—which stay together as internal units that can be activated when needed."[1]

Seeking to understand the genesis and, especially, the original function of vexatious brain-mind clusters leads us to the first principle of compassionate self-inquiry. Everything within us, no matter how distressing, exists for a purpose; there is nothing that shouldn't be there, troublesome and even debilitating though it may be. The question thus shifts from "How do I get rid of this?" to "What is this for? Why is this here?" In other words, we endeavor first to get to know these irksome aspects of ourselves and then, as best we can, to turn them from foes to friends.

The truth is, these disturbers of our peace have always been friends, strange though it may sound. Their origins were protective and beneficent and that remains their current aim, even when they seem to go about it in a misguided way.

We need not fear, avoid, reject, or suppress these "undesirables"; in fact, we merely delay our emancipation from them when we do. It isn't them but rather our desperate efforts to keep them at bay that levy the heaviest toll on our mental or physical well-being. Once we see these seeming inner antagonists for what they are and let them be, they tend to respond in kind and begin to let us be. Agency is gained not through resistance to ourselves but by way of acceptance and understanding.

Somewhat playfully, I call these apparent foes "stupid friends." If the adjective strikes you as harsh, feel free to substitute something with less pejorative charge, like "obtuse" or "stubborn." The wilderness guide and depth psychologist Bill Plotkin even honors them with the term "loyal soldiers," after the Japanese military men who, as late as the 1970s, were found hiding in the Philippine jungle, unaware that World War II had long ago ended. All I mean by "stupid" is that these parts cannot learn new tricks: they refuse to get the memo that the circumstances under which they first came along no longer exist, and we are no longer helpless children in peril.

Their reason for being, mind you, is anything but stupid. Although they cause us pain now, they first came along to save us. Their presence is in fact an unmistakable sign of the deep intelligence of the human bodymind. And fortunately, healing does not require their disappearance, only their realignment—or perhaps their reassignment. What matters is that we, rather than they, are in the lead.

———————

Over the years I have performed many acts of commission or omission for which healthy remorse was—or would have been—an appropriate response. I have lied, neglected duties, and been harsh to people. In the wake of such behaviors, I would hope for myself that I'd feel a proportionate degree of regret that would prompt me to be accountable: to rectify matters as much as possible, to restore trust, and to think twice before conducting myself that way again. This kind of healthy remorse goes hand in hand with self-knowledge, having a moral compass, and prosocial values; we might even call it Nature's way of bringing us back to our interconnected nature. I doubt any of us would want to live in a world where people were incapable of it.

But there is an unhealthy kind of guilt: a chronic conviction that we are innately blameworthy and should expect, or even deserve, punishment or reproach. In this dim light our faults and failings become evidence of our irredeemable lowliness rather than invitations to grow and to do better. This type of guilt, or the fear of it, often strangles a robust "no," smothering self-assertion: the prospect of others' disapproval or disappointment triggers the intolerable conviction that we are bad, wrong, inexcusable.

Left unchecked, it augurs physical or mental distress, as we have witnessed in stories throughout this book. Many people suffer a corrosive, automatic guilt and shame if they so much as contemplate letting others down, treating their own needs as valuable, or acting on their own behalf.

At its worst, there is a bone-deep guilt that makes a person feel culpable for even being here. Such existential guilt predates language and conscious awareness. I touched on this feeling in myself not long ago during a therapeutic psilocybin session.[†] Lying on the couch, I experienced what a patient of mine once described as "double-mindedness." On the one hand, I knew exactly who and where and when I was, and whom I was with; on the other, the dominant experience as I gazed up at the counselor's kind face was that she was my mother and I a one-year-old infant. I heard myself say, sobbing, "I'm so very sorry I've made your life so hard." I was being shown myself at my life's inception: a baby already bearing responsibility for the suffering around him and flooded with shame and guilt at being the source of it.

Chronic guilt, like the rest of the mind's "stupid friends," is just a guardian past its prime. How so? What possible role could this debilitating, self-shaming stance have played in preserving our safety? Think of it as harm reduction. When the adult world requires, even if inadvertently, that an infant or child suppress parts of her true self—her own desires, feelings, and preferences—she cannot risk noncompliance lest the indispensable attachment relationship be compromised or threatened. She must develop within herself some sturdy enforcement mechanisms to preempt the anxiety of disappointing, or being cut off from, the caregiver. Guilt is one of the most reliable of these inner invigilators. The child's self-expression is curtailed, yes, but above all the

---

†   Psilocybin, a.k.a. "magic mushrooms." I'll have more to say about psychedelic modalities in chapter 31.

relationship with the parent is preserved. For survival, attachment trumps authenticity, as at that age it must.

Most chronic guilt is obsessively single-minded, knowing only one stimulus and exactly one response. The stimulus is that you, child or adult, wish to do something for yourself that may disappoint someone else. This could be a true misdeed, such as stealing or behaving in a way that violates a moral principle; far more often, however, it's nothing more than a desire to act in accordance with an innate impulse, from asserting your boundaries to expressing a negative feeling to even *having* that feeling. Making no distinction, guilt hurls at you the same epithet for all of them: *selfish*. Caught in a time warp, this overstaying friend cannot discern between then and now: it interprets every present-day interaction—be it with a spouse, child, parent, friend, doctor, neighbor, stranger—through the filter of your earliest relationships.

Guilt speaks in the voice of tightly coiled implicit memory circuits, making it incapable of and impervious to reason. It can't help being there, and we cannot get rid of it by force. Even by obeying its dictates we shake it off only temporarily—it is sure to raise its clamor again soon. Our acquiescence, and our trap, derives from the fact that we fear guilt, loathe it, are eager to be rid of it. *Yes, I'll comply,* we plead. *Anything to make you go away.*

Recognizing guilt for the well-meaning friend it is—doggedly faithful to a fault—we can make room for it. Engaging it in cordial conversation without believing its self-devaluing message, we realize we are talking to a very young and innocent creature. Understanding this opens space for compassion toward the inner blame-monger. One might even, with time, feel gratitude for its devotion: we can now listen to the one-note song of warning, *Don't be selfish,* but consciously decide for ourselves whether or not we want to dance to its tune. *Yes, thank you, I hear what you're saying, and thanks for sharing. You're welcome to stick around, but I will let my adult intelligence judge whether I am really hurting someone else or merely respecting my authentic self. This is my show, not yours.* When we give guilt a seat at the table, it no longer needs to ransack the entire house.

Guilt's ornery downstairs neighbor is self-accusation. The internationally celebrated photographer Nan Goldin had long berated herself for her years of addiction, having been dependent on many substances, particularly opiates. "Every morning I wake up in hell," she told me, "waking up to self-condemnation. And then I'm taking two hours to get up because it's so awful." Our conversation took place during a Compassionate Inquiry session she had requested.

"If this were a trial," I asked, "and you were the defendant, what would the prosecution have to say about you?"

Nan didn't miss a beat. "That I've missed years of my life—I don't have many more years to go. That I've spent most of my adult life addicted to drugs, and I, as a result, know nothing. My knowledge is very limited. I didn't look in the mirror and deal with myself. So much has been lost." This from a creative dynamo who had never stopped producing fierce and distinctive art, exhibiting internationally to great acclaim.

"What's the verdict here?" I asked. "Because you've done all those things, that makes you what?"

"Worthless, defective." Nan had moved seamlessly from the roles of plaintiff, prosecutor, and accused to that of hanging judge.

She also said that when she accuses herself of being worthless and defective, she notices a tightness in her throat and a pressure in her torso. At this point in the process I generally ask whether such physical sensations are new phenomena. "No, deeply familiar," Nan replied. "The choked voice and this pressure here, they're familiar feelings." This is a prototypical response: there is nothing new under the sun, or in the shadows, as it were.

"What about the sense you have of yourself as worthless and defective. How familiar is that?"

"Very, very, very."

"And how far does it go back?"

"At least to when I was nine. Or maybe even before—I was told my mother had panic attacks when I was little." In other words, the core beliefs that Nan used to label herself, and their physiological embodiment, well predated her "wasted decades" spent in addiction. They were conceived long before the period about which the self-slandering voice castigated her each morning.

Unless their emotional distress can be shared with and validated by attuned adults, children's necessary developmental narcissism disposes them to take everything personally. It is natural that they should believe that when bad things happen—when life hurts them, when the environment is stressed, the parents unhappy or ill—it is because *they* are culpable, unworthy, defective.

Less obvious is that this belief, too, has a protective function. When a young person's universe is in turmoil—when things fall apart and the center cannot hold, to channel Yeats[†]—there are two working theories the child could adopt. One is that her little world is terribly awry and misshapen, her parents incapable or unwilling to love and care. In other words, she is unsafe. The other, which wins out virtually every time, is that she—the child—is flawed. Helen Knott depicts this process in her eloquent account of intergenerational trauma, sexual violence, and

---

†   W. B. Yeats's 1919 poem "The Second Coming."

addiction:‡ "I was so convinced that I was to blame, and because of that, I remained silent." She could not have been convinced otherwise: acknowledging that those on whom one depends are incapable of meeting one's needs would be a devastating blow to a young person. Thus self-blame, like guilt, is an unflagging protector. Believing that the deficiency is ours gives us at least a modicum of agency and hope: maybe, if we just work hard enough, we can earn the love and care we need.

Self-accusation is the relentless whip that spurs so many perfectionists and high achievers to buckle down, do more, be better. As with guilt, there is no bargaining, reasoning, or arguing with this booming but callow voice. It needs to be acknowledged, seen for what it is, and gently put in its place.

Once, at a group workshop in Budapest, I worked with a young German woman who carried inside her an entity she called her "inner Adolf Hitler," full of world-destructive rage. She hated and feared this part of her, as if it were literally the Führer's ghost haunting her. She experienced herself as being personally, devastatingly connected with and even guilty for the genocide that had annihilated millions decades before she was born. When she allowed herself to sink into the full-body memory of it, her "Adolf" was revealed to be a distraught and scared two-year-old, enraged at being left alone for long periods in her crib. That rage protected her from feeling the terror and pain of abandonment that she had long ago buried and that kept her from situations in which she could again be vulnerable and wounded. Of course, it also kept her in miserable isolation from which she sought relief in addiction.

"We are not all descendants of Nazis," Edith Eger, the Auschwitz survivor and therapist author, writes, "but we each have a Nazi in us."[2] The inner fascist, which can seem so fearsome,

---

‡   I have cited Knott's book throughout this volume: *In My Own Moccasins: A Memoir of Resilience.*

turns out to be a frightened part of ourselves that we have long ago banished from awareness.

Realizing that vicious self-loathing, like guilt, first showed up to defend us from greater harm, and realizing, too, just how young this inner dictator is, gives us the chance to now receive it with curiosity, compassion, and even, possibly, with appreciation. Allowing it to exist, neither condoning nor condemning its lectern-pounding invective, relaxes its totalitarian hold.

When it comes to guilt, self-loathing, and so on, we can easily hear the voices: after all, they never stop talking. But there are other, more insidious ways that our inner exiles and protectors can manifest. These ways are more visible than audible: they show up in our behaviors, mood states, and mental processes. I am speaking of compensatory afflictions we covered earlier in the book, such as addiction and so-called mental illness. These dynamics, too—and recall, they are dynamic processes rather than solid "things"—can be worked with in a way that turns them from adversary to ally, instructor, or, at worst, an annoying acquaintance.

Nan Goldin, regretful as she is for the "wasted" decades, readily acknowledges that her escape into substance use rescued her when she first resorted to it at eighteen, during an extraordinarily painful time for her, the details of which she asked me not to divulge. "Literally, addiction saved my life," she told me. Without that solace, she acknowledged, she might have been driven to suicidal despair. She wishes only, as all do, that the consequences could have been less harsh. But what if we focused not on the harm but on the harm reduction?

"What if I came to you at age eighteen," I suggested, "and said, 'Okay, let's make a deal. I'm going to save your life. You need not kill yourself. I'm going to give you a way to escape pain that will allow you to live and create and still be alive in your sixties and have new vistas open to you, but you're going to have to pay a price.' Would I have your attention at least?" Nan nodded in assent. "If you make this deal," I continued, "you'll be able to do a lot of great creative work in the world. You'll be able to express truth and beauty and suffering—the genuine artist's life. But it's going to exact a price—a heavy price—in isolation, loss of relationships, of self-esteem, and physical health even if you do live to be sixty. You're going to surrender some possibilities, miss out on experiences. Is that a 'bargain' you, having endured abuse and other traumas, might have struck?" She nodded again without hesitation. Such are the unconscious "bargains" we all strike with these obtuse friends of ours, and rightly so: at the time, it may be the best deal we're going to get.

Jesse Thistle was embittered about his years as a drug addict and outlaw, until one of his elders set him right. "I went to her kitchen and I was bitching about being on the streets and all the horrible stuff that happened," he recalled. "Just horrible. I knew that she had a similar past as a heroin addict when she lived in Vancouver back in the sixties. I thought she would relate to me, and we could, like, bond over griping . . . And she scolded me. She said, 'How dare you. How dare you talk about your elders that way.'" Before Jesse could apologize, the woman continued. "She said, 'I'm not your elder, Jesse; those addictions were your elders. They were teaching you the importance of family. They were teaching you the importance of good health. The importance of human connection. The importance of perseverance. All those things are taught through addiction. All of them.' And so for me it was the great test, the great tribulation of my life. Almost like a rite of passage into a wisdom. It's given me such wisdom where I can see things that other people can't see. I have a different perspective. I'm not condoning addiction. I would have rather started twenty years ago having a family and potentially owning a house like all my other friends are now. But I have a vision and a way of seeing the world that they'll never get."

———

The conditions we group under the umbrella of mental and personality disorders can be seen as having their helpful dimensions, too. We alluded to this in chapter 18 with respect to finding meaning in these disturbances; now we can take it one step further and glimpse the possibility of an amicable coexistence, even a productive alliance. My son and co-author, Daniel, describes an example of that from his own life:

Being diagnosed in 2019 with cyclothymia, basically a mild form of bipolar disorder, was huge for me. Something about my life became coherent when I realized that the crazily productive streaks and depressive crashes aren't really opposites—more like conjoined twins—and that both have been trying to help me get through the world since childhood. The can't-stop-won't-stop mode is a little boy's brain in overdrive, trying to keep up and cut through the noise around him, while the emotional collapse is like a breaker switch installed to prevent my fuse box from exploding.

Thanks in part to the mood stabilizers I take, there's now someone home in between them, observing the ups and downs, knowing they're not me. Now, anytime I find myself in hypomanic turbo mode, all insomniac inspiration, or when I wake up feeling heavy and reluctant, I don't fight it or sweat it. Both states come bearing gifts: on the one hand, exhilaration and creative flow; on the other, the gift of rest, of embracing my limitations. Neither one ever takes over for long.

It's a big deal, I'm finding, to know that your mind is not your enemy.

"I don't remember my childhood," I've heard people say. "All these folks with their childhood horror stories . . . nothing I can recall explains why I behave the way I do." You, too, may have found yourself drawing a blank in the face of tale after tale of adverse upbringings presented throughout this book.

Many people, stymied by what they believe is a failure to remember, often wonder if this memory gap inhibits their healing. There are a couple of good reasons why the answer is an encouraging no. As we have said, the trauma is not what happened *to* us, but what happened *inside* us as a result. Peter Levine reminds us that "trauma is about broken connection. Broken connection to the body, broken connection to our vitality, to reality, and to others." That being the case, it's impossible to overstate that so long as we are alive and of sound mind, reconnection remains possible. We do not require the past for that, only the present. That's the first reason we need not despair of healing even if we can't connect the historical dots. We can always work with the here and now, even if the long ago is locked away.

But there is a second, more practical reason: *it isn't true* that we don't remember. Our memories show up every day in our relationship to ourselves and others, if we only know how to recognize them. Every time we are triggered—which is to say, caught up suddenly in an unwanted, puzzlingly overwrought emotional reaction—that is the past showing up: an echo of our childhood as we actually experienced it, if not how we consciously recall it. There are ways to retrieve such encoded memories by using present-moment emotions and body experiences to find their origins.[†]

The word "trigger" is itself a major clue. It has become something of a rhetorical cannonball, hurled back and forth by opposite sides in many a debate or confrontation, rarely deepening conversations and often ending them. Yet, on closer examination, it has much to teach us about ourselves. Consider: How big a part of a weapon is the trigger? Minuscule, really; perhaps the smallest visible component. The weapon also bears ammunition, explosive material, often a guidance system, and mechanisms for delivering the payload to its target with the desired force. If, when triggered, we focus our ire only on the external stimuli that set us off, we miss a golden opportunity to examine what ammunition and explosive charges we ourselves have been packing since childhood.

Let's briefly revisit the issue of the "happy childhood," which is so often professed regardless of later challenges with illness, addiction, or emotional afflictions. The point in accessing a more well-rounded history is not to engender self-pity, nor to wipe the genuinely good times from the record. It's this: to make peace with our inner tormentors, we have to first understand them against the backdrop of their origin stories. This is the compassion of context.

I was once asked to provide expert testimony in a murder case where the accused, a chronic alcoholic, having been interviewed by three psychiatrists, was reported to have grown up in a happy environment. Ten minutes into our jail-cell conversation he told me that his father had been a heavy drinker, his mother depressed. When he was four, his arm was broken and his hair

---

[†] Illustrated in practice with the forthright participation of the podcaster Tim Ferriss here: "Dr. Gabor Maté on How to Reframe a Challenging Moment and Feel Empowered, *The Tim Ferriss Show*, November 4, 2019, YouTube, https://www.youtube.com /watch?v=__JLFw2FtEQ.

set on fire by his brother; later he was bullied in school. It had never occurred to him—nor to the forensic specialists who had accepted his "happy" story without further inquiry—that the actual history might contradict, even debunk, his whitewashed recollections. Nor was he being insincere: it was all he knew. He was probably holding tight to certain genuinely pleasant moments, a curated slide show of memories that he had titled "My Happy Childhood."

The myth of the happy childhood doesn't require such obvious extremes for its cracks to show. Recall Dr. Erica Harris, self-confessed workaholic and a survivor of leukemia, a double lung transplant, and a life-threatening, drug-resistant, blood-borne infection. At one point in our conversation, she remarked: "I was blessed with what most people call a very happy, blessed childhood. We were well off financially, I had a ton of friends, and so I wasn't bullied—I didn't have any of those big life circumstances. But at age twelve I had a really hard time." A family conflict left her sad, confused, and bewildered. This, she believed, was when her traumatic wound was sustained.

Actually, the self-disconnect had occurred long before then, in her "very happy, blessed childhood," as revealed by my next question. It's one I regularly pose to clients and participants, and I'll now put it to you, the reader. Anyone whose conscious recall is of a happy childhood—a category that may range from innocuous to idyllic—and yet is confronting chronic illness, emotional distress, addiction, or struggles to be authentic, is particularly invited to engage with it:

When I felt sad, unhappy, angry, confused, bewildered, lonely, bullied, who did I speak to? Who did I tell? Who could I confide in?

Notice your answer, and also your feelings around it. If, as in Erica's case, the answer is "No one" or indicates anything other than the presence of a consistently available adult "someone," an early disconnect was surely at play. (A loving older sibling can in some ways stand in for a parent, but it is unlikely they can fully replace a parent. And even then it signals a disconnect from the adult caregiver.) No infant refrains from emoting to the parents precisely what he feels or from signaling when she requires help. The failure to do so later in childhood is a developmentally abnormal adaptation—for some a truly devastating one, which undergirds the woundings that follow.

Thus, the suppression of early sorrow is not limited to overt trauma or abuse. I have never treated or interviewed anyone with chronic physical illness or mental affliction who could recall sharing unhappy feelings openly and freely, without restraint, with their caregivers or any trusted adult. This is a feature of life that most happy-childhood memories filter out, for the simple reason that we have an easier time recalling what happened than remembering what did *not* happen but should have. The pleasant memories we do recall, though genuine, are two-dimensional, missing the depth and the fullness of the child's actual experience. Until we can reestablish a link to that inner third dimension, we lack the depth perception to see ourselves in our totality, and healing and wholeness are blocked.

For those still unmoved by this notion of "nobody to talk to" being traumatic, I'll illustrate the point via my conversation with Dr. Harris, who was not subjected to maltreatment, nor ever came close to it. I offered my customary thought experiment, encouraging her to step outside herself and imagine another child, namely her own, in a similar position. Our conversation, prototypical in my experience, went like this:

"If you, as a parent, found out that your kid had an emotional shock at age twelve such as you experienced, but didn't talk to you, how would you explain that?"

"That they didn't trust me."

"What does it feel like for a kid not to trust their parents?"

"That would be really terrible. It wouldn't feel safe and secure. Like you were on your own, very alone."

There, then, was Erica's "very happy, blessed childhood," as actually lived. And none of it means that her parents didn't love her or wouldn't have done anything in their power for her well-being. It means only that some essential disconnect had happened earlier in that relationship. It didn't begin all of a sudden when she was twelve, even if that's when it hit home for her.

Finally, people often make comparisons that unfairly denigrate their own experience. Though you may be justifiably grateful for your lot, the fact that others have suffered "more than" you does not diminish by one iota your own pain, nor erase its traces in your psyche. Levels of trauma are not to be evaluated, much less graded on a bell curve. You may, for example, have reassured yourself along the same lines as Erica did: "We were well off financially, I had a ton of friends, and so I wasn't bullied—I didn't have any of those big life circumstances." "And fortunate you were," I customarily interject. "But just imagine for a moment your little niece or nephew sobbing to you, 'I feel so sad and alone and confused and I'm afraid to tell Mommy or Daddy about it.' Would you, if you wished to be supportive, dismiss this little one with 'Come on, what's the problem here? Think of all the children who are having big life circumstances, like hunger or abuse or bullying. By contrast, you have nothing to complain about.' Is that what you'd say to them if you wanted them to know their feelings were safe to feel, that they were lovable no matter what?" I have yet to hear anyone respond in the affirmative: when I put it to them that plainly, they're finally able to hear in it the absurd double standard enforced against the self.

―――――――――

As we wrap up, a bedtime story:

Once upon a time, our wholeness was lost to us when our all-star team of inner friends—Guilt, Self-Hatred, Suppression, Denial, and the rest—came aboard to keep us safe. We were barely involved in the hiring process, and mostly we didn't notice them as they went about their business. Like a cadre of reality-TV design experts, they set about remodeling our personalities so that we'd make it out of childhood in one piece: beautifying certain rooms and boarding up others, installing alarms, locking the cellar door. But their success at keeping us intact required that we emerge into adulthood with core parts of ourselves walled off. They were good at their jobs.

After many years of living in this stuffy, segmented home, we came to long for a more spacious, better-ventilated existence. So we thanked the experts for their service, and sent them out for a well-deserved sandwich. And we devoted ourselves gently but diligently to a new task, the literal antidote to the psychic dismemberment required of us long, long ago: the task of remembering ourselves.

Chapter 31

Jesus in the Tipi: Psychedelics and Healing

The only cure I know is a good ceremony.
—Leslie Marmon Silko, *Ceremony*

One morning, not long ago, I was fired from my own retreat by a group of Shipibo shamans. The night before, in the steamy heat of the jungle, these men and women had known nothing about me; by dawn, they understood everything they needed to draw up my walking papers. They did so for the well-being of the health professionals who had flown from many parts of the world to work with me, and to my eternal benefit.

To get to the Temple of the Way of Light, you transfer in Lima for a ninety-minute flight to Iquitos in northeastern Peru. From there you travel down the surging Nanay River, an Amazon tributary, through the lush rain forest, intermittently floating past small villages on the bank's edge. Occasionally the river branches narrowly enough that you can touch the verdant tropical vegetation.

The day we arrive, it has been raining heavily. We don Wellingtons to trudge through the forest paths, where the reddish muck is deep in spots. More than once the footwear I've been given, several sizes too large, gets stuck, leaving me to rely on our Shipibo helpers to lift me, extract my captive boots, and ease me back into them again. After a forty-five-minute hike through the dense, drenched woodland, the track narrows as we climb a hill to reach our destination.

I have been invited to this place to lead a healing retreat for health care providers from four continents, from countries such as Romania, Britain, Australia, Brazil, Canada, and the United States. The attendees are psychotherapists, psychologists, psychiatrists, counselors, family doctors, and internists. There are twenty-four of us in all, that being the maximum occupancy of the maloca, the thatched communal hut where the ayahuasca ceremonies will take place. Many facilities in Peru and other countries in the Amazon basin offer such ceremonies, some in full good faith and integrity, others more interested in the dollars the tourist trade provides.[†] The Temple of the Way of Light is widely known as one of the better ones. It is run by an Englishman, Matthew, whose personal salvation owes much to the plant and the traditional practices around it. The shamans are Shipibo people native to Peru, as are the staff who assist in the ceremonial buildings and the dining and meeting halls. The temple staff work closely with the Aboriginal healers, taking care to honor their traditional ways while trying to provide a meaningful and digestible experience for their mostly neophyte Western clientele. There are usually some international volunteers as well.

I have been facilitating retreats that use the bitter drink brewed from the mystic ayahuasca plant for over a decade. These events combine the Amazonian tradition of *vegetalismo*, an ancient and highly sophisticated system of plant healing, with my Compassionate Inquiry therapeutic approach. The plant sessions are conducted by shamans at night; usually I attend, ingesting *la medicina* along with the participants. My work begins earlier in the

---

[†] Generally, the latter kind are the places you hear about in sometimes sensationalistic but regrettably factual news stories about the dangers of psychedelics. Really, though, these headlines are about what happens when potent medicine traditions are co-opted by the profit motive—which, needless to say, is not particularly indigenous to the Amazon.

day, helping people formulate their intentions for the ceremony. An intention might take the form of a thorny personal issue they want to illuminate, a difficult emotion they hope to explore, or an inner quality they wish to nurture with the medicine's help. The following day, I help them process and integrate whatever revelations, thoughts, emotions, visions, nightmarish apparitions or dreamlike wonders, sensations, physical discomforts, or sheer ennui they had experienced as the shamans chanted to the circle and performed their energetic healing.

Over the years I have become adept at this work of facilitation, helping people overcome depressions and addictions and to heal from physical conditions. For whatever reason, as others pass through ayahuasca's portal, I find myself highly attuned to the nature of their stumbling blocks and the nuances of their breakthroughs, intuitively able to guide them as they carry their new, fledgling insights back to their ordinary plane of consciousness. I am inspired and moved by the transformations to which I regularly bear witness, transformations that gratifyingly ripple outward into people's lives, far beyond a weeklong retreat.

When it comes to my own transformation, it's a different story. All my life, no matter what breakthroughs I've beheld or helped potentiate, a glum certainty has dominated my outlook on my own healing prospects. I have participated in many dozens of ayahuasca ceremonies without believing that much could happen for me, and usually find my pessimism rewarded: nary a vision or visitation, no ancestors or spirit animals, not even one deep thought, just some mild nausea and the wish that more were happening. To be sure, a handful of moving experiences have left me with deepened gratitude or appreciation for my life's many blessings, but for all that, even these positive encounters with the plant have not shifted my mind's wondrously stubborn Eeyore setting.

We enter the first ceremony, the twenty-four of us, joined by six Indigenous shamans—three *maestras* and three *maestros*—all five feet tall at the most, dressed in white, with belts and sashes of vivid colors. Each of us will be visited by each of them in turn: six personalized chants for each participant. Interspersed with periods of silence in the dark maloca—not counting the night creatures that chirp, ribbit, and hoot all around us—are hypnotic incantations in the Shipibo language's ancient cadences, at once gentle and powerful. Under the influence of the acrid brew, these chants can take on synesthetic qualities: some people see images, while others experience the syllables as body sensations or travel in their minds to long-buried memories. A few are like me, and experience the disconcerting absence of these things.

Each time a shaman sits in front of my mat, I steel myself, silently daring them to do their worst. Go ahead, I think, try to break through the barricades of *this* psyche. Knowing full well this is an unhelpful attitude doesn't deter that inner voice from speaking first and loudest. Predictably, nothing happens except the usual frustration and disappointment. (Which, I would point out if I were coaching someone else, is hardly "nothing." Any experience at all in such a ceremony can be rich with teachings if approached with compassion and curiosity: easier preached than practiced, evidently.) Much of the time I'm almost dissociated, barely conscious of the chants or the goodwill being directed at me. The next day, after the appropriate sleep and food, the group gathers and I do my usual laser-guided counseling. As people describe their experiences of agony or joy or confusion, I guide them to make sense of their visions and help them connect the plant's teachings to their own life histories. In my role as healer and teacher, I can easily leave behind all cynicism: the retreat is not about me. All is going well.

At lunch Matthew pulls me aside. The shamans want to meet with me, he says; the group of them has delegated two spokes-men to deliver a communal decision. Through an interpreter, they give me the news. "You have a dense, dark energy our *icaros*[†] cannot penetrate," they say. "That energy pervades the room, so it impairs our work with the others. We cannot have you there." Before I can respond, they add that I may not work with the group even in the daytime.

To say that I'm taken aback is an understatement. My ego is not liking this at all—haven't these people rearranged their lives to come from all over the world to the rain forest specifically to work with *me*? Surely there must be some workaround, some compromise. The shamans are unmoved. "Even during the day," they explain, "your energy would have a disturbing effect on the others, and more importantly, you would be absorbing their griefs and traumas. As a *médico*,[‡] you have obviously done that for so long, working with troubled people, and you have done noth-ing to clear that out of yourself. And, long before that, we all sense you must have suffered a big, big scare very early in your life; you haven't gotten over it yet. That is why your energy is so dense."

Until last night these shamans had never heard of me. Apart from knowing me to be a doctor, they are familiar neither with my origin story nor with the work I do in the world. And yet they have read me with absolute accuracy. Even through my dismay, I immediately feel and understand that they are right. "We can help you," they promise. Despite their assurances, I have strong doubts they will succeed. And yet it is not deference alone, nor blind faith, that impels me to follow their lead. Something in me, it seems, is relieved to be relieved of duty.

[†]   A Quechua term for the healing chants performed in ayahuasca ceremonies.

[‡]   Spanish for "doctor."

For the next ten days I am socially distanced, as it were, from the retreat. I remain isolated in my cabin, except for mealtimes in the hall, when I do not interact with the participants; they are, luckily, in the able hands of an American colleague of mine. Throughout my psychic quarantine, I meditate, read spiritual books, do yoga, walk the rain forest paths, and contemplate. Assorted mental and emotional reactions to my strange situation come and go. And every second night, in a ceremonial hut all to myself, one of the shamans pours me the medicine, then chants to me and only me in Shipibo for more than three hours. He blows smoke, waves his arms above me, lays hands on my chest or back. Mostly he chants in his native language, but at times he incants Catholic hymns in Spanish, invoking Espíritu Santo, Santa María, and Jesús over my Hebraic head. His voice, now plumbing low baritone depths, now an insistent nasal tenor or keening falsetto, is indescribably supple and beautiful. In the murky dark of the maloca, this small man looms like a giant. Each day I feel myself lighter, my mind less preoccupied. Still, for the first four of those ceremony nights, no visions come, no deep experiences, only a growing sense of ease and gratitude.

The fifth and final ceremony over—so I think—with the anticipated non-results, I nevertheless feel cleansed and thankful. Via the interpreter Publio, I converse jovially with the maestro. Abruptly, mid-sentence, I throw myself on the mat—or rather, I should say, I am thrown facedown with sudden, involuntary force. At long last, the medicine is driving the bus and I am its helpless passenger. I am finally, indisputably, blessedly not in control.

Later they tell me I remained prone for nearly two hours. To me it might have been two days; in the vision's vortex, there was no sense of time. All the while, cross-legged, still, and silent, Publio and the shaman sat vigil next to me. I need not, indeed cannot, describe what I experienced, but I remember the transcendent joy of it.

What I can articulate is what I saw at the very end. On a sky-screen of deep blue, outlined in giant cloudlike wisps of letters, was spelled *B O L D O G*: the Hungarian word for "happy." The vision and the inner peace evoked with it came from beyond thought—even, I'd venture, beyond my subconscious mind.[†] It was both beyond me and deeply a part of me, connecting whatever I'd previously thought of as "I" to something mysterious, transcendent, awesome. That same state—spacious and aware, unfragmented, free from self-concern—infuses my awareness now as I revisit the experience and ponder its lessons (which I will return to in the next chapter).

The reader might wonder what happened with the health professionals who had traveled so far to engage in the plant work under my guidance. I'm pleased to report that most of them did famously well. My co-leader acquitted himself admirably. And for all their understandable disappointment, and contrary to my fears of a mutiny, people appreciated that I was modeling for them a willingness to care for myself. This may have been the teaching these overworked, compassion-fatigued, wounded healers most needed; certainly the shamans thought so. The temple had hosted many Europeans and North Americans, but never a group of medical workers, and the Shipibo healers reported afterward that, to their own surprise, they had never worked with such a "heavy bunch." "As healers ourselves," they said, "we must face all the pains and traumas people bring to us, but we take care of ourselves: we regularly clear those energies out of our bodies and souls, so they do not accumulate and burden us. We expected you *médicos* to have done the same for yourselves. But no, we found, you came here weighed down by the griefs and heavy energies you have all been absorbing for years and years."

---

†   I usually think, even dream, in English.

I spoke recently with a physician who was at the retreat, a specialist in his late fifties who holds a high medical position in the Canadian Armed Forces. Often his patients suffer from a combination of physical injuries and PTSD. "I'm finding so much joy in my work now," he told me. "I had been tired, cynical. After thirty-two years I couldn't wait to retire. Now I look forward to connecting with people at a real level, rather than in a shallow, artificial medical way." I have heard similar reports from many of the others of how much they had gained from the shamans giving "Dr. Gabor" the pink slip.

The morning after I read the Hungarian word for "happy" in the azure sky, Publio asked the shaman how he saw my journey. The *maestro* smiled. "Oh," he said, "Dr. Gabor was communing with God."

Sometime after the 2009 publication of my book on addiction, *In the Realm of Hungry Ghosts*, I began to receive inquiries about what I knew regarding the therapeutic use of ayahuasca. At the time, the answer was "Nothing," just as I knew nothing about the potential of psychedelics in general to promote well-being. Though I'd always been keen to investigate ways of healing outside the Western medical model, I initially found these inquiries bothersome. I didn't want to learn about anything so strange and new, so "out there." Nor could I imagine how a psychedelic substance could help anyone overcome addiction, or help heal PTSD, or decondition the ingrained patterns of self-suppression that so often contribute to illness.

Since then I have developed deep respect for the synergistic power of psychedelics allied with the insights and practice of modern psychology. "Respect" may be too mild a word—"reverence" hits closer to the mark. Over the years I have worked with people struggling with drug use and sex addiction, people facing cancer, degenerative neurological illness, depression, PTSD, anxiety, and chronic fatigue, as well as those seeking wholeness, meaning, and an experience of their true selves. In all cases, people have sought liberation from ingrained, habitual, constrictive patterns. I have witnessed people looking for their vulnerable and fully alive child selves, for their parents, for love, for God, for truth, for community, for Nature. I can't say that everyone found everything they were seeking. What I can say is that most people took major steps forward on their way to authenticity and found significant liberation from their limiting or even deadening mind patterns and behaviors.

One man in his thirties, a first responder in British Columbia, wrote to me, "Since my first ayahuasca experience several months ago, I have been experiencing that shift in my consciousness daily. My presence within myself and with others, including animals, is different. I see everything I've done from a completely new perspective and live it. I am able to see the difference I make to ease pain in others, and to help them see themselves in a different light." A real estate broker from New York who attended one of our retreats struck a similar chord: "In my day-to-day capitalistic pursuits, I often meditate now on ways that I might help other people in a deeper way." And a woman whose life had been blighted by chronic pain and addiction, the template for which had been a history of childhood sexual abuse, wrote, "Today I stand in awe of life's blessings and the sacred and precious nature of life. I never understood it until now."

To be sure, before spiritual transcendence, the psychedelic experience may first penetrate to the most hidden recesses of torment in the psyche. "Tonight I experienced my fetal pain, and then I gave it up to the heavens," a young man reported after a plant ceremony. "I had been asking the medicine to take me there, to my deepest, most fundamental suffering, but it hadn't.

All of a sudden tonight I was there, feeling myself in the womb, and feeling the harshest pain I think I've ever felt. It was awful. It consumed me fully. I stayed with it for as long as I could because I knew this is what I needed to experience. Then I came out of it, and without hesitation, I released that pain to the heavens. From the worst feeling I can recall, I was now experiencing one of the most joyful."

Michael Pollan's book *How to Change Your Mind: What the New Science of Psychedelics Teaches Us About Consciousness, Dying, Addiction, Depression, and Transcendence* has opened many eyes to the healing possibilities of psychedelics. "People are hungry for something," the bestselling author told me. "It's very hard to say what it is, but people are certainly looking for a spiritual dimension to their lives, it seems to me. Also, we have very high levels of mental illness: people are suffering in all sorts of ways, and the mental health treatments available are completely inadequate, not up to the job."

Pollan acknowledged that he had been startled by the reception that greeted his book—named as one of the ten best of the year by the *New York Times*—from within the medical world. "I thought there would be a lot of resistance from psychiatry, from people who work in mental health care," he said. "But they know how empty the cupboard is, how empty the medicine cabinet is, of effective drugs, effective healing modalities. This renaissance of psychedelic medicine is coming along at a time when it's much more urgently needed than I ever imagined when I wrote the book." His survey covered traditional ceremonial plants such as ayahuasca, peyote, tobacco, and mushrooms; it also included modern human-made substances such as the psychedelic LSD (or acid) and MDMA (the psychoactive drug popularly known as ecstasy, E, or Molly), both of which are increasingly studied in therapeutic settings, with encouraging results.

We often equate the word "psychedelic" with terms like "mind-altering," but a glance at its etymology gets us closer to the mark. The British psychiatrist Humphry Osmond, who coined the word from the Greek words *psyche*, for "soul," and *deloun*, "to reveal, to make visible," meant it to indicate "mind-manifesting." In other words, not altering or even "expanding" the mind, but revealing consciousness to itself.[†] The therapeutic use of psychedelics requires the proper setting and the right intention and guidance. This is absolutely crucial: absent these conditions, the use of psychedelics can too often lead to a *Sorcerer's Apprentice* nightmare scenario. Conversely, in adeptly led sessions and in safe circumstances, psychedelics can uncover and bring acceptance to pain and sorrows people have tried desperately to escape all their lives and, too, reveal the peace, joy, and love at the core of being alive, qualities often buried under the edifice of the conditioned personality.

Readers interested in the research and science behind the resurgence of psychedelic therapies in our time can consult Pollan's comprehensive volume or the many scientific studies continually being published internationally.[1] I'll say here only that after over a decade of experience as participant, physician, and healer, I have been more than impressed with the possibilities, which are rooted in the mind-body unity we have explored. I have seen people recover from addictions of all kinds, including pornography, cigarettes, alcohol, and drugs; from mental health challenges such as depression and anxiety; and from physical conditions such as multiple sclerosis and rheumatic diseases.

Recall Mee Ok, from chapter 5—the traumatized, sexually abused Korean adoptee in Boston with the diagnosis of advanced

---

[†] Another word—coined more recently and applicable to plant medicines only—is "entheogenic," which literally means "becoming divine with."

scleroderma, unable without assistance to move her painfully "mummified" body, as she called it. Moribund, beyond the help of Western medicine, she at one point longed for death as the only conceivable release from suffering. One evening, on her own, Mee Ok took some ayahuasca she had somehow obtained. That night, for the first time in months, she was able to rise from her bed, stand, and walk on her own. The experience was transformative. "Instead of seeing myself as Mandy[†] and as identifying with my physical body," she told me, "meaning my demographics, my race, my gender, and all of that, the plant helped me to see a deeper core to myself that would still be there after you stripped away all of those elements."[‡]

Mee Ok has since attended one of my retreats and has received other forms of therapy and physical treatment. As I mentioned in chapter 5, she is now independently mobile, physically active, and currently writing her autobiography. "Before, when I was very sick," she recalled, "I saw everything, as all of life just having happened to me. 'This is my fate; I'm going to die. I have no voice in this.' And I've never had a voice . . . When I saw that there was a reason behind all of that, then I could search for meaning. That was a big conceptual shift for me. I realized that all of those traumas I've experienced in my life could be meaningful and that I could choose the life I am meant to live. And so these traumas were also manageable, whereas before, I couldn't even access them. I couldn't remember a lot of my childhood. The ayahuasca did slowly open up a lot of those memories and

---

[†] Mandy was Mee Ok's Anglicized name. Part of her reclaiming of herself has been reclaiming her original Korean name. She has now taken on the surname Icaro to honor her connection to the medicine.

[‡] Desperate as Mee Ok was and helpful as her experience proved to be, *I never recommend anyone ingesting the plant on their own.* Ayahuasca, more even than most psychedelic plants, is best experienced in a ceremonial context with trusted practitioners. This is for safety, and also for the integrity of the tradition itself, in which the plant is seen as one part of a rich body of practices, not to be consumed ad hoc, especially by newcomers to its ways.

all those things I had forgotten about: who I was as a child, and who I really am."

I spoke with Mee Ok's Boston family doctor, who confirmed the medical history and the recovery, which she herself, the physician, was at a loss to explain. Yet from the perspective of body-mind science, there is nothing miraculous or even perplexing about it. Once Mee Ok reconnected with her authentic self—in her case with the aid of a plant, but the principle generalizes—she was able to divest from the trauma-confined personality. She began to free herself from the conditioned set of beliefs, behaviors, and emotions, and hence from the physiological responses these dictated. Her body—nervous system, immune system, and tissues—followed her lead, along pathways we have described.

Beyond the realm of healing, many have found psychedelics to be transformational teachers. Certainly, in their original contexts, plant medicines were and are consulted for far more than cures and pain relief: shamans consulted the spirits of these plants for community guidance, for divination of hunting and weather patterns, to commune with ancestors and help make peace between warring factions, and, most elementally, simply to know and learn their ways. Each plant—including many flowers, bushes, and trees that wouldn't be considered psychedelic by our standards—is thought to have its own wisdoms to impart, with its own curriculum that can take years of dedicated practice to absorb. The anthropologist Wade Davis is fulsome in his appreciation. "I always tell young people that our parents were so frightened of these substances, you know, that they'd scream at us, 'Don't take this. You'll never come back the same!' But that was the whole blessed point. In that sense, I am very open about how catalytic these substances have been in my life and how valuable they are. One thing I know is that these medicines allowed me to understand our connection to the natural world in a way that never in a million years could have happened just by reading books."

How can psychedelics exert such potent transformative effects? Through the mind-body unity we have been exploring and through their power to access the unconscious, where, hidden from awareness, many of the emotions and motivations driving our lives reside. Sigmund Freud once said that dreams are the royal road to the unconscious. Psychedelics may be said to be an even more direct route. Dr. Rick Doblin, founder and executive director of the Multidisciplinary Association for Psychedelic Studies, has spearheaded the drive for the investigation of psychedelic treatment modalities. "There is a membrane between conscious mind and unconscious mind," Doblin told me when we spoke recently, "between what we are paying attention to and what we are thinking and feeling on deeper levels. Psychedelics open up that membrane so that more emerges. Each substance does it in a different way. It both connects you to parts of yourself that have been suppressed or ignored, but also you can see the wider world beyond yourself, beyond your ego self." He drew an analogy to the Copernican revolution of the 1600s. "We tend to believe with our ego that we are the center of the universe," he explained. "Psychedelics displace that and we see that we are part of something enormously bigger than any individual and that this unity goes back in time and forward in time. They can take us out of our habitual patterns. When you are no longer looking at things from the perspective of the 'I,' you feel a newly released potential and sense of connection."

Plant substances and synthetic psychedelics are not "drugs" in the medical sense of the word. A pill like the antidepressant Prozac, or the easily accessible aspirin or codeine, is meant to change your biological state—your physiology—so long as you are taking it. Depending on circumstances, that may or may not be a good thing, but such pharmaceutical treatments are not designed to get at root causes and unconscious dynamics. Psychedelic medicines are not intended to be taken daily to keep you in a state of altered physiology. Ideally, they can help facilitate your entry into a renewed relationship with yourself and the world, long after you have ingested them, whether in ceremony, as with ayahuasca, or in a therapeutic session, as with MDMA. In a real way, these experiences retune the brain's emotional apparatus. I was not surprised, for example, by a recent study showing that psychedelic use reduced the odds of men perpetrating intimate-partner violence.[2]

All that said, I am no psychedelic evangelist. Contrary to the fond imaginings of some enthusiasts, neither plant-based nor manufactured psychedelic medicines will, on their own, transform health care or human consciousness at large. That will have to await vast-scale social change, not least the broadening of the mainstream medical ideology. For all they can offer, at present psychedelic treatments are esoteric, expensive, and time-intensive. They are bound to remain beyond most people's reach for both practical and cultural reasons. But we would be negligent to exclude them, to ignore their healing potential for many endemic conditions in the face of which Western medicine finds itself largely helpless.[†]

Wondrous as their effects can be, for our purposes plant medicines and other mind-manifesting substances are not only interesting in themselves but also powerful ambassadors for the bodymind principles that modern science is only now catching

---

†   Like many others, I'm confident that the studies now being pursued will prove that, even on strict economic grounds, such treatments can be cost-effective—consider, for example, the lifetime expense of keeping someone on medication for something like PTSD.

up to. The lessons they transmit testify to the indomitability of the human spirit and the possibility of unlocking its potency, with or without substances and no matter what life has thrown at us. We now know that on every continent, seemingly in every recorded era, people have availed themselves of the apothecary called Earth to promote healing, wisdom, and spiritual realization, and indeed to transmit culture down through the generations.

Psychedelic medicine came to exert a major influence in the life of one of the last great Native American warrior leaders to challenge the relentless, genocidal expansion of settler colonialism in the American Southwest. After his inevitable defeat and his people's humiliating confinement to ever-shrinking reservations, the brilliant Comanche chief Quanah Parker turned to spiritual pathways for solace. He worked with the desert cactus peyote, as a forerunner of what later became the Native American Church. Typical of Indigenous practices, he wasn't interested in religion but in spirituality. "The white man goes into his church and talks *about* Jesus," he once said, "but the Indian goes into his tipi and talks *to* Jesus."[3]

After my "communion with God" in the Peruvian jungle, I had a felt sense of what Quanah Parker had meant.

Chapter 32

My Life as a Genuine Thing: Touching Spirit

Ultimately your greatest gift to the world is being who you are—both your gift and your fulfillment.
—A. H. Almaas, *Being and the Meaning of Life*

Until my clear-blue-sky moment in the Peruvian jungle in 2019, spirituality had existed for me mostly as rumor, theory, or concept—or as a vague longing, both wistful and wishful. Though I had consumed shelves of books, and could even speak articulately on the subject, I had never myself been subject to a direct encounter with such storied states as wonder, mystery, or "the peace that passeth all understanding." My faith in humanity's potential for genuine, revelatory transformation, while sincere, had come to me largely secondhand; I could not trace this faith to any experience of my own. It certainly didn't derive from any deistic belief or devotional practices of the organized religious kind. That said, what I learned in Peru gave experiential substance to these inklings of possibility. It went beyond belief and spoke to the essence of healing.

Literal beliefs aside, to the shaman's unsurprised observation that "Dr. Gabor was communing with God," I can only say amen. Something transcendent *did* take place that morning: an overdue rendezvous with that in me which is beyond the "me" I've subscribed to for so long. I touched into a space where I was aware of myself as an expanse of consciousness, unmoored from my identity's self-confining biographical ballast. The medicine under the shaman's guidance—and, just as important, my days of inner preparation—had left me open to information so outside my usual frames of reference that I didn't imagine I could ever access it. Shakespeare's Hamlet knew this kind of knowledge: "There are more things in heaven and Earth, Horatio, / Than are dreamt of in your philosophy."†

Looking back, I see that the experience did not so much instill new beliefs in me, as it did relax and unfasten my personality's militant *un*belief, which can be every bit as fundamentalist as the theistic certainties of ultra-religious sects. The actor and activist Ashley Judd has a terrific phrase for this leap of nonliteral faith: "surrendering to a God you don't believe in."

The first thing I learned in Peru—and here I mean direct learning, not stacking more facts on the woodpile of knowledge—is that healing is outside the thinking mind's wheelhouse. For one thing, the mind by its nature is a house divided: our personalities contradict themselves constantly. In my case, part of me always held out hope, even if a theoretical kind, that I might someday, somehow, have an "enlightenment" moment, the big-ticket aha, while another part was stowed away, stoking cynicism and pessimism. Spirit, by contrast, is one with itself. Our minds, our learned knowledge, can store healing principles worth remembering and can even help lead us toward experiences that heal. There will come a time, if we wish to go "all the way," when these trusty protectors have to recuse themselves at the door and allow a less sophisticated, more vulnerable element, stripped of armored certainties, to enter.

---

† Act I, scene 5. In Shakespeare's time, "philosophy" could refer to rational, scientific thought.

Second, I learned that I could not have planned this. Quite the reverse: the entire set of events that brought me to that moment laid waste to every plan I'd made. My entry into the realm of spirit could take place only once I had given up the illusion of control and submitted completely to the way things were. My willingness to have my agenda undermined was my buy-in, the ante required of me to sit at the table of mystery.

Third, and closely related, was that I had to do several difficult things: surrender my identity as leader or healer; put aside my habit of helping others without sparing time or energy for my own transformation; and accept whatever personal diminishment I feared would result from stepping away from my expected role. The biggest challenge was to see past the resentful protests of my threatened ego: "I can't let these people down; they came all this way to work with *me*." My identity, the persona I had clung to all my life, had been subverted utterly. All it could do was negotiate its terms of surrender.

Life in its wisdom had put me in a position where I had no control. My only choice was to let go and trust—trust others, trust myself, and, most of all, trust the direction my life had suddenly taken—or not. Making the affirmative choice, which may not have been my selection in earlier moments, opened up the possibility of a powerful healing experience, a touch of grace. I won't say my letting go *caused* the healing—that's not how grace works, as far as I can tell—but it was a prerequisite. I just happened to finally be ready, at age seventy-five, to do so.

Not everyone will, or ought to, work with shamans or psychotropic plants; relatively few people are likely to even have such an opportunity. That doesn't matter. My particular experience, though under unusual circumstances, was suffused with the universal healing principles that guide this book's exploration, and which are available to all: the acceptance, the shedding of identity, the choosing to trust the inner guidance against the remonstrations of the conditioned mind, and the genuine agency that springs paradoxically from the willingness to give up rigid control. If I can do it, I am convinced that anyone can—anyone, that is, who commits to their healing and allows it to instruct them rather than the other way around.

My experience with the shamans in Peru also taught me something about what healing is not. For years I had retained a fixed idea that to heal I'd have to go through some monumental cathartic release, as I've seen happen for others, or perhaps travel back in time in some way, to relive or redeem the difficult past. Yes, it can take that form, but not necessarily. Once again, it is not the past that has to change (or can change), only our present relationship to ourselves. As I lay prone on the mat—I'm told I both laughed and sobbed at various times—I was profoundly aware that my infancy had occurred in just the way it had, that nothing will ever alter that, that my grandparents will never not have gone to their deaths. I also knew that none of that could interfere with or diffuse the peace that was my birthright and essence, ever present and ever possible. Not just mine: everyone's. It was beyond acceptance. In that moment, present to how it is and must be, I knew there was nothing to accept—except in the sense of gladly receive.

Even before Peru, it had dawned on me, if only through observation and intuition, that there is more to being human than meets the eye—or as the spiritual master Eckhart Tolle has quipped, "than meets the I." We are part of, and endowed with, something greater than the egoic mind, with its baked-in sense of separateness, can comprehend, much less prove. "No one has ever touched a soul or seen one in a test-tube," the founder of behaviorist psychology John Watson wrote in 1928—and so far as the five senses are concerned, he was correct. But we in the West are playing with a less-than-full sensory deck: our senses have been stripped, to borrow from Dylan,[†] of more subtle ones that spiritual adepts and Indigenous cultures have always cultivated. "We live in a world that is split," the Buddhist meditation teacher Jack Kornfield told me, "and so our psyche is split. We make money by going to work, and we take care of our bodies in the gym, and we maybe take care of our psyche a little bit in therapy, and we do the arts when we go to a concert, and we do the sacred by going to church or synagogue or mosque or something like that. They're all in compartments, as if the sacred was somehow separate from the work that we do, or the music that we make."

One of the earliest and, for many, most challenging steps in programs like Alcoholics Anonymous is to entrust one's life to the care of a higher power, whatever one understands that term to mean. Whether we know it or not, we all seek our higher power. The longing manifests in many ways: our desire to belong; our drive to know our purpose in life; the urge to escape the limitations of our conditioned, self-centered personalities; our taste for transcendent experiences. Unfortunately, in our culture we are taught to seek fulfillment by filling ourselves with evanescent externals. It cannot be done, for what we are missing within cannot be replaced from without. The emptiness dogging us emanates from the places where we have lost contact with our deepest selves. A. H. Almaas, whom I'm fortunate to call a mentor, calls these broken connections "holes." "Allowing ourselves to tolerate the holes and go through them on the other side is more difficult now, because everything in society is against this.

---

†   In his 1965 song "Mr. Tambourine Man."

Society is against essence. Everybody around you, wherever you go, is trying to fill holes, and people feel very threatened if you don't try to fill yours the same way."[1]

"I don't see society as an enemy," he clarified when we spoke. "It's more like society is asleep. It just doesn't know. Some knowledge of it may arise through religion, where there is at least an awareness that there is more to us than the usual physical thing. The spiritual drive wakes up in a human being at some point. It's mysterious when it wakes up: sometimes it wakes up by itself; sometimes it's triggered by something happening outside, by listening to somebody or reading a book. When the spiritual drive or curiosity wakes up, that's when one yearns to find out more about what a human being is beyond the limitations society normally understands, recognizes, and tries to enforce."

Spirituality defies both description and prescription. Countless pathways are out there; some of these resonate more than others for different people. I've tried as much extended meditation as my restless mind can tolerate. One time I sat in speechless contemplation for ten days; never again. It turns out it's not my way, even though I experienced some benefits at the time. Yoga, brief meditation sessions, the occasional psychedelic experience, contemplative silence, reading the spiritual classics of many faiths and disciplines, and listening to the contemporary masters have all helped as I stumble my way toward deeper truths. Some seekers choose none of the above, finding their way to their rapprochement with spirit via wholly self-mapped, even accidental byways. The point is not the big aha, but the arising—sudden or gradual, however it comes—of the consciousness that holds the mind but doesn't mistake itself for its contents. My colleague the physician Will Cooke, who in his work with addicted people in the Appalachian-adjacent region of Southern Indiana has seen his share of spiritual openings, described to me "this spark inside of everyone, that shimmering self waiting to be revealed, that's just cluttered and stacked with all this stuff that life has stuck to them, and they can't shine. But if we pull that away a little bit at a time and reveal who they are, it's always something beautiful."

The yearning for spirit was summed up by the American journalist and broadcaster Michael Brooks shortly before his untimely death at age thirty-six in the summer of 2020. Brooks, who has been widely mourned for his heart, humor, and commitment to truth and justice at home and internationally, had been delving more deeply into spiritual work. His sister, Lisha, has quoted him as having remarked, the day before he died, on a growing awareness of spirit: "I am feeling a spaciousness inside me, like outer space or the ocean." In words that crystallize the endeavor of getting real and returning to ourselves, he then stated his commitment to nurturing and expanding this felt sense. "I'd like to work in the coming weeks," he wrote, "on the mechanics of what it means to continue *separating myself from the stuff that separates me from me*. I want to remember the inner."

Ashley Judd has forged her own unique path to healing. One of the first women to call out the film mogul Harvey Weinstein for his inveterate sexual predations, Judd had long carried the early imprints of life in a family rife with alcoholism and unprocessed grief. For her, the grace that allowed her to surrender to a God she "didn't believe in" arose in part from an intimate encounter with the natural world. "I was sitting in a creek in the Great Smoky Mountains National Park," she recalled when we talked, "and all the butterflies were coming down the creek, and the sun was glinting off the water, and I just knew that everything was okay. It was one of those epiphanic moments where time was suspended and I was okay, and I was alone, and I might always be alone, but everything was all right." Even when old stuff arises,

Judd says the memory of that moment remains alive for her in a way that fortifies her dedication to the healing path, and can even lighten the proceedings. "There can be some humor," she said, chuckling. "I kicked its ass before. I'll be okay."

"I'll be okay" is also the message the Canadian Olympic cyclist and skater Clara Hughes found in her encounter with Nature. Having been the only athlete in history to win multiple medals at both the Summer and Winter Olympics—six altogether—Hughes had created for herself a new and busy career as a speaker and teacher, and a new identity as the bearer of healing and inspirational messages to others. Following her own painful struggles with deep depression, she came to an awakening. "I realized I was getting stuck," the vibrant forty-seven-year-old told me. "I was repeating everything. 'This is not healthy,' I felt. It's not me. I needed to get a life . . . In 2017, March 22, I quit everything. I stopped public speaking, I quit the board of directors that I was on, I just stopped, and started walking." Following her inner voice, she embraced a new passion: long-distance hiking, a pursuit that gives a whole new meaning to the title of this final section, "Pathways to Wholeness." She has spent about six months of each year in the last three years walking.

Among their many salutary effects, these extended pilgrimages bring Hughes into the present moment in a way that aligns perfectly with the will to heal. "When I walk," she said vibrantly, "there is no tomorrow. Yesterday is gone . . . there is only here, now. I listen to the forest speak, the mountains, the water. I hear their voices. Trees become family. Rocks become living beings that you know, and you're happy to see." Walking has also instilled in her a new sense of what it means to be resilient. "I know without a doubt that I can breathe through anything, every single difficult thing that surfaces. In whatever headspace that may come to me in my day . . . I can sit, and I can write, I can draw,

I can garden, I can do the dishes. I can bring myself back to my breath, and I'm okay. And I'm going to be okay, and it's me." I was glad she said the part about drawing and gardening, since few of us will ever journey into the wild in quite so epic a way as she has. But any activity that brings us back to our own nature— which is, of course, but one expression of Nature writ large— unencumbered by gadgets and digital obsessions, can be a fount of refreshment.

Nature played a major role in V's recovery from metastatic uterine cancer, following multiple surgeries and chemotherapy. "I used to be horrified by Nature," the writer and activist told me, "until I got very, very sick, and then I heard—I heard the Mother calling me to come to the country. It was like, 'you need to come.'" It began with a solitary potted tree outside the window of her hospital room. "I fell in love with that tree," she said, smiling at the recollection. "I was so sick at that point. I had lost thirty pounds, I didn't know if I was going to make it, and I was looking at that tree, saying to myself, 'Oh my God, I'm going to have to look at this tree every day as I anticipate death?' And that first day that tree just started to speak to me . . . And I was like, *Wow! I don't think I've ever seen what leaves are* . . . And the next day it was like, *Bark!* And the next day it was like, *Trunk!* Literally, I didn't want people to talk to me anymore, I didn't want people to come near me—just let me be with this tree; this tree and I are having something amazing happen here. The last day that I was in that room, the tree blossomed, white blossoms. That was the beginning of my transformation."

None of this is news to the world's Indigenous peoples; oneness with Nature has been a pillar of such cultures since forever. Even through the brutal displacement of North America's original

Nations from the life-giving lands that were part and parcel of their identities, the awareness of belonging to this planet has never been lost. In fact, according to the Navajo activist, artist, and ceremonial leader Pat McCabe, known as Woman Stands Shining, it is a lifeline, a fount of resilience and strength. "The first thing that comes to my heart," she told me, "is that we have a commitment to Earth. It's not just a commitment, though—it's a mad love affair with this Earth. And we have a capacity and a role in helping Her and all the rest of the life to thrive. It's not part of the modern world paradigm. Everything is so individualistic, individual achievement, and even anthropocentric, right? Totally self-oriented. When you are part of that larger community, Earth, and you are accountable to this mad romance with birds and fish and trees and mountains and sky, you have more to compel you, to guide you."

In my interviews for this book, I was struck by how often people would bring up their experience with and reverence for Indigenous traditions—an esteem I have come to share through my interactions with Native healers and elders in both South and North America, whether sitting in ceremony in a Peruvian maloca, a Colombian hut, or in a sweat lodge in Alberta. I am grateful to the communities who have welcomed me, an outsider from the "settler" side of the neocolonial divide, into their places and given me a taste of their ways—as much of a taste as one dropping in from the dominant culture can be given, anyway.

If we see Native wisdom not as something to be consumed but rather as a rich trove of traditions about ways of living and dying that deserve and demand our humble curiosity and respect, its broad, unitary perspective could round out the dualistic, biological focus of the Western medical mentality. Indigenous traditions are themselves fighting for survival, but they can still offer a salutary, equal complement to Western medicine's scientific wizardry. They can also be a necessary corrective to the latter's failure to honor our emotional, social, communal, and spiritual needs.

Helen Knott likens being in the sweat lodge to returning to the womb. "Our healing," she told me, "must include that piece of humility where you ask for help and recognize that you can't do everything on your own, that just on your own you could be a pitiful creature as a human being. Suffering from this human condition, trying to find our way, that sweat lodge takes us back to our origins—in the belly of our Mother Earth. Being able to let things go, and to lie on the earth and to just *be* there. The lodge is always a powerful place." When the large, heated rocks are hauled into the pit in the middle of the sweat lodge, participants welcome them as "grandmothers and grandfathers." This is not metaphor; it is profound understanding and clear seeing, far clearer and wiser than most of us are schooled in. Do we not all come from the earth that spawned those rocks, as from the water that is poured over them before the prayers and the chants begin? Would we not, if we could see things that way, think twice before despoiling and pillaging that which creates and sustains us? In the Western world, at great cost to ourselves, we have long lost touch with this unity that Indigenous cultures recognize and honor.

The part-Lakota psychiatrist and physician Lewis Mehl-Madrona[†] is experienced in both high-tech emergency medicine and in the traditional healing methods of his people. In his view, both have their place, and he would not want to do without either one. Like me, he has seen the miracles both can bestow. "For a Native American, a healing is a spiritual journey," he writes. "As most people intuitively grasp (except maybe doctors, who are

---

[†]   Former medical director at the Center for Complementary Medicine, University of Pittsburgh Medical Center, and currently on the faculty of the family medicine residency program at Eastern Maine Medical Center, affiliated with the University of New England.

trained to disbelieve the idea), what happens to the body reflects what is happening in the mind and the spirit. People *can* get well. But before a person can do so, he or she must often undergo a transformation—of lifestyle, emotions, and spirit—besides making the necessary shifts in the physical body."[2]

"In the Lakota idea," Mehl-Madrona told me when we met to discuss this book and the possibility of collaborating in some healing events, "we need to celebrate and support people who are ill because they're the canaries in the mine. They're the ones who are showing us that our society is out of balance, and we need to thank them for taking that on and doing it for the rest of us. All of us need to participate in their healing, because if not for them, where would we be? We're all responsible for whatever ails them. We have the responsibility to contribute to their healing for everybody's benefit." What a bracing old/new thought: a society in which all have responsibility for the health of all, where the illness is seen as the manifestation of shared experience. A culture like ours has much to learn from ones that take our biopsychosocial nature as a given.

I had to laugh when Mehl-Madrona then pointed out another distinction between Western medical attitudes and his grandparents' Indigenous tradition. One of his teachers, a famed American physician, lectured to his coed medical school class: " 'Boys,' he said—he couldn't get around the idea that there were women in the class—'Boys, life is a relentless progression toward death, disease, and decay. The job of a physician is to slow the rate of decline.' And I was really shocked, because my great-grandmother always taught us that you should die healthy 'so you can party on the other side.' She didn't really believe that you had to be sick to die. She didn't connect sickness and death. For her, death was like your time is up, and sickness is just something you may have to go through."

"How old was she when she died?" I asked.

"In her mid-nineties, and in good health. It's a funny story: one evening she told everyone that she was going to die that night. And she said, 'It's my time. My time is up.' Then my mother, who was trying very hard to be modern, said, 'Nonsense, you're very healthy.' 'That has nothing to do with dying,' my great-grandmother replied. And in the morning, she was dead."

It's not a question of romanticizing Native ways, nor of aping Indigenous practices. But we can and must overcome what Wade Davis furiously calls "cultural myopia," the sense that "other peoples are failed versions of ourselves. Or that they are ancient, vestigial creatures, destined to fade away, quaint and colorful humans who wear feathers. These are living, dynamic people who have something to say."

———————

Although my own experience of healing took place in the jungle, and Clara Hughes's in wide-open spaces, I have seen people coming home to themselves even in the claustrophobically confined and, far too often, less-than-humane precincts of prisons. Some of the gentlest people I've met have been lifers in Canadian or American prisons who have courageously confronted their past. Many others working with such people have shared with me that same heartfelt impression.

Thanks to my work in addiction, I have been invited to speak to incarcerated populations—in other words, to the most traumatized and marginalized in our culture. I will not forget what Rick, a lifer in California's notorious San Quentin State Prison, told me. He had been through a volunteer-led transformational program that took him for a deep dive into the self, beginning with a childhood that featured every category of adverse childhood experience: an alienated and violent adolescence, and a drug-addled young adulthood that culminated in a killing. He was now thirty years older, a smallish, thin Black man with gray stubble and thinning hair. He was hoping to apply for parole. We were sitting in a meeting room, along with about a dozen of his confreres, of various ages. "This group," he said, "made me think about my actions and helped me to stop running, to stand up and face those inner demons I had always run away from. I have learned to love myself and to know that there are people who care out there."

I wondered what he would want the parole board to know about him. "Well," Rick pondered, "at that time in my life I was separated from me. I didn't even know who I was. I didn't respect myself, so I couldn't respect no one else. I didn't love myself, so I didn't have no love for anybody else. But after doing this time, really stopping and looking at my life as a genuine thing, and with the love for myself and understanding that for me love is every-thing . . . love is opening me up to everything outside of me. What I'm doing for myself, learning about me, I'm learning about ev-eryone else, too. I'm not different from everybody else. If I touch spirit, I'm not separated. If you do let me out of here, this is the kind of work I want to do when I get out. I'm ready. I want to go home, but even if they don't let me go home, I already know who I am and what I want to do." Every one of the five compassions we looked at earlier was shimmeringly present in Rick's words.

"There is only one common rule valid in finding your special truth. It is to learn to listen patiently to yourself, to give yourself a chance to find your own way which is yours and nobody else's," wrote the psychologist and visionary Wilhelm Reich.[3]

Listening for our "special truth" is among the most daunting of challenges amid the clamor of our increasingly noisy world—

a world that isolates even as it discourages healthy solitude. The quest is age-old. George Bernard Shaw's play *Saint Joan* depicts the heroic life and death of the young peasant girl Joan of Arc, whose visions and "voices" inspired her to lead the armed revolt against the English occupation of fifteenth-century France. "Oh, your voices, your voices," the French king Charles VII says at one point to Joan with envy and frustration. "Why don't the voices come to me? I am king, not you." "They do come to you," Joan replies, "but you do not hear them. You have not sat in the field in the evening listening for them. When the angelus rings you cross yourself and have done with it; but if you prayed from your heart and listened to the thrilling of the bells in the air after they stop ringing, you would hear the voices as well as I do."

Among the challenges of healing ourselves personally and of bringing healing to our troubled world is being still long enough to allow our true selves, that "still small voice" we read of in the King James Bible, or as the Hebraic Tanakh describes it, that "soft murmuring sound," to be heard.[†] The ancient and modern practices of mindfulness encourage and allow space for that voice to emerge, by separating us from and enabling us to observe the cacophonous traffic in our minds without being seduced, overwhelmed, or intimidated by it.

Mindfulness practices have also had the documented benefits of reducing inflammation, reprogramming epigenetic functioning, promoting the repair of telomeres, reducing stress hormone levels, and encouraging the development of healthier brain circuitry.[4] Mindfulness even reduced the disease progression in patients with ALS:[5] the mind-body unity in action once again.

When we observe ourselves with compassionate curiosity instead of judgment, perhaps we can also learn to drop our

---

[†]   I Kings 19:12.

prejudgments—also known as prejudices—against others. A most encouraging study comes from Israel/Palestine, site of ongoing hatred and conflict. Over three hundred Jewish students from grades three to five were exposed to a mindfulness and compassion-based social-emotional program. Six months later, and despite a flare-up of violent hostilities, these students showed "significantly reduced" prejudice toward and negative stereotyping of Palestinians.[6]

I interviewed several leading mindfulness practitioners; each attested that their practice has led them, and others, to greater compassion and acceptance of fellow humans. "I would never bet against the human heart," the psychologist and Buddhist meditation teacher Rick Hanson† told me.

————————

The present book's title employs the word "myth" in its everyday, contemporary sense. "That's just a myth," we might say to an agitated friend peddling the conspiracy theory du jour. "There's no proof." But this pejorative use of the word actually puts us at odds with most of cultural history. Until very recently, myth was seen as a fount of knowledge, a portal to spirit, and one of the fundaments of any healthy culture. It may well be that this original notion of myth can serve as a gateway into the world of healing, reconnecting us with eons of human wisdom and fostering a mindset where nothing is isolated happenstance and where meaning can be made from any of life's raw materials. It is a potent antidote to the dualistic thinking that fantasizes mind and body to be separable. In the world of myth, everything is connected: one of many real-world truths that mythic thinking can help us face.

Myth is a collective expression of one of the most uniquely

—————————————————————————————

†   Author, most famously, of *Buddha's Brain: The Practical Neuroscience of Happiness, Love, and Wisdom.*

human qualities: imagination. Far from magical thinking or denialism, imaginative thinking allows us to see beyond appearances and tap into core insights into what wholeness and wellness mean. "When we lose myth," the American storyteller, author, and *Living Myth Podcast* host Michael Meade told me, "we know less. We know less about ourselves, we know less about illness, and thus we know less about healing." What, then, I asked, could a return to mythic imagination tell us about wholeness and healing? "An illness stops us in our course, and then can be a wake-up call, if we allow the body to teach us what's going on," he replied. We have witnessed that in these chapters many a time.

The mythic and the prophetic are closely linked. On the societal scale, we could move toward wholeness if we were willing to heed the warnings our collective afflictions, from cancer to COVID-19, are sounding about how we live. Mythic thinking might help us enshrine and enact the scientific principle that our health derives from connection—to our essence, to each other, and to a culture that honors these interrelationships.

Older understandings of myth also spring from a deep connection to (or oneness with) Nature, which is perhaps why myth-making in the positive sense comes to us so naturally. As Wade Davis put it when we spoke, "For most of human history, our relationships with the natural world had been based on metaphors." Mountains are symbols of strength and constancy; rivers embody change, flow, even life itself. These meanings have profound consequences for how we live, for how we see the world and our place in it. They are the marks of a culture that knows how to read, and heed, Nature's signs.

Michael Meade has a beautiful phrase for the kind of collective knowing that dates back as long as we've been around: "a thought in the heart." My own heart resonates with the thought that—despite all apparent evidence to the contrary—there is in all of us an essential aspect that cannot be extinguished. This society, in its spiritually dormant state of immaturity and denial, blocks our awareness of it, supplanting it instead with qualities, activities, goods, and beliefs that cannot possibly satisfy. As individuals we are unable to see our own beauty or perfection; as members of a collective, we miss how we are all made of, indeed interwoven within, the same divine fabric—if you prefer, you can substitute words like "eternal," "ancient," "more-than-human," or "soul" for "divine."

Touching spirit, to use the phrase of Rick from San Quentin, can only enliven the healing journey.

Chapter 33

Unmaking a Myth:
Visioning a Saner Society

At intervals can be seen a glimpse of truth,
that daylight of the human soul.

—Victor Hugo, *Les Misérables*

What will it take to unmake the myth of normal? How can we possibly hope to disassemble such a vast agglomeration of culturally manufactured misperceptions, prejudices, blind spots, and health-killing fictions—especially when they serve the interests of a world order intent on its own continuance, even unto self-destruction?

The truth is, I don't know. In some ways I'm more comfortable describing the problem than charting a course out of it. I have my own convictions and hunches, especially about the obstacles to a better world, but that doesn't equal a detailed blueprint for something new. Even to the extent that I have strong beliefs about how things ought to look, it seems less than fitting to use the final chapter of this book on trauma and healing to get on a soapbox. And yet, as we bring this inquiry to its conclusion, I do feel a responsibility to offer some sort of alternate vision to the toxic culture I've been depicting.

What I can say with confidence, as a physician and healer, is that for our society to right itself and chart a course toward maximum health, certain conditions will have to be met. And it will take some key changes or shifts to create those conditions. They all derive from the core principles of this book: biopsychosocial medicine, disease as teacher, the primacy of both attachment and authenticity, and, above all, fearless self-inquiry, here on a social scale. None of these shifts is sufficient in itself, but as far as I can tell, they are all necessary. They may not fully come to pass without significant social-political transformation, but they are easy to grasp, and it is well within our power to work toward them.

A few years ago, as I was researching this book, I spoke with Noam Chomsky, father of modern linguistics, philosopher, activist, and cultural critic. I asked this intellectual luminary, who has called himself a "tactical pessimist and strategic optimist," if he still remains on the positive side of what is to come. Chomsky smiled. "You've got to be an optimist, otherwise you might just as well commit suicide. So yes, of course, I'm an optimist. You try to do what you can to correct things; whether it can be done or not, we don't know. It's the slogan Gramsci made famous: 'pessimism of the intellect, optimism of the will.'† There is no other choice." I would also call it the optimism of heart and soul, which are the birthplace of will. These nonrational parts of ourselves know things about human potential and the nature of life that are untouchable by even the smartest intellect.

Before engaging in any major reforms toward a more trauma-aware, health-friendly society, we'll want to look into our own hearts and minds to make sure we're approaching these daunting tasks from a place of possibility. The problems facing the world are challenging enough without adding our own stresses stemming from our habitual coping patterns. Are we seeing things *creatively* or *reactively*? Automatic reactions are, after all, the specialty of the traumatized personality, which is the ultimate

---

†   Antonio Gramsci, the Italian philosopher, linguist, and antifascist activist.

hammer that only sees nails. Creativity, meanwhile, is about something more fundamental: it starts with seeing that we *can* create, and then has a feel for what *wants* to be created. It is a facet of authenticity, a close cousin of authorship.

One can create only from a perspective that says, "Something is possible here, no matter how things may look." There are plenty of grounds for this kind of optimism based on what we know about human nature and needs, and about the resilience and mysterious healing powers of the body and mind. We can also take sustenance from the knowledge that each of us is one of a growing community of people who are seeing through the status quo and envisioning alternatives to it.

Such an attitude necessarily involves patience and perspective, and a healthy tolerance for both the real and the ideal.

If we're out to see things as they are, we must be willing—even hungry—to shed our illusions. We have to welcome being disillusioned—perhaps even, as Alanis Morissette does in the chorus of one of her hit singles, thank it.[‡] Commonly we speak of disillusionment ruefully as an experience to be avoided, akin to disappointment or a sense of having been betrayed. And it does carry a cost: we may have to let go of something we've come to value, or a perspective or attitude we've taken refuge in. What we see less easily, however, is the cost of refusing. As I often ask people, "Would you prefer to be *illusioned* or *dis*illusioned?" Would we rather engage with the world as it really is or only as we wish it were? Which approach brings more suffering in the end?

I grew up during the period of Stalinist oppression in my homeland, Hungary, though as an idealistic little Communist I was oblivious to its nature. I recall my heart swelling with pride to be living in a system dedicated to freedom, equality, and the

---

‡   The song is 1998's "Thank U."

kinship of humankind. At school assemblies I would leap to my feet on cue, eagerly joining my classmates in rhythmic applause and chants whenever the principal mentioned "Party" and "Leader." My parents and teachers knew better than to burst my ideological bubble: a careless dissenting word escaping a child's lips could mean harassment, loss of livelihood, even imprisonment. Then, one morning in late October 1956, our building shook to the thunder of artillery. A few days of liberty granted by the evanescent triumph of the Magyar uprising against the dictatorship, followed by its swift and bloody suppression, opened my twelve-year-old eyes. The Soviet Army I had long idolized, the fighting force that had saved my infant life, was suddenly the enemy. Not long after, on a rainy November night, my brother, parents, and I trudged across the muddy Austrian border, leaving behind our life in Hungary forever. That was my first disillusionment; more followed. In the wake of the horrors of the Vietnam War and the unconscionable lies used to justify it, I learned that the American empire, which in my adolescent mind had displaced the Soviet one as the new shining city on the hill, was as cruelly and rapaciously self-centered as its rival. I had to arrive as well at the heartrending realization that the dream that had been a balm to my soul, that of a triumphant Jewish national rebirth in my people's ancestral biblical home, had been achieved by imposing a nightmare on the Palestinian inhabitants of the land, a nightmare that continues to this day.[1] When the truth struck home, I was once again astonished that my imagined universe could have been such a distorted version of the real one. Visiting the West Bank and Gaza, I wept every day for two weeks.

I say all this not to enroll you, the reader, in my particular political views; only to indicate that, for each of us, there may be things about our "normal," including our sense of who we are and the nature of our society, that we are reluctant to let go of. My serial disillusionments were painful at the time, to be sure: they meant leaving something behind, something I had cherished and built a part of my world around. And yet I would not trade the freedom that has accompanied each relinquishing of illusion for the comforts I had to give up. When a false belief falls away, after the ache of loss and sense of being unmoored subsides, I have noticed that something in me relaxes, no longer tasked with squaring circles and holding together impossible contradictions. Ignorance may bring a blissed-out tranquility, but that is not true bliss; on the collective level, it can result in great and wide suffering. We do ourselves and the world a profound service when we endeavor to dissolve our illusions and open ourselves to the truths they conceal.

"Not everything that is faced can be changed," James Baldwin wrote, "but nothing can be changed until it is faced."[2]

A willingness to be disillusioned means confronting denial, one of the central buttresses of the status quo and a major barrier to imagining or seeking a transformed world. After all, were we to alter our worldview enough to see the state of things for what it is and what it is costing us, we would no longer consent to it so easily. "We live in a country in which words are mostly used to cover the sleeper, not to wake him up"—another penetrating observation from Baldwin that could accurately describe almost any place on earth.[3]

"The world forgets easily, too easily, what it does not like to remember," wrote Jacob Riis almost a hundred years earlier in *How the Other Half Lives*, his account of the squalidity of tenement life in late-nineteenth-century New York. This culture is a master at forgetting its past and obscuring the sordid aspects of its present.

Anyone anticipating that the global corporate capitalist system might one day face the truth of its own nature and fundamentally transform itself is in for a long and frustrating wait. Nor will its academic institutions or media be eager to give up their role as its ideological enablers. As Joan Didion remarked about the latter, for journalists "what 'fairness' has often come to mean is a scrupulous passivity, an agreement to cover the story not as it is occurring but as it is presented, which is to say as it is manufactured."[4] That leaves it up to each of us, as individuals and as groups, to seek out and support alternative sources of knowledge, to expose ourselves to uncertainty, to enter into the points of view of others, whether we agree with them or not, to listen to people doing hard activist work on the ground, to stay alert to the many tendrils the myth of normal extends to keep itself normalized. This would represent a new kind of citizenship, one arising from the needs and demands of the moment.

A Trauma-Conscious Society

It's hard to think of any collective domain where greater trauma awareness and insight into the nature of healing would not make a positive difference. I want to focus in these last pages on a few key ones.

The implications of a society being trauma-literate could be immense. Since trauma is the core dynamic undergirding so much ill health, we need to develop the eyes and ears to spot it to begin with. Some see encouraging signs: my colleague Bessel van der Kolk goes so far as to assert that "we are on the verge of becoming a trauma-conscious society."[5] I do not share that optimism in the short term, because that consciousness is still far from penetrating the decisive institutions of our culture. But I agree there is a recent sea change in the public's recognition of trauma's prevalence and significance in our lives. Many people, both lay and professional, are hungry to understand it. We see that in the long-term bestseller status of Bessel's foundational text and the gratifyingly impressive success of books like Dr. Bruce Perry's *What Happened to You?*, co-written with Oprah Winfrey. As too, if I may use it as an example, in the viral success of a film documenting my work, *The Wisdom of Trauma*, which was eye-opening in this regard even for me—it was seen by four million people in over 220 countries within two weeks of its release in June 2021.[†]

Trauma Awareness: Medicine

A trauma-informed medical system, for starters, could help heal and prevent suffering on a scale and in ways inspiring to envision. Such a system would revamp how health care is delivered, aligning itself with the latest scientific findings. Published almost every week in leading science journals, these findings have yet to make much of a dent in mainstream medical thinking. In this book we have cited many already, and more appear regularly.[6]

At present there remains powerful resistance to trauma awareness on the part of the medical profession—albeit a resistance more subliminal than deliberate, more passive than active. In the dozens of interviews I conducted with medical colleagues for this book, including recent graduates, virtually none of them recalled being taught about the mind-body unity or the profusely documented relationship between, for example, trauma and mental illness or addictions—let alone the links between adversity and physical disease. We doctors pride ourselves on what we call evidence-based practice while ignoring vast swaths of evidence that call into question central tenets of our dogma.

Then there is the highly stressed and often emotionally wounding or numbing impact of medical education, an experience reported by so many of my medical interviewees. "I was totally

---

[†]   The film can be viewed at https://wisdomoftrauma.com.

traumatized in my first year of medical school," a well-known colleague told me. "It was teaching by terror, as in intimidating us to learn when we're already highly motivated to learn." "It's an abusive system; it's a traumatic system," my friend the Colorado psychiatrist Will Van Derveer said. "Residents [doctors] are killing themselves." His words brought to mind the study I mentioned in chapter 4 showing that the telomeres of physicians in training frayed more rapidly than those of other young people their age. Aside from the health dangers to these health care professionals themselves, trauma unawareness impedes them from recognizing the imprints of painful life experiences in others. Thus, unwittingly, they perpetuate a system that ignores and even compounds the real problem. A harried existence and the time constraints imposed, especially by fee-for-service models, inhibit physicians from delving into their patients' life histories, even when they are inclined to do so. Residents gave me heartbreaking accounts of listening to patients' personal stories with the effect of almost immediate symptom relief, only to be denigrated by their specialist mentors. Medical students find themselves criticized for not working fast enough. I interviewed Oregon physician Pamela Wible, whose own painful trajectory has led her to work in preventing suicide among doctors. "Never in my wildest dreams," Wible confessed, "did I think that after jumping through all the hoops of medical education I'd end up funneled into seven-minute office visits, and be treated as a factory worker, and be expected to treat my patients as widgets." A trauma-informed medical system would have care for the emotional health of its students and practitioners.

And yet, there are positive developments. Some medical schools are introducing elements of empathy training, and in Canada, there have been initiatives to acquaint medical students with

Indigenous history and traditions. Pediatrician Nadine Burke Harris, a well-known trauma awareness advocate and now the surgeon general of California, is introducing screening for adverse childhood experiences into public health programs in her state. In an interview held before her appointment to the post, she expressed an optimism that mirrors Bessel van der Kolk's. "Believe it or not," she told me, "it's going better than I'd hoped. I think we are looking at incremental milestones that need to happen over thirty or forty years' time, but a lot of groundwork is taking place." For his part, Will Van Derveer has initiated a popular trauma-focused training for fellow psychiatrists, subscribed to by colleagues from around the world. And Pam Wible has pioneered a community-based approach that respects the body-mind unity and helps empower people to be active agents in their health care. "Medicine," she told me, "is a calling and it's a soul's purpose." She has now created a way to follow that call.

Trauma Awareness: The Law

Can we next imagine a trauma-informed legal apparatus, one that could earn its title of "correctional system"? Such a system would have to dedicate itself to actually correcting things in a humane way, a far cry from what we have now. In North America, and in many parts of the world, the current model should more accurately be called a "trauma-punishing-and-inducing system." Despite the documented fact that a large number of prison inmates committed their crimes out of dynamics originating in severe childhood suffering, legal training leaves the average lawyer or judge even more woefully trauma-ignorant than their medical counterparts. True to its other customary name, morally speaking, ours is a *criminal* justice system.

A trauma-informed legal system would not justify or excuse

harmful behavior. Rather, it would replace nakedly punitive measures with programs designed to rehabilitate people and not to further traumatize them. "All us criminals start out as normal people just like anyone else, but then things happen in life that tear us apart, that make us into something capable of hurting other people," writes the academic and former inmate Jesse Thistle. "That's all any of the darkness really is. Love gone bad. We're just broken-hearted people hurt by life."[7] "Unlike in some other countries, here prison is not designed to rehabilitate you," he told me. "It's designed to mess you up so that you'll continue with high rates of recidivism, that's what I think."

Dr. Nneka Jones Tapia, a psychologist, is a former prison guard and currently the managing director of Chicago Beyond and Justice Initiatives. As a Black woman, she knows institutionalized racial trauma well. She spoke to me of resilience and the creation of a trauma-informed justice system. "We tend to reduce people to their behaviors: 'You're a murderer, you're a robber, you're a thief.' But we are not our worst behavior. I have had the blessing to see that everyone who is incarcerated has strengths and they have the capability of loving, if only we gave them the opportunity. It's not just people that need the healing. It's the system that has to be indicted and transformed."

Trauma Awareness: Education

Because trauma affects kids' ability to learn, a trauma-informed educational system would train teachers to be well versed in the science of development. Education in such a system would encourage an atmosphere where emotional intelligence is valued as highly as intellectual achievement. We would no longer evaluate kids based on performance goals that still mostly reflect and bestow social and racial advantage, but would provide settings where all were encouraged to thrive. "School programs could be designed to support healthy social and emotional development," writes teacher and school psychologist Maggie Kline. "When students feel safe, the regions of the brain for language, thinking, and reasoning are enhanced."[8] Teacher training would recognize signs and signals of children's "acting out" as pleas for help or markers of emotional pain, rather than viewing them as bad behaviors to be suppressed or as cause for punishment or exclusion.

Beyond schooling, the potential implications of my friend Raffi Cavoukian's vision of an entire society that honors the irreducible needs of children (see chapter 9) are both vast and simple. I leave it to you, the reader, to imagine what our world would look like if we placed young people's well-being in the forefront. What would it mean for parenting and for support for parenting, for childcare and education, for the economy, for what products we sell and buy, for what foods we sell and prepare, for the climate, for the culture? What if our intention, as parents, as educators, as a society, was to raise children in touch with their feelings, authentically empowered to express them, to think independently and be prepared to act on behalf of their principles?

A healthy society would also strive to close the largely artificial generation gap that makes it difficult for parents to relate to their kids and vice versa. As discussed in an earlier section on peer orientation (chapter 13), the natural human arrangement has a strong communal dimension, and the adult community is meant to work together to hold space for the development of the young. That does not mean lording it over our kids, nor dictating every aspect of their lives, only that we reclaim responsibility for creating and maintaining the container for their growth. And we must also remember that parents need each other, and that we all need the presence of life-tested elders; in a world that's committed to health, child-rearing and intergenerational transmission of values and culture wouldn't be an isolating task.

———————

In the last decades, in many countries around the world, people—adults and children in the millions—have mobilized to force into the political conversation critical issues such as environmental justice, Indigenous rights, women's rights, gender justice, racial equity, and police reform. One such person is Greta Thunberg, the teenage climate activist, who, describing her autism as her "superpower," has contributed greatly to her generation's awareness of climate change. "Many ignorant people still see it as an 'illness,' or something negative," she said on Twitter. "When the haters go after your looks and differences, it means they have nowhere left to go. And then you know you are winning." Her own example illustrates the healing power of meaningful engagement. Prior to her climate campaign, she divulged, she had "no energy, no friends and I didn't speak to anyone. I just sat alone at home, with an eating disorder."[9]

Inspired by figures like Thunberg and countless others whose names we may never know, we can revisit our list of the four *A*'s I laid out in chapter 26 that promote healing—*authenticity, agency, anger,* and *acceptance*—and add two more that are required for the pursuit of broad transformational change: *activism* and *advocacy.* The last two are socially meaningful ways of synthesizing the previous four, with some added ingredients—solidarity, collective thinking, and connection—to help counter capitalism's atomizing effects.

Part of advocacy is to use whatever privilege we may have to amplify the voices of those to whom society denies a voice; part of activism is organizing groups of people to demand necessary change. Both express a healthy, necessary "no," often accompanied by a resounding "yes"—for example, to a concrete policy goal like Medicare for All in the United States or long-overdue justice for First Nations people in Canada. These two bonus A's are not, and cannot be, individual pursuits. I visited Zuccotti Park in New York City, in September 2011, the site of the Occupy Wall Street protests against inequality. Flawed and evanescent as that movement proved to be, I was struck by the enthusiasm, solidarity, and sheer energy of the crowd as they found a collective outlet for forwarding their vision of a just society. Often blocked from being expressed, that latent energy is within us all.

The photographer Nan Goldin, whose addiction to opiates we touched on in chapter 15, has waged more than a private struggle for recovery: she has engaged in both personal and collective activism against Purdue Pharma, the corporation that helped generate the opioid overdose crisis that has claimed hundreds of thousands of lives. Purdue reaped vast profits from its drug OxyContin, which it marketed as a less addictive opioid painkiller, suppressing evidence to the contrary. Goldin's friends in AA had advised against her going public, saying it would destroy her sobriety. "It turned out to be the best choice I ever made," she told me.

Her particular crusade has been directed against the Sacklers, the family that controls Purdue. Goldin's fame as an artist gave her a platform to raise her banner, especially since the Sacklers have cultivated a reputation as art benefactors. "I knew their names from going to museums," she said, "and I always thought of them as benevolent art philanthropists with great taste." Another salutary disillusionment, I thought. "And then I found out," Goldin continued, "about their involvement with the opiate crisis, their profiting off the suffering of hundreds of thousands of people, their complete callousness and inhumanity." Fueled by outrage at what she discovered, Goldin induced some of the world's most prestigious museums, including the Met in New York, to stop accepting money from the Sacklers and to eliminate their self-laundering logo from their buildings. The Sackler Institute of Graduate Biomedical Sciences at NYU's medical school has also dropped the family name.

I asked Goldin why she saw her decision to engage in public activism as the best choice she ever made. Her answer speaks to the health rewards of the two added *A*'s of *activism* and *advocacy*. "You need something bigger than yourself," she replied without hesitation. "For me what's bigger than myself is other people suffering. And that's a situation I can help rectify. The politics of this moment are bigger than any individual, the way the world is right now. Trying to find a way to impact that, that's my power, that's what I fight about. It helps keep me sober." As Goldin found, standing up to a toxic system can help us find a place to stand within ourselves.

It is never redundant to remind ourselves that the Chinese phrase for "crisis" is a compound of symbols for "danger" and "opportunity."

We have seen how people with debilitating and even life-threatening pathology can learn from their illnesses and transform their lives. If the same principle were applied on a societal scale, the climate crisis would be an opportunity to examine the dominant perceptions and practices of a culture on a path of self-destruction. The COVID-19 experience, which, ironically enough, has done much to *unmask* many unflattering facts about our ways of life, is a powerful reminder of the interconnections between all life-forms; of our true nature rooted in our relationship to one another; of the inequities of a system in which the most socially vulnerable are left most open to attack by a deadly virus; of how the slogan "We are all in this together" is a sad fiction when it comes to the economic ravages and windfalls of the public health catastrophe that has marked this decade for all time.

And speaking of crises, there could be no more damning indictment of a system than that its young people, stalked as they are by anxieties about human-made climate change, distrust adults and governments en masse.[10] The inimitable Greta Thunberg put it with devastating simplicity at a youth summit in Milan held in September 2021: "Build Back Better. Blah, blah, blah. Green economy. Blah blah blah. Net zero by 2050. Blah, blah, blah. This is all we hear from our so-called leaders. Words that sound great but so far have not led to action. Our hopes and ambitions drown in their empty promises."[11] Unfettered greed, inauthenticity, and disconnection have driven us to such a dark place that it falls to young people to wake us up to what this toxic culture has perpetrated and ignored for so long.

───────────

Prior to his trial for war crimes, the master engineer of Nazi genocide SS Lieutenant Colonel Adolf Eichmann was certified as "normal" by several psychiatrists—"more normal, at any rate than I am," one of them was said to have exclaimed according to Hannah Arendt's classic account.[12] "Another," Arendt reported, "had found that Eichmann's whole psychological outlook, including his relationship with his wife and children, his mother and father, his brothers and sisters and friends, was 'not only normal but most desirable.'"

This is what the American psychiatrist Robert J. Lifton has termed "malignant normality." Many of the greatest crimes have been and continue to be perpetrated by people in leadership positions who are deemed to be the epitome of normal in their respective societies, whether it's the production of toxic and climate-altering chemicals or, say, the imposition of policies that lead to mass starvation in countries far away. Hundreds of thousands of Iraqi children died of malnutrition in the 1990s because of U.S. sanctions.[13] America's then–U.N. ambassador Madeleine Albright declared that "the price is worth it," in an interview seen by millions. As we now know, and as anyone could have known then, there was no credible justification for such heartless cruelty. Albright subsequently became the first woman secretary of state and remains highly respected, especially in liberal circles.[†] One is reminded of Victor Hugo's withering phrase for such figures: "the barbarians of civilization."

As it turns out, it is often individuals who defy conventional normality who are the healthy ones. The psychologist Abraham Maslow made the investigation of self-actualization—the attainment of authentic satisfaction not based on external valuations—his life's work. "A study of people healthy enough to be self-actualized," he wrote in a widely read paper, "revealed that they were not 'well-adjusted' (in the naïve sense of approval of and identification with the culture)." These healthy people, suggested Maslow, had a complex relationship with their "much less healthy culture." Neither conformists nor automatically reflexive rebels, such men and women expressed their unconventionality in ways that kept them true to their inner values, without hostility but not without fight, when that was called for. "An inner feeling of detachment from the culture was not necessarily conscious but was displayed by almost all . . . They very frequently seemed to be able to stand off from it as if they did not quite belong to it."[14]

As we saw earlier, the antidote to the hypnotizing influence of

---

†   Albright, who died in March 2022, would later publicly regret making that statement. She never did renounce the policies it justified.

normality is authenticity: finding meaning in one's inner experience, unobscured by societally promulgated fictions—prime among them what Daniel Siegel calls "the lie of the separate solo self." That falsehood is the ultimate abnormality. From where I stand, a life devoted to seeing through such a traumatizing nontruth, dwelling and creating outside its bounds, is a life lived well.

It all starts with waking up: waking up to what is real and authentic in and around us and what isn't; waking up to who we are and who we're not; waking up to what our bodies are expressing and what our minds are suppressing; waking up to our wounds and our gifts; waking up to what we have believed and what we actually value; waking up to what we will no longer tolerate and what we can now accept; waking up to the myths that bind us and the interconnections that define us; waking up to the past as it has been, the present as it is, and the future as it may yet be; waking up, most especially, to the gap between what our essence calls for and what "normal" has demanded of us.

We are blessed with a momentous opportunity. Shedding toxic myths of disconnection from ourselves, from one another, and from the planet, we can bring what is normal and what is natural, bit by bit, closer together. It is a task for the ages: one that can redeem the past, inspire the present, and point to a brighter, healthier future.

It is our most daunting challenge and greatest possibility.

Acknowledgments

No book springs forth fully formed from its author, like Athena from the head of Zeus. This one surely didn't. It bears the imprint of hundreds of scientists, researchers, physicians, thinkers, and authors, to say nothing of the many medical colleagues and professionals of various disciplines who generously shared with me their time and expertise, along with hundreds of ex-patients and other laypeople who openheartedly and trustingly spoke to me of their travails, struggles, and triumphs. While the interpretations, formulations, and presentation are fully my responsibility, along with any mistakes, I can claim no personal ownership of the truths I have tried to convey.

My New York literary super-agent, Laurie Liss, came along just as this book project emerged after a long period of near-frozen hibernation, and helped nurse it back to life, from proposal stage to fruition, through times of despondence to confident creativity. She also brought together the ideal team of English-language publishers in the U.S., U.K., and Canada. Much thanks to Megan Newman of Avery, Louise Dennys and Martha Kanya Forstner of Knopf in Toronto, and Joel Rickett of Ebury in London for enthusiastically seeing the possibilities in this work right from the beginning, and for continuing to do so despite some overreaching and trudging down blind alleys by the authors at times. I am grateful, too, for their incisive editing notes throughout and their forbearance as the authors repeatedly lurched from churlishness to appreciation as the truth of their bracing critiques hit home. The reader has much to thank them for. I must also acknowledge Rick Meier, Nina Shield, and Hannah Steigmeyer for their editorial contributions. Of this valiant crew my special thank-you to my dear friend

Louise Dennys, who took on the brunt of guiding the revision of the manuscript during its most crucial phase and with whom I was, on many days, in almost 24/7 communication.

Helping with the research in its crucial early states was the diligent Estella Kuchta, in which regard I must also mention the unfailingly helpful staff at the Library of the College of Physicians and Surgeons of B.C., most particularly Karen Shaw-Karvelson. I owe gratitude as well to Professor Peter Prontzos, who for years steered essential research data in my direction. Katherine Abegg and Jordan Stanger-Ross were kind enough to cast early eyes on the book proposal, sharpening it with their astute reflections.

Laura Kassama of Virtual Squirrel and Elsa DeLuca transcribed hundreds of hours of interviews. Thank you both.

Stephanie Lee, my ever-considerate and efficient manager, kept me grounded as best she could by saying no on my behalf, organizing my many activities, and protecting time to work on this book.

For my acknowledgment of the indispensable collaboration of my co-writer Daniel, please see the Author's Note at the beginning of this volume. What is not described there is the sheer pleasure of working with my son on this, the first of two books we have contracted to write together. The next one, *Hello Again: A Fresh Start for Adult Children and Their Parents*, will be even more of a partnership, one I look forward to.

Finally, I return to the person to whom this work is dedicated: my wife, Rae, who, well beyond moral and emotional support through thick and thin—and often the stress was thick while the confidence was thin—provided, through many hours and through many repeated iterations of each chapter, much-needed critique and the most honest feedback, not always graciously received but eventually, almost always heeded. Much to the reader's benefit.

Gratitude to all.

Gabor Maté

DANIEL THANKS: Mom, Aaron, and Hannah, for thinking I could do it and insisting I should—I'm as lucky a son and sibling as they come; Laurie Liss, for your solidarity and sagacity from the first to the last; Eric Adams, Stan Byrne, Jeremy Gruman, Anna Guest, Katie Halper, Michael R. Jackson, Dashaun Justice Simmons, and Jordan and Ilana Stanger-Ross and family, for loving friendship and encouragement under every imaginable circumstance and some unimaginable ones; my brilliant musical theater collaborators—especially but not limited to Will Aronson, Victoria Clark, Max Friedman, Hannah Kohl, Fred Lassen, Kent Nicholson, and Marshall Pailet—for teaching me everything I know about playing nice with others (now let's get these dang musicals made, dang it!); my theater agent Sarah Douglas for believing in my voice all these years; Scott Kouri, for hearing me better than I ever could. Much appreciation as well to a couple of supremely incisive cultural commentators, Stephen Jenkinson and Matt Christman, whose eloquent irreverence in speaking faithfully to the moment's many madnesses was both a balm during the plague times and an invigorating invitation to clearer thought and bolder delivery.

Special thanks to all those I met at Estación Migratoria Las Ajugas in Mexico City. The kindness and fortitude of these men—hailing from Cuba, Ecuador, Haiti, Uganda, Venezuela, and throughout the "Global South"—got me through an unexpected, COVID-extended stay in summer 2021 that forever reconfigured my sense of normal. I also owe a huge debt of thanks to my heroes and angels "on the outside," including: Roberto Banchik at Penguin Random House México; Louise Dennys at Knopf Canada; John Ralston Saul; and Jorge Kanahuati and Katherine Abegg, most especially.

Kat, beyond those harrowing few weeks, I can't express how much your insight, companionship, allegiance, and unsparing truthfulness have meant to me throughout this book's long lifespan, and nourished what ended up on these pages. Thank you.

Finally, thanks to Dad: for inviting me to play with you, for sticking with it through the more-than-occasional bump, and for trusting me with your magnum-est opus yet while giving me space to contribute to your contribution to the world. It's been the opportunity of my lifetime to finally get to put words in your mouth, and a true joy besides. Proud of you, Pop.

Notes

Introduction

1. Respectively, *Scattered Minds: The Origins and Healing of Attention Deficit Disorder*; *When the Body Says No: The Cost of Hidden Stress*; *In the Realm of Hungry Ghosts: Close Encounters with Addiction*; and, with Dr. Gordon Neufeld, *Hold On to Your Kids: Why Parents Need to Matter More Than Peers*. These are the Canadian and U.K. titles. In the U.S. the ADD book is titled *Scattered: How Attention Deficit Disorder Originates and What You Can Do About It*, and *When the Body Says No* is subtitled *Exploring the Stress-Disease Connection*.

2. Morris Berman, *The Twilight of American Culture* (New York: W. W. Norton, 2001), 64–65.

3. Thom Hartmann, *The Last Hours of Ancient Sunlight: The Fate of the World and What We Can Do About It Before It's Too Late* (New York: Three Rivers Press, 2000), 164.

4. Christine Buttorff et al., *Multiple Chronic Conditions in the United States* (Santa Monica, CA: RAND Corporation, 2017).

5. "Nearly 7 in 10 Americans Take Prescription Drugs, Mayo Clinic, Olmsted Medical Center Find," Mayo Clinic, news release, June 19, 2013, https://newsnetwork.mayoclinic.org/discussion/nearly-7-in-10-americans-take-prescription-drugs-mayo-clinic-olmsted-medical-center-find/.

6. Carly Weeks, "Up to Half of Baby Boomers Will Have High Blood Pressure Soon, Report Warns," *Globe and Mail*, April 3, 2013.

7. Alvaro Alonso and Miguel Hernán, "Temporal Trends in the Incidence of Multiple Sclerosis: A Systematic Review," *Neurology* 71, no. 2 (July 8, 2008), doi: 10.1212/01.wnl.0000316802.35974.34.

8. Calum MacLeod, "Obesity of China's Kids Stuns Officials," *USA Today*, January 9, 2007, https://usatoday30.usatoday.com/news/world/2007-01-08-chinese-obesity_x.htm.

9. "Mental Health by the Numbers," National Alliance on Mental Illness, https://www.nami.org/mhstats.

10. "The Size and Burden of Mental Disorders in Europe," ScienceDaily, September 6, 2011, https://www.sciencedaily.com/releases/2011 /09/110905074609.htm. Source: European College of Neuropsycho-pharmacology.

11. Brett Burstein et al., "Suicidal Attempts and Ideation Among Children and Adolescents in US Emergency Departments, 2007–2015," *JAMA Pediatrics* 173, no. 6 (April 2019): 598–600, https://doi.org/10.1001 /jamapediatrics.2019.0464, cited in Carly Cassella, "Child Suicide Attempts Are Skyrocketing in the US, and Nobody Knows Why," ScienceAlert, April 11, 2019, https://www.sciencealert.com/us-children-are -facing-a-mental-health-crisis-as-suicidal-ideations-climb.

12. Samira Shackle, " 'The Way the Universities Are Run Is Making Us Ill': Inside the Student Mental Health Crisis," *Guardian*, September 27, 2019.

13. Hui Cao et al., "Prevalence of Attention-Deficit/Hyperactivity Disorder Symptoms and Their Associations with Sleep Schedules and Sleep-Related Problems Among Preschoolers in Mainland China," *BMC Pediatrics* 18, no. 1 (February 19, 2018): 70.

14. Caroline Hickman et al., "Young People's Voices on Climate Anxiety, Government Betrayal and Moral Injury: A Global Phenomenon," preprint submitted to the *Lancet*, September 2021, https://papers.ssrn .com/sol3/papers.cfm?abstract_id=3918955.

15. "CDC Continues to Support the Global Polio Eradication Effort," Centers for Disease Control and Prevention, March 18, 2016, https://www.cdc .gov/polio/updates/?s_cid=cs_404.

Chapter 1: The Last Place You Want to Be

1. As summarized by Dr. Bessel van der Kolk in his foreword to Peter Levine, *Trauma and Memory: Brain and Body in a Search for the Living Past* (Berkeley, CA: North Atlantic Books, 2015), xi.

2. Levine, *Trauma and Memory*, xx.

3. John Bowlby, *Separation: Anxiety and Anger* (New York: Basic Books, 1973), 12.

4. Bessel van der Kolk, *The Body Keeps the Score: Brain, Mind, and Body in the Healing of Trauma* (New York: Penguin, 2014), 43.

5. Levine, *Trauma and Memory*, xxii.

6. Peter Levine, *Healing Trauma Study Guide* (Boulder, CO: Sounds True, 1999), 5.

7. Clyde Hertzman and Tom Boyce, "How Experience Gets Under the Skin to Create Gradients in Developmental Health," *Annual Review of Public Health* 31 (April 21, 2010): 329–47.

8. Mark Epstein, *The Trauma of Everyday Life* (New York: Penguin, 2013), 17.

9. Levine, *Healing Trauma Study Guide*, 7.

10. Levine, *Healing Trauma Study Guide*, 7.

11. Tara Westover, *Educated: A Memoir* (New York: HarperCollins, 2018), 111.

12. Rollo May, *The Courage to Create* (New York: W. W. Norton, 1975), 100.

13. Gershen Kaufman, *Shame: The Power of Caring* (Rochester, VT: Schenkman Books, 1980), 20.

14. Elizabeth Wurtzel, "Elizabeth Wurtzel Confronts Her One-Night Stand of a Life," *New York*, January 6, 2013.

15. *Dhammapada: The Sayings of the Buddha*, trans. Thomas Cleary (New York: Bantam Books, 1995), 7.

16. Eva Hoffman, *Time* (London: Profile Books, 2009), 7–8.

Chapter 2: Living in an Immaterial World

1. Candace Pert, *Molecules of Emotion: Why You Feel the Way You Feel* (New York: Touchstone, 1997), 30.

2. M. Wirsching et al., "Psychological Identification of Breast Cancer Patients Before Biopsy," *Journal of Psychosomatic Research* 26, no. 1 (1982): 1–10.

3. S. Greer and T. Morris, "Psychological Attributes of Women Who Develop Breast Cancer: A Controlled Study," *Journal of Psychosomatic Research* 19, no. 2 (April 1975): 147–53.

4. Sandra P. Thomas et al., "Anger and Cancer: An Analysis of the Linkages," *Cancer Nursing* 23, no. 5 (November 2000): 344–48.

5. A. J. Wilbourn and H. Mitsumoto, "Why Are Patients with ALS So Nice," presented at the ninth International ALS Symposium on ALS/MND, Munich, 1998.

6. Theresa Mehl, Berit Jordan, and Stephan Zierz, " 'Patients with Amyotrophic Lateral Sclerosis (ALS) Are Usually Nice Persons'—How Physicians Experienced in ALS See the Personality Characteristics of Their Patients," *Brain Behavior* 7, no. 1 (January 2017).

7. Frank J. Penedo et al., "Anger Suppression Mediates the Relationship Between Optimism and Natural Killer Cell Cytotoxicity in Men Treated for Localized Prostate Cancer," *Journal of Psychosomatic Research* 60, no. 4 (April 2006): 423–27.

8. Edna Maria Vissoci Reiche, Sandra Odebrecht Vargas Nunes, and Helena Kaminami Morimoto, "Stress, Depression, the Immune System, and Cancer," *Lancet Oncology* 5, no. 10 (October 2004): 617–25. The authors write: "These notions could explain the increased occurrence of lymphatic and hematological malignant diseases, and of melanomas seen in a cohort of 6,284 Jewish Israelis who lost an adult son. The incidence of cancer was increased in the parents of accident victims and in war-bereaved parents, compared with that in non-bereaved members of the population. Accident-bereaved parents also had an increased risk of respiratory cancer."

9. J. Li et al., "The Risk of Multiple Sclerosis in Bereaved Parents: A Nationwide Cohort Study in Denmark," *Neurology* 62, no. 5 (March 9, 2004: 726–29.

10. A. Roberts et al., "PTSD Is Associated with Increased Risk of Ovarian Cancer: A Prospective and Retrospective Longitudinal Cohort Study," *Cancer Research* 79, no. 19 (October 1, 2019): 5113–120. September 5, 2019, https://doi.org/10.1158/0008-5472.CAN-19-1222.

11. Premal H. Thekar et al., "Chronic Stress Promotes Tumor Growth and Angiogenesis in a Mouse Model of Ovarian Carcinoma," *Nature Medicine* 12, no. 8 (August 12, 2006): 939–44; published online July 23, 2006, https://doi.org/10.1038/nm1447.

12. Saskia L. Mol et al., "Symptoms of Post-Traumatic Stress Disorder After Non-Traumatic Events: Evidence from an Open Population Study," *British Journal of Psychiatry* 286 (June 2005): 494–99.

13. S. Weiss, "The Medical Student Before and After Graduation," *Journal of the American Medical Association* 114 (1940): 1709–18.

14. Dr. Jeff Rediger, medical director at McLean Hospital, Harvard, personal communication.

15. Ahmed Tawakol et al., "Relation Between Resting Amygdalar Activity and Cardiovascular Events: A Longitudinal and Cohort Study," *Lancet* 389, no. 10071 (February 25, 2017): 834–45.

16. N. Slopen et al., "Job Strain, Job Insecurity, and Incident Cardiovascular Disease in the Women's Health Study: Results from a 10-Year Prospective Study," *PLoS ONE* 7, no. 7 (2012): e40512, https://doi.org/10.1371/journal.pone.0040512.

17. Esme Fuller-Thomson et al., "The Link Between Childhood Sexual Abuse and Myocardial Infarction in a Population-Based Study," *Child Abuse and Neglect* 36, no. 9 (September 2012): 656–65, https://doi.org/10.1016/j.chiabu.2012.06.001.

18. D. Baumeister et al., "Childhood Trauma and Adulthood Inflammation: A Meta-Analysis of Peripheral C-Reactive Protein, Interleukin-6 and Tumor Necrosis Factor-α," *Molecular Psychiatry* 21, no. 5 (May 2016): 642–49.

Chapter 3: You Rattle My Brain

1. George L. Engel, "The Clinical Application of the Biopsychosocial Model," *American Journal of Psychology* 137, no. 5 (May 1980): 535–44.

2. George L. Engel, "The Need for a New Medical Model: A Challenge for Biomedicine," *Science* 196, no. 4286 (April 8, 1977): 129–36.

3. Bessel van der Kolk, *The Body Keeps the Score: Brain, Mind, and Body in the Healing of Trauma* (New York: Penguin, 2014), 80.

4. Richard Grant, "Do Trees Talk to Each Other?," *Smithsonian*, March 2018, https://www.smithsonianmag.com/science-nature/the-whispering-trees-180968084.

5. Daniel Siegel, *Pocket Guide to Interpersonal Neurobiology: An Integrative Handbook of the Mind* (New York: W. W. Norton, 2012), xviii.

6. N. J. Johnson et al., "Marital Status and Mortality: The National Longitudinal Mortality Study," *Annals of Epidemiology* 10, no. 4 (May 2000): 224–38.

7. J. C. Coyne and A. DeLongis, "Going Beyond Social Support: The Role of Social Relationships in Adaptation," *Journal of Consulting and Clinical Psychology* 54, no. 4 (August 1986): 454–60, cited in T. E. Robles and J. K. Kiecolt-Glaser, "The Physiology of Marriage: Pathways to Health," *Physiology and Behavior* 79, no. 3 (August 2003): 409–16.

8. "There's quite a bit of research linking relationship conflict to different types of physiological responses, such as increased release of stress hormones, inflammation, changes in appetite regulation, and immune functioning," said Veronica Lamarche, a professor of social psychology at the University of Essex. "A Bad Marriage Can Seriously Damage Your Health, Say Scientists," *Guardian*, July 16, 2018, https://www.theguardian.com/lifeandstyle/2018/jul/16/a-bad-marriage-is-as-unhealthy-as-smoking-or-drinking-say-scientists.

9. J. M. Gottman and L. F. Katz, "Effects of Marital Discord on Young Children's Peer Interaction and Health," *Developmental Psychology* 25, no. 3 (1989): 373–81.

10. Constance M. Weil and Shari L. Wade, "The Relationship Between Psychosocial Factors and Asthma Morbidity in Inner City Children with Asthma," *Pediatrics* 104, no. 6 (December 1999): 1274–80.

11. N. Yamamoto and J. Nagano, "Parental Stress and the Onset and Course of Childhood Asthma," *BioPsychoSocial Medicine* 9, no. 7 (March 2015), https://doi.org/10.1186/s13030-015-0034-4.

12. P. F. Coogan et al., "Experiences of Racism and the Incidence of Adult-Onset Asthma in the Black Women's Health Study," *CHEST Journal* 145, no. 3 (March 2014): 480–85.

13. T. E. Seeman and B. S. McEwen, "Impact of Social Environment Characteristics on Neuroendocrine Regulation," *Psychosomatic Medicine* 58, no. 5 (September–October 1996): 459–71.

14. A. Hughes et al., "Elevated Inflammatory Biomarkers During Unemployment: Modification by Age and Country in the UK," *Epidemiology and Community Health* 69, no. 7 (July 2015): 673–79, https://doi.org/10.1136/jech-2014-204404.

15. P. Butterworth et al., "The Psychosocial Quality of Work Determines Whether Employment Has Benefits for Mental Health: Results from a Longitudinal National Household Panel Survey," *Occupational and Environmental Medicine* 68, no. 11 (November 2011): 806–12, https://doi.org/10.1136/oem.2010.059030.

16. J. Holt-Lunstad et al., "Social Relationships and Mortality Risk: A Meta-analytic Review," *PLoS Medicine* 7, no. 7 (July 27, 2010), https://doi.org/10.1371/journal.pmed.1000316.

17. Thich Nhat Hanh, *Buddha Mind, Buddha Body* (Berkeley, CA: Parallax Press, 2007), 25.

Chapter 4: Everything I'm Surrounded By

1.   As an editorial in the journal *Nature* acknowledged in 2010, "For all the intellectual ferment of the past decade, has human health truly benefited from the sequencing of the human genome? A startlingly honest response can be found [in the publication's current issue], where the leaders of the public and private efforts, Francis Collins and Craig Venter [American geneticist and physician who captained the Human Genome Project and director of the National Institutes of Health and leading biochemist and entrepreneur, respectively], both say 'not much.'" "Has the revolution arrived?" *Nature* 464 (March 31, 2010): 674–75.

2.   Martha Henriques, "Can the Legacy of Trauma Be Passed Down the Generations?" *BBC Future*, March 26, 2019, https://www.bbc.com/future/article/20190326-what-is-epigenetics.

3.   Moshe Szyf et al., "Maternal Programming of Steroid Receptor Expression and Phenotype Through DNA Methylation in the Rat," *Frontiers in Neuroendocrinology* 26, nos. 3–4 (October–December 2005): 139–62.

4.   Frances A. Champagne et al., "Maternal Care Associated with Methylation of the Estrogen Receptor-1b Promoter and Estrogen Receptor-Alpha Expression in the Medial Preoptic Area of Female Offspring," *Endocrinology* 147, no. 6 (June 2006): 2909–15.

5.   Lei Cao-Lei et al., "DNA Methylation Signatures Triggered by Prenatal Maternal Stress Exposure to a Natural Disaster: Project Ice Storm," *PLoS ONE* 9, no. 9 (September 19, 2014), https://doi.org/10.1371/journal.pone.0107653.

6.   Wendy Leung, "Pregnancy Stress During 1998 Ice Storm Linked to Genetic Changes in Children After Birth, Study Suggests," *Globe and Mail*, September 30, 2014.

7.   Ali B. Rodgers et al., "Paternal Stress Exposure Alters Sperm MicroRNA Content and Reprograms Offspring HPA Stress Axis Regulation," *Journal of Neuroscience* 33, no. 21 (May 2013): 9003–12.

8.   Marilyn J. Essex et al., "Epigenetic Vestiges of Developmental Adversity: Childhood Stress Exposure and DNA Methylation in Adolescence," *Childhood Development* 84, no. 1 (January 2013): 58–57.

9. Nada Borghol et al., "Associations with Early-Life Socio-Economic Position in Adult DNA Methylation," *International Journal of Epidemiology* 41, no. 1 (February 2012): 62–74.

10. April D. Thames et al., "Experienced Discrimination and Racial Differences in Leukocyte Gene Expression," *Psychoneuroendocrinology* 106 (August 2019): 277–83.

11. April D. Thames, "Racism Shortens Lives and Hurts Health of Blacks by Promoting Genes That Lead to Inflammation and Illness," The Conversation, October 17, 2019, https://theconversation.com/study -racism-shortens-lives-and-hurts-health-of-blacks-by-promoting-genes -that-lead-to-inflammation-and-illness-122027.

12. Kathryn K. Ridout et al., "Physician-Training Stress and Accelerated Cellular Aging," *Biological Psychiatry* 86, no. 9 (November 1, 2019): 725–30.

13. Elissa S. Epel et al., "Accelerated Telomere Shortening in Response to Life Stress," *Proceedings of the National Academy of Sciences* 101, no. 49 (December 7, 2004): 17312–15, https://www.pnas.org/content/101/49 /17312.

14. Amanda K. Damjanovic et al., "Accelerated Telomere Erosion Is Associated with a Declining Immune Function of Caregivers of Alzheimer's Disease Patients," *Journal of Immunology* 179, no. 6 (September 15, 2007): 4249–54.

15. David H. Chae et al., "Discrimination, Racial Bias, and Telomere Length in African-American Men," *American Journal of Preventative Medicine* 46, no. 2 (February 2014): 103–11.

16. Arline T. Geronimus et al., "Do US Black Women Experience Stress-Related Accelerated Biological Aging?," *Human Nature* 21, no. 1 (March 10, 2010): 19–38.

17. Tonya L. Jacobs et al., "Intensive Meditation Training, Immune Cell Telomerase Activity, and Psychological Mediators," *Psychoneuroendocrinology* 36, no. 5 (June 2011): 664–81; Gene H. Brody et al., "Prevention Effects Ameliorate the Prospective Association Between Nonsupportive Parenting and Diminished Telomere Length," *Prevention Science* 16, no. 2 (February 2015): 171–80, https:// doi.org/10.1007/s11121-014-0474-2; and Dean Ornish et al., "Effect of Comprehensive Lifestyle Changes on Telomerase Activity and Telomere Length in Men with Biopsy-Proven Low-Risk Prostate Cancer: 5-Year

Follow-Up of a Descriptive Pilot Study," *Lancet Oncology* 14, no. 11 (October 2013): 1112–20, https://doi.org/10.1016/S1470-2045(13)70366-8.

Chapter 5: Mutiny on the Body

1. Karen Crouse, "Venus Williams Says She Struggled with Fatigue for Years," *New York Times,* September 1, 2011.

2. "Autoimmune Disease Rates Increasing," Medical News Today, https://www.medicalnewstoday.com/articles/246960.php; Jean-Francois Bach, "Why Is the Incidence of Autoimmune Diseases Increasing in the Modern World?," *Endocrine Abstracts* 16, S3.1 (2008).

3. Moises Velasquez-Manoff, "Educate Your Immune System," *New York Times,* June 3, 2016.

4. Sarah Knapton, "Crohn's Disease in Teens Jumps 300 Percent in 10 Years Fuelled by Junk Food," *The Telegraph,* June 18, 2014.

5. Eric I. Benchimol et al., "Trends in Epidemiology of Pediatric Inflammatory Bowel Disease in Canada: Distributed Network Analysis of Multiple Population-Based Provincial Health Administrative Databases," *American Journal of Gastroenterology* 112, no. 7 (July 2017): 1120–34, https://doi.org/10.1038/AJG.2017.97.

6. Grace Rattue, "Autoimmune Disease Rates Increasing," *Medical News Today,* June 22, 2012, https://www.medicalnewstoday.com/articles/246960.php.

7. Robin McKie, "Global Spread of Autoimmune Disease Blamed on Western Diet," *The Guardian,* January 9, 2022.

8. Arndt Manzel et al., "Role of 'Western Diet' in Inflammatory Autoimmune Disease," *Current Allergy and Asthma Reports* 14, no. 1 (January 2014): 404, doi: 10.1007/s11882-013-0404-6. ("The association between diet and the risk of developing inflammatory autoimmune diseases was proposed as early as 50 years ago . . . no definite associations between dietary factors and autoimmune diseases have so far been firmly established.")

9. In this condition not all the facts are unfavorable toward women; in men the same condition tends to be more severe and more likely to be fatal. Christine Peoples, "Gender Differences in Systemic Sclerosis: Relationship to Clinical Features, Serologic Status and Outcomes," *Journal of Scleroderma and Related Disorders* 1, no. 2 (May–August 2016): 177–240.

10. Sarah-Michelle Orton et al., "Effect of Immigration on Multiple Sclerosis Sex Ratio in Canada: The Canadian Collaborative Study," *Journal of Neurology, Neurosurgery and Psychiatry* 81, no. 1 (January 2010): 31–36.

11. Melinda Magyari, "Gender Differences in Multiple Sclerosis Epidemiology and Treatment Response," *Danish Medical Journal* 63, no. 3 (March 2016).

12. Paul H. Black, "Stress and the Inflammatory Response: A Review of Neurogenic Inflammation," *Brain, Behavior, and Immunity* 16, no. 6 (December 2002): 622–53.

13. C. H. Feldman et al., "Association of Childhood Abuse with Incident Systemic Lupus Erythematosus in Adulthood in a Longitudinal Cohort of Women," *Journal of Rheumatology* 46, no. 12 (December 2019): 1589–96.

14. R. Coelho et al., "Childhood Maltreatment and Inflammatory Markers: A Systematic Review," *Acta Psychiatrica Scandinavica* 129, no. 3 (March 2014): 180–92; Huang Song et al., "Association of Stress-Related Disorders with Subsequent Autoimmune Disease," *Journal of the American Medical Association* 319, no. 23 (June 19, 2018): 2388–400.

15. Andrea Danese et al., "Childhood Maltreatment Predicts Adult Inflammation in a Life-Course Study," *Proceedings of the National Academy of Sciences of the United States of America* 104, no. 4 (January 23, 2007): 1319–24.

16. George F. Solomon and Rudolf H. Moos, "The Relationship of Personality to the Presence of Rheumatoid Factor in Asymptomatic Relatives of Patients with Rheumatoid Arthritis," *Psychosomatic Medicine* 27, no. 4 (July 1965): 350–60.

17. C. E. G. Robinson, "Emotional Factors and Rheumatoid Arthritis," *Canadian Medical Association Journal* 77, no. 4 (August 15, 1957): 344–45.

18. Alex J. Zautra et al., "Examination of Changes in Interpersonal Stress as a Factor in Disease Exacerbations Among Women with Rheumatoid Arthritis," *Annals of Behavioral Medicine* 19, no. 3 (Summer 1997): 279–86.

19. G. S. Philippopoulos et al., "The Etiologic Significance of Emotional Factors in Onset and Exacerbations of Multiple Sclerosis," *Psychosomatic Medicine* 20, no. 6 (November 1958): 458–73.

20. Varda Mei-Tal et al., "The Role of Psychological Process in a Somatic Disorder: Multiple Sclerosis," *Psychosomatic Medicine* 32, no. 1 (January–February 1970): 67–85.

21. Gary M. Franklin et al., "Stress and Its Relationship to Acute Exacerbations in Multiple Sclerosis," *Journal of Neurologic Rehabilitation* 2, no. 1 (March 1, 1988): 7–11.

22. L. Briones et al., "The Influence of Stress and Psychosocial Factors in Multiple Sclerosis: A Review," conference paper, in *Psychotherapy and Psychosomatics* 82, suppl. 1 (September 2013): 1–134.

23. "In the last half-century, the prevalence of autoimmune disease . . . has increased sharply in the developed world," reported Moises Velasquez-Manoff in "Educate Your Immune System" (*New York Times*, June 5, 2016). "Many, like Type 1 diabetes and celiac disease, are linked with specific gene variants of the immune system, suggesting a strong genetic component. But their prevalence has increased much faster—in two or three generations—than it's likely the human gene pool has changed."

    Many theories have been advanced for the sharp rise in autoimmune cases, including the so-named hygiene hypothesis. According to this notion, industrialization and prosperity have led to lifestyles that prevent human beings from being exposed to microorganisms that would have trained our immune systems to be hardier, more resilient. "The implication is that, by delaying exposure to once-common infections, improvements in societal hygiene may increase the prevalence of autoimmune diseases." Velasquez-Manoff, "Educate Your Immune System." For all we know, there may be some truth to that view—but surely it cannot explain the dramatic rise over a few decades: Has the hygienic state of Danish women, for example, really changed that much in the past quarter century?

24. Huang Song et al., "Association of Stress-Related Disorders with Subsequent Autoimmune Disease," *Journal of the American Medical Association* 319, no. 23 (June 19, 2018): 2388–400.

25. Idam Harpaz et al., "Chronic Exposure to Stress Predisposes to Higher Autoimmune Susceptibility in C57BL/6 Mice: Glucocorticoids as a Double-Edged Sword," *European Journal of Immunology* 43, no. 3 (March 2013): 258–769.

26. Deborah Talbot, "What's It Like Living with Lupus," Elemental, July 13, 2018, https://elemental.medium.com/what-its-like-living-with-lupus -8doc2efcbe5e.

Chapter 6: It Ain't a Thing

1. Except for some specific malignancies, no major breakthroughs have been made in cure or prevention. Little has changed since Gina Kolata reported in 2009 that in over half a century, cancer death rates had "barely budged," falling by only 5 percent between 1950 and 2005. The major improvements were the results of smoking cessation, not medical advances as such. Gina Kolata, "Advances Elusive in the Drive to Cure Cancer," *New York Times*, April 21, 2009.

2. Gabor Maté, *When the Body Says No: The Cost of Hidden Stress* (Toronto: Knopf Canada, 2003; published in the United States with the subtitle *Exploring the Stress-Disease Connection*), chapter 18.

3. Michelle Kelly-Irving et al., "Childhood Adversity as a Risk for Cancer: Findings from the 1958 British Birth Cohort Study," *BMC Public Health* 13, no. 1 (August 19, 2013): 767, https://bmcpublichealth .biomedcentral.com/articles/10.1186/1471-2458-13-767.

4. Holly R. Harris et al., "Early Life Abuse and Risk of Endometriosis," *Human Reproduction* 3, no. 9 (September 2018): 1657–68.

5. M. Watson et al., "Influence of Psychological Response on Breast Cancer Survival: 10-Year Follow-Up of a Population-Based Cohort," *European Journal of Cancer* 41, no. 12 (August 2005): 1710–14.

6. Janine Giese-Davis et. al., "Decrease in Depression Symptoms Is Associated with Longer Survival in Patients with Metastatic Breast Cancer," *Journal of Clinical Oncology* 29, no. 4 (February 1, 2011): 413–20.

7. This cervical cancer study is cited in Jane G. Goldberg, ed., *Psychotherapeutic Treatment of Cancer Patients* (New York: Routledge, 1990), 45.

8. Frank J. Penedo et al., "Anger Suppression Mediates the Relationship Between Optimism and Natural Killer Cell Cytotoxicity in Men Treated for Localized Prostate Cancer," *Journal of Psychosomatic Research* 60, no. 4 (April 2006): 423–27.

9. Ann L. Coker et al., "Stress, Coping, Social Support, and Prostate Cancer Risk Among Older African American and Caucasian Men," *Ethnicity and Disease* 16, no. 4 (Autumn 2006): 978–87.

10. Meghan O'Rourke, "What's Wrong with Me?" *New Yorker*, August 19, 2013.

11. Paige Green McDonald et al., "A Biobehavioral Perspective of Tumor Biology," *Discovery Medicine* 5, no. 30 (December 2005): 520–26.

12. David Smithers, "Cancer: An Attack on Cytologism," *Lancet* 279, no. 7228 (March 10, 1962): 493–99.

Chapter 7: A Traumatic Tension

1. Susan Sontag, *Illness as Metaphor and AIDS and Its Metaphors* (New York: Picador, 2001), 55. The essay originally appeared in the *New York Review of Books* in 1978.

2. Jonathon Cott, *Susan Sontag: The Complete Rolling Stone Interview* (New Haven: Yale University Press, 2013). The original interview was published October 1979.

3. Marcia Angell, "Disease as a Reflection of the Psyche," *New England Journal of Medicine* 312 (June 13, 1985): 1570–72.

4. "From Irritated to Enraged: Anger's Toxic Effect on the Heart," Harvard Heart Health, December 6, 2014, https://www.health.harvard.edu/heart -health/from-irritated-to-enraged-angers-toxic-effect-on-the-heart.

5. Geoffrey H. Tofler et al., "Triggering of Acute Coronary Occlusion by Episodes of Anger," *European Heart Journal: Acute Cardiovascular Care*, February 2015, https://doi.org/10.1177/2048872615568969.

6. "Keep Calm, Anger Can Trigger a Heart Attack!," ScienceDaily, February 24, 2015, https://www.sciencedaily.com/releases/2015/02 /150224083819.htm.

7. I cite this verbatim from a first-person account of her breast cancer diagnosis by a Montreal woman, published in the *Globe and Mail*. I no longer have the date of the article, which appeared sometime between 2004 and 2007. It's exactly the dynamic noted by Lydia Temoshok.

8. Andrew W. Kneier and Lydia Temoshok, "Repressive Coping Reactions in Patients with Malignant Melanoma as Compared to Cardiovascular Disease Patients," *Journal of Psychosomatic Research* 28, no. 2 (1984): 145–55, https://doi.org/10.1016/0022-3999(84)90008-4.

9. James J. Gross and Robert W. Levenson, "Emotional Suppression: Physiology, Self-Report, and Expressive Behavior," *Journal of Personality and Social Psychology* 64, no. 6 (June 1993): 970–86.

10. Lydia Temoshok, Letter to the Editor, *New York Times*, September 6, 1992.

11. Susan Sontag, *As Consciousness Is Harnessed to Flesh: Journals and Notebooks, 1964–1980*, ed. David Rieff (Farrar, Straus and Giroux, 2012), 313.

Chapter 8: Who Are We Really?

1. Alfie Kohn, *No Contest: The Case Against Competition*, rev. ed. (Boston: Houghton Mifflin, 1992), 13.

2. Marshall Sahlins, *The Western Illusion of Human Nature* (Chicago: Prickly Paradigm Press, 2008), cited by Darcia Narvaez in "Are We Losing It? Darwin's Moral Sense and the Importance of Early Experience," in *The Routledge Handbook of Evolution and Philosophy*, ed. Richard Joyce (New York: Routledge, 2017), 328.

3. Jack D. Forbes, *Columbus and Other Cannibals: The Wétiko Disease of Exploitation, Imperialism, and Terrorism* (New York: Seven Stories Press, 1992), 49.

4. François Ansermet and Pierre Magistretti, *Biology of Freedom: Neural Plasticity, Experience, and the Unconscious*, trans. Susan Fairfield (New York: Other Press, 2007), 8.

5. Jean Liedloff, *The Continuum Concept: In Search of Happiness Lost*, rev. ed. (1985; Boston: Da Capo Press, 1975), 24.

6. "Probably all humans lived in such bands until at least a few tens of thousands of years ago, and probably most still did as recently as 11,000 years ago." Jared Diamond, *The World Until Yesterday: What We Can Learn from Traditional Societies* (New York: Penguin Books, 2012), 14.

7. Frans de Waal, *The Age of Empathy: Nature's Lessons for a Kinder Society* (New York: Broadway Books, 2010), 25.

Chapter 9: A Sturdy or Fragile Foundation

1. Cavoukian has worked with some of the world's leading developmental experts to create the Raffi Foundation for Child Honouring. Officially, the foundation may have been Raffi's first foray into advocacy, but it was far from the first time he had contemplated what children require and deserve, as his famous 1980 song about the need for love in a family illustrates.

2. Antonio R. Damasio, *Descartes' Error: Emotion, Reason and the Human Brain* (New York: G. P. Putnam's Sons, 1994), 128.

3. Jean Liedloff, *The Continuum Concept: In Search of Happiness Lost*, rev. ed. (1985; Boston: Da Capo Press, 1975), 37.

4. Jack P. Shonkoff et al., "An Integrated Scientific Framework for Child Survival and Early Childhood Development," *Pediatrics* 129, no. 2 (February 2012): 1–13.

5. The seminal psychologist and researcher Allan Schore writes: "The mother is implicitly shaping her infant's unconscious mind, which as Freud observed develops before the conscious mind"; and "the essential adaptive right-brain functions of interdependence, social connection, and emotion regulation emerge out of early attachment experience." Allan Schore, *The Development of the Unconscious Mind* (New York: W. W. Norton, 2019), 33, 57.

6. Stanley I. Greenspan and Stuart Shankar, with Beryl I. Benderly, "The Emotional Architecture of the Mind," in Raffi Cavoukian et al., *Child Honouring: How to Turn This World Around* (Homeland Press, 2006), 5.

7. Gordon Neufeld, "The Keys to Well-Being in Children and Youth: The Significant Role of Families," keynote address, delivered at the European Parliament, Brussels, November 13, 2012, https://neufeldinstitute.org /wp-content/uploads/2017/12/Neufeld_Brussels_address.pdf.

8. Maia Szalavitz and Bruce D. Perry, *Born for Love: Why Empathy Is Essential—and Endangered* (New York: William Morrow, 2011), 5.

9. J. Maselko et al., "Mother's Affection at 8 Months Predicts Emotional Distress in Adulthood," *Journal of Epidemiology and Community Health* 65, no. 7 (2011): 621–25.

10. Jordan Peterson, *12 Rules for Living: An Antidote to Chaos* (Toronto: Random House Canada, 2018), 141.

11. Jaak Panksepp and Lucy Biven, *The Archaeology of Mind: Neuroevolutionary Origins of Human Emotions* (New York: W. W. Norton, 2012), 386.

Chapter 10: Trouble at the Threshold

1. Thomas Verny, *Pre-Parenting* (New York: Simon and Schuster, 2003), 159–60.

2. In the 2011 documentary *Zeitgeist III: Moving Forward*, directed by Peter Joseph.

3. In the 2016 documentary *In Utero*, directed by Kathleen Man Gyllenhaal, https://www.inuterofilm.com/stephen_gyllenhaal.

4. Laurie Tarkian, "Tracking Stress and Depression Back to the Womb," *New York Times*, December 4, 2004.

5. Catherine Lebel et al., "Prepartum and Postpartum Maternal Depressive Symptoms Are Related to Children's Brain Structure in Preschool," *Biological Psychiatry* 80, no. 11 (December 1, 2016): 859–68.

6. Claudia Buss et al., "High Pregnancy Anxiety During Mid-Gestation Is Associated with Decreased Gray Matter Density in 6–9-Year-Old Children," *Psychoneuroimmunology* 35, no. 1 (January 2010): 141–53.

7. D. Kinney et al., "Prenatal Stress and Risk for Autism," *Neuroscience and Biobehavioral Reviews* 32, no. 8 (October 2008): 1519–32.

8. Sonja Entringer et al., "Fetal Programming of Body Composition, Obesity, and Metabolic Function: The Role of Intrauterine Stress and Stress Biology," *Journal of Nutrition and Metabolism* 2012: 632548; published online May 10, 2012, https://doi.org/10.1155/2012/632548.

9. Sonja Entringer et al., "Prenatal Stress, Development, Health and Disease Risk: A Psychobiological Perspective," *Psychoneuroendocrinology* 62 (December 2015): 366–75.

10. Sonja Entringer et al., "Stress Exposure in Intrauterine Life Is Associated with Shorter Telomere Length in Young Adulthood," *Proceedings of the National Academy of Sciences* 108, no. 33 (August 16, 2011).

11. Jill M. Goldstein, "Impact of Prenatal Maternal Cytokine Exposure on Sex Differences in Brain Circuitry Regulating Stress in Offspring 45 Years Later," *Proceedings of the National Academy of Sciences* 118, no. 15 (April 13, 2021), https://doi.org/10.1073/pnas.2014464118.

12. Maartie Zijlman et al., "Maternal Prenatal Stress Is Associated with the Infant Intestinal Microbiota," *Psychoneuroendocrinology* 53 (March 2015): 233–45.

13. C. Liu et al., "Prenatal Parental Depression and Preterm Birth: A National Cohort Study," *BJOG: An International Journal of Obstetrics and Gynecology* 123, no. 12 (November 2016): 1973–82, https://doi.org/10.1111/1471-0528.13891.

14. "Fetal Scans Confirm Maternal Stress Affects Babies' Brains,"

MediBulletin Bureau, March 27, 2018, https://medibulletin.com/fetal
-scans-confirm-maternal-stress-affects-babies-brains/.

15. Frederica P. Perera et al., "Prenatal Polycyclic Aromatic Hydrocarbon
(PAH) Exposure and Child Behavior at Age 6–7 Years," *Environmental
Health Perspectives* 120, no. 6 (June 1, 2012): 921–26.

16. Jane E. Allen, "Prenatal Pollutants Linked to Later Behavioral Ills,"
ABC News, March 12, 2012, https://abcnews.go.com/Health/w
_ParentingResource/prenatal-pollutants-linked-childhood-anxiety-adhd
/story?id=15974554.

17. Of course, environmental pollution affects virtually everyone, through
chemicals in our food and daily environment whose effects have not
been adequately investigated, if at all. What news we do have is far from
reassuring, as a large number of potentially harmful chemicals have
been identified in the umbilical cord blood samples in both Canada and
the United States, as in Europe and Asia. Moreover, in a sane society, it
would not be up to underfunded researchers to prove that some chemical
is harmful to fetus, child, and adolescent—it would be up to those who
introduce such substances into our air, earth, food supply, and the very
bloodstreams of pregnant women to show that it is not.

18. See, for example, Malidoma Patrice Somé, *Ritual, Magic and Initiation in
the Life of an African Shaman* (New York: G. P. Putnam's Sons, 1994), 20.
See also the documentary *What Babies Want*, https://www.youtube.com
/watch?v=-3mtFRjEVWc.

Chapter 11: What Choice Do I Have?

1. Susan J. McDonald et al., "Effect of Timing of Umbilical Cord
Clamping of Term Infants on Maternal and Neonatal Outcomes,"
Cochrane Database of Systemic Reviews 7 (July 11, 2013), https://doi
.org/10.1002/14651858.CD004074.pub3.

2. Anne Fadiman, *The Spirit Catches You and You Fall Down: A Hmong Child,
Her American Doctors, and the Collision of Two Cultures* (New York: Farrar,
Straus and Giroux, 1997; paperback edition, 2012), 74.

3. See, for example, Michael Klein et al., "Relationship of Episiotomy to
Perineal Trauma and Morbidity, Sexual Dysfunction, and Pelvic Floor
Relaxation," *American Journal of Obstetrics and Gynecology* 171, no. 3
(October 1994): 591–98.

4. Ties Boerma et al., "Global Epidemiology of Use of and Disparities in Caesarean Sections," *Lancet* 392, no. 10155 (October 2018): 1341–48.

5. Boerma, "Global Epidemiology."

6. Obstetric Care Consensus, "Safe Prevention of the Primary Cesarean Delivery," *Obstetrics and Gynecology* 123, no. 3 (March 2014): 693–711.

7. Cited by Suzanne Hope Suarez, "Midwifery Is Not the Practice of Medicine," *Yale Journal of Law and Feminism* 5, no. 2 (1992).

8. Sarah J. Buckley, "Hormonal Physiology of Childbearing: Evidence and Implications for Women, Babies, and Maternity Care," Childbirth Connection Programs, National Partnership for Women and Families, Washington, D.C., January 2015.

9. Ilana Stanger-Ross, *A Is for Advice: The Reassuring Kind* (New York: William Morrow, 2019), 23–24.

10. Buckley, "Hormonal Physiology of Childbearing."

11. World Health Organization, "Evidence Shows Significant Mistreatment of Women During Childbirth," news release, October 9, 2019, https://www.who.int/news/item/09-10-2019-new-evidence-shows-significant-mistreatment-of-women-during-childbirth.

12. Jesse Feith, "Indigenous Woman Records Slurs by Hospital Staff Before Her Death," *Montreal Gazette,* September 30, 2020, https://montrealgazette.com/news/local-news/indigenous-woman-who-died-at-joliette-hospital-had-recorded-staffs-racist-comments.

13. Jean Liedloff, *The Continuum Concept: In Search of Happiness Lost*, rev. ed. (1985; Boston: Da Capo Press, 1975), 58.

Chapter 12: Horticulture on the Moon

1. Emily Oster, "The Data All Guilt-Ridden Parents Need," *New York Times*, April 19, 2019, https://www.nytimes.com/2019/04/19/opinion/sunday/baby-breastfeeding-sleep-training.html (published as "Baby's First Data" in the print edition on April 20, section SR 1).

2. Lloyd deMause, ed., *The History of Childhood: The Untold Story of Child Abuse* (New York: Peter Bedrick Books, 1988), 53.

3. Jordan R. Peterson, *12 Rules for Life: An Antidote to Chaos* (Toronto: Random House Canada, 2018), 144.

4. Ashley Montagu, *Touching: The Human Significance of Skin*, 3rd ed. (New York: Harper and Row, 1986), 296.

5. D. W. Winnicott, *Through Pediatrics to Psycho-Analysis: Collected Papers* (Abingdon, UK: Brunner-Routledge, New York: 1992), 99.

6. Montagu, *Touching*, 42.

7. Adrienne Rich, *Of Woman Born: Motherhood as Experience and Institution* (New York: W. W. Norton, 1995), 31.

8. Lane Strathearn et al., "What's in a Smile? Maternal Brain Responses to Infant Facial Clues," *Pediatrics* 122, no. 1 (July 2008): 40–51.

9. John H. Kennell et al., "Maternal Behavior One Year After Early and Extended Post-Partum Contact," *Developmental Medicine and Child Neurology* 16, no. 2 (April 1974): 172–79.

10. Darcia Narvaez, *Neurobiology and the Development of Human Morality: Evolution, Culture, and Wisdom* (New York: W. W. Norton, 2014), 29–30.

11. Jean Liedloff, *The Continuum Concept: In Search of Happiness Lost*, rev. ed. (1985; Boston: Da Capo Press, 1975), 97.

12. As documented, for example, by Charles C. Mann in his bestselling book *1491: New Revelations of the Americas Before Columbus* (New York: Knopf, 2005).

13. Stacy Schiff, *The Witches: Salem, 1692* (London: Weidenfeld and Nicholson, 2015), 45.

14. Peterson, *12 Rules for Life*, 139.

15. Robert D. Sage and Benjamin S. Siegel, "Effective Discipline to Raise Healthy Children," *Pediatrics* 142, no. 6 (December 2018).

16. Manisha Aggarwal-Schifellite, "How Spanking May Affect Brain Development in Children," *Harvard Gazette*, April 12, 2021, https://news.harvard.edu/gazette/story/2021/04/spanking-children-may-impair-their-brain-development/.

17. "Breastfeeding: Achieving the New Normal," editorial, *Lancet* 387 (January 30, 2016): 404.

18. Craig A. McEwen and Bruce S. McEwen, "Social Structure, Adversity, Toxic Stress, and Intergenerational Poverty: An Early Childhood Model," *Annual Review of Sociology* 43, no. 1 (August 2017): 445–72.

19. Allan Schore, *Affect Regulation and the Origin of the Self: The Neurobiology of Emotional Development* (Mahwah, NJ: Lawrence Erlbaum Associates, 1994), 378.

20. Claire Cain Miller, "The Relentlessness of Modern Parenting," *New York Times*, December 25, 2018, A1.

21. Emily Oster, "Don't Worry, Baby," *New Yorker*, June 3, 2019.

22. Miranda Bryant, " 'I Was Risking My Life': Why One in Four US Women Return to Work Two Weeks After Childbirth," *Guardian*, January 27, 2020.

23. Colin M. Turnbull, *The Forest People* (London: Chatto and Windus, 1961), 113.

24. Darcia Narvaez, "Allomothers: Our Evolved Support Systems for Mothers," *Psychology Today*, May 12, 2019, https://www.psychologytoday .com/ca/blog/moral-landscapes/201905/allomothers-our-evolved -support-system-mothers.

25. NBC News, May 15, 2020.

26. Robert D. Putnam, *Bowling Alone: The Collapse and Revival of the American Community* (New York: Simon and Schuster, 2000), 27.

27. Rich, *Of Woman Born*, 53–54.

Chapter 13: Forcing the Brain in the Wrong Direction

1. James Garbarino, *Raising Children in a Socially Toxic Environment* (San Francisco: Jossey-Bass, 1995), 2.

2. Garbarino, *Raising Children in a Socially Toxic Environment*, 5.

3. Natalie Angier, "Ideas and Trends: The Sandbox; Bully for You—Why Push Comes to Shove," *New York Times*, May 20, 2001.

4. D. Clark, "Frequency of Bullying in European Countries, 2018," Statista, October 7, 2021, https://www.statista.com/statistics/1092217/bullying-in -europe/.

5. Cited in Timothy Singham, "Concurrent and Longitudinal Contribution of Exposure to Bullying in Childhood Mental Health: The Role of

Vulnerability and Resistance," *JAMA Psychiatry*, published online October 4, 2017, https://doi.org/10.1001/jamapsychiatry.2017.2678.

6. Bridgette Watson, "They Killed Him for Entertainment: Carson Crimeni's Father Speaks Out Against Bullying," CBC News, February 26, 2020, https://www.cbc.ca/news/canada/british-columbia/darrel-crimeni -bullying-awareness-1.5477247.

7. Gordon Neufeld, "The Keys to Well-Being in Children and Youth: The Significant Role of Families," keynote address, delivered at the European Parliament, Brussels, November 13, 2012.

8. Joel Bakan, *Childhood Under Siege: How Big Business Targets Children* (New York: Free Press, 2011), 6.

9. Joel Bakan, "Kids and the Corporation," in *Child Honouring: How to Turn This World Around*, ed. Raffi Cavoukian and Sharna Olfman (Salt Spring Island, BC: Homeland Press, 2006), 190.

10. Georgia Wells et al., "Facebook Knows Instagram Is Toxic for Teen Girls, Company Documents Show," *Wall Street Journal*, September 14, 2021, https://www.wsj.com/articles/facebook-knows-instagram-is-toxic-for -teen-girls-company-documents-show-11631620739.

11. Shimi Kang, *The Tech Solution: Creating Healthy Habits for Kids Growing Up in a Digital World* (New York: Viking, 2020), ch. 1.

12. John S. Hutton et al., "Associations Between Screen-Based Media Use and Brain White Matter Integrity in Preschool-Aged Children," *JAMA Pediatrics* 174, no. 1 (2020).

13. Mari Swingle, *i-Minds: How and Why Constant Connectivity Is Rewiring Our Brains and What to Do About It* (New Society, 2019), 11, 185.

14. Allana Akhtar, "The World Health Organization Just Released Screen- Time Guidelines for Kids. Here's How Some of the World's Most Successful CEOs Limit It at Home," *Business Insider*, April 25, 2019, https://www.businessinsider.com/how-silicon-valley-ceos-limit-screen -time-at-home-2019-4.

15. James Garbarino, *Children and Families in the Social Environment* (New York: Routledge, 1992), 11.

16. Jasper Jackson, "Children Spending More Time Online Than Watching TV for the First Time," *Guardian*, January 26, 2012, https://www .theguardian.com/media/2016/jan/26/children-time-online-watching-tv.

17. William Doyle, "Why Finland Has the Best Schools," op-ed, *Los Angeles Times*, March 18, 2016, https://www.latimes.com/opinion/op-ed/la-oe -0318-doyle-finnish-schools-20160318-story.html.

18. Alfie Kohn, *No Contest: The Case Against Competition: Why We Lose in Our Race to Win* (Boston: Houghton Mifflin, 1992), 25.

Chapter 14: A Template for Distress

1. Siddhartha Mukherjee, "Same but Different: How Epigenetics Can Blur the Line Between Nature and Nurture," *New Yorker*, May 2, 2016.

2. Michael E. Kerr and Murray Bowen, *Family Evaluation: An Approach Based on Bowen Theory* (New York: W. W. Norton, 1988), 30.

3. Thomas Merton, *The Seven Storey Mountain: An Autobiography of Faith* (Boston: Mariner Books, 1999), 362.

4. Erich Fromm, *The Sane Society* (New York: Henry Holt, 1955), 79.

5. Aldous Huxley, *Brave New World* (New York: HarperCollins, 2014), 244.

6. Cited in Noelle McAfee, *Julia Kristeva* (New York: Routledge, 2004), 108.

7. Merton, *The Seven Storey Mountain*, 148.

8. Neil Postman, *Amusing Ourselves to Death: Public Discourse in the Age of Show Business*, 20th anniversary ed. (New York: Penguin Books, 2008), 128.

9. Ezra Klein, "Noam Chomsky's Theory of the Good Life," transcript, April 23, 2021, https://www.nytimes.com/2021/04/23/opinion/ezra-klein -podcast-noam-chomsky.html.

Chapter 15: Just Not to Be You

1. "Overdose Death Rates," National Institute on Drug Abuse, https://www .drugabuse.gov/drug-topics/trends-statistics/overdose-death-rates.

2. Roni Caryn Rabin, "Overdose Deaths Reached Record High as the Pandemic Spread," *New York Times*, November 17, 2021, https://www .nytimes.com/2021/11/17/health/drug-overdoses-fentanyl-deaths.html.

3. Nora D. Volkow and T. K. Li, "Drug Addiction: The Neurobiology of Behavior Gone Awry," *Neuroscience* 5 (December 2004): 963–70.

4. F. Zhou et al., "Orbitofrontal Gray Matter Deficits as Marker of Internet Gaming Disorder: Converging Evidence from a Cross-Sectional and

Prospective Longitudinal Design," *Addiction Biology* 24, no. 1 (January 2019): 100–109, https://doi.org/10:1111/adb.12750.

5.   Kyle S. Burger and Eric Stice, "Frequent Ice Cream Consumption Is Associated with Reduced Striatal Response to Receipt of an Ice Cream–Based Milkshake," *American Journal of Clinical Nutrition* 94, no. 4 (April 2012): 810–17, https://doi.org/10.3945/ajcn.111.027003.

6.   "Definition of Addiction," American Society of Addiction Medicine, https://www.asam.org/quality-care/definition-of-addiction.

7.   Keith Richards with James Fox, *Life* (New York: Back Bay Books, 2011), 322.

8.   P. A. Harrison, J. A. Fulkerson, and T. J. Beebe, "Multiple Substance Use Among Adolescent Physical and Sexual Abuse Victims," *Child Abuse and Neglect* 21, no. 6 (June 1997): 529–39.

9.   Hannah Carliner et al., "Childhood Trauma and Illicit Drug Use in Adolescence: A Population-Based National Comorbidity Survey Replication," *Journal of the American Academy of Child and Adolescent Psychiatry* 55, no. 8 (August 2016): 701–8.

Chapter 16: Show of Hands

1.   Vincent J. Felitti et al., "The Relationship of Adult Health Status to Childhood Abuse and Household Dysfunction," *American Journal of Preventive Medicine* 14 (1998): 245–58.

2.   Vincent J. Felitti and Robert Anda, "The Lifelong Effects of Adverse Childhood Experiences," chapter 10, in *Chadwick's Child Maltreatment: Sexual Abuse and Psychological Maltreatment,* vol. 2, 4th ed. (St. Louis, MO: STM Learning, 2014), 207.

3.   Gene H. Brody et al., "Parenting Moderates a Genetic Vulnerability Factor in Longitudinal Increases in Youths' Substance Use," *Journal of Consulting and Clinical Psychology Association* 77, no. 1 (February 2009): 1–11; among other studies, such as, for example, Marcello Solinas et al., "Prevention and Treatment of Drug Addiction by Environmental Enrichment," *Progress in Neurobiology* 92, no. 4 (December 2010): 572–92.

4.   I first cited this statement by Dr. Perry in my book on addiction, *In the Realm of Hungry Ghosts.*

5.   Gail Dines, *Pornland: How Porn Has Hijacked Our Sexuality* (Boston: Beacon Press, 2010), 57.

6. Jaak Panksepp et al., "The Role of Brain Emotional Systems in Addictions: A Neuro-Evolutionary Perspective and New 'Self-Report' Animal Model," *Addiction* 97, no. 4 (May 2002): 459–69.

7. Louis Cozolino, *The Neuroscience of Human Relationships: Attachment and the Developing Social Brain* (New York: W. W. Norton, 2006), 115.

Chapter 17: An Inaccurate Map of Our Pain

1. Kay Redfield Jamison, *Touched with Fire: Manic-Depressive Illness and the Artistic Temperament* (New York: Free Press, 1994), 193.

2. I dispensed fully with this issue of twin and adoption studies in an appendix to my book on addiction. In short, I argue that these ostensibly pristine cases of "different environments, same health problems" are so blind to the environmental factors *contained in their experimental design*— maternal stress during pregnancy and the trauma of separation from birth mother, to cite two obvious examples—as to be invalid, no matter what mental or physical condition we are talking about. A link to that appendix is posted at this book's website, https://drgabormate.com/book/the-myth -of-normal, for the benefit of the curious or unconvinced. The professional reader may further consult the psychologist Jay Joseph's comprehensive work *The Trouble with Twin Studies: A Reassessment of Twin Research in the Social and Behavioral Sciences* (Routledge, 2016).

3. "Because the troubled mind has been perceived in terms of diverse religious, scientific, and social beliefs of discrete cultures, the forms of madness from one place and time in history often look remarkably different from the forms of madness in another," notes Ethan Watters in his book *Crazy Like Us: The Globalization of the American Psyche* (New York: Free Press, 2020), 5.

4. Cited in Robert Whitaker, *Anatomy of an Epidemic: Magic Bullets, Psychiatric Drugs, and the Astonishing Rise of Mental Illness in America* (New York: Broadway Books, 2010), 274.

5. American Psychiatric Association, "Chair of DSM-5 Task Force Discusses Future of Mental Health Research," press release, May 3, 2013.

6. For example, by the psychologist Irvin Kirsch, recently associate director of the program in placebo studies and a lecturer in medicine at the Harvard Medical School. "It now seems beyond question that the traditional account of depression as a chemical imbalance in the brain is

simply wrong," Kirsch wrote in his own extensive review of the scientific literature, *The Emperor's New Drugs: Exploding the Antidepressant Myth*, cited in Marcia Angell, "The Epidemic of Mental Illness: Why?," *New York Review of Books*, June 23, 2011. (Dr. Angell is the former editor of the *New England Journal of Medicine*.)

7. Richard L. Morrow et al., "Influence of Relative Age on Diagnosis and Treatment of Attention-Deficit/Hyperactivity Disorder in Children," *Canadian Medical Association Journal* 184, no. 7 (April 17, 2012): 755–62.

8. "Oppositional Defiant Disorder," Mayo Clinic, https://www.mayoclinic.org/diseases-conditions/oppositional-defiant-disorder/symptoms-causes/syc-20375831.

9. J. E. Khoury et al., "Relations Among Maternal Withdrawal in Infancy, Borderline Features, Suicidality/Self-Injury, and Adult Hippocampal Volume: A 30-Year Longitudinal Study," *Behavioral Brain Research* 374 (November 18, 2019): 112139, https://doi.org/10.1016/j.bbr.2019.112139.

10. John Read et al., "Child Maltreatment and Psychosis: A Return to a Genuinely Integrated Bio-Psycho-Social Model," *Clinical Schizophrenia and Related Psychoses* 2, no. 3 (October 2008): 235–54.

11. Thomas Bailey et al., "Childhood Trauma Is Associated with Severity of Hallucinations and Delusions in Psychotic Disorders: A Systematic Review and Meta-Analysis," *Schizophrenia Bulletin* 44, no. 5 (2018): 1111–22.

12. Richard Bentall, "Mental Illness Is a Result of Misery, Yet Still We Stigmatize It," *Guardian*, February 26, 2016.

13. Martin H. Teicher and Jacqueline A. Samson, "Annual Research Review: Enduring Neurobiological Effects of Childhood Abuse and Neglect," *Journal of Child Psychology and Psychiatry* 57, no. 3 (March 2016): 241–66.

14. R. C. Lewontin, *Biology as Destiny: The Doctrine of DNA* (New York: Harper Perennial, 1991), 30.

15. W. Thomas Boyce, *The Orchid and the Dandelion: Why Some Children Struggle and How All Can Thrive* (London: Allen Lane, 2019), 11.

16. E. Fox and C. B. Beevers, "Differential Sensitivity to the Environment: Contribution of Cognitive Biases and Genes to Psychological Wellbeing," *Molecular Psychiatry* 21, no. 12 (2016): 1657–62.

17.   Louis Menand, "Acid Reflux: The Life and High Times of Timothy Leary,"
      New Yorker, June 26, 2006.

Chapter 18: The Mind Can Do Some Amazing Things

1.   A. H. Almaas, *The Freedom to Be* (Berkeley, CA: Diamond Books, 1989), 85.

2.   Douglas F. Watt and Jaak Panksepp, "Depression: An Evolutionarily
      Conserved Mechanism to Terminate Separation Distress? A Review
      of Aminergic, Peptidergic, and Neural Network Perspectives,"
      Neuropsychoanalysis 11, no. 1 (January 1, 2009): 7–51.

3.   Noël Hunter, *Trauma and Madness in Mental Health Services* (New York:
      Palgrave Macmillan, 2018), 5.

4.   The psychologist and research scientist Stephen Porges posits the concept
      of *neuroception*, the brain's unconscious assessment of security. "This
      automatic process," he writes, "involves brain areas that evaluate cues of
      safety, danger, and life threat." "The perception of safety," he suggests, "is
      the turning point in the development of relationships for most mammals."
      This is particularly true for human beings, with our long formative period of
      helpless dependency. Stephen W. Porges, *The Pocket Guide to the Polyvagal
      Theory: The Transformative Power of Feeling Safe* (New York: W. W. Norton,
      2017), 19; and Stephen W. Porges, *The Polyvagal Theory: Neurophysiological
      Foundations of Emotions, Attachment, Communication, Self-Regulation*
      (New York: W. W. Norton, 2011), see especially chapter 1.

5.   Helen Knott, *In My Own Moccasins: A Memoir of Resilience*
      (Saskatchewan, Canada: University of Regina Press, 2019), 96.

6.   This quote by Robin Williams was reported to have been sourced from a
      video interview I have not been able to view directly. But he reveals much
      about his childhood loneliness and inner torments in almost similar words
      in this YouTube interview with James Lipton: https://www.dailymotion
      .com/video/x640jf8.

7.   In a Swedish study looking at hundreds of thousands of subjects, the risk
      of Parkinson's disease was nearly three times as great in those who had
      experienced depression, and even greater in those with severe depression.
      Helena Gustafsson et al., "Depression and Subsequent Risk of Parkinson
      Disease," *Neurology* 84, no. 24 (June 16, 2015): 2422–29. Another review
      concluded that chronic emotional stress also elevates the risk for the
      disease, possibly by damaging dopamine cells in certain parts of the brain:

Atbin Djamshidian and Andrew Lees, "Can Stress Trigger Parkinson's Disease?," *Journal of Neurology, Neurosurgery, and Psychiatry* 85, no. 8 (August 2014): 879–82.

8. Schizophrenia Working Group, "Biological Insights from 108 Schizophrenia-Associated Genetic Loci," *Nature* 511 (2014): 421–27.

9. "Dissociation," writes the psychiatrist Mark Epstein, "offers immediate protection from the traumas of life." Mark Epstein, *The Trauma of Everyday Life* (New York: Penguin, 2014), 84.

10. Knott, *In My Own Moccasins*, 24.

11. Theo Fleury, *Playing with Fire* (New York: HarperCollins, 2010), 25.

12. A recent study showed that prolonged use of antipsychotics in *adults* results in a diminished thickness of the cerebral cortex, the brain's executive apparatus. "The prefrontal cortex doesn't get the input it needs and is being shut down by drugs," a leading researcher told the *New York Times*. "That reduces the psychotic symptoms. It also causes the prefrontal cortex to slowly atrophy." Aristotle N. Voineskos et al., "Effects of Antipsychotic Medication on Brain Structure in Patients with Major Depressive Disorder and Psychotic Features: Neuroimaging Findings in the Context of a Randomized Placebo-Controlled Clinical Trial," *JAMA Psychiatry* 77, no. 7 (July 1, 2020): 674–83.

13. Russell A. Barkley, *Attention-Deficit Hyperactivity Disorder: A Handbook for Diagnosis and Treatment* (New York: Guilford Press, 1990), 103.

14. Jaak Panksepp, "Can PLAY Diminish ADHD and Facilitate the Construction of the Social Brain?," *Journal of the Canadian Academy of Child and Adolescent Psychiatry* 16, no. 2 (May 2007): 57–66.

15. For example, Liliana J. Lengua et al., "Pathways from Early Adversity to Later Adjustment: Tests of the Additive and Bidirectional Effects of Executive Control and Diurnal Cortisol in Early Childhood," *Development and Psychopathology*, 2019, https://doi.org/10.1017/S0954579419000373; also Jens C. Pruessner et al., "Dopamine Release in Response to a Psychological Stress in Humans and Its Relationship to Early Maternal Care: A Positron Emission Tomography Study Using [11C]Raclopride," *Journal of Neuroscience* 24, no. 11 (March 17, 2004): 2825–31.

16. Bruce D. Perry and Maia Szalavitz, *The Boy Who Was Raised as a Dog (And Other Stories from a Child Psychiatrist's Notebook): What*

Traumatized Children Can Teach Us About Loss, Love, and Healing (New York: Basic Books, 2006), 51.

17. The study by Nicole M. Brown, M.D., and her colleagues analyzed data from the 2011 National Survey of Children's Health and was presented on May 6, 2014, at the Pediatric Academic Societies' annual meeting in Vancouver, B.C. It was reported in ScienceDaily, May 6, 2014: "Study Finds ADHD and Trauma Often Go Hand in Hand."

18. Stanley Coren, "Can Dogs Suffer from ADHD?," *Psychology Today*, January 9, 2018, https://www.psychologytoday.com/us/blog/canine -corner/201801/can-dogs-suffer-adhd.

19. John Bowlby, *Attachment*, 2nd ed. (New York: Basic Books, 1982), 377.

20. Bruno Etain et al., "Childhood Trauma Is Associated with Severe Clinical Characteristics of Bipolar Disorders," *Journal of Clinical Psychiatry* 74, no. 10 (October 2013): 991–98.

The study does not imply, and neither do I, that childhood adversity "causes" bipolar disorder. It is, however, a contributing factor, especially to the condition's severity.

Chapter 19: From Society to Cell

1. János Selye, *The Stress of Life*, rev. ed. (New York: McGraw-Hill, 1978), 370.

2. Zachary M. Harvanek et al., "Psychological and Biological Resilience Modulates the Effects of Stress on Epigenetic Aging," *Translational Psychiatry* 11 (2021), https://doi.org/10.1038/s41398-021-01735-7.

3. E. R. De Kloet, "Corticosteroids, Stress, and Aging," *Annals of the New York Academy of Sciences* 663 (1992): 357–71.

4. Yuval Noah Harari, *Sapiens: A Brief History of Humankind* (Toronto: McClelland & Stewart, 2014), 314.

5. BBC interview, "Blair Calls for Lifestyle Change," 2006, cited in Ted Schrecker and Clare Bambra, *How Politics Makes Us Sick: Neoliberal Epidemics* (New York: Palgrave Macmillan, 2015), 29.

6. Phillip Inman, "IMF Boss Says Global Economy Risks Return of Great Depression," *Guardian*, January 17, 2020.

7. David Lao, "Almost 9 out of 10 Canadians Feel Food Prices Are Rising Faster Than Income: Survey," *Global News*, December 16, 2019.

8.   Vancity, "Report: B.C. Women Are Financially Stressed, Stretched and Under-Resourced," press release, March 17, 2018, based on the province-wide survey "Money Troubled: Inside B.C.'s Financial Health Gender Gap."

9.   Schrecker and Bambra, *How Politics Makes Us Sick*, 42.

10. John Ralston Saul, "The Collapse of Globalism," *Harper's*, March 2004.

11. Ashild Faresjö et al., "Higher Perceived Stress but Lower Cortisol Levels Found Among Young Greek Adults Living in a Stressful Social Environment in Comparison with Swedish Young Adults," *PLoS ONE* 8, no. 9 (September 16, 2013), https://doi.org/10.1371/journal.pone.0073828.

12. Sonia J. Lupien et al., "Child's Stress Hormone Levels Correlate with Mother's Socioeconomic Status and Depressive State," *Biological Psychiatry* 48, no. 10 (November 15, 2000): 976–80.

13. Tara Siegel Bernard and Karl Russell, "The Middle-Class Crunch: A Look at 4 Family Budgets," *New York Times*, October 3, 2019.

14. Wade Davis, "The Unravelling of America," *Rolling Stone*, August 6, 2020, https://www.rollingstone.com/politics/political-commentary/covid-19-end-of-american-era-wade-davis-1038206/.

15. Morris Berman, *The Twilight of American Culture* (New York: W. W. Norton, 2001), 64–65.

16. Bernard and Russell, "The Middle-Class Crunch."

17. William T. Gallo et al., "Involuntary Job Loss as a Risk Factor for Subsequent Myocardial Infarction and Stroke: Findings from the Health and Retirement Survey," *American Journal of Industrial Medicine* 45, no. 5 (May 2004): 408–16; and W. T. Gallo et al., "The Impact of Late Career Job Loss on Myocardial Infarction and Stroke: A 10 Year Follow Up Using the Health and Retirement Survey," *Journal of Occupational and Environmental Medicine* 63, no. 10 (October 2006): 683–87.

18. Matthew E. Dupre et al., "The Cumulative Effect of Unemployment on Risks for Acute Myocardial Infarction," *Archives of Internal Medicine* 172, no. 22 (December 2012): 1731–37.

19. Louis Uchitelle, "Job Insecurity of Workers Is a Big Factor in Fed Policy," *New York Times*, February 27, 1997.

20. Schrecker and Bambra, *How Politics Makes Us Sick*, 53.

21. Ben Stein, "In Class Warfare, Guess Which Class Is Winning," *New York Times*, November 26, 2006, https://www.nytimes.com/2006/11/26/business/yourmoney/26every.html.

22. David Marchese, "Ben and Jerry's Radical Ice Cream Dreams," *New York Times*, July 29, 2020.

23. Joseph E. Stiglitz, *The Price of Inequality: How Today's Divided Society Endangers Our Future* (New York: W. W. Norton, 2013), xlviii–xlix.

24. Rupert Neate, "Billionaires' Wealth Rises to $10.2 Trillion amid Covid Crisis," *Guardian*, October 7, 2020.

25. *Star* editorial board, "Billionaires Get Richer While Millions Struggle. There's a Lot Wrong with This Picture," *Toronto Star*, September 21, 2020.

26. Martin Gilens and Benjamin I. Page, "Testing Theories of American Politics: Elites, Interest Groups, and Average Citizens," *Perspectives on Politics* 12, no. 3 (September 2014): 564–81.

27. Paul Krugman, "Why Do the Rich Have So Much Power?," *New York Times*, July 8, 2020.

28. James Reid, *Alienation* (University of Glasgow Publications, 1972), 5.

Chapter 20: Robbing the Human Spirit

1. David Brooks, "Our Pathetic Herd Immunity Failure," *New York Times*, May 6, 2021.

2. Karl Marx, *Economic and Philosophical Manuscripts*, trans. T. B. Bottomore, in Erich Fromm, *Marx's Concept of Man* (London: Continuum, 2004), 83.

3. Bruce Alexander, *The Globalization of Addiction: A Study in Poverty of the Spirit* (New York: Oxford University Press, 2008), 58.

4. Tony Schwartz and Christine Porath, "Why You Hate Work," *New York Times*, June 1, 2014.

5. Charles Duhigg, "Wealthy, Successful, and Miserable," *New York Times*, February 21, 2019, https://www.nytimes.com/interactive/2019/02/21/magazine/elite-professionals-jobs-happiness.html.

6. Awais Aftab, "Meaning in Life and Its Relationship with Physical, Mental, and Cognitive Functioning: A Study of 1,042 Community-Dwelling Adults Across the Lifespan," *Journal of Clinical Psychiatry* 81, no. 1 (2020).

7. John T. Cacioppo and Stephanie Cacioppo, "The Growing Problem of Loneliness," *Lancet* 391, no. 10011g (February 3, 2018): 426–27.

8. American Psychological Association, "Social Isolation, Loneliness, Could Be Greater Threat to Public Health Than Obesity," ScienceDaily, August 5, 2015, www.sciencedaily.com/releases/2017/08/170805165319.htm.

9. Denise Aydinonat et al., "Social Isolation Shortens Telomeres in African Gray Parrots," *PLoS ONE* 9, no. 4 (2014): e93839, https://doi.org/10.1371/journal.pone.0093839.

10. Nicole K. Valtorta et al., "Loneliness and Social Isolation as Risk Factors for Coronary Heart Disease and Stroke: Systematic Review and Meta-analysis of Longitudinal Observational Studies," *Heart* 102, no. 13 (2016), https://heart.bmj.com/content/102/13/1009.

11. Dhruv Kullur, "Loneliness Is a Health Hazard, but There Are Remedies," *New York Times*, December 22, 2016.

12. Vivek H. Murthy, *Together: The Healing Power of Human Connection in a Sometimes Lonely World* (New York: Harper Wave, 2020), 98.

13. Tim Kasser et al., "Some Costs of American Corporate Capitalism: A Psychological Exploration of Value and Goal Conflicts," *Psychological Inquiry* 18, no. 1 (March: 2007): 1–22.

Chapter 21: They Just Don't Care If It Kills You

1. Russell Brand, "Edward Snowden: The Worst Conspiracies Are in Plain Sight," YouTube video, April 16, 2021, https://www.youtube.com/watch?v=eozAJfbP3gg&t=23s.

2. Belinda S. Lennerz et al., "Effects of Dietary Glycemic Index on Brain Regions Related to Reward and Craving in Men," *American Journal of Clinical Nutrition* 98, no. 3 (September 2013): 641–47.

3. Ashkan Afshin et al., "Health Effects of Dietary Risks in 195 Countries, 1990–2017: A Systemic Analysis for the Global Burden of Disease Study 2017," *Lancet* 393, no. 10184 (May 11, 2019): 1958–2017.

4. American Heart Association, "180,000 Deaths Worldwide May Be Associated with Sugary Soft Drinks, Research Suggests," ScienceDaily, March 19, 2013, https://www.sciencedaily.com/releases/2013/03/130319202144.htm.

5. "Mexico Obesity: Oaxaca Bans Sales of Junk Food to Children," BBC News, Aug. 6, 2020, https://www.bbc.com/news/world-latin -america-53678747.

6. "Mexico Takes Title of 'Most Obese' from America," *Global Post*, July 28, 2013, https://www.cbsnews.com/news/mexico-takes-title-of-most-obese -from-america.

7. Susan Greenhalgh, "Making China Safe for Coke: How Coca-Cola Shaped Obesity Science and Policy in China," *British Medical Journal* 364 (January 9, 2019): k5050, https://doi.org/10.1136/bmj.k5050.

8. "Statistics on Obesity, Physical Activity, Diet, England, 2020," National Health Service, May 5, 2020, https://digital.nhs.uk/data-and-information /publications/statistical/statistics-on-obesity-physical-activity-and-diet /england-2020.

9. Ted Schrecker and Clare Bambra, *How Politics Makes Us Sick: Neoliberal Epidemics* (New York: Palgrave Macmillan, 2015), 32.

10. Nicholas Kristof, "Drug Dealers in Lab Coats," *New York Times*, October 18, 2017.

11. In 2014, on the fiftieth anniversary of the U.S. surgeon general's landmark report exposing the ill effects of manufactured tobacco, the same office issued an update. "The tobacco epidemic was initiated and *has been sustained* by the aggressive strategies of the tobacco industry, which has deliberately misled the public on the risks of smoking cigarettes."

12. "Smoking and Tobacco Use: Fast Facts," Centers for Disease Control and Prevention, https://www.cdc.gov/tobacco/data_statistics/fact_sheets /fast_facts/index.htm.

13. Sheila Kaplan, "Biden Plans to Ban Cigarettes with Menthol," *New York Times*, April 29, 2021.

14. Milton Friedman, "Your Greed or Their Greed?," *Phil Donahue Show*, YouTube, uploaded July 14, 2007, https://www.youtube.com/watch ?v=RWsx1X8PV_A.

15. Milton Friedman, "The Social Responsibility of Business Is to Increase Its Profits," *New York Times*, September 13, 1970.

16. Andrea Wulf, *The Invention of Nature: The Adventures of Alexander von Humboldt, the Lost Hero of Science* (London: John Murray, 2015), 5.

17. William J. Ripple et al., "World Scientists' Warning of a Climate Emergency," *BioScience* 70, no. 1 (January 2020): 8–12.

18. Nick Watts et al., "The 2018 Report of the *Lancet* Countdown on Health and Climate Change: Shaping the Health of Nations for Centuries to Come," *Lancet* 392, no. 10163 (December 8, 2018): 2479–514.

19. "More Than 200 Health Journals Call for Urgent Action on Climate Crisis," *Guardian*, September 6, 2021; and Robert Lee Holtz, "Action on Climate Change Is Urged by Medical Journals in Unprecedented Plea," *Wall Street Journal*, September 6, 2021.

Chapter 22: The Assaulted Sense of Self

1. Malcolm X, as told to Alex Haley, *The Autobiography of Malcolm X* (1964; New York: Ballantine Books, 2015), 56.

2. Jean-Paul Sartre, *Anti-Semite and Jew: An Exploration of the Etiology of Hate* (1948; New York: Schocken Books, 1995), 53–54.

3. "Ken Hardy on the Assaulted Sense of Self," Psychotherapy Networker, YouTube video, 2016, https://www.youtube.com/watch?v=i26A5oec UWM.

4. Helen Knott, *In My Own Moccasins: A Memoir of Resilience* (Saskatchewan, Canada: University of Regina Press, 2019), 200–201.

5. David H. Chae et al., "Racial Discrimination and Telomere Shortening Among African-Americans: The Coronary Artery Risk Development in Young Adults (CARDIA) Study," *Health Psychology* 39, no. 3 (March 2020): 209-19.

6. Ta-Nehisi Coates, *Between the World and Me* (New York: Spiegel & Grau, 2015), 27–28.

7. Clyde Hertzman and Tom Boyce, "How Experience Gets Under the Skin to Create Gradients in Developmental Health," *Annual Review of Public Health* 31, no. 1 (April 2010): 329–47.

8. David T. Lackland, "Racial Differences in Hypertension: Implications for High Blood Pressure Management," *American Journal of the Medical Sciences* 348, no. 2 (August 2014): 135–38.

9. American Academy of Allergy, Asthma, and Immunology, "Black Children Six Times More Likely to Die of Asthma," press release, March

4, 2017, https://www.aaaai.org/about-aaaai/newsroom/news-releases /black-children-asthma.

10. The Baldwin citation is from a panel discussion moderated by Nat Hentoff, broadcast in 1961 on WBAI-FM radio and subsequently published with the title "The Negro in American Culture," in *CrossCurrents* 11, no. 3 (Summer 1961): 205–224.

11. Amy Roeder, "America Is Failing Its Black Mothers," *Harvard Public Health,* Winter 2019, https://www.hsph.harvard.edu/magazine /magazine_article/america-is-failing-its-black-mothers.

12. Brad N. Greenwood et al., "Physician-Patient Racial Concordance and Disparities in Birthing Mortality for Newborns," *Proceedings of the National Academy of Sciences* 117, no. 35 (September 1, 2020): 21194–200, https://doi.org/10.1073/pnas.1913405117.

13. Cristina Nova and Jamila Taylor, "Exploring African Americans' High Maternal and Infant Death Rates," Center for American Progress, February 1, 2018, https://www.americanprogress.org/issues/early -childhood/reports/2018/02/01/445576/exploring-african-americans -high-maternal-infant-death-rates.

14. Arline Geronimus et al., " 'Weathering' and Age Patterns of Allostatic Load Scores Among Blacks and Whites in the United States," *American Journal of Public Health* 96, no. 5 (May 2006): 826–33.

15. "Lifespan of Indigenous People 15 Years Shorter Than That of Other Canadians, Federal Documents Say," Canadian Press, January 23, 2018, https://www.cbc.ca/news/health/indigenous-people-live-15-years-less -philpott-briefing-1.4500307.

16. Roland Dyck et al., "Epidemiology of Diabetes Mellitus Among First Nations and Non–First Nations Adults," *Canadian Medical Association Journal* 182, no. 3 (February 23, 2010): 249–56.

17. L. Kirmayer, "Suicide Among Canadian Aboriginal People," *Transcultural Psychiatric Research Review* 31 (1994): 3–57.

18. Michael Marmot, *The Health Gap: The Challenge of an Unequal World* (New York: Bloomsbury, 2015), 12.

19. Sonia J. Lupien et al., "Child's Stress Hormone Levels Correlate with Mother's Socioeconomic Status and Depressive State," *Biological Psychiatry* 48, no. 10 (November 15, 2000): 976–80.

20. In Dennis Raphael, ed., *Social Determinants of Health: Canadian Perspectives*, 3rd ed. (Canadian Scholars Press, 2016), xiii.

21. Alex Soth, "The Great Divide," *New York Times*, September 5, 2020, https://www.nytimes.com/interactive/2020/09/05/opinion/inequality -life-expectancy.html.

22. M. Lemstra et al., "Health Disparity by Neighborhood Income," *Canadian Journal of Public Health* 97, no. 6 (November 2006): 435–39.

23. For example, Joan Luby et al., "The Effects of Poverty on Childhood Brain Development: The Mediating Effect of Caregiving and Stressful Life Events," *JAMA Pediatrics* 167, no. 12 (December 2013): 1135–42.

24. J. R. Swartz et al., "An Epigenetic Mechanism Links Socioeconomic Status to Changes in Depression-Related Brain Function in High-Risk Adolescents," *Molecular Psychiatry* 22, no. 2 (February 2017): 209–224.

25. Dennis Raphael et al., *Social Determinants of Health*, 2nd ed., 13. (Raphael here is recycling facetious advice that has been circulating for some years.) https://thecanadianfacts.org/The_Canadian_Facts -2nd_ed.pdf.

26. Michael Marmot and Eric Brunner, "Cohort Profile: The Whitehall II Study," *International Journal of Epidemiology* 34, no. 2 (April 2005): 251–56; and Aline Dugravot et al., "Social Inequalities in Multimorbidity, Frailty, Disability, and Transitions to Mortality: A 24-Year Follow-Up of the Whitehall II Cohort Study," *Lancet Public Health* 5, no. 1 (January 1, 2020): e42–50.

27. Richard Wilkinson, *The Impact of Inequality: How to Make Sick Societies Healthier* (New York: New Press, 2005), 58.

28. Robert Sapolsky, "The Health-Wealth Gap," *Scientific American*, November 2018, https://www.scientificamerican.com/index.cfm /_api/render/file/?method=inline&fileID=123ECD96-EF81-46F6 -983D2AE9A45FA354.

Chapter 23: Society's Shock Absorbers

1. Haider J. Warraich, "Why Men and Women Feel Pain Differently," *Washington Post*, May 15, 2021.

2. "Female Smokers Are Twice as Likely as Male Smokers to Develop Lung

Cancer," ScienceDaily, December 2, 2003, https://www.sciencedaily.com
/releases/2003/12/031202070515.htm.

3. Margaret Altemus et al., "Sex Differences in Anxiety and Depression
    Clinical Perspectives," *Frontiers in Neuroendocrinology* 35, no. 3 (August
    2014): 320–30.

4. Franck Mauvois-Jarvis et al., "Sex and Gender: Modifiers of Health,
    Disease, and Medicine," *Lancet* 396, no. 10250 (August 22, 2020): 565–82.

5. In the United States, for example, being Black or Hispanic and being
    female create more risk for autoimmune disease than either factor alone.
    A 1964 study on systemic lupus in New York in the *American Journal of
    Public Health* reported that "the morbidity and mortality rates were highest
    among Negroes, followed in descending order by the rates for Puerto
    Ricans and other whites" (Morris Siegel, "Epidemiology of Systemic
    Lupus Erythematosus: Time Trend and Racial Differences, *American
    Journal of Public Health* 54, no. 1 [January 1964]: 33–43). Fifty years later,
    that racial differential persisted. "By and large, SLE is more frequent and
    more severe with higher disease activity and more damage accrual in
    non-Caucasian populations (Hispanics, African descendants and Asians)
    than in Caucasians" (L. A. Gonzalez et al., "Ethnicity in Systemic Lupus
    Erythematosus [SLE]: Its Influence on Susceptibility and Outcomes,"
    Lupus 22, no. 12 [October 2013]: 1214–24). Being female and Indigenous
    on either side of the 49th parallel also elevates the risk—in Canada, for
    example, rheumatoid arthritis affects Indigenous people at a rate three
    times higher than the national average (Stephen Hunt, "Arthritis Affects
    Indigenous People at a Rate Three Times Higher Than Average," CBC
    News, November 5, 2018, https://www.cbc.ca/news/canada/calgary
    /indigenous-rates-arthritis-higher-than-average-1.4892319). Women,
    of course, predominate in these statistics: among Aboriginal women,
    the rheumatoid arthritis ratio is not three but *six* times elevated over
    men ("Rheumatoid Arthritis and the Aboriginal Population—What
    the Research Shows," JointHealth Insight, September 2006, https://
    jointhealth.org/programs-jhmonthly-view.cfm?id=19&locale=en-CA).

6. A 2021 World Health Organization study reported that one in four
    women and girls around the world have been assaulted by a male partner.
    If nonpartner violence is factored in, the WHO estimates that "about a
    third of women aged 15 or older—between 736 million and 852 million—
    will experience some form of sexual or physical violence in their lifetime."

The rates, according to the WHO paper, would be significantly higher were other forms of abuse factored in, such as online violence and sexual harassment. Liz Ford, "Quarter of Women and Girls Have Been Abused by a Partner, Says WHO," *Guardian*, March 9, 2021.

7. Melanie A. Hom et al., "Women Firefighters and Workplace Harassment: Associated Suicidality and Mental Health Sequelae," *Journal of Nervous and Mental Disease* 205, no. 12 (December 2017): 910–17.

8. Catherine E. Harnois and João L. Bastos, "Discrimination, Harassment, and Gendered Health Inequalities: Do Perceptions of Workplace Mistreatment Contribute to the Gender Gap in Self-Reported Health?," *Journal of Health and Social Behavior* 59, no. 2 (2018): 283–99.

9. Julie Holland, *Moody Bitches* (New York: Penguin Press, 2015), 30.

10. Elaine D. Eaker et al., "Marital Status, Marital Strain, and Risk of Coronary Heart Disease or Total Mortality: The Framingham Offspring Study," *Psychosomatic Medicine* 69, no. 6 (July–August 2007): 509–13.

11. Suzanne G. Haynes et al., "Women, Work and Coronary Heart Disease: Prospective Findings from the Framingham Heart Study," *American Journal of Public Health* 70, no. 2 (February 1980): 133–41.

12. Gillian Friedman, "Jobless, Selling Nudes Online, and Still Struggling," *New York Times*, January 12, 2021, https://www.nytimes.com/2021/01/13/business/onlyfans-pandemic-users.html.

13. Gail Dines, *Pornland: How Porn Has Hijacked Our Sexuality* (Boston: Beacon Press, 2010), xi.

14. Emer O'Hanlon, "Porn Lies Behind Cuts and Bruises of Rough Sex Fad," *Irish Independent*, August 2, 2020, https://www.independent.ie/opinion/comment/porn-lies-behind-cuts-and-bruises-of-rough-sex-fad-39416367.html.

15. Mary Wollstonecraft, *A Vindication of the Rights of Woman* (New York: Vintage Classics, 2014), 65.

16. Andrea Dworkin, *Intercourse* (1987; New York: Basic Books, 2007), 112.

17. Janice K. Kiecolt-Glaser et al., "Spousal Caregivers of Dementia Victims: Longitudinal Changes in Immunity and Health," *Psychosomatic Medicine* 53 (1991): 345–62.

18. Rachel M. Radin et al., "Maternal Caregivers Have Confluence of Altered Cortisol, High Reward-Driven Eating, and Worse Metabolic Health,"

PLoS ONE 14, no. 5 (May 10, 2019): e0216541, https://doi.org/10.1371 /journal.pone.0216541.

19. Jessica Grose, "Mothers Are the 'Shock Absorbers' of Our Society," *New York Times*, October 14, 2020, https://www.nytimes.com/2020/10/14 /parenting/working-moms-job-loss-coronavirus.html.

20. Caroline Criado Perez, *Invisible Women: Exposing Data Bias in a World Designed for Men* (London: Chatto & Windus, 2019), 73.

21. Kate Manne, *Down Girl: The Logic of Misogyny* (New York: Oxford University Press, 2018), 130.

Chapter 24: We Feel Their Pain

1. Anthony Brooks and Grace Tatter, "Surviving Family Politics at Thanksgiving," *On Point*, WBUR, November 27, 2019, https://www.wbur .org/onpoint/2019/11/27/family-politics-thanksgiving.

2. Kevin B. Smith et al., "Friends, Relatives, Sanity, and Health: The Costs of Politics," *PLoS One* 14, no. 9 (September 2019), https://journals.plos .org/plosone/article?id=10.1371/journal.pone.0221870.

3. Elissa Epel, "Stressed Out by Politics? It Could Be Making Your Body Age Faster, Too," *Quartz*, March 16, 2017, https://qz.com/931355/telomeres -and-cell-aging-nobel-prize-for-medicine-winner-elizabeth-blackburn -and-elissa-epel-explain-how-trump-is-aging-our-cells/.

4. Steven Stosny, "He Once Called It 'Election Stress Disorder.' Now the Therapist Says We're Suffering from This," *Washington Post*, February 6, 2017, https://www.washingtonpost.com/news/inspired-life /wp/2017/02/06/suffering-from-headline-stress-disorder-since-trumps -win-youre-definitely-not-alone/?noredirect=on.

5. Alice Miller, *For Your Own Good: Hidden Cruelty in Child-Rearing and the Roots of Violence* (1983; New York: Farrar, Straus and Giroux, 1990), 65.

6. Sue Gerhardt, *The Selfish Society* (London: Simon and Schuster, 2011), 46.

7. Jim Coyle, "For Stephen Harper, a Stable Upbringing and an Unpredictable Path to Power," *Toronto Star*, October 8, 2015, https://www .thestar.com/news/insight/2015/10/04/for-stephen-harper-a-stable -upbringing-and-an-unpredictable-path-to-power.html.

8. "An Emotional Justin Trudeau Cries Discussing the Death of Gord

Downie," *Global News*, YouTube, October 18, 2017, https://www
.youtube.com/watch?v=YMCaDvah6No.

9. Jonathan Kay, "The Justin Trudeau I Can't Forget," *Walrus*, September
    29, 2015.

10. Claudia Wallis, "Of Psychopaths and Presidential Candidates,"
    Scientific American Mind, guest blog, August 12, 2016, https://blogs
    .scientificamerican.com/mind-guest-blog/of-psychopaths-and
    -presidential-candidates/.

11. Jane Mayer, "Trump's Boswell Speaks," *New Yorker*, July 26, 2016.

12. Amy Chozick, "Clinton Father's Brusque Style, Mostly Unspoken but
    Powerful," *New York Times*, July 20, 2015.

13. Megan Twohey, "Her Husband Accused of Affairs, a Defiant Clinton
    Fought Back," *New York Times*, October 3, 2016.

14. David Brooks, "The Avalanche of Distrust," *New York Times*, September
    13, 2016.

15. George Lakoff, *The Political Mind* (New York: Penguin Books, 2008), 76.

16. Randy Rainbow (@randyrainbow), "G'night, mom and dad. See you in
    the morning. ♥," Twitter, August 11, 2020, 10:17 p.m., https://twitter.com
    /randyrainbow/status/1293386210388381696.

17. See, for example, "Stephen Kicks Off a *Late Show*'s Obama-Rama
    Extravagama with a Special Obamalogue," *The Late Show with Stephen
    Colbert*, CBS, YouTube video, https://www.youtube.com
    /watch?v=RmtCV-U8wwo.

Chapter 25: Mind in the Lead

1. Aeschylus, *Agamemnon*, in *The Orestia*, translated by Robert Fagles (New
    York: Penguin, 1979), 109.

2. Edith Eva Eger, *The Choice: Embrace the Possible* (New York: Scribner,
    2017), 280.

Chapter 26: Four *A*'s and Five Compassions

1. Kelly Turner, *Radical Remission: Surviving Cancer Against All Odds* (New
    York: HarperOne, 2014), 45.

2. Henning Krampe et al., "The Influence of Personality Factors on Disease Progression and Health-Related Quality of Life in People with ALS," *Amyotrophic Lateral Sclerosis* 9, no. 2 (May 2008): 99–107.

3. Henriët van Middendorp et al., "Effects of Anger and Anger Regulation Styles on Pain in Daily Life of Women with Fibromyalgia: A Diary Study," *European Journal of Pain* 14, no. 2 (February 2010): 176–82.

4. Helen Knott, *In My Own Moccasins: A Memoir of Resilience* (Saskatchewan, Canada: University of Regina Press, 2019), 240.

5. Thomas Merton, *The Seven Storey Mountain: An Autobiography of Faith* (Boston: Mariner Books, 1999), 362.

Chapter 27: A Dreadful Gift

1. Nancy A. Shadick et al., "A Randomized Controlled Trial of an Internal Family Systems–Based Psychotherapeutic Intervention on Outcomes in Rheumatoid Arthritis: A Proof-of-Concept Study," *Journal of Rheumatology* 40, no. 11 (November 2013): 1831–41.

2. Aleksandr Solzhenitsyn, *Cancer Ward* (New York: Vintage Classics, 2017), 89.

Chapter 28: Before the Body Says No

1. Richard C. Schwartz, *Introduction to the Internal Family Systems Model* (Trailheads Publications, 2001), 54.

2. A. H. Almaas, *The Freedom to Be* (Diamond Books, 1989), 12.

3. Cited in Thich Nhat Hanh, *The Heart of the Buddha's Teaching* (New York: Broadway Books, 1998), 45.

4. János Selye, *The Stress of Life*, rev. ed. (New York: McGraw-Hill, 1978), 419.

Chapter 29: Seeing Is Disbelieving

1. Bruce H. Lipton and Steve Bhaerman, *Spontaneous Evolution: Our Positive Future (And a Way to Get There from Here)* (Carlsbad, CA: Hay House, 2009), 38–39.

2. Jeffrey M. Schwartz and Sharon Begley, *The Mind and the Brain: Neuroplasticity and the Power of Mental Force* (New York: ReganBooks, 2002).

Chapter 30: Foes to Friends

1.   Richard Schwartz, *Introduction to the Internal Family Systems Model* (Trailheads Publications, 2001), 67–68.

2.   Edith Eger, *The Gift* (New York: Scribner, 2020), 156.

Chapter 31: Jesus in the Tipi

1.   For example, on ayahuasca: José Carlo Bouso et al., "Ayahuasca, Technical Report 2021," International Center for Ethnobotanical Education, Research and Service, December 2021, https://www.iceers.org/ayahuasca -technical-report/.

2.   Michelle S. Thiessen et al., "Psychedelic Use and Intimate Partner Violence: The Role of Emotion Regulation," *Journal of Psychopharmacology*, 2018, https://doi.org/10.1177/0269881118187.

3.   S. C. Gwynne, *Empire of the Summer Moon: Quanah Parker and the Rise and Fall of the Comanches* (New York: Scribner, 2010), 314.

Chapter 32: My Life as a Genuine Thing

1.   A. H. Almaas, *Elements of the Real in Man* (Diamond Books, 1987), 26.

2.   Lewis Mehl-Madrona, *Coyote Medicine: Lessons from Native American Healing* (New York: Simon and Schuster, 1997), 16–17.

3.   Wilhelm Reich, *The Murder of Christ: The Emotional Plague of Mankind* (New York: Farrar, Straus and Giroux, 1953), 174–75.

4.   For example, Quinn A. Conklin et al., "Meditation, Stress Processes, and Telomere Biology," *Current Opinion in Psychology* 28 (2019): 92–101; D. Bergen-Cico et al., "Reductions in Cortisol Associated with Primary Care Brief Mindfulness Programs with Veterans with PTSD," *Med Care* 52, no. 12, suppl. 5 (December 2014): S25–31; and A. M. Gallegos et al., "Mindfulness-Based Stress Reduction to Enhance Psychological Functioning and Improve Inflammatory Biomarkers in Trauma-Exposed Women: A Pilot Study," *Psychological Trauma* 7, no. 6 (November 2015): 525–32.

5.   Francesco Pagnini et al., "Mindfulness, Physical Impairment and Psychological Well-Being in People with Amyotrophic Lateral Sclerosis," *Psychology and Health* 30, no. 5 (October 2014): 503–17, https://doi.org /10.1080/08870446.2014.982652.

6. Rony Berger et al., "Reducing Israeli-Jewish Pupils' Outgroup Prejudice with a Mindfulness and Compassion-Based Social Emotional Program," *Mindfulness* 9, no. 2 (December 2018), https://doi.org/10.1007/s12671-018-0919-y.

Chapter 33: Unmaking a Myth

1. For people who might find this assertion surprising, I recommend the works of such Israeli historians as Ilan Pappe, Simha Flapan, Benny Morris, Tom Segev, and Avi Shlaim, or of American Jewish scholars like Norman Finkelstein; for example, Pappe's seminal work, *The Ethnic Cleansing of Palestine* (Oneworld, 2006). Or the reports of the indomitable Gideon Levy in the Israeli paper *Haaretz*. Or for a Palestinian view, the illuminating book of personal memoir and history by Rashid Khalidi, *One Hundred Years' War on Palestine: A History of Settler Colonialism and Resistance, 1917–2017* (New York: Picador, 2020).

2. James Baldwin, "As Much Truth as One Can Bear," *New York Times Book Review*, January 14, 1962.

3. Baldwin, "As Much Truth as One Can Bear."

4. The Joan Didion citations are from an obituary of the late writer: Sian Cain and Edward Helmore, "Joan Didion, American Journalist and Author, Dies at 87," *Guardian*, December 23, 2021.

5. Bessel van der Kolk, *The Body Keeps the Score: Brain, Mind, and Body in the Healing of Trauma* (New York: Penguin, 2014), 349.

6. For example, a study that crossed my desk just as I was writing this chapter: Nina T. Rogers, Christine Power, and Snehal M. Pinto Pereira, "Child Maltreatment, Early Life Socioeconomic Disadvantage and All-Cause Mortality: Findings from a Prospective British Cohort," *BMJ Open* 11 (2021): e050914, https://doi.org/10.1136/bmjopen-2021-050914.

7. Jesse Thistle, *From the Ashes* (Toronto: Simon & Schuster Canada, 2019), 260.

8. Maggie Kline, *Brain-Changing Strategies to Trauma-Proof Our Schools* (Berkeley, CA: North Atlantic Books, 2020), 2.

9. Alison Rourke, "Greta Thunberg Responds to Asperger's Critics: 'It's a Superpower,'" *Guardian*, September 2, 2019.

10. Caroline Hickman et al., "Young People's Voices on Climate Anxiety, Government Betrayal and Moral Injury: A Global Phenomenon,"

preprint submitted to the *Lancet*, September 2021, https://papers.ssrn
.com/sol3/papers.cfm?abstract_id=3918955.

11. Damian Carrington, "'Blah, Blah, Blah': Greta Thunberg Lambasts
Leaders over Climate Crisis," *Guardian*, September 28, 2021.

12. Hannah Arendt, "Eichmann in Jerusalem—I," *New Yorker*, February 16,
1963.

13. According to an April 11, 2021, *New York Times* editorial, the number of
Iraqi children who died as a result of U.S. sanctions in the 1990s was
500,000. The interview in which Albright made the statement was aired
on CBS's *60 Minutes*, May 12, 1996. Albright later wrote, "I had fallen
into a trap and said something I did not mean, regretting having seemed
'cold-blooded and cruel.'" Apart from her regret about how she came
across, neither she nor any U.S. official responsible for the sanctions ever
apologized for the deaths of the children.

14. Abraham Maslow, "Resistance to Acculturation," *Journal of Social Issues*
1 (Fall 1951): 26–29.

Index

Page numbers in *italics* refer to illustrations.

The Bible
Is for
Living

Dick Barton

Christmas 2009

The Bible Is for Living

A Scholar's Spiritual Journey

PHILIP J. KING

Biblical Archaeology Society
Washington, DC

STAFF FOR *The Bible Is for Living*
Steven Feldman *Managing Editor*
Heather Metzger *Production Manager*
Bonnie Mullin *Administrative Editor*

AURAS DESIGN
Jinna Hagerty *Layout*
Rob Sugar *Design*
Sharri Wolfgang *Cover Design*

BIBLICAL ARCHAEOLOGY SOCIETY
Susan Laden *Publisher*
Hershel Shanks *Editor*

Unless otherwise noted, quotations from the Bible are from the
New Revised Standard Version. Emphases within quotations are the author's.

Library of Congress Cataloging-in-Publication Data

King, Philip J.
The Bible is for living: a scholar's spiritual journey / Philip J. King.
p. cm.
Includes bibliographical references.
ISBN 978-0-9796357-9-3
1. Bible--Criticism, interpretation, etc. I. Title.

BS511.3.K57 2008
220.6--dc22
2008033897

Table of Contents

To the McGuire Family—
Kevin, Ana María, Philip, Elena

Preface

AMIDST MY LIFELONG BIBLICAL UNDERTAKINGS, I often wanted to write a popular book, convinced that the Bible has much to say to modern life. My desire to do so was reinforced by a recent encounter. I stopped to chat briefly with a homeless person just released from jail, now out on probation. Because of behavioral misconduct, the consequence of heroin addiction, he was consigned several times during incarceration to the isolation unit (the "hole"). In response to my concern about coping with boredom in seclusion, surprisingly he acknowledged that he was never bored—he spent all his time reading the Bible. The only regret was his lack of background essential for a better understanding of the Bible's meaning. This book, *The Bible Is for Living*, is the result of that chance meeting in Harvard Square, Cambridge.

The book's title sets the motif; my emphasis is on the practical value of the Scriptures for everyday living. It is the book I always wanted to write, but I felt it would be better done at the end of one's academic career than at the beginning. Time is required to move from the theoretical to the practical; scholarly requirements are more easily acquired than the experiences of life. At this point in my life, after years in the field excavating and a long time in the library researching, I think I am now ready to write that book on the Scriptures for everyday life. This is but one person's review of life.

I am indebted to my teachers and colleagues at home and abroad, from whom I have learned much. In retrospect, I would say it was Professor G. Ernest Wright of Harvard University to whom I am most grateful; it was his dedication to Bible and archaeology that had such a formative influence on me.

In the immediate preparation of this book, several showed interest and gave encouragement. In the last analysis, however, four people have placed me in their debt: Richard McBrien, University of Notre Dame, read the manuscript carefully and made valuable suggestions; Kristen Vagliardo, Harvard Semitic Museum, assisted me every step of the way with her computer expertise and her biblical knowledge; Sandra Schneiders, Graduate Theological Union, who at my request so generously and promptly compiled an annotated bibliography on biblical spirituality; and finally, Lawrence Boadt, editor and publisher of the Paulist Press and leading biblical scholar, who was readily available with professional advice and sage suggestions. It was he who convinced me that the age of eighty-three is not an impediment to authoring a final book. You can make you own judgment whether he was right.

MARCH 26, 2008

Introduction

Scientific Study of the Bible

The life of a biblical scholar is an exalted but arduous profession. Expending practically all of one's waking hours in intimate contact with the biblical text is indeed a privilege. For my part, I have spent most of my adult life researching, lecturing, and excavating, all in connection with the Bible, concentrating on the Iron Age (ca.1200–586 BCE). Many years are required to gain competence in the biblical languages (Hebrew, Aramaic, Greek), as well as other ancient and modern languages needed for scholarly research. These are only prerequisites. Then follows the study of the ancient Near East—its history, geography, culture, and archaeology, to mention a few of the cognate disciplines. Like all ancient literature, the biblical text is sometimes ambiguous, tendentious, or unintelligible; at such times, ancillary studies, especially archaeology, may assist in clarifying, supplementing, or correcting the biblical text.

Archaeology and the Bible

Archaeology, too, has its innate limitations: the unearthed artifacts are frequently mute, ambiguous, or anonymous, subjecting them to a variety of interpretations. Modern archaeology is not a treasure hunt; its objective is the reconstruction of history and culture. Archaeological method embraces many specialties, both scientific and humanistic, and their confluence leads to sound interpretation. Archaeology does not "prove" the Bible—the Bible is a book of faith.

None of this is to suggest that the Bible is so arcane that only specialists hold the key for unlocking its treasures:

Surely, this commandment that I am commanding you today is not too hard for you, nor is it too far away. It is not in heaven, that you should say, 'Who will go up to heaven for us, and get it for us so that we may hear it and observe it?' Neither is it beyond the sea, that you should say, 'Who will cross to the other side of the sea for us, and get it for us so that we may hear it and observe it?' No, the word is very near to you; it is in your mouth and in your heart for you to observe." (Deuteronomy 30:11–14)

Modern Approaches to the Bible

Despite the advances achieved in biblical studies during the last half century, the Bible is still the best known and least understood book in literature. Since the Bible is conditioned by time and place, the first requisite is to situate the text in its own historical, social, and cultural context. In interpreting ancient literature, particularly the Bible, it is imperative to bear in mind the worldview of the biblical writers: It is far removed from present-day political, economic, and social values. One must prescind from Western thought patterns, and adjust to the Semitic way of thinking. Instead of analyzing narratives, the biblical writers tell stories; the Bible is *story*, not history. To state this fact is not to diminish the reliability and authenticity of the Bible; its significance lies elsewhere—the Bible is a book of faith, calling for complete commitment. It is a personal challenge in every generation. Do not search the Bible for ready answers to the problems of life; it does not necessarily provide immediate responses for every inquiry.

The Bible and Ancient Texts

Ancient texts are fascinating, but they were composed when the understanding of issues like sexuality and parental discipline was quite different. For example, filial insubordination is included in the list of offenses punishable by stoning, which is a form of capital punishment. The parents of an incorrigible son ("a stubborn and rebellious son; he is a glutton and a drunkard") shall have him brought out to the elders at the gate. "Then all the men of the town shall stone him to death" (Deuteronomy 21:18–21). The stoning of Stephen, a leader in the early Jerusalem church, attests that this form of capital punishment continued into New Testament times.

Excising texts out of their historical and cultural context leads to serious distortion. Quarrying the Bible for proof-texts is just as erroneous; the Bible is not a mine of proof-texts to "shoot down" the adversary. To quote a biblical text in order to "prove" the error of a certain modern practice (ethos) is faulty hermeneutics (methodology of interpretation).

Mythology in the Bible

"Myth" is a disarmingly simple word—common in ordinary conversation but ambiguous in scholarly research. Ernst Cassirer's definition of myth is "a symbolic form of expression together with art, language, and science."[1] One hesitates to label the Genesis creation stories "myths" in popular lectures; invariably many in the audience automatically think "fable." Myth is not a synonym for fable; in fact quite the opposite. The problem of defining myth in ancient and modern literature is exacerbated by the fact that the word has a long history in which its meaning has evolved over the centuries. Definitions of literary myth abound, although they do not all agree. So that we shall be on the same page, I offer a definition from *Webster's Third New International Dictionary* (unabridged):

A story that is usually of unknown origin and at least partially traditional, that ostensibly relates historical events usually of such character as to serve to explain some practice, belief, institution, or natural phenomenon, and that is especially associated with religious rites and beliefs.[2]

John McKenzie, noted biblical scholar, pointed out that "myth is the most apt form for the expression of transcendental reality."[3] The word "myth" is absent from the Old Testament, and appears only five times in the New Testament (all but one time in the pastoral epistles). In each of these, myth has a pejorative (fictional) sense, for example: "I [Paul] urge you [Timothy] ... to remain in Ephesus so that you may instruct certain people not to teach any different doctrine, and not to occupy themselves with myths and endless genealogies that promote speculations rather than the divine training that is known by faith" (1 Timothy 1:4). The remaining four references can be found in 1 Timothy 4:7; 2 Timothy 4:4; Titus 1:14; 2 Peter 1:16.

Ancient Near Eastern mythology has influenced the Old Testament. The closest parallel to the Genesis creation story is the Mesopotamian creation myth, *Enuma elish*; the title comes from its opening words, meaning "When on high." The Old Testament has been influenced by ancient Near Eastern mythology, but it is in no way a carbon copy. Its differences are attributable to the transforming power of the Yahwistic faith. The use of mythical language and imagery in the Old Testament has been recognized since the recovery of the mythological literature of the ancient Near East in the nineteenth century.

Creation/Cosmogony

Genesis (1:1–2:4a) opens with a well-known and much-misconstrued description of creation, a dominant biblical theme. The problem arises from a failure to differentiate between a scientific treatise and a religious discourse. Some basic principles of interpretation may help to grasp the nature of the biblical account of creation. Modern science is no help in understanding the Bible's description of creation, which is pre-modern, and at the same time without any pretense at modern science. Just as the creation text made religious sense to the original readers, it is our responsibility to make religious sense of the text for ourselves and our contemporaries. Since the biblical account of creation is a religious document, and not a scientific description, the accounts are not to be understood literally, nor are they to be harmonized. (It just won't work.) The following guidelines may illuminate the problem and lead to a solution.

Efforts to reconcile biblical cosmogony with modern science confuse two different forms of mental activity. Religious treatises are not founded upon abstract reasoning. Important differences distinguish the ancient Near Eastern and the modern Western conceptions of creation. The ancient Near Eastern account is narrated as a drama, based upon traditional ancient Near Eastern lore, and consequently is not to be taken literally. The Bible's portrayal of the ancient Israelite view of the world is borrowed from ambient cultures, especially the Ugaritic Baal epic and Babylonian *Enuma elish*, which describes how the god

Marduk became the king of the gods and the principal god of Babylon.

Cosmogony, distinguished from cosmology, which studies the physical universe at large, is any theory concerning the origins and evolution of the universe. The word derives from the Greek *kosmos*, "universe," and the root of *gìnomai*, "to come about."

According to the worldview (*Weltanschauung*), the earth was the center of the universe and the heavenly bodies encircled the earth. Water surrounded the earth, both above and below, and the firmament retained the water in place. The firmament was a solid vault upon which the heavenly luminaries were attached. The sky and the heavenly bodies constituted the upper firmament; from the lower firmament, springs and rivers flowed upward to earth. Water provided the support and survival of plant and animal life.

Before Nicolaus Copernicus (died 1543) formulated the solar system in heliocentric terms, that is, that the earth and other planets revolve around the sun, the earth was thought to be at the center of the universe (geocentric terms). The ancient Israelites and their neighbors understood the universe as being composed of three levels: the heavens, the earth, and the regions under the earth.

Names for God

In the ancient Near East, special significance was attached to personal names, which revealed not only the identity, but also the character of persons. To know the name was to know something of the person; the name expressed something of the essence of the one named. Every personal name commanded respect, and especially the name of God. The divine name was God's self-revelation in history; it is also the name by which the Deity could be approached.

Yahweh is the most important name for God in the Hebrew Bible. Eager to know God's personal name when the Israelites would make inquiry, Moses asked God directly, "What shall I say to them?" The divine response was enigmatic, "I am who I am" (*'ehyeh 'asher 'ehyeh*) (Exodus 3:14). YHWH, pronounced "Yahweh," is a tetragrammaton (a four-letter word); its origin is uncertain, and out of respect it is conventionally translated "Lord," ("adonay"), which is substituted for the tetragrammaton and is used exclusively of Yahweh. Yahweh is derived from the imperfect form of the Hebrew verb "to be," expressing the causative: "he who causes [something] to exist."

El and Elohim are parallel and interchangeable terms meaning God. Elohim (plural in form) is the most common word for God in the Hebrew Bible. El, meaning "power, might," is one of the most frequent names for the God of Israel; it is also the title of the head of the Canaanite pantheon. "Elohim," another of the most frequent names for God in the Old Testament, is plural in form (considered a plural of majesty), but it may also be used with reference to a single divine being. It designates the one God of Israel.

Other references to the God of Israel are often defined by a genitive, as in the following examples: YHWH *sebaoth* (Yahweh [God] of hosts), is plural in form and may refer to the armies of Israel, to the heavenly bodies, or to hosts in the sense of enemies; *El Shaddai* (the One of the cosmic mountain, an ancient title of the Deity); *El Elyon* (God most high; the exalted One); *El Olam* (God the eternal; the everlasting God); *El Berit* (God of the covenant). The title "Bull (*'abbir*) of Jacob," a divine epithet, played an important role in ancient Near Eastern religions, including the religion of Israel. Names of animals were often transferred to deities; in the case at hand, the bull, respected for its strength and fertility, was conferred upon Yahweh and translated "the Mighty One of Jacob." "Jacob" was a term of endearment for the chosen people of Yahweh. The earliest appearance in the Bible of this epithet is in Genesis 49:24—"Yet his [Joseph's] bow remained taut, and his arms were made agile by the hands of the Mighty One [literally, the 'Bull'] of Jacob."

Relationship between the Testaments

The Bible makes sense to the degree the reader bears in mind that the Old Testament (Hebrew Scriptures) and the New Testament form an organic unity. There is hardly a single page of the New Testament without an allusion to the Old Testament. With respect to biblical interpretation, a caveat is in order: the New Testament is not necessarily a commentary on the Old Testament, that is to say, Jesus is not to be found on every page of the Old Testament. The Old Testament text is not simply shining in reflected glory; it has rich meaning in its own right. Without the Old Testament, the New Testament is a superstructure suspended in midair. There is both continuity and discontinuity between the Testaments. Jesus is the unifier of the Bible, both Old Testament and New Testament; for example, consider the two great commandments—love of God (Deuteronomy 6:5), and love of neighbor (Leviticus 19:18). These two Old Testament injunctions are combined in the New Testament: "You shall love the Lord your God with all your heart, and with all your soul, and with all your mind, and with all your strength ... You shall love your neighbor as yourself" (Mark 12:30–31; Matthew

22:37–39). Another example is the crucifixion when, in his final agony, Jesus cried out: "Father, into your hands I commend my spirit." (Luke 23:46). This prayer is taken from Psalm 31:5—"Into your hand I commend my spirit." Again, Jesus cried from the cross with a loud voice, praying the words of Psalm 22:1: "*Eli, Eli lema sabachthani?*" ("My God, my God, why have you forsaken me?") (Matthew 27:46; Mark 15:34). Likewise, the prerogatives of the ancient Israelites described in Exodus 19:6 are fittingly applied to the people of the New Testament—"But you are a chosen race, a royal priesthood, a holy nation" (1 Peter 2:9).

The Bible is not a dead letter, but a living Word; to fulfill that definition, the Word must be *lived*. The Bible is replete with lived experiences, not abstract generalizations; the conceptual world of the Bible is concrete, not abstract. The Bible is not the "golden rule"; sinners are everywhere in evidence. After King David had Uriah the Hittite killed by setting him "in the forefront of the hardest fighting," the prophet Nathan confronted him with a story about a rich man who exploited a poor man. David reacted vehemently against such patent injustice. At that point Nathan indicted David with the immortal words: '*attah ha'ish* ("you are the man!") (2 Samuel 12:7).

Instead of plaster-of-Paris or stained-glass-window saints, the Bible features real people, along with all of our foibles. To transfigure human beings (whether in the biblical, political, or ecclesiastical realms) is contrary to nature, and also runs counter to the incarnation of Jesus, who was also human, and by exception, without sin: "We have one who in every respect has been tested as we are, yet without sin" (Hebrews 4:15). Why is it—God became man, and some men want to become God?

[1] Ernst Cassirer, *Language and Myth*, trans. Susanne Langer (New York: Dover Publications, 1953), 8.

[2] Philip Babcock Gove, ed., *Webster's Third New International Dictionary* (unabridged) (Springfield, MA: Miriam-Webster Inc., 1993), 1497.

[3] John McKenzie, "Aspects of Old Testament Thought," in *The New Jerome Biblical Commentary*, ed. by R. Brown, J. Fitzmyer, and R. Murphy (Englewood Cliffs, NJ: Prentice Hall, 1990), 1290.

CHAPTER ONE

A Triad of Virtues: Faith, Hope, Love

IT IS REMARKABLE HOW FREQUENTLY the famous triad—faith, hope, and love—appears in the New Testament Letters: "Therefore, since we are justified by faith, we have peace with God through our Lord Jesus Christ, through whom we have obtained access to this grace in which we stand; and we boast in our hope of sharing the glory of God ... and hope does not disappoint us, because God's love has been poured into our hearts" (Romans 5:1–5). "And now faith, hope, and love abide, these three; and the greatest of these is love" (1 Corinthians 13:13). "We have heard of your faith in Christ Jesus and of the love that you have for all the saints, because of the hope laid up for you in heaven" (Colossians 1:4–5). "Remembering before our God and Father your work of faith and labor of love and steadfastness of hope in our Lord Jesus Christ" (1 Thessalonians 1:3). These are sometimes called "theological virtues" because they are divine gifts and God is their principal object. Not really separate virtues, faith, hope, and love are communal gifts of the Spirit. And they are basic to being "in right relation" to God and neighbor.

Faith: Commitment to Life

Abraham: Our Father in Faith

The "call" of Abraham initiated a series of episodes culminating in the events of Jesus' death and resurrection. Abraham is not merely the ancestor of Jesus; he is also the father of our faith. He is the paradigm for the person of faith. When Abraham heard the voice of Yahweh, it demanded extraordinary courage to respond. When a person determines to follow the divine call, that obedience may cost even one's life.

Abraham (with his wife Sarah) was asked to do something practically unheard of in the ancient world—to leave everything and travel to a new land. He set out upon his journey of faith from the Mesopotamian city of Haran, his ancestral home, en route to the land of Canaan. Genesis 11 starts on a dismal note— the "tower of Babel" story. The people are so divided they are incapable of extricating themselves from their self-made chaos. Then in chapter 12, Yahweh directed Abraham: "Go from your country and your kindred and your father's house to the land that I will show you" (Genesis 12:1). Despite that extraordinary command, the spontaneity of Abraham's response is expressed with majestic simplicity: *wayyelek* ("and he went") (Genesis 12:4). It required incredible generosity for Abraham to follow God in the formidable trials throughout his life.

Biblical Faith

Biblical faith is not a series of propositions either believed or rejected. It is not simply intellectual assent; rather it is a total commitment of life, an engagement of the entire person. Faith is the consequence of a hard-fought struggle in the context of innate human weaknesses: loving, envying, lusting, deceiving, failing, and a host of others. Faith is that trust in God which leads us to follow Yahweh in whatever situation we may find ourselves. Dietrich Bonhoeffer, a notable Protestant theologian, learned that adhering to the divine will may be extremely costly. His fierce opposition to Adolph Hitler and the Nazis climaxed in his hanging in 1945.

Abraham is not described in the Bible as a glorified hero, but as a weak human being, constituted of real flesh and blood. To dehumanize biblical figures is a serious disservice leading to distortion; rendering them surreal puts them beyond the reach of human imitation. The divine call comes to fallible humanity, seldom to spiritual superstars.

Faith is described rather than defined in the Bible. The Hebrew Bible does not actually have a noun equivalent to our English word "faith." However, the transitive verb *he'emin*, from which our well-known word "amen" is derived, means simply to be certain about something or someone. New Testament faith (*pistis*) is not unlike that of the Old Testament; in both cases faith is essentially a response to God. A commitment that must be continually renewed is what renders faith complete. The greatest resource in troublesome times is faith, a trust in and dependence upon God.

In consideration of Abraham's faith, Genesis 15 adds an important note: "And he believed the Lord; and the Lord reckoned it to him as righteousness" (verse 6), that is, it expresses the right attitude of humankind toward God. It is what Yahweh expects Abraham to do. The New Testament (Romans 4:1–25; Galatians 3:6–9; Hebrews 11:8–12) makes Abraham's faith a model for Christians.

Abraham's Inspiring Obedience

Genesis 22 should be considered in conjunction with Genesis 15:6, inasmuch as both are about biblical faith. With restraint and simplicity, Genesis 22 relates the story of Abraham's heroic act of faith; out of obedience he was prepared to sacrifice Isaac, his firstborn. The key to the incident is: "God *tested* Abraham" (Genesis 22:1). He was directed to take "his son, his only son, the son whom he loved" and offer him as a holocaust on a hill. En route, Abraham carried the dangerous objects—the fire and the knife—while his son Isaac carried the less-threatening wood, a manifestation of the father's solicitous love for his son. "And they went on together," apparently in painful silence, although it would not be difficult to imagine their private thoughts as they approached the place of holocaust. As Abraham was about to plunge the knife into his son, an angel of God called to Abraham, "Do not lay your hand on the boy ... for now I know that you fear God, since you have not withheld your son, your only son from me" (Genesis 22:12). Faith is magnificently portrayed in this story of Abraham being *tested* by God. This story of Abraham and Isaac attests that faith is a journey, even when the way is not clear.

Faith in the New Testament

In response to the question of Thomas (the "doubter"), Jesus makes it certain that he is the focus of Christian faith in the New Testament—"I am the way, and the truth, and the life. No one comes to the Father except through me" (John 14:6). In addition, John tells us that his Gospel was written "so that you may come to believe that Jesus is the Messiah, the Son of God, and that through believing you may have life in his name" (John 20:31).

"Affirmations of Faith"

Certain Psalms are classified as "affirmations of faith" because they forcibly express a firm trust in God. Psalm 23, a masterpiece of simplicity and beauty, is an "affirmation of faith" in God's loving care. The Psalm is a diptych wherein God's servant is portrayed under the figures of a shepherd solicitous for his sheep, and a munificent host anxious for his guest. On his pilgrimage through life, the psalmist asks for absolutely nothing—"The Lord is my shepherd, I shall not want" (Psalm 23:1). The Psalm begins and ends on a note of profound gratitude for the immeasurable goodness of God. Verses 4 and 5 make it evident that the psalmist had many bitter experiences in the course of life. He alludes in verse 4 to the treacherous ravines where the wild beasts and marauders lurk; in verse 5 he calls attention to his enemies. The Psalm closes with the assurance that divine goodness and kindness (*hesed*) will pursue the psalmist all the days of his life.

No one has described the faith of Abraham more concisely than the author of the Letter to the Hebrews:

By faith Abraham obeyed when he was called to set out for a place that he was to receive as an inheritance; and he set out, not knowing where he was going. By faith he stayed for a time in a land he had been promised, as in a foreign land, living in tents, as did Isaac and Jacob, who were heirs with him of the same promise. For he looked forward to the city that has foundations, whose architect and builder is God. By faith he received power of procreation, even though he was too old—and Sarah herself was barren—because he considered him faithful who had promised. (Hebrews 11:8–11)

5

Yahweh: The Hope of Israel/ Christ Jesus: Our Hope

Faith and hope are inseparable virtues in the Bible; in both Old Testament and New Testament an atmosphere of hope permeates the Bible. However, no single word is adequate to express the reality of biblical hope. "Let us hold fast to the confession of our hope (Greek, *elpis, elpidos*) without wavering, for he who has promised is faithful (Greek, *pistos*)" (Hebrews 10:23).

Throughout the Old Testament, God is acknowledged as the "hope of Israel" (Jeremiah 14:8). The motive for hope in the Old Testament is the past deeds of Yahweh; in the New Testament it is the resurrection of Jesus Christ. "By his great mercy he has given us a new birth into a *living hope* through the resurrection of Jesus Christ from the dead" (1 Peter 1:3). In the words of Paul, God can be called simply the "God of hope" (Romans 15:13).

Hope in the New Testament

In the New Testament, the concept is most fully developed in the Pauline Letters, especially Romans. In addition, the theology of hope appears in these passages: 1 Thessalonians 2–5; 1 and 2 Corinthians; Galatians; Philippians; and Philemon, as well as John 13:33, 36. The Letter to the Hebrews declares: "We have this hope, a sure and steadfast *anchor* of the soul" (Hebrews 6:19). This image symbolizing hope was often used in the New Testament world.

Today's world is in a desperate situation, not unlike the tragic conditions of Israel's final days, witnessed by the eighth century BCE Prophets (Isaiah, Amos). A message of hope was desperately needed then, and it assuredly is needed now. The Northern Kingdom (Israel) was on the verge of collapse, and the Southern Kingdom (Judah) was not far behind. Despite the turbulence of their times, the eighth-century prophets preached a message of hope.

Amos' harsh severity and Micah's stern proclamations may obscure their assurances of hope, nonetheless they are there. The message of hope is more transparent in Isaiah, while Hosea proclaims the words of hope more loudly. He proclaimed the possibility of a "new beginning" after the judgment. He underscored God's new saving acts in all ages, and this is precisely the message today's world needs to hear. It is no wonder that Hosea is regarded as the "prophet of hope," just as, in the New Testament, John is the "evangelist of hope." When Paul speaks of "hoping against hope" (Romans 4:18), he is emphasizing the extraordinary trust that Abraham invested in the promises God had bestowed upon him. The Pauline Letters encompass the broadest use of the words for "hope" and the most developed concept of this virtue.

Hope and Faith

The connection between hope and faith is very close. "Faith is the assurance of things *hoped* for, the conviction of things not seen" (Hebrews 11:1). "Through him [Christ] you have come to trust in God, who raised him from the dead and gave him glory, so that your faith and hope are set on God" (1 Peter 1:21). Rightly, 1 Peter is called the letter of hope.

As mentioned, Hebrew lacks a word corresponding to "hope." In both the Old Testament and New Testament, no single word is adequate for expressing the reality of *hope* which is translated by several Hebrew words. Hope is closely related to *trust* in God. Hope is a relational word, and our relationship with God is the ultimate basis for hope. Hope is confident expectation of what is to come; the Exodus, the Sinai Covenant, and the Conquest of Canaan are the grounds for Israel's confidence in God. "And now, O Lord, what do I wait for? My hope is in you" (Psalm 39:7). "For surely I [Yahweh] know the plans I have for you, says the Lord, plans for your welfare and not for harm, to give you a future with hope" (Jeremiah 29:11). True hope is always directed to God.

The Syro-Ephraimite War

The Civil War which engaged the Northern and Southern Kingdoms, also known as the Syro-Ephraimite War, may have been the occasion for Hosea's frequent messages of hope. This war, which pitted the Southern Kingdom of Judah against a coalition composed of Damascus (Syria) and Israel (Ephraim), was fought to pressure Judah into joining Damascus and Israel so as to prevent the expansion of the Assyrian empire. It was a tumultuous time—the collapse of the Northern Kingdom was imminent; the Assyrian imperialists were on their relentless march westward. Internecine warfare is the most heinous form of hostility; no animosity can match the enmity between family members and close neighbors, as the Jews and Samaritans of Jesus' time attest. The Israelites of the North and the Judahites of the South, kinsfolk and acquaintances, nurtured the same degree of hostility toward each other. In contrast, according to Hosea's oracle of salvation, "Yet the number of the people of Israel shall be like the sand of the sea, which can be neither measured nor numbered...The people of Judah and the people of Israel shall be gathered together [reunited]" (Hosea 1:10–11).

"The Door of Hope"

Hosea 2:14–23 is another salvation oracle, expressed in the language of courtship; it is a promise of reconciliation and renewal of covenant. The setting is the wilderness (*midbar*), understood not simply as a geographical region, but as an idyllic age. The desert represents the time when Israel was closest to God. Hosea develops this proclamation in terms of his own marital experience (marriage–divorce–remarriage).

In developing the theme of a "second exodus" as part of this salvation oracle, Hosea refers to the valley of Achor as the "door of hope." "Achor," the Hebrew word for "trouble," refers to the wilderness area three miles west of the Dead Sea and identified with the modern el-Buqeah ("the valley plain"). In this desert region Achan and his family were put to death by stoning, followed by burning, in the time of Joshua, for disregarding the command of Yahweh to take no spoils from Jericho. Because of Achan's transgression, Israel failed in its military attack on the city of Ai. After Achan's death, the Israelites succeeded in conquering the land of Canaan.

In the Iron Age (1200–538 BCE), the Buqeah served as an access route from the land of Moab (in Transjordan) to Jerusalem. Hence Hosea could refer literally to the valley of Achor (the Buqeah) as the "door of hope." The Valley of Achor, once an obstacle to the Israelites' entry into the Promised Land, was to become a gateway, a "door of hope." *Petah tiqvah*, Hebrew for "door of hope," is the name of a modern city on Israel's coastal plain, located 12 miles from Tel Aviv. Settled in 1878 by observant

Jews from Jerusalem, Petah Tikva (modern spelling) was the first Jewish village in Palestine. When the State of Israel was established in 1947 following the Holocaust (*Shoah*), quite naturally the title chosen for Israel's national anthem was *Ha-tiqvah* ("the hope").

Salvation Oracles

Hosea 11:10–11, an additional promise of hope, represents Yahweh's calling home the weary people of Israel. "They shall go after the Lord, who roars like a lion; when he roars, his children shall come trembling from the west. They shall come trembling like birds from Egypt, and like doves from the land of Assyria; and I will return them to their homes, says the Lord."

The final announcement of salvation (Hosea 14:2–9) brings the Book of Hosea to a close. This oracle makes it clear that a great tragedy (perhaps the surrender of the Northern Kingdom in 722–721 BCE) had already happened. Now, Yahweh desired to make a new covenant to achieve national restoration. As the first step in covenant renewal, Hosea summoned the wayward people to return (*shub*) to their original relationship with Yahweh. The verb *shub* ("to return") and the substantive *teshubah* ("a return") have profound theological implications in Hosea; they require repentance and reorientation (changing the course) of one's life. Repentance and acknowledgment of sin are the basic requirements for redemption. The redeemed Israelites are prepared to place their trust in Yahweh alone. Reliance on international treaties with the Assyrians and other treacherous neighbors was to no avail, and military might had also been futile. The same irony is present today, when nations seek peace by arming themselves mightily; the more sophisticated the weaponry, the more the arms race escalates. Yahweh alone, who has a special concern for the "little people" of society—in this case the parentless Israelites, or "orphans"—can help these helpless people. Yahweh, the loving parent, has come to the aid of ancient Israel. With unshakeable faith, Hosea knew that what Yahweh had done in the "first exodus" Yahweh would do again in the "second exodus." Hosea was convinced that people needed only to have confidence in the love and mercy of God. In our day, that conviction is still the best antidote to discouragement and despair.

The Gospel Today

Through daily visits to a local coffee house, I have come to know several people—good people—some of whom have experienced many personal tragedies along life's bumpy journey. Chatting with them over coffee, I have become more aware of the addictions that plague them. Each conversation ends with their voicing the conviction that hope alone is their sole anchor. "Truly the eye of the Lord [that is, "divine providence"] is on those who fear him, on those who *hope* in his steadfast love (*hesed*)" (Psalm 33:18).

Psalms of Hope

The Psalter (Book of Psalms) will be treated in more detail below, but in the context of "hope," it is worthwhile to consider briefly four Psalms (among others) that address the issue of hope. These Psalms (25, 31, 39, 130) are included under the category of "individual laments/complaints." This genre is the most frequent type in the Psalter. It may seem ironic that the Psalter is known in Hebrew as *Seper Tehillim* ("Book of Praises"), despite the fact that laments outnumber praises. Perhaps there are more occasions in life to lament than to praise; after all, the Book of Psalms mirrors life. Individual psalms cannot be rigidly squeezed into a category, but certain of their characteristics define laments. Invariably, they include a description of the lament/complaint that is distressing the psalmist, followed by a prayer for help, a profession of confidence in God, and a promise to praise God.

"Lead me in your truth, and teach me, for you are the God of my salvation; for you I *wait* (*"hope"*) all day long" (Psalm 25:5). This Psalm is a prayer for deliverance from enemies.

"Love the Lord, all you his saints. The Lord preserves the faithful, but abundantly repays the one who acts haughtily. Be strong, and let your heart take courage, all you who wait [*"hope"*] for the Lord" (Psalm 31:23–24). This Psalm, composed by a person in deep distress, emphasizes God's faithfulness and steadfast love (*hesed*), echoing the prophet Jeremiah in his "Confessions." Because it is so easy for us to lose our first fervor and initial enthusiasm, the psalmist encourages us always to be faithful. Christians, especially, cherish Psalm 31 because, according to Luke 23:46, it is the source of Jesus' prayer on the cross: "Into your hand I commend my spirit" (see Psalm 31:5).

"And now, O Lord, what do I *wait* for? My *hope* is in you" (Psalm 39:7). (In due course I shall make the distinction between the primary Hebrew roots for *wait* and *hope*.) The psalmist is suffering alone and in silence; the nature of his pain is not divulged. We all have our own reason to make this Psalm *our* prayer; and with the psalmist, each can declare confidently: "My hope is in God (and God alone)."

Christians, especially, can resonate with the psalmist, who was suffering in silence, and praying alone, as alluded to in the story of Philip and the Ethiopian eunuch: "Now the passage of the scripture that he [the eunuch] was reading was this: 'Like a sheep he was led to the slaughter, and like a lamb silent before its shearer, so he does not open his mouth'" (Acts 8:32). This verse is taken from the prophet Isaiah in his description of the Suffering Servant of Yahweh. "He was oppressed, and he was afflicted, yet he did not open his mouth; like a lamb that is led to the slaughter, and like a sheep that before its shearers is silent, so he did not open his mouth" (Isaiah 53:7). Like the psalmist, we must live with *hope* in a hopeless world.

"My soul *waits* for the Lord more than those who watch for the morning, more than those who watch for the morning. O Israel, *hope* in the Lord! For with the Lord there is steadfast love, and with him is great power to redeem" (Psalm 130:6–7). This is one of the seven Penitential Psalms featured in the lenten liturgy of the medieval church. Known as "De Profundis" (Out of the Depths) from its introductory words, this Psalm is a prayer for the departed faithful. "Depths" refers to the "deep waters," or the "waters of chaos," or the "abode of the dead." The psalmist is in profound distress, until he resolves to hope in Yahweh, and at the same time appealing for divine mercy. The Hebrew verb *yahal*, "to hope," is synonymous with "to wait." It has been observed that *yahal* suggests a waiting characterized by expectant *hope*.

"You Shall Love the Lord Your God with All Your Heart, and with All Your Soul, and with All Your Mind, and with All Your Strength...You Shall Love Your Neighbor as Yourself" (Mark 12:30–31)

Love dominates the relationship between God and humanity. It is said that "love [charity] is the grandest theme of Scripture," the virtue that pervades the Bible. Love includes the relationships of friendship, sex, covenant, loyalty, kindness, mercy. A rich vocabulary in both Hebrew (Old Testament) and Greek (New Testament) underscores the variety of meanings of love. The following are Hebrew words for "love," each with a slightly different connotation: The word for "womb" is *rehem*, and the adjective is *rahum*, denoting the kind of love a mother has for her child. Designating "loving kindness," the adjective *rahum* is used in the Bible only of God. "Can a woman forget her nursing child, or show no compassion (*merahem*) for the child of her womb? Even these may forget, yet I [Yahweh] will not forget you" (Isaiah 49:15). Nowhere in the Old Testament, except in Jeremiah 31:20, is Yahweh's love for the people of Israel so sensitively expressed. "Is Ephraim [the Northern Kingdom of Israel] my dear son? Is he the child I delight in? As often as I speak against him, I still remember him. Therefore I am deeply moved for him; I will surely have mercy (*rahem 'arahamenu*) on him, says the Lord." In a classic profession of faith, we read: "The Lord, the Lord, a God merciful (*rahum*) and gracious" (Exodus 34:6).

A general verb for "love" in the Old Testament is *'aheb*, meaning "to choose someone to love"; the cognate noun is *'ahaba*, "love." It is used frequently to describe the attraction of one person to a member of the opposite sex. There are many examples: "Jacob loved Rachel" (Genesis 29:18); "Michal loved David" (1 Samuel 18:20); Amnon loved Tamar (2 Samuel 13:1). Isaac brought Rebekah into his mother Sarah's tent, "and she became his wife; and he loved her [sexual connotation]" (Genesis 24:67). One of my favorite biblical verses is Isaiah 41:8, where Yahweh refers to Abraham as *'ohabi*, "my [dearly beloved] friend." In sum, *'ahaba* is love pure and simple.

The indestructibility of God's love for his people is nowhere so sympathetically portrayed as in the prophet Hosea: "When Israel was a child, I loved him [*'ohabehu*, election verb]; out of Egypt I called [*qara'ti*, election verb, "to summon into a relationship"] my son" (Hosea 11:1). The prophet describes poignantly the love of a father for his son (here, it is Yahweh's love for Ephraim [Israel]).

The Sinai covenant is called a covenant of love—"Know therefore that the Lord your God is God, the faithful God who maintains covenant loyalty with those who love him (*'ohabayw*) and keep his commandments" (Deuteronomy 7:9).

Hesed, the Untranslatable Virtue

Hesed, appearing 250 times in the Hebrew Bible, is the principal term for expressing God's relationship to Israel; also, it is the quality of life most desirable in a person. Often translated "loving kindness," "steadfast love," "mercy," the Hebrew word *hesed* is actually untranslatable. These English equivalents do not express all the nuances included in *hesed*. For that reason, we shall use the Hebrew form throughout, while suggesting the implications behind it in specific contexts. *Hesed* corresponds in both importance and meaning to agape in the New Testament. I was fortunate early in my academic career to have come under

15

the influence of Harvard professor G. Ernest Wright, my mentor, from whom I learned so much about both Biblical Archaeology and the Bible. With regard to the Bible, I gained from him a great insight into the meaning of "the Bible for the modern age." That is especially true with regard to *hesed*, Wright's favorite biblical virtue. He never tried to define *hesed*, but he described it in an inspiring way:

> [It concerns] a great-hearted person, usually one older or superior to me in some way, who for some mysterious reason ... does a gracious, loving deed, or shows a special favor to me. Each of us is what he is today ... because of such gracious gifts of love, friendship, assistance, which we did not deserve and had no right to expect. In most cases there can be no question of repayment. We can only learn the art of humble, grateful acceptance. Yet such an act of love pulls me to the giver of love. A bond is created, and I am led to respond in love. The gift of the giver implants a loving response in me. Love then is both a gift and a response. And to betray the bond thus created is instinctively felt to be the most heartless, faithless, and scandalous of personal actions ... The relationship between God and the people in the Bible is of this type. *Hesed* is what God has done to us ... and is what we owe him in return.[1]

The Hebrew *hen* and the Greek *charis* may be rendered "grace" or "favor." It is the outpouring of goodness and kindness that expects no return. Normally one-directional love, it is the generous act. They bear some relationship to *hesed*, except that *hesed* is always two-directional.

The key verse in Hosea reads: "For I desire steadfast love (*hesed*) and not sacrifice (*zebah*), and knowledge (*da'at*) of God rather than burnt offerings (*'olot*)" (Hosea 6:6). Hosea draws a poetic parallel between the two substantives *hesed* and *da'at*, with one defining the other.

All that has been said thus far about *hesed* is applicable to *da'at* ("knowledge"), which far transcends intellectual apprehension. It is knowledge of the heart, far more than knowledge of the mind. To know God is to respond in faithful love. The verb *yada'*, used in reference to close personal relations, means "to know" in the sense "to experience," "to realize," "to appreciate." Older translations of the Bible referred to marital relations as partners *knowing* each other. In the context of marriage, "to know" is an apt description. It is a knowledge possessed only in a personal relationship that involves the entire existence of the knower. To "know God" (*da'at 'elohim*) is to respond to God in faithful love. Hosea's lesson for the community of Israel is: love and loyalty are preferred to sacrificial meals. In other words, integrity of life is more important than ritual sacrifices. In the New Testament, at the arrest of Jesus, Peter disclaimed any "knowledge" of Jesus, protesting "I do not know the man [Jesus]" (see Matthew 26:69–75). That denial was tantamount to saying: "This person means absolutely nothing to me; he has no claim on my devotion."

The *Shema'*

From pre-Christian times to the present, devout Jews have recited, morning and evening, the great profession of faith, known as the *Shema'* (imperative of the Hebrew verb "to hear"). In this context, it really means "to hear first and then to obey"; a love to be expressed by obedience to the commandments. Both the rabbis and Jesus regarded this concise summary as the heart of the Law. "Hear (*shema'*) O Israel: The Lord is our

God, the Lord alone. You shall love (*'ahabta*) the Lord your God with all your heart, and with all your soul, and with all your might" (Deuteronomy 6:4–5). On an equal plane is the second great commandment: "You shall love (*'ahabta*) your neighbor as yourself" (Leviticus 19:18); "to love" meaning "to be useful," "to be helpful." No narcissism intended here! We are not asked to *feel* love, but to *do* love.

Jesus and the Neighbor

Jesus taught a Jewish lawyer what it means to be a generous neighbor by recounting the story of the "Good Samaritan" (Luke 10:25–37). In New Testament times, Samaritans were members of an ethno-religious community resident in the district of Samaria, the central hill country of Palestine. Despite a common heritage, the Jews (especially the Pharisees) and the Samaritans had sharp differences, particularly concerning the relative sanctity of Jerusalem/Zion and Mount Gerizim, as well as the interpretation of the Torah. When Jesus sent forth the twelve apostles, he instructed them: "Enter no town of the Samaritans" (Matthew 10:5). When Jesus cleansed ten lepers, only the Samaritan, not the Jewish priest or the Levite, returned to express gratitude, and the Samaritan was a "foreigner" (*allogenes*), that is, "not of the house of Israel" (Luke 17:18).

The evangelist Luke recounts that when a traveler was beaten and robbed, a passing Samaritan demonstrated mercy and compassion. After a Jewish priest and a Levite had passed by, oblivious of the man who fell prey to robbers, a Samaritan came along, and was "moved with pity." He dressed the victim's wounds, pouring in oil and wine; he then brought him to an inn and cared for him. Jesus asked the lawyer: "Which of these three, do you think, was a neighbor to the man who fell into the hands of the robbers?" The lawyer answered: "The one who showed him mercy (*eleos*)." Jesus said to him: "*Go and do likewise*" (Luke 10:36–37).

This parable of mercy is even more poignant when we realize that Jews and Samaritans hated each other as only close neighbors can. No one has to be reminded of the long-lasting enmity when family members have a falling out. It is much easier to love someone seldom seen than one encountered regularly at home or at the workplace. The antipathy existing far too long between the Jews and the Arabs in the Middle East is a parade example. An equally hostile environment prevails among the Muslim branches (Shiites, Sunnis, Kurds) in Iraq; sectarian violence is tearing them apart.

Jesus' attitude is always inclusive and nondiscriminatory. A major problem dividing Americans recently centers on immigration; rhetoric shouts down reason. This and similar problems are not easy to resolve, but then the gospel lesson, specifically the story of the Good Samaritan, was never meant to be easy.

The New Testament and Love

No New Testament writer is associated with the word "love" (*agape*) more than John, the apostle of love, especially in his First Letter [Exhortation]. The second section of this Letter (1 John 3:11–5:12) deals with the obligation of mutual love; Christians must love one another. The following are selected texts about *agape* from this First Letter of John: "We know love (*agape*) by this, that he [Jesus] laid down his life for us—and we ought to lay down our lives for one another" (1 John 3:16). "Beloved, let us love one another, because love is from God; everyone who loves

19

is born of God and knows God. Whoever does not love does not know God, for God is love (*agape*)" (1 John 4:7–8). "God is love (*agape*), and those who abide in love abide in God, and God abides in them" (1 John 4:16). "We love (*agapomen*) because he first loved us. Those who say, 'I love God,' and hate their brothers or sisters, are liars" (1 John 4:19–20). The centrality of *love* in the Johannine writings (the Fourth Gospel and the Three Letters) could not be stated more clearly.

John 3:16 is often referred to as "a miniature Gospel"—"For God so loved the world that he gave his only Son, so that everyone who believes in him may not perish but may have eternal life." Jesus' new commandment requires that his disciples love one another: "I give you a new commandment, that you love one another. Just as I have loved you, you also should love one another. By this everyone will know that you are my disciples, if you have love for one another" (John 13:34–35). The disciples' mutual love should be the same as Jesus' love for them. Johannine love is not an abstract emotion, but the concrete acts of love that are the underpinnings of society.

Greek has four verbs expressing the primary senses of "love"—*stergo* and *erao* are not found in the New Testament; *phileo* and *agapao* are. In John's Gospel the latter two are used synonymously. During a resurrection appearance in Galilee, Jesus asked Simon Peter three times: "Simon, son of John, do you love me?" After the third inquiry, Peter, slightly offended, answered: "You know that I love you" (John 21:15–17). In Jesus' first two questions, the verb is *agapao*; the third time, the verb is *phileo*, the most common word for "love." In each of Peter's responses, the verb is *phileo*. The difference between these two verbs is inconsequential.

Luke's instruction on the love of one's enemies is classic—"Love your enemies, do good to those who hate you, bless those who curse you, pray for those who abuse you" (Luke 6:27–28). Most of us can attest this is more easily said than done, and it may take a very long time to realize.

Paul and Love

The apostle Paul has bequeathed the most elegant portrayal of love in his great discourse (1 Corinthians 13:1–13). He lists the charisms (tongues, prophecy, knowledge, faith, self-sacrifice) that have value only when informed by love (13:1–3). Paul then enumerates the positive qualities of love, defining each by what it does or does not do (13:4–7). Paul proclaims the permanence of love and its superiority over other virtues (13:8–13). Of faith, hope, and love, the greatest gift is love.

[1] G. Ernest Wright, *The Rule of God* (Garden City, NY: Doubleday, 1960), 119–120.

CHAPTER TWO

Addressing God in Prayer

Attributes of God

In the Bible, the attributes of God are, in reality, all words portraying relations among persons. Israel's greatest liturgical confession, composed solely of the divine attributes, appears in Exodus 34:6–7:

> The Lord passed before him [Moses], and proclaimed, "The Lord, the Lord, a God merciful (*rahum*) and gracious (*hannun*), slow to anger, and abounding in steadfast love (*hesed*) and faithfulness (*'emet*), keeping steadfast love (*hesed*) for the thousandth generation, forgiving iniquity and transgression and sin, yet by no means clearing the guilty, but visiting the iniquity of the parents upon the children and the children's children, to the third and the fourth generation."

Here we have a valuable insight into the complexities of the divine character: God is generous and forgiving on the

one hand; on the other, God will not pardon covenant violations, but will impose sanctions on the community of Israel in
future generations. How to solve the apparent contradiction in
the divine nature? There is no easy answer, except to point out
that seven attributes support the positive side, and only two
the negative side.

"Merciful" (*rahum*) is an adjective used only in relation to
God. As already suggested, this is the kind of loving solicitude
that a mother manifests toward the child in the womb (*rehem*).
"Gracious" (*hannun*), suggesting unmerited favor, is kindness
that expects nothing in return. Again, the adjective *hannun* is
used only of God. "Slow to anger" is the literal equivalent of
"long-nosed" in Hebrew. The Hebrew term (*'ap*) denoting "anger"
means "nostril," thought to be the locale of anger; it may be associated with angry snorting. (God's abiding *hesed*, "steadfast love,"
has already been discussed in chapter 1.) "Faithfulness" (*'emet*)
suggests God's total reliability and is defined as abiding *hesed*; it
is the longevity of love. *Hesed* and *'emet* often appear together in
the Bible, as in the Christological formula found in the Prologue
of the Fourth Gospel: "The glory as of a father's only son, full
of *grace and truth*" (John 1:14); "grace and truth came through
Jesus Christ" (John 1:17). The Hebrew verb to "forgive" is *nasa',*
very common in the Old Testament; literally it means "to lift up,"
"to carry." God lifts the burden of sin, and herein is the root of
forgiveness. A caveat—God will not acquit the guilty, but will
impose sanctions.

Anger in the Bible

The frequent references to anger, human and divine, in the Old
and New Testaments can be a source of bewilderment to the

faithful who read the Bible for edification. Only an informed appreciation of biblical times and the people's mentality can restore confidence in the Word of God. The Hebrews were people of their own generations; they were part of the cultural legacy of the ancient Near East.

Some solve the problem of God's anger by recourse to an outmoded and erroneous thesis—that the God of the Old Testament is an angry God, and the God of the New Testament is a loving God. That supposition is fallacious; both Testaments attest to the presence of both human and divine anger. How then to resolve the problem? The following perceptions may be helpful.

The ancient peoples of the Bible conceived of God in human terms. The attribution of human behavior and characteristics to nonhumans is called anthropomorphism; the ascription of human feelings and emotions to nonhumans is known as anthropopathism. The biblical writers always speak of Yahweh in terms of human traits.

Anger is as much of a human emotion as love; it is but one feature of God's person. The epithet "the living God" suggests the measure of commonality existing between God and human beings. In contrast to lifeless deities, Yahweh is characterized as "the living God."

The great profession of faith that we have just read, the only one in the Old Testament composed solely of the divine attributes, places anger in distinctive relationship with the other divine qualities. Also, it reveals much about the character of God:

The Lord passed before him [Moses], and proclaimed, "The Lord, the Lord, a God merciful and gracious, slow to anger, and abounding in steadfast love and faithfulness, keeping steadfast love for the thousandth generation, forgiving iniquity and transgression and sin, yet by no means clearing the guilty, but visiting the iniquity of the parents upon the children and the children's children, to the third and the fourth generation." (Exodus 34:6–7)

God's anger was kindled against Moses when he attempted to defect from his commission to lead the Israelites out of Egypt. "But he [Moses] said, 'O my Lord, please send someone else.' Then the anger of the Lord was kindled against Moses" (Exodus 4:13–14).

The anger of the Lord was ignited whenever the Israelites rebelled and rejected Yahweh. "Now when the people complained in the hearing of the Lord about their misfortunes [in the wilderness], the Lord heard it and his anger was kindled" (Numbers 11:1). Yahweh's anger was a response to sin; there was a direct connection between Yahweh's anger and sin. "They [Israelites] angered the Lord at the waters of Meribah, and it went ill with Moses on their account" (Psalm 106:32).

The words of the psalmist regarding the duration of divine anger are encouraging. "For his anger is but for a moment; his favor is for a lifetime" (Psalm 30:5).

Divine wrath is related to covenant violations; it was the covenant that cemented the relationship between God and the people of Israel. The principal cause for divine anger was Israel's failure to observe the terms of the covenant.

The New Testament offers some admonitions about divine anger. "But I [Jesus] say to you that if you are angry with a brother or sister, you will be liable to judgment" (Matthew 5:22).

"Whoever believes in the Son has eternal life; whoever disobeys the Son will not see life, but must endure God's wrath" (John 3:36).

The Psalms: The Bible in Miniature

The Psalter (Book of Psalms) is a summary of all the themes in the Bible. It is also known as the prayerbook of Jesus; as an observant Jew, he prayed the Psalms daily. Many people, even though they may not read the Bible regularly, do have some familiarity with the Psalms. As mentioned earlier, Dietrich Bonhoeffer, a Protestant theologian, was notable for his opposition to the Nazis, which resulted in his execution. From his prison cell in May 1943, he wrote: "I am reading the psalms daily, as I have done for years. I know them and love them more than any other book in the Bible."[1] Dag Hammarskjold, secretary-general of the United Nations, always took three items with him on his travels around the world—the Psalms, the New Testament, and the United Nations Charter. They were recovered from his briefcase after the plane crash that took his life in September 1961. He understood that the Psalter conveys God's will for justice, righteousness, and peace among all peoples and nations. When David Jacobsen, an American held hostage in Lebanon, was released in November 1986, he gave a message to those still confined, "a message that served me [Jacobsen] well." It is the final verses of Psalm 27—"I believe that I shall see the goodness of the Lord in the land of the living. Wait for the Lord; be strong, and let your heart take courage; wait for the Lord!" (Psalm 27:13–14). One further example: in March 1977, the Soviet government released Anatoly Shcharansky, a young Jewish mathematician and leader of the "refuseniks," who had spent the previous nine years in Soviet prisons and work camps. Shortly before his release, Shcharansky's guards confiscated his copy of the Psalms. He protested, lying in the snow and refusing to move, until his Book of Psalms was returned. He relates that in prison, from morning to evening, he read and studied all 150 Hebrew Psalms.

Types of Psalms

Our English word "psalm" is derived from Greek *psalmos*, meaning a "song accompanied by a stringed instrument." Biblical scholars have identified a variety of literary forms among the Psalms—basically, hymns of praise, laments (complaints), and thanksgivings. The Book of Psalms is designated in Hebrew as *tehillim*, "praises," despite that "laments" outnumber "praises" in the Psalter. Again, it may be that there are more occasions to lament than to praise in the course of every life. The basic idea behind the verb "to praise" is to speak well of someone or something. Most praise in the Bible is corporate, a summons to praise Yahweh, demonstrated by the continuous use of the verb *hll*, "to praise" in the plural form. The happiness of acknowledging God's greatness is to be shared by all people (Psalm 65:1–2).

Hymns of praise are tripartite in structure, consisting of an invocation, reasons for praise, and a final note of praise. Laments begin with a plea to Yahweh for help and are followed by a description of the psalmist's suffering, such as illness, persecution, or sin.

The Psalms as Prayers

The Psalter teaches one to pray, and at the same time contains prayers readily adaptable to our present needs. The Psalms, essentially poetic prayers, are not only a record of past events but a living voice speaking of the present human condition. Every mood of the human heart is expressed in the Psalms: complaint and praise, repentance and sinlessness, pessimism and optimism, sorrow and joy, hate and love. Who has not experienced these contradictory emotions! The Psalms do relate to every life, ancient and modern, since they are intensely human. I suspect that the Roman Breviary, an adaptation composed in large measure of psalms, is unfortunately a "turn off" for many readers because of the frequent emotional shifts in the course of each day's recitation. It is unrealistic to think one can be joyful at one moment and sorrowful at the next. At the same time, it is helpful to remember that the Psalms are liturgical compositions, composed for worship, and not simply isolated prayers.

Selected Psalms

Psalm 1, the prologue to the entire Psalter, answers the question of how life is to be lived. It contrasts the two ways of life: the way of the righteous (verses 1–3), a life that makes the love of *torah* (God's instruction to Israel) the basis for one's existence; and the way of the wicked (verses 4–5), a life lived apart from Yahweh, which is empty and meaningless. The two ways are reminiscent of the wide and narrow gate in the Gospel of Matthew: "Enter through the narrow gate; for the gate is wide and the road is easy that leads to destruction, and there are many who take it. For the gate is narrow and the road is hard that leads to life, and there are few who find it" (Matthew 7:13–14).

The organizing principle of this introductory Psalm is *torah*, the basic term for "law" in the Hebrew Bible, connoting instruction, guidance, direction, but definitely not legalism. The placement of this Psalm at the beginning of the Psalter indicates that the whole work is a book of instruction (*torah*).

Three clauses in Psalm 1 form a synonymous parallelism: the "wicked who walk" (follow their own advice rather than divine guidance); the "sinners who stand" (share the sinners' way of life); and the "scoffers who sit" (refuse to accept divine instruction). These wrongdoers are the antitheses of the righteous. To "delight" and to "meditate" on *torah* is not merely a cognitive exercise but also has an affective dimension. This Psalm calls for lifetime study, not merely casual reading. The godly person is compared with a well-watered, luxuriant tree, whereas the wicked person is like worthless chaff blown away by the wind.

Psalm 117, the shortest of the Psalms, is a classic example of the hymn of praise. It opens and closes with an invitation to praise: *halelu-yah*, "praise Yah (Yahweh)." The middle portion, introduced by the Hebrew word *ki*, "for," gives the reasons for praise—Yahweh's *hesed*, "steadfast love," and *'emet*, "faithfulness" toward Israel.

Psalm 27. The psalmist's longing for the temple—"to live in the house of the Lord all the days of my life" (Psalm 27:4)—makes Psalm 27 a personal favorite. Psalm 27:7–14 is an individual lament; it begins with a cry for help: *shema'*, "Hear, O Lord"; then it follows the complaint detailing the present problem; afterward a statement of trust ensues; finally a declaration of praise. The psalmist has been unjustly accused and consequently has become an outcast even from his family because he is considered guilty. He is lonely and forsaken. In contrast, the Psalm ends with a conviction of faith, hope, and courage: "I believe that I shall see the goodness of the Lord in the land of the living. Wait for the Lord; be strong, and let your heart take courage; wait for the Lord!" (verses 13–14).

Psalm 34 is classified as an individual thanksgiving, consisting of three principal parts. It opens with a hymn praising Yahweh, and at the same time inviting others to join in (verses 1–3). The second part (verses 4–10) is a testimony to Yahweh's goodness. In the third section (verses 11–22), the psalmist assumes the didactic role of the Wisdom teacher, expounding on the meaning of the "fear of Yahweh." Thanksgivings resemble hymns of praise in that they elaborate all the good things Yahweh has done. This is the Hebrew way of saying "thank you." Our "thank you" does not have an equivalent in biblical Hebrew, although it does in modern Hebrew.

Psalm 137, an individual lament accompanied by a community concern, has been described as a Psalm of love and hate: love for Jerusalem, hate for enemies (Babylonians and Edomites), who rejoiced over the destruction, in 586 BCE, of Jerusalem and the temple. This is considered a beautiful Psalm—"By the rivers of Babylon [Tigris and Euphrates]—there we sat down and there we wept when we remembered Zion [Jerusalem]" (verse 1)—except for the third and final section (verses 7–9), where a blessing is pronounced on Israel's enemies: "Happy shall they be who take your little ones and bash them against the rock!" (verse 9).

"It is monstrously simple-minded to read the cursings in the Psalms with no feeling except one of horror at the uncharity of the poets."[2] Simply to charge such cruelty to the conventions of the ancient world seems to be myopic; our own society can match many of these pitiless practices. We should not assume a position superior to the psalmist, as though inhumanity and hatred are alien to us.

It has been observed: "We are not asked to *condone* the hatred, but let us not *condemn* it too quickly, until we have *examined* ourselves on forgiveness." We must *hear* the psalmist. Instead of judging the Psalm, we should allow the Psalm to judge us.

It is improper use of Scripture to pick-and-choose verses as the liturgy does, specifically regarding Psalm 137. That sounds much like manipulation of the Word of God, and is akin to proof-texting [see Introduction]. It would be more beneficial to ask ourselves: Who made the Babylonians and Edomites that way? Perhaps we, too, at times have been the cause of other people's rage and cursing. To pray is to offer ourselves with all of our shortcomings—anger, violence, vengeance, enmity, revenge—to God, with the assurance that God loves us just as we are. No one who understands Psalm 137 feels the need to apologize for its candid content.

Psalm 139 is comparable to Psalm 137 in terms of the imprecations visited on the enemies at the conclusion of each of these Psalms. It is said that Psalm 139 is one of the most profound statements of personal religion in the Psalter. This hymn begins on a note of intimacy with God, with the psalmist expressing wonderment at the omniscience and omnipresence of Yahweh. "O Lord, you have searched me and known me. You know me when I sit down and when I rise up [this comprises one's whole life]; you discern my thoughts from far away" (verses 1–2). Some are shocked at the violence and anger vented at the conclusion of Psalm 139, so they "piously" excise the final six verses. Since anger and violence are a part of life, they are to be confronted in prayer. Biblical scholar Roland Murphy pointed out that we are not to assume a superior attitude, as though we knew nothing of hatred and violence in our own lives. In the concluding verses, the psalmist, acknowledging his own proclivities to sin, requests: "Search me, O God, and know my heart; test me and know my thoughts. See if there is any wicked way in me, and lead me in the way everlasting" (verses 23–24). Now we know the answer to the question: Do the Psalms relate to our everyday life? Yes, because they are intensely human.

Psalm 103. Few Psalms match the warmth and beauty of Psalm 103; in the form of a hymn, it is an individual thanksgiving, probably for the recovery from illness (verse 3). The association of forgiveness and healing of sickness is a common motif in the Bible. Recall Mark 2:10–11, describing Jesus' healing of a paralytic: "'So that you may know that the Son of Man has authority on earth to forgive sins'—he said to the paralytic—'I say to you, stand up, take your mat and go to your home.'" Healing is an outward sign of forgiveness.

The psalmist calls upon us to praise and then gives the reason for praise. Few passages in the Old Testament cause us to experience the certainty that "God is love" as Psalm 103; for example, "The steadfast love (*hesed*) of the Lord is from everlasting to everlasting on those who fear him" (verse 17). The psalmist chooses the imperative of the verb "to bless" (*barak*) for "to praise." Recall what C.S. Lewis said: "The psalmists in telling everyone to praise God are doing what all do when they speak of what they care about."[3] The great profession of faith in Exodus 34:6–7, composed solely of the divine attributes, is featured in Psalm 103:8–18, with its emphasis on Yahweh's kindness and graciousness. Yahweh is desirous of restoring, instead of destroying, the sinner; the persistence of divine forgiveness is illustrated in the father-son relationship (verse 13), a common analogy in biblical Israel and the ancient Near East, based on the compassion of a father.

The transitoriness of human existence in contrast to eternal love is vividly portrayed in terms of the grass and the flowers (verse 15) which are swept away by the sirocco (east wind), but the *hesed* of Yahweh is forever (verses 17–18). Yahweh takes human nature into account, and perhaps may be too understanding of human frailty. This Psalm deepens our appreciation of Yahweh's forgiving love, and offers an added incentive to keep "covenant" with Yahweh.

Anytime we are overwhelmed by discouragement, guilt, depression, despair, we can turn to Psalm 103; there is no better antidote. Also, any person who erroneously perceives the God of the Old Testament as a God of wrath and vengeance should meditate on Psalm 103.

"Pray Then in This Way" (Matthew 6:9)

The Old Testament is replete with references to prayer, and many of these appear in the New Testament. The essence of the mutual commitment between God and people is manifest in the biblical concept of *berit* ("covenant"). Authentic prayer is always a matter of the heart. "When you [the exiles in Babylon] call upon me [Yahweh] and come and pray to me, I will hear you. When you search for me, you will find me; if you seek me with all your heart, I will let you find me, says the Lord, and I will restore your fortunes" (Jeremiah 29:12–14).

Prayer is one of the dominant themes binding the Old Testament and New Testament. This is evident in the prayer life of Jesus, who was nurtured on the prayers of the Old Testament. Biblical prayer is an unmistakable expression of the covenant relationship obligating God and people. Since, by definition, the covenant is central to both Testaments, prayer is a leading biblical theme. In addition to the Psalms, many other prayers, long and short, fill the Scriptures.

For our purposes, the biblical vocabulary for prayer may be reduced basically to two words, one in the Old Testament, the other in the New Testament. The common verb "to pray" in the Old Testament is *hithpallel* (Hebrew), and the noun is *tepilla*. In the New Testament the verb "to pray" is *proseuchomai* (Greek), and the noun is *proseuche*.

Essentially, prayer is a personal and reciprocal relationship between God and people. The Bible emphasizes the simplicity of prayer. As already noted, the Psalter is the prayerbook of the Bible, and the two pillars supporting all forms of prayer are praise and petition. Also, the Psalms are the model of both individual and collective prayer. Biblical prayer deals with the basic issues of everyone's daily life. Prayer indicates people's dependence on God, who is concerned for them and is prepared to assist them. In other words, prayer is comparable to a dialogue between friends who enjoy a trusting relationship with each other.

A brief analysis of selected prayers in the Bible will clarify these points.

Prayer of Intercession

While Moses was separated from the people, atop Mount Sinai, they did not know what happened to him. When the Israelites, in Moses' absence, sinned at Sinai by fashioning the golden, or molten (made of liquid metal), calf, "Moses implored the Lord his God, and said: 'O Lord, why does your wrath burn hot against your people, whom you brought out of the land of Egypt with great power and with a mighty hand? ... Turn from your fierce wrath; change your mind and do not bring disaster on your people.' ... And the Lord changed his mind about the disaster that he planned to bring on his people" (Exodus 32:11–14).

Hannah's Prayer of Thanksgiving

Hannah's thanksgiving prayer for the birth of Samuel, here, in part: "My heart exults in the Lord; my strength is exalted in my God ... There is no Holy One like the Lord, no one besides you; there is no Rock like our God ... He raises up the poor from the dust; he lifts the needy from the ash heap, to make them sit with princes and inherit a seat of honor" (1 Samuel 2:1–10).

David's Praise of God

David's response to the prophet Nathan's oracle about the promise of dynasty: "You are great, O Lord God; for there is no one like you, and there is no God besides you, according to all that we have heard with our ears ... For you, O Lord of hosts, the God of Israel, have made this revelation to your servant, saying, 'I will build you a house'; therefore your servant has found courage to pray this prayer to you" (2 Samuel 7:22–27).

Solomon's Prayer

At Gibeon the Lord appeared to Solomon in a dream by night; and God said, "Ask what I should give you"..."Give your servant therefore an understanding mind [*leb shomea'*, literally, "a listening heart"] to govern your people, able to discern between good and evil; for who can govern this your great people?"...

God said to him, "Because you have asked this and have not asked for yourself long life or riches, or for the life of your enemies, but have asked for yourself understanding to discern what is right, I now do according to your word." (1 Kings 3:5–12)

Solomon's prayer at the dedication of the Temple is one of the great prayers of the Bible (1 Kings 8:22–53). The major portion of this prayer requests Yahweh to attend to supplications offered in or toward the Temple. Seven petitions are described: the oath of innocence, military defeat, drought, a variety of plagues, a foreign pilgrim, military campaign, captivity.

Jeremiah's Prayer

Prayer is concerned with the immediate problems of daily life. "You will be in the right, O Lord, when I [Jeremiah] lay charges against you; but let me put my case to you. Why does the way of the guilty prosper? Why do all who are treacherous thrive? ... But you, O Lord, know me; you see me and test me—my heart is with you" (Jeremiah 12:1–3).

Jesus' Prayers

In the New Testament, prayer is the personal relationship with God through Jesus Christ. "On that day you will ask nothing of me. Very truly, I tell you, if you ask anything of the Father in my name, he will give it to you" (John 16:23). The outlook on prayer established in the Old Testament also characterizes the New Testament. Jesus is both a model and teacher of prayer, and is depicted as one who prays. "In the morning, while it was still very dark, he [Jesus] got up and went out to a deserted place, and there he prayed" (Mark 1:35). "He [Jesus] would withdraw to deserted places and pray" (Luke 5:16). "He [Jesus] went out to the mountain to pray; he spent the night in prayer to God" (Luke 6:12). The New Testament calls attention to Jesus teaching about prayer. "When Jesus saw the crowds, he went up the mountain; and after he sat down, his disciples came to him. Then he began to speak, and taught them" (Matthew 5:1–2).

The Beatitudes

Then follow the Beatitudes, pronouncements associated with the Sermon on the Mount (Matthew 5–7) and the Sermon on the Plain (Luke 6:20–49). These collections of Jesus' teachings usually begin with "blessed" (in the sense of "happy" or "satisfied"). In Matthew's version (Matthew 5:3–12), the nine Beatitudes concern the spiritual and ethical nature of the people of the kingdom; for example, "Blessed are the poor in spirit." Jesus portrays the ideals expected of his followers. In Luke's version (Luke 6:20–23), the four Beatitudes refer to socioeconomic conditions, not the spiritual state; for example, "Blessed are you who are poor." For the most part, the Sermon on the Plain in Luke is paralleled in the Sermon on the Mount in Matthew. There are both resemblances and differences between them, but most readers are probably more familiar with Matthew's version of the Sermon on the Mount, which includes what has come to be known as the "Lord's Prayer."

The Lord's Prayer

The Lord's Prayer ("Our Father") appears in both a Matthean (6:9–13) and a Lucan (11:2–4) form. The Lord's Prayer, filled with allusions to the Old Testament, is a paradigm of how the disciples should pray. Jesus' prayer shares terminology with the Talmud (collection of ancient Rabbinic writings), as well as some theological concepts taught by Jewish leaders in the early centuries.

"Whenever you pray, do not be like the hypocrites; for they love to stand and pray in the synagogues and at the streetcorners, so that they may be seen by others ... Whenever you pray, go into your room and shut the door and pray to your Father who is in secret ... When you are praying do not heap up empty phrases as the Gentiles do; for they think that they will be heard because of their many words" (Matthew 6:5–7). "Pray then in this way: 'Our Father in heaven, hallowed be your name. Your kingdom come. Your will be done, on earth as it is in heaven. Give us this day our daily bread. And forgive us our debts, as we also have forgiven our debtors. And do not bring us to the time of trial, but rescue us from the evil one'" (Matthew 6:9–13; see Luke 11:2–4). The opening words of the Lord's Prayer, "Our Father," express the unique relationship between God and those who pray.

Luke's Gospel

Luke's Gospel is best-known as the gospel of prayer. Luke portrays Jesus at prayer more frequently than the other evangelists (writers of the four Gospels). This is one of the ways in which his disciples are to follow him. Luke tells us that Jesus prayed at the critical moments in his life: at his baptism (3:21); when choosing the twelve (6:12); at his transfiguration (9:28–29); in Gethsemane (22:41–45); at the crucifixion (23:46).

Notice that Luke's Gospel begins and ends in the temple. At the beginning, the people are assisting at the incense-offering. Zechariah the priest, father of soon-to-be-born John the Baptist and husband of Elizabeth, is offering the incense in the temple. At the end, the eleven, after witnessing the ascension, "were continually in the temple blessing God" (Luke 24:53).

Only Luke informs us that John the Baptist used to teach his disciples how to pray. Luke alone describes the disciples' requesting Jesus to teach them to pray: "He was praying in a certain place, and after he had finished, one of his disciples said to him, 'Lord, teach us to pray'" (Luke 11:1). The Acts of the Apostles is a continuation of the Gospel of Luke. In Acts, when the seven (the first deacons) were appointed to serve at table (that is, to feed the hungry), this was done to permit the twelve (apostles) to participate in prayer and "serving the word" (Acts 6:4). Prayer was as important in the life of the apostles as the "ministry of the word," that is, the preaching of the gospel.

John's High Priestly Prayer

The crescendo of John's Gospel is reached in the "high priestly prayer" (John 17:1–26). The last supper closes with this prayer in which Jesus prays for himself (verses 1–5), then for the disciples who are with him and who will continue his presence in the world (verses 6–19), and finally for the next generation who will believe through the witness the disciples give to Jesus (verses

20–26). The substance of Jesus' prayer is that the unity between God and Jesus may be shared by the disciples with him and with one another. It is a prayer focused on the theme of unity. British scholar C.H. Dodd has summarized John 17 superbly:

> Finally it rises into prayer; for it is only in the language of prayer that the last truths of religion find fitting expression. I [Dodd] will quote a few phrases from the prayer: "For their sake I consecrate myself, that they too may be consecrated in the truth ... that they may all be one, as you, Father, are in me, and I in you, that they may be in us ... made perfectly one." I [Dodd] will not attempt to comment on that. It is the conclusion of the whole matter.[4]

Prayer in Paul's Letters

Prayer is prominent in Paul's Letters, especially the thanksgiving prayer that introduces each of the letters, as well as the blessing at the conclusion. "May the God of steadfastness and encouragement grant you to live in harmony with one another, in accordance with Christ Jesus" (Romans 15:5). "And this is my prayer, that your love may overflow more and more with knowledge and full insight to help you to determine what is best, so that in the day of Christ you may be pure and blameless" (Philippians 1:9–10). "May the God of peace himself sanctify you entirely; and may your spirit and soul and body be kept sound and blameless" (1 Thessalonians 5:23). "May the Lord of peace himself give you peace at all times in all ways. The Lord be with all of you" (2 Thessalonians 3:16).

[1] Dietrich Bonhoeffer, *Letters and Papers From Prison* (New York: Collier Books, 1953), 40.

[2] C.S. Lewis, *Reflections on the Psalms* (New York: Harcourt, Brace, and World, 1958), 25.

[3] C.S. Lewis, *Reflections on the Psalms* (New York: Harcourt, Brace and World, 1958), 95.

[4] C.H. Dodd, *About the Gospels* (Cambridge: Cambridge University Press, 1958), 40.

CHAPTER THREE

Covenant and Hospitality

"I Will Be Their God, and They Shall Be My People" (Jeremiah 31:33)

Covenant (*berit*), a dominant biblical theme, is an agreement between parties outlining mutual rights and obligations. More precisely, it is a paramount metaphor for the relationship between God and people. Biblical covenants are modeled on international treaties throughout the ancient Near East, principally Hittite treatises (1400–1200 BCE) and Assyrian treaties (750–650 BCE). They are divided into suzerainty treaties (between overlord and vassal) and parity treaties (among equals). In the Hebrew Bible, covenants were made with Noah (Genesis 9:8–17), Abraham (Genesis 15:9–20), Moses (Exodus 19–24), David (2 Samuel 7:16), as well as the "new covenant" announced by Jeremiah (Jeremiah 31:31–34). The history of the Bible can be summarized by the sequence of covenant-making, covenant-breaking, covenant-remaking. Divine forgiveness is boundless.

Covenant with Noah

Then God said to Noah and to his sons with him, "As for me, I am establishing my covenant with you and your descendants after you, and with every living creature that is with you, … never again shall all flesh be cut off by the waters of a flood and never again shall there be a flood to destroy the earth." God said, "This is the sign of the covenant that I make between me and you and every living creature that is with you, for all future generations; I have set my bow in the clouds, and it shall be a sign of the covenant between me and the earth. When I bring clouds over the earth, and the bow is seen in the clouds, I will remember my covenant." (Genesis 9:8–15)

Abrahamic Covenant

When Yahweh established his covenant with Abraham, he said: "Bring me a heifer three years old, a female goat three years old, a ram three years old, a turtledove, and a young pigeon" (Genesis 15:9). In the eighteenth century BCE, a donkey, a puppy, and a goat were considered acceptable sacrifices for *cutting* a covenant. The Hebrew idiom for "making a covenant" is *karat berit* (literally, "cutting a covenant"). Genesis describes a rite of covenant-making in which Abraham cut in two a heifer, a goat, and a ram; subsequently a smoking fire pot and a flaming torch, both representing God, passed between those pieces. Anyone who violated the covenant would incur the same fate as the sacrificed animals (Genesis 15:9–19). Parallels to this covenant rite appear among the Amorites (a West Semitic people) who slew donkeys, goats, and puppies. Sacrificing an animal to ratify a treaty between two parties probably gave rise to the Hebrew idiom, *karat berit*, "to cut a treaty."

Genesis 17:1–14, the covenant of circumcision, offers another impression of the covenant from a different source than Genesis 15:9–20; it is really a theological reflection on Genesis 15:9–20. The practice of circumcision was widespread in antiquity, although its origin and purpose are uncertain. In biblical times, Israelites, Ammonites, Moabites, and Edomites were circumcised, but not so the Akkadians, Assyrians, and Babylonians. The non-Semitic Philistines did not practice circumcision, whence the Israelites disparaged them with the disdainful epithet "uncircumcised." An Israelite father circumcised his infant son eight days after birth (Genesis 17:12; Leviticus 12:3). As an indication of the antiquity of circumcision, in early Israel the rite was performed with a flint or stone knife (Exodus 4:25; Joshua 5:2–3). Children of Israel's neighbors were more apt to undergo circumcision during childhood or at puberty, instead of eight days after birth. Even uncircumcised adults had to undergo circumcision to become members of the community, as they do today. Jewish males are circumcised in a ceremony known as *brit milah*, "the covenant of circumcision." *Bris* is the Ashkenazic (Hebrew name for German) pronunciation and abbreviated name for a *brit milah*. Only a circumcised male is qualified to participate in the Passover ritual (Exodus 12:48–49). For the Israelites, circumcision was a sign of covenant-kinship between Yahweh and Israel (Genesis 17:10–14).

Yahweh addressed Abraham: "I will establish my covenant between me and you, and your offspring after you throughout their generations, for an everlasting covenant ... Every male among you shall be circumcised. You shall circumcise the flesh of your foreskin, and it shall be a sign [a tangible sign making covenant a public record] of the covenant between me and you" (Genesis 17:7–12).

Covenant on Mount Sinai

Exodus 19–24 describes God's covenant with Israel on Mount Sinai. "On the third new moon after the Israelites had gone out of the land of Egypt, on that very day, they came into the wilderness of Sinai" (Exodus 19:1). Mount Sinai is an imposing granite range at the southern end of the Sinai Peninsula, with Jebel Musa (Mount of Moses) as its highest peak at 7,500 ft. It was an awe-inspiring spectacle; however, the location of Sinai cannot be determined with certainty. "Then Moses went up to God; the Lord called to him from the mountain" (Exodus 19:3). Moses was the mediator of covenant relations between God and the people.

The Ten Commandments (Hebrew, "Words") follow in Exodus 20:1–17, and are paralleled in Deuteronomy 5:6–21. These unconditional laws are the essence of covenant obligations toward God and neighbors. They are apodictic laws (categorical imperatives) in contrast to casuistic (conditional) laws. Yahweh is described as a "jealous God," demanding exclusive allegiance (Exodus 20:5). The first five Commandments deal with Israel's relationship with God; the latter five, concerned with neighborly conduct, are not unique among ancient collections of law. It is clear that to serve God also means to serve one's neighbor. Hammurabi, the most important king of the first (Amorite) dynasty of Babylon, reigned in the first half of the eighteenth century BCE. His code of laws demonstrates a considerable concern for justice. The Ten Commandments are prescriptions for the execution of the one great commandment of love, and their aim is to claim all people completely for God.

Then follows a collection of civil and religious ordinances, called the Book of the Covenant (Exodus 21–23). Among them is one, which is frequently cited and mostly misunderstood: "If any harm follows [from a fight], then you shall give life for life, eye for eye, tooth for tooth, hand for hand, foot for foot, burn for burn, wound for wound, stripe for stripe" (Exodus 21:23–25). This ordinance is known as the *lex talionis*, "law of retaliation," whereby the punishment agrees with the offense. The purpose of this law is not to require vengeance, but to restrict it. Compare Matthew 5:38–39: "You have heard that it was said, 'An eye for an eye and a tooth for a tooth.' But I say to you, 'Do not resist an evildoer. But if anyone strikes you on the right cheek, turn the other also.'"

Another law, with particular application to North America, concerns the timely and critical issue of immigration: "You shall not oppress a resident alien (*ger*); you know the heart of an alien, for you were aliens in the land of Egypt" (Exodus 23:9). This is a complex and emotionally-laden human condition that must be considered with great empathy, especially when whole families are involved. Nothing would be more devastating to the commonwealth than the dispersement of families. Americans, especially, should be sensitive to the knotty question of immigration since it has figured in the lineage of all Americans. I find the Bible to be a reliable guide in helping to deal with all aspects of immigration, especially the love of neighbor.

Exodus 24 records the solemn sealing of Yahweh's covenant with Israel. The ratification of the Sinai covenant includes two rituals: sprinkling of blood (verses 3–8) and a ritual banquet

47

(verses 1–2, 9–11). The *nephesh* ("life," "spirit"), which belongs to God, resides in the blood; consequently, injunctions regulating the use of blood, outside of sacrifice, are restrictive. The sprinkling of blood signifies the covenant bond; Yahweh and the Israelites became blood relatives. Sacrificial blood was thought to have the sacramental power to bring together two parties in covenant. Moses splashed blood on the altar, representing Yahweh's participation in the rite, and then he sprinkled blood on the people, saying, "See the blood of the covenant that the Lord has made [cut] with you in accordance with all these words" (Exodus 24:8).

Covenants were often ratified by a common meal. At the banquet scene, the guests "saw the God of Israel ... God did not lay his hand on the chief men of the people of Israel; also they beheld God, and they ate and drank [of the sacrificial meal]" (Exodus 24:9–11). In antiquity, it was assumed that to see God would result in immediate death. See below for the allusions to the Eucharist in the ratification of the Sinai covenant.

Davidic Dynasty

By bringing the ark of the covenant to Jerusalem, David endeavored to relate his newly established kingdom to the divine promises revealed in the Sinai covenant. The dynastic oracle of David (2 Samuel 7:1–17) enumerates the elements of this promissory covenant. The first centers on the ambiguous Hebrew word *bayit*, "house," which may also be translated "temple" or "dynasty." David wanted to build the temple for Yahweh, just as Yahweh wished to establish an everlasting dynasty for David and his successors (verse 11). Solomon, not David, eventually constructed the temple. The oracle also specified that sin on the part of a Davidic heir would not result in Yahweh's everlasting love (*hesed*) being forfeited. In sum, this passage is fundamental to Israelite, Jewish, and Christian royal messianism.

Jeremiah's New Covenant

Jeremiah 31:31–34, the new covenant, is one of the most profound and stirring passages in the Bible; it is also a landmark in Old Testament theology, as well as the "gospel before the gospel." Jeremiah's portrayal of Israel's restoration in the vision of a new covenant is a staggering act of faith because it was proclaimed at a time of culminating tragedy, when the land and the city (Jerusalem) had been decimated and the people exiled. The new covenant forms part of Jeremiah's Book of Consolation (Jeremiah 30–33), so-called because of the hopeful words contained therein. This new covenant, accentuating the inwardness of personal religion as well as individual responsibility, was founded on Yahweh's initiative and forgiveness.

Listed among the qualities of the new covenant are the following: it will endure in perpetuity; its law will be inscribed in the heart, not merely on stone tablets; love and faith will dominate; there will be forgiveness of sin, but not sinlessness. "I will be their God, and they shall be my people" (Jeremiah 31:33) is the basic formula of the new covenant. This prophecy influenced the writers of the New Testament: for example, 2 Corinthians 3:2–18; Hebrews 8:6–11; Matthew 26:28; Mark 14:24. Jesus recalled Jeremiah's words on the evening before he died, when he said to his disciples at table: "This cup is the new covenant in my blood" (1 Corinthians 11:25; Luke 22:20). The Christian church understands its members to be people of the new covenant.

The "New" Covenant

"This Is My Blood, of the Covenant" (Mark 14:23)

There is organic unity between Sinai and the Cenacle (the upper room where the last supper took place), as the following texts attest. "Moses took the blood and dashed it on the people, and said, 'See the blood of the covenant that the Lord has made with you in accordance with all these words'" (Exodus 24:8). Compare "This is my blood of the covenant, which is poured out for many for the forgiveness of sins" (Matthew 26:28; Mark 14:23). Paul (1 Corinthians 11:23–26; see Luke 22:15–20) records the words of Jesus: "This cup is the new covenant in my blood," reflecting the "new covenant" in Jeremiah 31:31–34. The cup is associated with the covenant in Matthew, Mark, Luke, and Paul. In the synoptics (Matthew, Mark, Luke) the last supper was a Passover meal. The evangelists and Paul interpret Jesus' death in the framework of the Passover. At the last supper Jesus identified the cup of wine as covenant or new covenant. John's Gospel lacks a historical narrative of the last supper, but the new commandment of love in this Gospel—"I give you a new commandment, that you love one another. Just as I have loved you, you also should love one another" (John 13:34)—pertains to the nature of covenant.

The Lord's Supper

Paul is the only New Testament writer to use the designation "Lord's supper" (1 Corinthians 11:20), commemorating Jesus' last meal with his disciples. The Eucharist (*eucharistia*, "thanksgiving") is the rite of the Lord's supper, although the word "Eucharist" does not occur in the New Testament. It is the renewal of covenant and recalls the obligations the members of the church owe to God and neighbor. The Eucharist was combined with a meal (*agape*) taken in common with the members of the Christian community. The *agape* ("love" in the New Testament), preceding the celebration of the Eucharist and signifying the communal meal of the early Christians, provided religious companionship and the opportunity to assist the destitute, as well as the social outcasts, such as tax-collectors and prostitutes. Paul criticized the members of the community at Corinth for certain abuses and lack of decorum that obscured the purpose of the *agape* (1 Corinthians 11:17–34). In the Hebrew Bible, the reign of God at the end of time is depicted as a festive meal.

Catholic and most Protestant theology differ in the interpretation of the Eucharist: Catholics understand literally the phrases "this is my body" and "this is my blood," convinced that translations such as "represents" or "symbolizes" do not convey the realism of the words. Thomas Aquinas, Doctor of the Church, declared that the Eucharist is a mystery "no theological explanation can hope to master."

"Whoever Welcomes You Welcomes Me" (Matthew 10:40)

Hospitality in the Old Testament

Living in the wilderness makes sojourners (*gerim*) vitally aware that hospitality is necessary for survival. The "sojourner" ("stranger," "alien") is a person dwelling in a place other than his own home or home country. "You shall not oppress a resident alien (*ger*); you know the heart of an alien (*ger*), for you were aliens (*gerim*) in the land of Egypt" (Exodus 23:9). Hospitality is rooted in the realization that people are obligated to help one another. Loners cannot survive for long in the desert.

Hospitality was preferred to fasting as a way of serving God, as the prophet Isaiah declares when distinguishing false and true worship. The fast that God desires consists in reaching out to those who are in need: "Is not this the fast that I choose? ... Is it not to share your bread with the hungry, and bring the homeless poor into your house?" (Isaiah 58:6–7).

Ancient Near Eastern hospitality emphasized the proper treatment of guests. The Hebrew Bible has no single word for "hospitality," but real-life examples abound therein. "Hear my prayer, O Lord, and give ear to my cry ... For I am your passing guest, an alien (*ger*), like all my forebears" (Psalm 39:12). Abraham and Sarah extended prodigious hospitality to "three men" who visited them at Hebron, as "Abraham sat at the entrance of his tent in the heat of the day" (Genesis 18:1). Anyone standing at the tent of a stranger was obviously seeking hospitality. Abraham responded instinctively: he greeted them courteously, bowing down to the earth; he brought water for washing their dust-covered feet.

Foot washing was emphasized in biblical times, which explains why archaeologists have recovered foot baths from several sites. Not only a convention of hospitality in antiquity, it was also a necessity since the people walked barefoot, in sandals, or in slippers with turned-up toes. In addition to Abraham's providing water for the foot washing of the three strangers (Genesis 18:4), Laban, a member of Abraham's ancestral family, supplied water for Abraham's servant "to wash his feet and the feet of the men who were with him" (Genesis 24:32).

Abraham also invited his three guests to rest under the tree, prepared a lavish meal, including meat, and stood beside them while they ate. Guests were offered freshly baked bread as a sign of hospitality and honor to the guest. Bread (even today) is never cut, but always broken. Abraham was the exemplary host, manifesting prodigal generosity. Curiously, Abraham served no wine to his visitors, even though Hebron is a grape-producing region. Notice, too, that Sarah stayed in the tent because women do not sit with male guests. This narrative reflects a deep and childlike faith: God was very personal to Abraham and Sarah. If you read this episode carefully, you will find several hints as to the identity of the "three men" (Genesis 18:1–15).

In biblical times the people ate three daily meals, noticeably different in quantity. Breakfast was meager, simply bread or fruit. The midday meal was light, just bread, grain, olives, and figs. The principal meal was eaten in the evening, after sunset, with the whole family participating. The economic status of the household determined the amount of the food consumed. The meal was basically a one-pot stew served in a common bowl and sopped up with bread. Ordinarily prepared with lentils or other vegetables, the pottage was seasoned with herbs. The average family ate meat only on festive occasions.

I witnessed the following scene being reenacted many times in the Middle East. When excavating or traveling, so often we would be invited to share the hospitality of the local people in the villages or in the desert. Nothing was too good for the guests. I observed situations where, despite our protestations, we were served the only food in the house or tent. Should you find yourself in the same situation, never refuse the proferred generosity; to do so would be considered an insult. Nowadays, when one is invited to dine in a village or camp setting, a special bond is created between host and guest, and at the same time a moral obligation is incurred. On the occasion of a common meal, friendships were often sealed. In my experience, Arabs especially are keenly aware of the sacramental value of sharing meals.

Hospitality in the New Testament

Table fellowship and other forms of hospitality are more evident in Luke's Gospel than elsewhere in the New Testament. Many scenes in this Gospel are set at dinner tables, whereas in Matthew's Gospel they take place on mountain tops. A certain severity evident in Matthew is lacking in Luke, the scribe of the kindness of Christ. In that vein, for the sheer pleasure of reading, Luke's Gospel surpasses the other three.

Five stories found exclusively in Luke's Gospel accentuate the theme of hospitality: the parable of the Good Samaritan (Luke 10:25–37; mentioned above), the prodigal son (Luke 15:11–32), the rich man and Lazarus (Luke 16:19–31), the story of Zacchaeus (Luke 19:1–10), and the Emmaus story (Luke 24:13–35).

Luke narrates the story of a Pharisee who invited Jesus to dine with him but withheld the customary amenities (foot washing, a kiss, anointing the head). At the same time, a penitent woman was also present, and she extended these courtesies to Jesus out of her "great love" (Luke 7:36–50).

The First Letter of Paul to Timothy lists the qualifications required of those who aspire to be bishops: "A bishop must be above reproach, married only once, temperate, sensible, respectable, hospitable" (1 Timothy 3:2).

The requirements detailed on the occasion of the "judgment of the nations" are quite personal: "I was hungry and you gave me food, I was thirsty and you gave me something to drink, I was a stranger and you welcomed me, I was naked and you gave me clothing" (Matthew 25:35). All these come under the rubric of hospitality.

Jesus as Host, Guest, and Servant

At meals Jesus carried out a variety of roles—host, guest, servant. Jesus said to one of the leading Pharisees who had invited him: "When you give a luncheon or a dinner, do not invite your friends or your brothers or your relatives or rich neighbors, in case they may invite you in return, and you would be repaid" (Luke 14:12–13).

"Levi [the tax collector] gave a great banquet for him [Jesus] in his house; and there was a large crowd of tax collectors and others sitting at the table with them" (Luke 5:29). "A dispute also arose among them [the apostles] as to which one of them was to be regarded as the greatest. But he said to them, '... Rather the greatest among you must become like the youngest, and the leader like one who serves ... But I [Jesus] am among you as one who serves'" (Luke 22:24–27).

At times, Jesus dined with Pharisees, with sinners, and with the crowds, as on the occasion of the multiplication of the loaves (Luke 9:16). In practice, the readers of the Gospel are to see themselves at various times in the roles of host, guest, and servant. Incidentally, the feeding of the 5,000 is the only miracle story to appear in all four Gospels.

The New Testament describes the itinerant Jesus as dependent upon hospitality for his sustenance and lodging. "From there he [Jesus] set out and went away to the region of Tyre. He entered a house and did not want anyone to know he was there" (Mark 7:24). "While he [Jesus] was at Bethany in the house of Simon the leper, as he sat at the table, a woman came with an alabaster jar of very costly ointment of nard" (Mark 14:3).

"As they [the disciples] went on their way, he [Jesus] entered a certain village, where a woman named Martha welcomed him into her home" (Luke 10:38). "When Jesus was going to the house of a leader of the Pharisees to eat a meal on the sabbath, they were watching him closely" (Luke 14:1). "When Jesus came to the place [of the sycamore tree], he looked up and said to him, 'Zacchaeus [a wealthy tax collector in Jericho], hurry and come down; for I must stay at your house today'" (Luke 19:5). "Six days before the Passover Jesus came to Bethany, the home of Lazarus, whom he had raised from the dead. There they gave a dinner for him. Martha served, and Lazarus was one of those at the table with him" (John 12:1–2).

Hospitality was assumed in the sending forth of the apostles: "Whatever town or village you enter, find out who in it is worthy, and stay there until you leave. As you enter the house, greet it" (Matthew 10:11–12). "Remain in the same house, eating and drinking whatever they provide, for the laborer deserves to be paid. Do not move about from house to house" (Luke 10:7).

Whereas a common meal was often the occasion of sealing friendship, sometimes it was just the opposite. A covenant was concluded between Isaac and Abimelech, king of the Philistines, which ended a dispute over wells and deflected enmity between the parties. "So he [Isaac] made them [Abimelech, Ahuzzath his adviser, and Phicol, the commander of his army] a feast, and they ate and drank" (Genesis 26:30). An example of the opposite—the psalmist, in his sickness, was embittered by an erstwhile friend who reviled him: "Even my bosom friend in whom I trusted, who ate of my bread has lifted the heel against me" (Psalm 41:9). At the last supper Jesus cited these words in reference to Judas, also a "treacherous" friend (John 13:18).

Ancient banquets consisted of two principal courses: the eating course (*deipnon*) was followed by the drinking course (*symposion*). Each began with a blessing over the food and wine. At the institution of the Lord's supper, Luke makes clear the separation between the two by inserting "and he did the same with the cup, *after supper*" (Luke 22:20).

When the prophets of Israel envisioned a new age of peace and righteousness, they pictured Yahweh hosting a lavish banquet for all people. The paterfamilias hosted the family banquet; the king hosted the royal banquet; Yahweh hosted the eschatological (messianic) banquet. Isaiah described two such copious feasts: "On this mountain [Mount Zion in Jerusalem] the Lord of hosts will make for all peoples a feast of rich food, a feast of well-aged wines, of rich food filled with marrow, of well-aged wines strained clear" (Isaiah 25:6). Isaiah supplied an additional invitation to the messianic banquet for all peoples—the banquet of the kingdom of God: "Everyone who thirsts, come to the waters; and you that have no money, come, buy and eat! Come, buy wine and milk without money and without price" (Isaiah 55:1). Luke emphasized the messianic banquet ("kingdom of God") at the last supper—"I [Jesus] have eagerly desired to eat this Passover with you before I suffer; for I tell you, I will not eat it until it is fulfilled in the kingdom of God" (Luke 22:15–16).

CHAPTER FOUR

Holiness and Humility

"You Shall Be Holy, For I the Lord Your God Am Holy" (Leviticus 19:2)

Nature of Holiness

Holiness is that indefinable quality originating in God and distinguishing the Deity from all creation. "Who is like you, O Lord, among the gods? Who is like you, majestic in holiness, awesome in splendor, doing wonders?" (Exodus 15:11). "There is no Holy One (*qadosh*) like the Lord, no one besides you; there is no Rock (*sur*) like our God" (1 Samuel 2:2). Creatures are called holy in a derivative sense—they are intimately related to God. People are considered holy (*qadosh*) because God dwells in their midst. "For I am the Lord your God; sanctify yourselves therefore, and be holy, for I am holy" (Leviticus 11:44–45; see also 19:2; 20:26). People, places, and things may be holy by association with God. Mount Sinai, for example, is holy because God appeared there in fire to bequeath the Ten Commandments (Exodus 19:23).

Holiness (*qodesh*), the most important component in the character of the Deity, entails the separation of the sacred from the profane. Indicative of its significance, the Hebrew root *qdsh* occurs 850 times in the Old Testament. It is found especially in the Holiness Code (Leviticus 17–26) of the Torah (Pentateuch), a corpus of laws regulating both liturgy and ethical conduct, such as cultic prescriptions, sexual conduct, and civil damages. Separation, otherness, and withdrawal are synonyms for holiness. The moral dimension of Yahweh's holiness is evident from the various ethical and ritual commands found in Leviticus 19. Interspersed throughout this chapter is the oft-repeated injunction and central theme of Leviticus: "You shall be holy, for I the Lord your God am holy," with slight variations (Leviticus 19:2). People must emulate Yahweh's holiness by observing the commandments. In Psalm 99, a hymn praising Yahweh's holiness, each stanza concludes with an almost identical refrain: "The Lord, who is holy" (verses 3, 5, 9). Both the Psalms and Isaiah frequently refer to God as "the Holy One."

The concept of holiness is at the heart of the theology of the prophet Isaiah. The Israelites are referred to as they "who have forsaken the Lord, who have despised the Holy One of Israel," a title frequent in Isaiah, but seldom in other prophetic books (Isaiah 1:4). Additional examples: "Let the plan of the Holy One of Israel hasten to fulfillment, that we may know it" (Isaiah 5:19). "For they [Israelites] have rejected the instruction (*torah*) of the Lord of hosts, and have despised the word of the Holy One of Israel" (Isaiah 5:24).

Commissioning of Isaiah

The account of Isaiah's commissioning to the prophetic office is one of the classic passages in the Bible (Isaiah 6:1–3). It came at a time of international crisis: in 742 BCE, the year King Uzziah (Azariah) of Judah died; leprosy had curtailed his very successful reign. Imperial Assyria was casting a menacing shadow over the Southern Kingdom (Judah), which was eventually devastated during the Assyrian campaign in 701 BCE. Isaiah experienced a vision of divine transcendence, related in the first person. The imagery, initially the Jerusalem temple, is transformed into a heavenly scene, set in the throne room of the celestial court.

Isaiah saw the glory (*kabod*) of God, that is, God's external manifestation. Seraphim (literally, "burning ones"), guardians of the temple precincts and snakelike in appearance, with six wings, "with two they covered their faces, with two they covered their feet [a euphemism for genitals], and with two they flew" (Isaiah 6:2). They cried out, "Holy, holy, holy," the awesome trisagion (*qedusha*, literally, the three holys), emphasizing that Yahweh is the font of all holiness. The "smoke" emanated from the temple's incense and burnt offerings. Aware of his own unworthiness in the presence of Divinity, Isaiah was terrified. At that point, burning coals from the incense altar touched his lips, and his sin was forgiven. In response to Yahweh's question, "Whom shall I send?" Isaiah replied spontaneously, "Here am I; send me" (verse 8). His unhesitating rejoinder contrasts with Jeremiah's demurring response to his divine call: "I do not know how to speak, for I am only a boy" (Jeremiah 1:6).

Call of Moses

The call of Moses (Exodus 3:1–2) is couched in a theophany (appearance of God) in the vicinity of "the mountain of God," called Horeb (verse 2), but better known as Sinai. While herding the sheep of his father-in-law, Jethro (also called Reuel), Moses catches sight of fire flaming out of a bush (*seneh*, alluding to the name Sinai), but the bush is not burned. In the Old Testament, fire is frequently a symbol for a manifestation of God. As Moses approached the bush to get a better view, God called out from the bush, directing him to come no closer and to remove his sandals, "for the place on which you are standing is holy ground" (verse 5) by reason of its association with and consecration to God. "Holy" is the operative word; God's presence makes all the difference. Terrified, Moses veiled his face, so as not to gaze upon Divinity. In this same encounter God disclosed the divine name to Moses: "I am who I am" (*'ehyeh 'asher 'ehyeh*, causative form of Hebrew verb *hyh*, "to be," from which the name Yahweh is derived). For the remainder of the wilderness wandering, the Israelites complained, Moses interceded, and God provided.

Holiness in Hosea

The prophet Hosea describes the holiness of Yahweh's love, which includes both mercy and judgment, as analogous to a father's love for his small child, as well as to an owner's kindness to his ox where the example shifts to animals (Hosea 11:4). Hosea 11:1–9 is a mountain peak of biblical spirituality—nowhere else is the profundity of divine love so sensitively portrayed. The father's warm and tender feelings toward his son are expressed poignantly in terms of parental nurturing, such as teaching the child to walk, ... taking the child up in his arms, ... lifting the child to his cheeks, ... and bending down to feed the child (Hosea 11:3–4).

Hosea portrays the inner struggle between wrath and love within the heart of Yahweh. Ephraim (the Northern Kingdom of Israel) had rejected its God and deserved to be punished; at the same time, Yahweh was yearning for his people. The unmerited love and mercy of God trumped divine wrath, resulting in

Yahweh's radical change of heart. "How can I [Yahweh] give you up, Ephraim? How can I hand you over, O Israel? ... I will not execute my fierce anger; I will not again destroy Ephraim; for I am God and no mortal ('*is*), the Holy One (*qadosh*) in your midst, and I will not come in wrath" (Hosea 11:8–9). God's holiness is conceived as redemptive love.

The Temple of Jerusalem

In the ancient world, a temple served as a visible symbol of the Deity's presence. The Jerusalem temple, built by King Solomon, was first and foremost the dwelling place or house (*bayit*) of Israel's God; in addition, it was part of the administrative structure of Jerusalem. The presence of God rendered the temple a holy place. The temple was the most holy place in Israel because the divine Presence dwelled there. It was not a place of public worship; worshipers were confined to the courtyards surrounding the temple.

The Bible (1 Kings 6–7) provides a detailed description of the temple construction and its appurtenances; however, much of the architectural terminology relating to the temple eludes us today. Rectanglar and tripartite in structure, the temple's constituent parts are the '*ulam* or portico; the *hekal* or nave, where most of the priestly functions took place; and the *debir* or innermost chamber overlaid with pure gold, known as the Holy of Holies (the most holy place), where Yahweh resided. The layout of the Jerusalem temple indicated the degrees of holiness. As one moved away from God's presence, the intensity of holiness diminished. Only on Yom Kippur (Day of Atonement) did the high priest enter the Holy of Holies; it was a fast day (and still is), reminding the people of Israel (and present-day Jews) of Yahweh's holiness and their sinfulness.

The Nazirite Vow

A person, male or female, could consecrate oneself to God for a specific period of time: this was known as taking the vow of a nazirite (from Hebrew *nazar*, to separate). The requirements are stated in Numbers 6:1-21—to refrain from intoxicants, from cutting one's hair, and from contact with corpses. "All their days as nazirites they are holy (*qados*) to the Lord" (Numbers 6:8), that is, they enter a state of holiness. The strongman Samson is the earliest biblical example of a nazirite (Judges 13:2–7). Although not explicitly named as such, Samuel also was a nazirite (1 Samuel 1:11). The word "nazirite" does not appear in the New Testament, nor was Jesus a nazirite.

Holy Times

In addition to holy places (spatial holiness) and holy people, there are holy times (cultic calendar). The following are among the principal holy times:

Pesach **(Passover).** Passover (*Pesach*) is the most widely observed Jewish holiday, commemorating the exodus of the Israelites from Egypt. The message of this festival is freedom in every aspect of life: to think, believe, and pray as one chooses. The *seder* is a Passover meal celebrated on the first night of Passover.

Shavu'ot **(Weeks).** *Shavu'ot*, "Weeks," occurs seven weeks or 50 days after Passover. For that reason, it is also called Pentecost (Greek for 50), well-known from the Christian feast of the same name. *Shavu'ot* was an agricultural festival, marking the end of the barley harvest and the beginning of the wheat-ripening season.

Sukkot **(Booths).** The word *sukkot* is Hebrew for booths, and this seven-day festival is known as the festival of Booths or the feast of Tabernacles. Commemorating the 40-year wandering of the Israelites in the wilderness when they lived in temporary dwellings, or booths, today observant Jews erect a *sukkah* (singular of *sukkot*, booth or tent) where they live for seven days (Leviticus 23:42–43). Historically, *Sukkot* is a harvest festival. *Pesah* (Passover), *Shavu'ot*, and *Sukkot* mark the three festivals when the Israelites were obliged to make pilgrimages to the temple in Jerusalem.

Holiness in the New Testament

Hagios is the principal word for "holy" in the New Testament; *hieros* is rarely used for "holy." The New Testament concept of holiness is founded on the Old Testament, except that the cultic aspect of holiness is set aside, while the moral (ethical) component is emphasized. "Instead, as he who called you is holy, be holy yourselves in all your conduct; for it is written 'You shall be holy, for I am Holy'" (1 Peter 1:15–16). Superstitious rituals and false asceticism have no value (Colossians 2:20–23). But, "As God's chosen ones, holy and beloved, clothe yourselves with compassion, kindness, humility, meekness, and patience. Bear with one another and, if anyone has a complaint against another, forgive each other" (Colossians 3:12–13). This is the definition of holiness in the New Testament: a lifestyle characterized by these virtues in every activity and in every relationship of daily life.

Also, the Hebrew prophets emphasize not merely ceremonial purity but interior holiness.

"Forgive, and You Will Be Forgiven" (Luke 6:37)

For most of us, forgiveness is not easy to effect. Instead of responding with mercy and pardon, we frequently harbor residual resentment and even revenge. The Bible has wise counsel, emphasizing both divine and human forgiveness. Hebrew has three basic terms for "forgiveness," but for our purposes, they are synonymous, making it unnecessary to specify technical distinctions. After Yahweh had proclaimed the sole confession, in the Old Testament, composed exclusively of the divine attributes, including God's graciousness in "forgiving iniquity and transgression and sin" (Exodus 34:7), Moses recited an intercessory prayer for the Israelites consequent upon their sinful behavior: "Although this is a stiff-necked people, pardon our iniquity and our sin, and take us for your inheritance" (Exodus 34:9).

Requests for Forgiveness

In Solomon's prayer of dedication of the temple addressed to Yahweh, he petitions multiple times for forgiveness; for example, "Forgive your people who have sinned against you, and all their transgressions that they have committed against you; and grant them compassion" (1 Kings 8:50). The divine response: "If my people ... turn from their wicked ways, then I will hear from heaven, and will forgive their sin and heal their land" (2 Chronicles 7:14).

And Daniel's prayer: "We do not present our supplication before you on the ground of our righteousness, but on the ground of your great mercies. O Lord, hear; O Lord, forgive; O Lord, listen and act and do not delay!" (Daniel 9:18–19). A call to repentance is a common prophetic theme: "Let the wicked forsake their way, and the unrighteous their thoughts; let them return to the Lord, that he may have mercy on them, and to our God, for he will abundantly pardon" (Isaiah 55:7). In praise of divine goodness, the psalmist writes: "who forgives all your iniquity, who heals all your diseases, who redeems your life from the Pit, who crowns you with steadfast love and mercy" (Psalm 103:3).

Included among divine blessings is the forgiveness of sin. A communal lament in time of distress affirms: "For you, O Lord, are good and forgiving, abounding in steadfast love to all who call on you" (Psalm 86:5). In a cry "from the depths" (*de profundis*), the psalmist prays: "But there is forgiveness with you [Yahweh], so that you may be revered" (Psalm 130:4).

Naaman, commander of the Syrian army, contracted leprosy, and was cured by the prophet Elisha. Profoundly grateful, Naaman wanted to present a gift to the God of Israel and to Elisha, but it was refused. Required in his official capacity to serve the king of Syria by worshiping Rimmon (epithet of the Syrian deity Hadad) in the temple, Naaman besought Yahweh's forgiveness for any future participation in non-Yahwistic rites. Elisha, understanding Naaman's predicament, said approvingly: "Go in peace" (2 Kings 5:19).

Yahweh forgives sinners by removing human sin: "The Lord is slow to anger, and abounding in steadfast love, forgiving iniquity and transgression" (Numbers 14:18; see Exodus 34:6–7).

Prophets and Forgiveness

In an atmosphere of hopeful expectation, Hosea exhorts: "Take words [prayers] with you and return to the Lord; say to him, 'Take away all guilt; accept that which is good, and we will offer the fruit of our lips'" (Hosea 14:2–3).

Note the Israelite community's confession of trust in Yahweh: "Who is a God like you, pardoning iniquity and passing over the transgression of the remnant of your possession?" (Micah 7:18). On the afternoon of Rosh Hashanah (New Year), Jews participate in a popular ritual known as *tashlik* (casting off). It involves walking to a body of water, reciting assigned prayers, and then casting bread crumbs into the water, a ceremony symbolizing the forgiveness of sins. "You will cast all our sins into the depths of the sea" (Micah 7:19).

Psalm 51, Prayer for Forgiveness

Have mercy on me, O God,
>according to your steadfast love;
according to your abundant mercy
>blot out my transgressions.
Wash me thoroughly from my iniquity,
>and cleanse me from my sin.
For I know my transgressions,
>and my sin is ever before me ...
You desire truth in the inward being;
>therefore teach me wisdom in my secret heart.
Purge me with hyssop, and I shall be clean;
>wash me, and I shall be whiter than snow ...

Psalm 51 is the well-known and moving prayer for forgiveness placed on the lips of an individual who is vitally aware of his own sinfulness and guilt, as well as being in dire need of God's mercy. This Psalm, an individual lament, may later have been modified to become the prayer of the community. Its use in the Jewish liturgy of Yom Kippur (Day of Atonement) and the Christian liturgy of Ash Wednesday illustrates how this Psalm has relevance for both communities down to this day. The superscription (heading) of the Psalm connects it with the sin and penitence of King David's adultery with Bathsheba and the murder of Uriah, the Hittite, followed by the confrontation between David and the prophet, Nathan (2 Samuel 11–12). In reality, Psalm 51 (known as the Miserere [have mercy]), has much more to do with God's character than with David's sins; divine mercy prevails over human sinfulness.

All of us can claim this Psalm for ourselves; everyone is in need of forgiveness. Israel's story, David's story, and our own story, if we are honest enough to acknowledge it, are assuredly a long list of human weaknesses and worse. In this connection, the Gospels, especially Mark, are quite candid in their indictment of Jesus' weak disciples: "Then all the disciples deserted him [Jesus] and fled" (Matthew 26:56). The First Letter to the Corinthians does not spare the early church, just as the media have not refrained from candid criticism of the contemporary church.

With reference to criticism, as a priest for sixty years I wish the Catholic hierarchy would divest itself of royal robes and inflated titles. Pomposity and the gospel are incompatible. As a biblical scholar, I find such pretense irreconcilable with Jesus' instruction to his disciples: "But whoever wishes to become great among you must be your servant, and whoever wishes to be first among you must be slave of all. For the Son of Man [Jesus] came not to be served but to serve, and to give his life a ransom for many" (Mark 10:43–44).

Jesus alone is without sin: "We do not have a high priest who is unable to sympathize with our weaknesses, but we have one who in every respect has been tested as we are, yet without sin" (Hebrews 4:15). Consequently, Psalm 51 is about the rest of us.

Stories about Forgiveness

The Bible includes many examples of forgiveness. In the Jacob-Esau story (Genesis 33), the meeting with Esau that Jacob dreaded, fearful that Esau would kill him, ended in reconciliation, despite that Jacob acted obsequiously and Esau behaved patronizingly.

Miriam and Aaron rebelled against Moses out of jealousy, protesting that they should share equal authority with him. The humility of Moses contrasts with the assertiveness of his "power-hungry" siblings (Numbers 12:1–13).

From the cross, Jesus uttered those unforgettable words: "Father, forgive them; for they do not know what they are doing" (Luke 23:34). These words are a challenge in every age.

The writer of Acts was intent upon drawing a parallel between Stephen's death and that of Jesus. Both died unjustly and full of forgiveness. Stephen's words are comparable to Jesus': "While they were stoning Stephen [a leader in the early Jerusalem church], he prayed, 'Lord Jesus, receive my spirit.' Then he knelt down and cried out in a loud voice, 'Lord, do not hold this sin against them.' When he had said this, he died" (Acts 7:59–60).

Paul, too, manifested the same forgiving spirit. "At my [Paul's] first defense no one came to my support, but all deserted me. May it not be counted against them!" (2 Timothy 4:16). Jeremiah's description of the new covenant, one of the profoundest passages in the Bible, ends: "I [Yahweh] will forgive their iniquity, and remember their sin no more" (Jeremiah 31:34). Divine forgiveness derives from the loving nature of God. Unwillingness to forgive others is an obstacle to one's own forgiveness. "If you forgive others their trespasses, your heavenly Father will also forgive you; but if you do not forgive others, neither will your Father forgive your trespasses" (Matthew 6:14–15). "Forgive, and you will be forgiven" (Luke 6:37).

The story of the "prodigal son" (Luke 15:11–32), a parable of mercy, is too well known to be repeated, except to underscore the son's return (that is, his repentance) and the father's compassion (that is, his forgiveness). The magnanimous father is the hero of this story; he transcended the son's personal insult of requesting the "share of the property that will belong to me" (15:12). This parable's purpose is to project a merciful God as father and forgiver. Over 200 times Jesus called God "Father."

In the Old Testament, God is presented as a father, and also as a mother, acting with tenderness and compassion. "You were unmindful of the Rock [God] that bore you; you forgot the God who gave you birth" (Deuteronomy 32:18). "As a mother comforts her child, so I will comfort you; you shall be comforted in Jerusalem" (Isaiah 66:13). The parable of the prodigal son is the *locus classicus* (model) of the forgiveness of the sinner; not surprisingly, it appears only in the Gospel of Luke, the scribe of the kindness of Christ.

Summary

The three synoptic Gospels (Matthew 9:1–8; Mark 2:1–12; Luke 5:17–26) describe the healing of the paralytic at Capernaum and Jesus' words to the handicapped man: "Take heart, son; your sins are forgiven" (Matthew 9:2). This healing confirms the assertion that the Son of Man (an Aramaic idiom pointing to Jesus' human nature) can forgive sins.

The Letters to the Colossians and the Ephesians both enumerate the virtues of the new life in Christ. "Bear with one another and, if anyone has a complaint against another, forgive each other; just as the Lord has forgiven you, so you also must forgive" (Colossians 3:13). "Be kind to one another, tenderhearted, forgiving one another, as God in Christ has forgiven you" (Ephesians 4:32).

The Lord's Prayer (Our Father) attests that divine forgiveness and human forgiveness are parallels. Words addressed to the Father: "Forgive us our debts, as we also have forgiven our debtors" (Matthew 6:12). "Forgive us our sins, for we ourselves forgive everyone indebted to us" (Luke 11:4).

In the Old Testament, forgiveness is related to atoning sacrifices: "He shall do with the bull just as is done with the bull of sin offering … The priest shall make atonement for them, and they shall be forgiven" (Leviticus 4:20). In the New Testament, forgiveness is associated with Jesus' death and resurrection: "Everyone who believes in him [Jesus] receives forgiveness of sins through his name" (Acts 10:43; see Luke 24:47; Colossians 1:14).

As we know all too well, forgiveness is never easy; it usually is a slow process, entailing a lifetime of forgiveness. When Peter asked Jesus: "How often should I forgive someone who sins against me? Seven times?" Jesus replied: "Seventy times seven!" (see Matthew 18:21–22); in other words—*Unlimited*!

"Whoever Wishes to Become Great Among You Must Be Your Servant" (Mark 10:43)

Hebrew *'ebed* and Greek *doulos* are non-technical terms usually translated "servant," more properly "slave." *'Ebed* generally expresses the relationship of the subordinate to the superior party in a covenant. *Diakonos*, "servant," connotes "one who renders personal help to others." Jesus used the verb, *diakoneo*, when he said: "Just as the Son of Man came not to be *served* but to *serve*, and to give his life a ransom for many" (Matthew 20:28). Writers of both Old Testament and New Testament acknowledge slavery as a normal social institution; nowhere is there an indication of the abolition of slavery. Generally, slaves in biblical times were well treated. Some English-language translators of the Bible tendentiously use "servant" in place of "slave," despite its inaccuracy, as a way of white-washing the concept.

The theme of service is prominent in the Bible because believers are called to a life of service. It stands at the center of biblical faith, inasmuch as it expresses the covenant relationship between God and believers. "Do not lag in zeal, be ardent in spirit, serve the Lord" (Romans 12:11). "You serve the Lord Christ ... Masters, treat your slaves justly and fairly, for you know that you also have a Master in heaven (Colossians 3:24; 4:1). Concerning the Thessalonians' reception of Paul's gospel: "The people of those regions report about us what kind of welcome we had among you, and how you turned to God from idols, to serve a living and true God" (1 Thessalonians 1:9). "James, a servant (*doulos*) of God and of the Lord Jesus Christ" (James 1:1).

Servants of Yahweh

Many of Israel's ancestors, including kings and prophets, are designated as servants of Yahweh. After the disaster of the golden calf, Moses implored Yahweh, invoking "Abraham, Isaac, and Israel, your servants" (Exodus 32:13). On the occasion of Moses' death, the writer of Deuteronomy records: "Then Moses, the servant of the Lord, died there in the land of Moab, at the Lord's command" (Deuteronomy 34:5). "Moses was one hundred twenty years old when he died" (Deuteronomy 34:7). So, too, with Joshua: "Joshua son of Nun, the servant of the Lord, died at the age of one hundred ten years" (Judges 2:8). On the occasion of God's covenant with David: "The word of the Lord came to Nathan: Go and tell my servant David: Thus says the Lord: 'Are you the one to build me a house to live in?'" (2 Samuel 7:4–5). When Yahweh appeared in a dream to Solomon at Gibeon by night, Solomon answered: "O Lord my God, you have made your servant king in place of my father David, although I am only a little child" (1 Kings 3:7).

In the New Testament, Paul, among others, is a "servant of Jesus Christ" (Romans 1:1). In the letter to the Philippians, Paul and Timothy are "servants of Christ Jesus" (Philippians 1:1).

Servant Songs

Second Isaiah (Isaiah 40–55) develops, in the course of four songs or oracles, the dominant theme of the servant of Yahweh, who is depicted as a mysterious figure who suffers vicariously. Because the servant is anonymous, Old Testament commentators conjecture endlessly about his identity, ranging from collective to individual interpretations. New Testament writers have no problem in seeing Jesus as the fulfillment of the servant songs.

The four servant songs, embedded in the text of Second Isaiah, may be an integral part of Second Isaiah, or they may have been added later. There are grounds for both opinions, but it does not change their meaning.

In the first servant song (Isaiah 42:1–4), Yahweh is the speaker who describes the person and mission of the anonymous servant. Many identifications for this servant have been proposed. The New Testament sees the fulfillment of the prophecy in Jesus, a suffering Messiah, a concept essentially alien to Judaism. Most Jews adopt the collective theory, that is, the servant is a historical or ideal Israel. He is God's "chosen" (election) one on whom God's favor rests; also, an agent of peace and nonviolence, who works gently and unobtrusively to bring justice to all nations.

On the occasion of Jesus' baptism by John in the Jordan, a voice came from the heavens: "This is my Son, the Beloved, with whom I am well pleased" (Matthew 3:13–17; Mark 1:9–11; Luke 3:21–22; John 1:29–34). These words are reminiscent of the opening of the first servant song: "Here is my servant, whom I uphold, my chosen, in whom my soul delights" (Isaiah 42:1; compare with Psalm 2:7). The words of the psalmist are an ancient formula of adoption. Baptism is a summons to assume the role of servant. The New Testament identifies Jesus at his baptism as the servant of Yahweh. The disciples, Peter, James, and John, who were present at Jesus' transfiguration, heard the same voice that Jesus heard at his baptism (Mark 9:2–8; see Matthew 17:1–8; Luke 9:28–36).

The second servant song (Isaiah 49:1–6) has the servant as the speaker, who describes his divine call and commission. Extending far beyond the confines of Israel, his mission reaches to the whole world. From their formation in the womb, the similarities between the servant's call and Jeremiah's are striking; each thought of his ministry as a failure. The servant is described as a "light to the nations," that is, an agent of divine salvation.

In the third servant song (Isaiah 50:4–9), the servant is again the speaker. This song, too, is reminiscent of Jeremiah's call (Jeremiah 1:4–10) and confessions (Jeremiah 11:18–23; 15:10–21; 17:14–18; 18:18–23; 20:7–18). The servant does not shrink from his vocation despite the violence and hostility directed against him. The servant, like Jeremiah, was subjected to persecution. Complete trust in God makes his submission possible. Note in this servant song (verses 4–6) the references to various bodily parts (tongue, ear, back, cheeks, face).

In the fourth servant song (Isaiah 52:13–53:12), Yahweh is speaker at the beginning and the end of the poem. In the intervening verses the kings of many nations are the speakers. Humiliation (suffering) and exaltation (triumph) are contrasted throughout this song; ultimately, exaltation is achieved through humiliation. The servant is portrayed as rejected and despised by his own people. The vicarious suffering of the sinless servant, endured in silence, counteracts the people's sins; this atoning work of the servant in the world predominates in Isaiah 53:1–12.

New Testament Use of Isaiah 53

Matthew sees Jesus as the servant of Yahweh, as he took upon himself our infirmities (Isaiah 53:4). "That evening they brought to him many who were possessed with demons; and he cast out the spirits with a word, and cured all who were sick. This was to fulfill what had been spoken through the prophet Isaiah, 'He took our infirmities and bore our diseases'" (Matthew 8:16–17).

This fourth servant song has never occupied a prominent place in Jewish theology. According to Jewish scholars, these references are to the sufferings of Israel in the world, whereas Christian scholars understand the references to Jesus, the suffering servant. Jesus is identified as the servant in Acts 8:32–35, where Isaiah 53:7–8 is cited: "Like a sheep he was led to the slaughter, and like a lamb silent before its shearer, so he does not open his mouth."

In Acts 8:26–40, Luke tells how the apostle Philip had a chance-meeting with an Ethiopian eunuch on the Jerusalem-Gaza road. Seated in his chariot, the eunuch was reading the prophet Isaiah. Philip inquired whether he understood what he was reading. The passage was: "Like a lamb that is led to the slaughter, and like a sheep that before its shearers is silent, so he did not open his mouth. By a perversion of justice he was taken away. Who could have imagined his future? For he was cut off from the land of the living, stricken for the transgression of my people" (Isaiah 53:7–8). The eunuch did not know whether the prophet (Isaiah) was speaking about himself or someone else. "Then Philip began to speak, and starting with this scripture, he proclaimed to him the good news about Jesus" (Acts 8:35).

Reflection on the four servant songs makes it clear why these texts are a perfect description of Jesus and his mission, as the New Testament writers assert. Jesus did not fulfill his messianic mission by identifying with the conquering kings of the Royal Psalms (Psalms 2, 18, 20–21, 45, 72, 101, 110, 144:1–11);

rather by conforming to the suffering servant (a mysterious figure) of Second Isaiah (Isaiah 40–55), where the mission of the servant is described so poignantly. When the New Testament writers searched for an appropriate paradigm of Jesus and his mission, they borrowed from the four servant songs. Jesus, too, regarded himself as their fulfillment.

Jesus the Servant

In his public life Jesus exemplified, both in word and deed, his role as servant. James and John approached Jesus and asked for personal preference in the kingdom: "They said to him, 'Grant us to sit, one at your right hand and one at your left, in your glory'" (Mark 10:37); the other disciples were indignant at such hubris. Jesus admonished them, saying that is how the world functions, but "It is not so among you; but whoever wishes to become great among you must be your servant, and whoever wishes to be first among you must be slave of all. For the Son of Man came not to be served but to serve, and to give his life a ransom for many" (Mark 10:43–45). In short, true primacy consists in service.

Jesus has given us many examples of service. In the course of the last supper, Jesus rose from the table, removed his cloak, girded himself with a towel, poured water in a basin, and began to wash his disciples' feet and dry them with the towel wrapped around him. After he had washed their feet, he put his cloak back on and reclined at table once more. He said to them:

Do you know what I have done to you? You call me Teacher and Lord—and you are right, for that is what I am. So if I, your Lord and Teacher, have washed your feet, you also ought to wash one another's feet. For I have set you an example, that you also should do as I have done to you.

Very truly, I tell you, servants are not greater than their master, nor are messengers greater than the one who sent them. For if you know these things, you are blessed if you do them. (John 13:12–17)

Another example, from the Gospel of John, of service to the community: Jesus identified with the good (Greek, *kalos*, "ideal" rather than "good") shepherd: "The good shepherd lays down his life for the sheep" (John 10:11).

The New Testament writers identify Jesus as the suffering servant not only at his baptism (Mark 1:11; John 1:34), but also in his miracles. As noted previously, "That evening they brought to him many who were possessed with demons; and he cast out the spirits with a word, and cured all who were sick. This was to fulfill what had been spoken through the prophet Isaiah, 'He took our infirmities and bore our diseases'" (Matthew 8:16–17). Matthew sees Jesus as the servant of Yahweh (Isaiah 53:4) as he took upon himself our infirmities.

When Jesus cured the infirm he strictly charged them not to publicize what he had done, in fulfillment of what had been said through the prophet Isaiah in the first servant song:

Here is my servant, whom I have chosen, my beloved, with whom my soul is well pleased. I will put my Spirit upon him, and he will proclaim justice to the Gentiles. He will not wrangle or cry aloud, nor will anyone hear his voice in the streets. He will not break a bruised reed or quench a smoldering wick until he brings justice to victory. And in his name Gentiles will hope. (Matthew 12:18–21; from Isaiah 42:1–4)

In several places in the New Testament, apart from the Gospels, the role of servant is attributed to Jesus. After Peter cured a crippled man at the entrance to the temple, he addressed the astonished onlookers, explaining "the God of Abraham, the God of Isaac, and the God of Jacob, the God of our ancestors has glorified [through resurrection and ascension] his servant (Greek, *pais*) Jesus, whom you handed over and rejected in the presence of Pilate, though he had decided to release him" (Acts 3:13). Ending his discourse, Peter said: "When God raised up his servant, he sent him first to you to bless you by turning each of you from your wicked ways" (Acts 3:26).

The Christian community refers twice to Jesus as holy servant (Acts 4:27, 30). In the Letter to the Philippians, Paul exhorts the believers: "though he was in the form of God, did not regard equality with God as something to be exploited, but emptied himself (*kenosis*), taking the form of a slave (*doulos*), being born in human likeness" (Philippians 2:6–7).

In the Letter to the Ephesians, the community is told that God "has put all things under his [Jesus'] feet and has made him the head over all things for the church, which is his body, the fullness of him who fills all in all" (Ephesians 1:22–23). Since Jesus was God's servant, it behooves us to assume a comparable role. Just as Jesus was identified as servant at baptism, so we are truly baptized to service.

In all the Old Testament covenants, the covenant partners committed themselves to a life of service. The verb *'abad* (to serve) is the most common word summarizing the covenant obligations of the Israelites to God. So, too, the Eucharist, which is the renewal of covenant, gives us Christians the opportunity to commit (or recommit) ourselves to a life of service to God and one another.

CHAPTER FIVE

"A Prophet to the Nations I Appointed You"

(JEREMIAH 1:5)

The Prophetic Role

The Book of Jeremiah lists the three classes of spiritual leaders in Old Testament times, each with a specific function: instruction (*torah*) for the priest, counsel (*'esa*) for the wise, and word (*dabar*) for the prophet (Jeremiah 18:18). The Hebrew word *nabi',* "prophet" (probable meaning: one who is called), is not a hereditary office, unlike king and priest. The prophet is essentially a religious intermediary to whom communications are transmitted through visions, dreams, and ecstasies. The New Testament uses the Greek word *prophetes* to translate the Hebrew *nabi'*.

The Jewish tradition divides the canon (list of religious writings deemed authoritative) into three parts; the second of the three divisions of the Hebrew Bible is *nebi'im* ("Prophets,"), in turn, subdivided into Former (Joshua–2 Kings) and Latter (Isaiah,

Jeremiah, Ezekiel, and the Book of the Twelve [Minor Prophets]). Prophecy flourished in monarchic Israel and Judah (ca. 1000–586 BCE). The historical and cultural context of Old Testament prophecy was the period of Israelite and Judahite monarchies, continuing through the exile (586–515 BCE), and into the early postexilic period (first half of the fifth century BCE). After the exile, prophetic influence appears to have waned.

The prophet is a person authorized to speak for another. "The Lord said to Moses, 'See, I have made you like God to Pharaoh, and your brother Aaron shall be your prophet. You shall speak all that I command you, and your brother Aaron shall tell Pharaoh to let the Israelites go out of his land'" (Exodus 7:1–2). Prophets came from many walks of life, and the calls of some were quite specific. "The Lord took me [Amos] from following the flock, and said to me, 'Go, prophesy to my people Israel. Now therefore hear the word of the Lord!'" (Amos 7:15–16). The purpose of this call was to authenticate Amos' words as legitimate prophetic words.

Both Old and New Testament prophets were spokespersons for God to their own generation. Prophecy is much more concerned with the here-and-now, and much less with the distant future; prophets were not forecasters. To concentrate on the distant future would be to miss much of the message for today. The value of the prophets for today's audience, as for their original audiences, is essentially in their message of repentance, judgment, and hope for salvation. Today, they serve us in two ways: by calling us to the same holy life to which they called their contemporaries; also, by depicting a near future shaped by God's purposes. However, in warning Israel that terrible things would happen if it continued on its faithless course, there was an element of predicting the future because so often the things they warned about actually occurred. Just as assuredly, modern-day prophets are in our midst, and we are invited to identify our own prophets and to listen to their words. Today's prophets are still not fully appreciated in society or in the church. It is often said that the function of the prophetic office is not to comfort the afflicted, as much as to afflict the comfortable.

The Book of Isaiah

Isaiah's Three Sections

Until recently, most scholars recognized the Book of Isaiah as a composite work consisting of three parts: chapters 1–39 (First Isaiah), chapters 40–55 (Second Isaiah), and chapters 56–66 (Third Isaiah); not independent collections, but organically related by themes such as the centrality of Jerusalem, the significance of the anointed (*meshiah*) ruler, and the holiness (*qodesh*) of God. Accordingly, the Book of Isaiah was composed and assembled over several centuries, beginning in the eighth century BCE. First Isaiah is attributed to an eighth century BCE Judahite prophet (named Isaiah); Second (Deutero) Isaiah is assigned to an anonymous prophet who lived in Babylon in the sixth century BCE; Third (Trito) Isaiah is ascribed to the postexilic period (after 539 BCE). Today, however, many scholars espouse the unity of Isaiah, on the basis of literary considerations, the development of major themes, as well as other features. The usage of the epithet—Holy One of Israel—can also serve as an argument in favor of one book. This title for God appears almost an equal number of times in both chapters 1–39 and 40–66.

Isaiah's Call

The vocation of the prophets and their mission attest to their trust in God. Isaiah's call, in the form of a vision, is one of the classic passages in prophetic literature (Isaiah 6:1–13). As mentioned, initially the scene takes place in the Jerusalem temple; then it is transformed into a heavenly setting. Yahweh the king is seated upon the throne. Recall this was a critical juncture in Israel's history—Uzziah, king of Judah, had died about 742 BCE, and Isaiah prophesied during the second half of the eighth century BCE, when two political events—the Syro-Ephraimite war and Assyrian threats on Jerusalem—traumatized the Southern Kingdom of Judah. Seraphim, fiery (Hebrew, *sarap*, "to burn") serpents guarded the throne. To recall, each had six wings: two to cover the face lest they look upon God; two to cover their "feet" (genitals), and two in preparation for flight. They joined in acclaiming "holy, holy, holy," that ineffable quality that differentiates Yahweh from all creation. Aware of his own unworthiness, Isaiah is symbolically purified by an ember touched to his lips, rendering him worthy to fulfill his prophetic vocation. When Yahweh inquired of the divine assembly (council of divine beings presided over by Yahweh) about who should be sent to carry out the prophetic mission, Isaiah answered the call spontaneously, unlike Moses who claimed to have a speech impediment (Exodus 4:10); Jeremiah who complained he was too young (Jeremiah 1:6); and Jonah, when told to go north, went in the opposite direction (Jonah 1:3). In fact, God calls each of us, but not everyone responds.

Some Themes of First Isaiah

Early in his ministry, the prophet Isaiah inveighed against the futility of empty ritual in his criticism of institutional religion (Isaiah 1:10–20). "When you stretch out your hands, I will hide my eyes from you; even though you make many prayers, I will not listen; your hands are full of blood. Wash yourselves; make yourselves clean ... seek justice, rescue the oppressed, defend the orphan, plead for the widow" (Isaiah 1:15–17).

Isaiah's description of Yahweh's universal reign of peace is one of the most moving passages of Isaiah (Isaiah 2:1–5). Too long to quote in its entirety, select verses need to be highlighted:

The mountain of the Lord's house shall be established as the highest of the mountains, and shall be raised above the hills; all the nations shall stream to it. Many peoples shall come and say, 'Come, let us go up to the mountain of the Lord, to the house of the God of Jacob; that he may teach us his ways and that we may walk in his paths.' For out of Zion shall go forth instruction (*torah*), and the word (*dabar*) of the Lord from Jerusalem. (Isaiah 2:2–3)

A classic verse follows: "They shall beat their swords into plowshares, and their spears into pruning hooks; nation shall not lift up sword against nation, neither shall they learn war any more" (Isaiah 2:4). Was there ever a time in history when this passage was more pertinent than the present? These words have been around a long time, but seldom heeded, especially today. Ultimately, warfare fails, whereas peace treaties, achieved through discussion and compromise, usually triumph. How many more combatants, not to mention innocent non-combatants, must die before present-day leaders are aroused from their stupor? "O my people, your leaders mislead you, and confuse the course of your paths" (Isaiah 3:12).

Having spent a good part of my professional life as an archaeologist in the Middle East, a battlefield for centuries, I became acquainted with many of the local people in countries such as Israel, Jordan, Syria, Egypt, Iraq, Yemen, Tunisia, Cyprus, Iran; I shudder to think how many of my local friends are deceased. Our own scholarly contribution to that desperate part of the world, in pursuit of the history and culture of the ancient Near East, is as nothing compared to theirs, except as evidence of the utter futility of war. Just about everything we and others accomplished in our excavations in Iraq has been destroyed. The only antidote to war is found in the Old Testament and New Testaments—love thy neighbor. That exhortation continues to bind each of us today, whether at home or abroad.

Song of the Vineyard

That Yahweh comes to judge his people is the theme of the unforgettable love song about the vineyard (Israel) in the Book of Isaiah. In both the Old Testament and New Testament, the image of the fruitful/fruitless vineyard is one of the prime metaphors for the people of God. This ballad was sung at the autumn festival celebrating the completion of the wine harvest. Although the vineyard was planted meticulously, it produced only wild grapes. The threat is that the people of God in their vineyard (the promised land) would be destroyed, just as a fruitless vineyard was demolished by the vintager (Isaiah 5:1–7). Isaiah 27:2–6 is opposite in meaning to Isaiah 5:1–7—the vineyard (Israel) will be restored. "On that day: A pleasant vineyard, sing about it! I, the Lord, am its keeper; every moment I water it. I guard it night and day so that no one can harm it; ... In days to come Jacob shall take root, Israel [the vineyard, that is, the people] shall blossom and put forth shoots, and fill the whole world with fruit."

"The Young Woman Is with Child"

Since Isaiah 7:14 is invoked in Matthew 1:23, its use in the New Testament is a much-discussed issue. It falls into the category of proof-text, so it is important to know how the Hebrew text reads: "The young woman (*ha'alma*) is with child and shall bear a son, and shall name him Immanuel [God is with us]." *Ha'alma* (a young marriageable woman) is not the technical term for a virgin (*betula*). The Septuagint (the Greek translation of the Old Testament) text reads *parthenos* (virgin, unmarried girl), whence "The virgin shall conceive and bear a son, and they shall name him Emmanuel" (Matthew 1:23). Scholars ordinarily identify the child (Isaiah 7:14) as either a son of King Ahaz, or a son of Isaiah and his wife. In the New Testament, Emmanuel ("God with us") is identified with Jesus; following the Septuagint, early Christian tradition understood the young woman (virgin) to be Mary, mother of Jesus (Matthew 1:23). An understanding of the Hebrew and Greek texts prevents tendentious use of the biblical text. A translation is never sufficient evidence; in the words of the Italian adage: *traduttori traditori* "translators are traitors."

The splendid poem in Isaiah describes the radically changed condition in the world when God, through his righteous king, will bring about universal peace and justice:

The wolf shall live with the lamb, the leopard shall lie down with the kid, the calf and the lion and the fatling together, and a little child shall lead them. The cow and the bear shall graze, their young shall lie down together;

and the lion shall eat straw like the ox. The nursing child shall play over the hole of the asp, and the weaned child shall put its hand on the adder's den. They will not hurt or destroy on all my holy mountain; for the earth will be full of the knowledge of the Lord as the waters cover the sea. (Isaiah 11:6–9)

Messiah, Messianism

The biblical concepts associated with the word "messianism" are difficult to define, as is the development of Israelite messianism over 2,000 years.

"Messiah" is derived from the Hebrew *mashiah*, denoting an anointed person, and is translated in Greek with *ho Xristos*, the Christ. The Hebrew noun *mashiah*, "anointed," is used particularly of kings and (high) priests. Yahweh's anointing of the king signifies the exclusive relationship between the God of Israel and the king. By way of exception, in Second Isaiah, the term *mashiah* is applied to the Persian king Cyrus: "Thus says the Lord to his anointed, to Cyrus" (Isaiah 45:1), who is commissioned to establish peace and liberty for God's people.

Some of the Old Testament prophecies concerned future Davidic kings. They announce a permanent change in the fortunes of the chosen people, achieved by God—war will come to an end, peace will be restored, exiles will be returned. A new era has begun. The principal figure in these prophecies is a descendant of King David. There was always the hope for an ideal Davidic king.

Isaiah 9:1–7 is an oracle of promise to Judah describing the prince of peace, the messiah: God's light in the darkness. There will be a new age, and a new ruler. Isaiah 11:1–9 describes the future peaceful kingdom; the principal attribute of its ruler is the equitable administration of justice. The prophet Isaiah proclaimed that the messiah was to be the light to the nations (49:6). The expectation of a future messiah was rooted in the dissatisfaction with the reigning kings.

Second Isaiah

Second Isaiah (chapters 40–55) is basically a message of hope, promise, and consolation; the redemption of the exiled people of Israel from Babylon is at hand. A new epoch coincides with the call of the prophet Second Isaiah (Isaiah 40:1–11). This call parallels that of First Isaiah, but they differ considerably in context and content. The opening words of Second Isaiah, "Comfort, O comfort my people, says your God," is the key to the whole prophecy; Jerusalem's warfare is ended. The exodus motif is one of the central themes in Second Isaiah: "In the wilderness prepare the way of the Lord, make straight in the desert a highway for our God. Every valley shall be lifted up, and every mountain and hill be made low; the uneven ground shall become level, and the rough places a plain" (Isaiah 40:3–4).

The message the prophet is to proclaim appears in Isaiah 40:6–11; it contrasts the transitoriness of all earthly things with the permanence of God's promise: "The grass withers, the flower fades; but the word of our God will stand forever" (verse 8).

The dominant motif of Second Isaiah is the new exodus; Israel's redemption is imminent, accompanied by great assurance—"Do not fear, for I am with you" (Isaiah 43:5). Exodus typology is used to reinforce divine assurances:

Do not fear (*'al-tira'*), for I have redeemed you; I have called you by name, you are mine. When you pass through the waters, I will be with you; and through the rivers, they shall not overwhelm you; when you walk through fire you shall not be burned, and the flames shall not consume you. For I am the Lord your God, the Holy One of Israel, your Savior. I give Egypt as your ransom, Ethiopia and Seba in exchange for you. Because you are precious in my sight, and honored, and I love you. (Isaiah 43:1–4)

Second Isaiah concludes with an eloquent invitation to the messianic banquet for all people; it is the banquet of the kingdom of God. "Everyone [wide-hearted universalism] who thirsts, come to the waters; and you that have no money, come, buy and eat! Come, buy wine and milk without money and without price ... Listen carefully to me, and eat what is good, and delight yourselves in rich food. Incline your ear, and come to me; listen, so that you may live" (Isaiah 55:1–3).

Creation and Redemption in Second Isaiah

God is the Lord of creation and redemption. All things belong to God because God created them, as affirmed by several passages in Isaiah. "Lift up your eyes on high and see: Who created these?" (Isaiah 40:26). "Have you not known? Have you not heard? The Lord is the everlasting God, the Creator of the ends of the earth" (Isaiah 40:28). "Thus says God, the Lord, who created the heavens and stretched them out, who spread out the earth, and what comes from it" (Isaiah 42:5). "For thus says the Lord, who created the heavens (he is God!), who formed the earth and made it" (Isaiah 45:18). God's creative activity goes far beyond creation in Genesis. After the world is besmirched by sin God will create a glorious new creation: "For I [Yahweh] am about to create new heavens and a new earth" (Isaiah 65:17).

"Thus says the Lord, the King of Israel, and his Redeemer, the Lord of hosts: I am the first and I am the last; besides me there is no god" (Isaiah 44:6). The Creator-God is also Israel's redeemer who buys it back from slavery. This refers to the first exodus; the liberation from Babylon is the new exodus, the dominant theme of Second Isaiah. The Judean exiles' journey homeward under the guiding hand of God is poignantly described in Isaiah 49:8–13; in part, "They shall not hunger or thirst, neither scorching wind nor sun shall strike them down, for he who has pity on them will lead them, and by springs of water will guide them. And I will turn all my mountains into a road, and my highways shall be raised up" (Isaiah 49:10–11). Those who return home after many trials can identify with these words of Isaiah.

God's role as creator-redeemer is summarized in Isaiah 43:1: "But now thus says the Lord, he who created you, O Jacob, he who formed you, O Israel: Do not fear, for I have redeemed you; I have called you by name, you are mine."

Basic to the New Testament message is the declaration that Jesus of Nazareth is the fulfillment of Israel's messianic hope. Through the death and resurrection of Jesus Christ, "who was handed over to death for our trespasses and was raised for our justification" (Romans 4:25), humankind has been restored to the friendship of God.

Third Isaiah

Turning to Third Isaiah (chapters 56–66), we encounter one of the most compassionate statements of the Scriptures, one of the strongest protests against exclusiveness. Eunuchs had originally been rejected from the community of Israel. Because of their respect for the human body as the creation of God, the Israelites were appalled at mutilation; hence eunuchs were denied full membership in the community. Henceforth, neither eunuchs, foreigners, nor the marginalized would be rejected; instead, participation would be available to all who believe and observe the commandments, regardless of national origin and social status.

Jerusalem's stark, black-marble memorial to the European Jews murdered in World War II derives its name, Yad Vashem (monument [*yad*]) and a name [*shem*]), from Isaiah 56:5: "I [Yahweh] will give, in my house and within my walls, a monument and a name better than sons and daughters; I will give them an everlasting name that shall not be cut off."

Mere external worship does not suffice with God. The genuine fast in terms of the Hebrew doctrine of righteousness is described thus: "Is not this the fast that I choose: to loose the bonds of injustice, to undo the thongs of the yoke, to let the oppressed go free, and to break every yoke? Is it not to share your bread with the hungry, and bring the homeless poor into your house; when you see the naked, to cover them, and not to hide yourself from your own kin?" (Isaiah 58:6–7). These are the uncompromising demands of social justice, of kindness and compassion, of love of neighbor. Note the similarities with the list of works of mercy in Matthew 25:35–36.

Isaiah 60–66 comprises a group of marvelous, eschatological (relating to ultimate destiny or purpose) poems, of which chapter 60 is one of the most elegant. It is too long to cite, but reading is not sufficient; serious reflection is required. Verses 17–18 provide a marvelous description of a land at peace, appropriate then and just as timely today. "Instead of bronze I will bring gold, instead of iron I will bring silver; instead of wood, bronze, instead of stones, iron. I will appoint Peace as your overseer and Righteousness as your taskmaster. Violence shall no more be heard in your land, devastation or destruction within your borders; you shall call your walls Salvation, and your gates Praise."

Isaiah 66:18–21 is one of the most expansive views of religion and humankind in the entire Old Testament. Again, it requires deep reflection, especially nowadays, when religion appears to be more divisive than unifying. Because of its ideological component, religion can be distorted to justify violence and exclusiveness. A cursory glance of history will reveal how many wars have been fought in the name of God, each side claiming to have the Deity on its side. Too many people of all religious traditions pretend to know God's will. Karl Barth warned of the danger in taking the mystery out of God. I think the most accurate definition of God is still *magnum mysterium*.

Other Major and Minor Prophets

Jeremiah the Prophet

More is known about Jeremiah than any other prophet. He fulfilled his prophetic ministry (about 627–580 BCE) during one of the most turbulent and tragic periods in the history of Israel. Jeremiah's most appealing attribute is his humanness, a quality with which every reader can identify. He was a timid, reluctant, rebellious, introspective person. He did not enjoy being condemned as a collaborationist and traitor for urging Judah to surrender to the Babylonians as a way of averting a worse fate.

Jeremiah was destined to be a prophet even before birth, when Yahweh had already known him and dedicated him.

Unlike Isaiah, his call did not come in the temple; it was a simple conversation between Yahweh and the prophet.

"Now the word of the Lord came to me saying, 'Before I formed you in the womb I knew you, and before you were born I consecrated you; I appointed you a prophet to the nations ...You shall go to all to whom I send you, and you shall speak whatever I command you'" (Jeremiah 1:4–7). Jeremiah was not eager to embrace the prophetic vocation; no wonder, it is never profitable to be a prophet. He, like Moses before him, had personal misgivings; both, for example, had speech impediments (Exodus 4:10; 6:12, 30; Jeremiah 1:6). To allay their anxiety, they were assured that Yahweh's abiding presence would sustain them. "Do not be afraid of them, for I am with you to deliver you, says the Lord" (Jeremiah 1:8).

Jeremiah's life, like Jesus' after him, was a veritable vale of tears. Few people suffered so greatly as they. The striking similarities between Jeremiah and Jesus were not lost on the author of Matthew's Gospel, unlike Mark and Luke's Gospels. "He [Jesus] asked his disciples this question: 'Who do people say that the Son of Man is?' And they said, 'Some say John the Baptist, others say Elijah, and still others say Jeremiah or one of the prophets'" (Matthew 16:13–14). Matthew's inclusion of Jeremiah's name is one of many significant differences among the evangelists. The Gospels are not photocopies; each has its own distinguishing features.

Jeremiah and Jesus

Both Jeremiah and Jesus were reared in small towns; both suffered grievously; both identified with the "little people" of society; both incurred the wrath of Jerusalem's civil and religious establishments; both foretold the destruction of Jerusalem and its temple.[1]

The Book of Jeremiah contains a series of candid laments, so-called confessions, in which this very sensitive prophet speaks in his own name. Unique in prophetic literature, these personal prayers reveal Jeremiah's inner feelings of anguish, self-doubt, bitterness, resentment; he even struggles with Yahweh. Those readers who may be shocked by the disarming frankness of these laments should bear in mind: "God does not make his call to his servants conditional upon their purging themselves of weakness … It is precisely in their weakness and frailty—even in their rebellion—that God calls his servants. So it was with Jeremiah; so it is through all the pages of scripture; and so it is today."[2]

The Prophet Micah

Micah, a younger contemporary of Isaiah, lived during the last quarter of the eighth century BCE, a period of political crisis and a time of economic pressure for the people of Judah. Micah foresaw the collapse of Jerusalem and the destruction of the temple; they were fulfilled when the Babylonians destroyed Jerusalem and the temple in 586 BCE. "Therefore because of you [wicked rulers, priests, and prophets] Zion [Jerusalem] shall be plowed as a field; Jerusalem shall become a heap of ruins, and the mountain of the house [the temple] a wooded height" (Micah 3:12).

Little is known of Micah's life, but his message of social justice was unmistakably clear. In answer to the question: what does God expect from the people for whom he has done so much, Micah's response epitomizes prophetic religion, underscoring the connection between believing and doing. "He has told you, O mortal (*'adam*, humankind) what is good; and what does the Lord require of you but to do justice (*mishpat*), and to love kindness (*hesed*), and to walk (*halak*) humbly with your God" (Micah 6:8). This triad constitutes one of the noblest utterances of Scripture, as well as a perfect summary of prophetic teaching. Two parts pertain to humankind; only one refers to God. There is no purpose in serving God if one does not also serve the neighbor. The Hebrew terms above are more easily described than defined, despite their frequency in the Hebrew Bible. Justice (*mishpat*) calls upon us to work for equality among all of our neighbors. Kindness (*hesed*) has to do with love, loyalty, and faithfulness, with particular concern for the poor and needy. "Walk (*halak*) humbly with God" describes a life lived in dependence upon God. In summary, "God is more interested in the way people live their daily lives than in their religious practices."[3]

The Prophet Amos

Amos was invoked as the role model of Martin Luther King, Jr. Biographical data on this eighth-century BCE prophet are incomplete; however, the Bible mentions he was a herdsman (Amos 1:1) and a dresser of sycamore trees (Amos 7:14). He preached in the Northern Kingdom of Israel where he was associated with the capital city of Samaria and the royal sanctuary at Bethel, from which he was expelled by the priest Amaziah (Amos 7:10–17). He was conversant with political developments not only in Israel, but also in neighboring nations. His prophetic ministry coincided with a peaceful era during the prosperous reigns of King Uzziah of Judah and King Jeroboam II of Israel.

Amos, the first prophet whose oracles and visions have been preserved in written form, preached divine judgment in a tone of harsh severity. Influenced by the tradition of the Mosaic covenant, with emphasis not on privilege but responsibility, Amos was profoundly disturbed by the rampant social injustice (greed and corruption) perpetrated by his contemporaries and compatriots, specifically the venal elite. Economic prosperity had created a social imbalance, resulting in two separate classes, the rich and the poor. The upper class exploited the weak and oppressed the poor by alienating their land, forced labor, and onerous taxes. Amos protested bitterly against this perversion of justice among his fellow Israelites. He went so far as to say, contrary to covenant tradition, that the "day of Yahweh" would not be a day of vindication, but one of inevitable doom. "Therefore because you trample on the poor you take from them levies of grain [heavy taxation], you have built houses of hewn stone [luxury homes], but you shall not live in them; you have planted pleasant vineyards, but you shall not drink their wine" (Amos 5:11).

Hosea, Prophet of Love

Hosea ("may Yahweh save") was more tenderhearted than the austere Amos. Again, biographical information about Hosea, the younger contemporary of Amos, is quite sparse. He married Gomer, who was either a temple prostitute or an unfaithful spouse. Their three children were given symbolic names: a son "Jezreel" ("God sows"), a daughter "Not-Pitied" (*Lo'-ruhamah*), and a second son, "Not-My-People" (*Lo'-'ammi*). The names foreshadowed the demise of the Northern Kingdom of Israel for its violation of the divine covenant.

Hosea was master of metaphor, appealing to flora and fauna to make his theological arguments. He describes the divine-human relationship in familial terms of father-son and husband-wife. Marital imagery symbolized for Hosea the covenant relationship between Yahweh and Israel. His sensitive and emotional nature, even his brokenheartedness, may be attributable in some degree to his own domestic tragedy.

Hosea was primarily concerned with Israel's religious apostasy, which was especially shocking owing to Yahweh's great love for Israel. No prophet was more profoundly cognizant of the depth of love, as well as its indestructibility, as Hosea chapter 11 bears witness. Whereas John is the evangelist of love in the New Testament, Hosea is the prophet of love in the Old Testament. Hosea preached hope of renewal, but only after the destruction of the nation and the repentance of the people. As an expression of hope in the future, he utilized the second exodus-conquest motif; what Yahweh had accomplished in the first exodus, he would achieve again. In the words of Yahweh: "Therefore, I will now allure her [Israel], and bring her into the wilderness, and speak tenderly to her. From there I will give her her vineyards, and make the Valley of Achor [literally, "valley of trouble"] a door of hope" (Hosea 2:14–15). As already stated, this treacherous valley, near Jericho, would be transformed into a "door of hope" (*petah tiqvah*), which, as we have noted earlier, is the name of the modern city of Petah Tiqva in Israel.

Ezekiel, the Prophet

Ezekiel, a contemporary of Jeremiah, was the first prophet to receive his call outside of Israel (Ezekiel 2:1–3:27); he was commissioned as a prophet in Babylon, where he had been taken into exile in 597 BCE. Both prophet and priest, Ezekiel met with considerable opposition during his lifetime. His final mandate was communicated in these words: "Mortal, all my [Yahweh's] words that I shall speak to you receive in your heart and hear with your ears; then go to the exiles, to your people, and speak to them. Say to them, 'Thus says the Lord God'; whether they hear or refuse to hear" (Ezekiel 3:10–11). A dynamic spokesperson for Yahweh, Ezekiel's prophecies are enigmatic, consisting of imagery, signs, visions, allegories, and metaphors. Because of his influence on postexilic religion (after 538 BCE), Ezekiel is known as the "father of Judaism."

The Book of Ezekiel, to say the least, is puzzling and complex, but a thoughtful reading brings some clarity. The prophet develops a variety of concepts, among them the temple and the liturgy. Also, the holiness of God, holy denoting one who completely transcends human understanding, is a major theme of Isaiah, Jeremiah, Hosea, and Ezekiel. "I [Yahweh] will sanctify my great name, which has been profaned among the nations, and which you have profaned among them" (Ezekiel 36:23). Additionally, no other prophet has emphasized so much the absolute majesty of God. The year 586 BCE, commemorating the destruction of Jerusalem at the hands of the Babylonians, signaled a turning point in the Book of Ezekiel. Before that fateful date, words of doom and judgment predominate (Ezekiel 1–24); after that, words of hope and consolation, promises of salvation and restoration, prevail (Ezekiel 33–48).

Ezekiel's classic vision of the dry bones and their reinvigoration (Ezekiel 37:1–14) represents his belief in a pending restoration by divine power. In this chapter, the concept that God makes the difference between life and death is vividly portrayed. The bones symbolize Israel in despair (exile); and the resurrection from the dead is the return of the people to their ancestral land. Humankind is dead until made alive by the indwelling Spirit (*ruah*) of God. God created; now God recreates. Many of us, I dare say, have found ourselves in desperate situations. Always remember, God still makes the difference between life and death, hope and despair.

Yahweh's presence among his people is the prime theme of the utopian vision in the closing chapters of Ezekiel (Ezekiel 40–48). It is an idealized picture of the restored community and the new temple. Ezekiel sees the glory (*kabod*) of the God of Israel return from the east and reenter the temple through the east gate (Ezekiel 43:1–5). Ezekiel's vision of the new Jerusalem ends with the famous apparition of a wonderful stream of water gushing from beneath the threshold of the temple, signifying Yahweh's renewed presence among the people (Ezekiel 47:12). In a land where existence was often hazardous, the people depended greatly on bread and water, the necessities of life.

The water in Ezekiel 47:1–12 is reminiscent of the living water (*hydor zon*) in the Gospel of John, set in the scene of Jesus and the woman of Samaria (John 4:7–15). The principal theological insight developed throughout this final vision is expressed cogently in Ezekiel 48:35: "And the name of the City [Jerusalem] from that time on shall be, *YHWH shammah* ("the Lord is there")." The new name indicates the new status of the City. The difference between life and death, hope and despair is the presence of God.

Ezekiel was a strong advocate of individual responsibility, as expressed in Ezekiel 18:1–32. At the beginning of this chapter, Ezekiel quotes a proverb to support the claim of the people that they were being penalized for the sins of their forebears, and not for their own. "The parents have eaten sour grapes, and the children's teeth are set on edge" (Ezekiel 18:2; see Jeremiah

31:29). We are all familiar with the too human tendency to blame others instead of ourselves. Both Jeremiah and Ezekiel reject this popular saying. The basic principle is already stated in Deuteronomy 24:16: "Parents shall not be put to death for their children, nor shall children be put to death for their parents; only for their own crimes may persons be put to death." This decree restricting punishment to the guilty party is cited in 2 Kings 14:6, concerning King Amaziah, son of Joash of Judah, who executed his father's assassins, but not their sons. Ezekiel 18:31 terminates this chapter on accountability with an invitation to repentance: "Get yourselves a new heart and a new spirit!"

Jonah the Prophet

Jonah is one of the better known books in the Hebrew Bible, but for the wrong reason, namely, Jonah and the "whale." But there is no whale in the book; the Hebrew text reads *dag gadol* ("big fish"). Jonah is remarkably different from other prophetic books; it is a short story *about* a prophet, who was reluctant, obstinate, petulant, and selfish. Yahweh mandated Jonah to prophesy in the great city of Nineveh, the capital of Assyria, which was responsible for destroying, in 721 BCE, the Northern Kingdom, thus becoming the traditional enemy of Israel.

Rejecting the call to go east to preach in Nineveh, he deliberately boarded a ship traveling west to the city of Tarshish, assumedly located in Spain. Although Tarshish occurs more than 30 times in the Bible, its location is uncertain, prompting several scholarly suggestions. Tarshish may refer to the Phoenician colony of Tartessus in southwest Spain, on the mouth of the Guadalqivir River, north of Cadiz. Tarsus, a large commercial city on the Cydnus River in southeast Asia Minor (modern Turkey),

and the birthplace of the apostle Paul, is the more probable location of Tarshish. For the Hebrews, it represented the far west.
Jonah tried to flee from his divine commission, but it is never
easy to run away from God.

Through the instrumentality of a big fish, Jonah was
rerouted to Nineveh, where, to his amazement, the Ninevites
responded to his message and immediately repented. "Jonah
began to go into the city, going a day's walk. And he cried out,
'Forty days more, and Nineveh shall be overthrown!' and the
people of Nineveh believed God; and they proclaimed a fast and
everyone, great and small, put on sackcloth" (Jonah 3:4–5).

Jonah was furious at the unexpected outcome because, in
accord with his vindictive and narrow-minded mentality, only
the Hebrew people were to be saved. Such exclusiveness calls to
mind the common Catholic pre-Vatican II view that "outside the
Church, no salvation." Jonah did not wish Yahweh to forgive the
Ninevites; he had completely forgotten about extending God's
boundless love and mercy to sinners. In fact, he was far more
bereft by the loss of his shady gourd plant (*qiqayon*) than for the
potential decimation of the Ninevites (Jonah 4:6).

The Book of Jonah prepares for the gospel, with its message of redemption for all, both Jews and Gentiles. The New
Testament utilizes in two Gospels the sign of Jonah:

Then some of the scribes and Pharisees said to him [Jesus],
"Teacher, we wish to see a sign from you." But he answered
them, "An evil and adulterous generation asks for a sign,
but no sign will be given to it except the sign of the prophet
Jonah. For just as Jonah was three days and three nights
in the belly of the sea monster (Hebrew, *dag gadol;* Greek,
en koilia tou ketous), so for three days and three nights the

Son of Man will be in the heart of the earth. The people of Nineveh will rise up at the judgment with this generation and condemn it, because they repented at the proclamation of Jonah, and see, something greater than Jonah is here!" (Matthew 12:38–41; see Luke 11:29–32)

The "sign of Jonah" is the person of Jonah and his preaching, as a consequence of which the Ninevites reformed their ways.[4]

Appropriately the Book of Jonah is read in the Jewish community on Yom Kippur (Day of Atonement); repentance and deliverance are the principal themes in the story of Jonah.

[1] Philip King, *Jeremiah: An Archaeological Companion* (Louisville: Westminster/John Knox Press, 1993), 7, note 7.

[2] Philip King, *Jeremiah: An Archaeological Companion* (Louisville: Westminster/John Knox Press, 1993), 6, note 6.

[3] Daniel J. Simundson, "Micah" in *New Interpreter's Bible*, vol. 7 (Nashville: Abingdon Press, 1996), 580.

[4] Joseph Fitzmyer, *The Gospel According to Luke X-XXIV*, The Anchor Bible (Garden City, NY: Doubleday, 1985), 933.

CHAPTER SIX

"Many Women Have Done Excellently, But You Surpass Them All"

(PROVERBS 31:29)

Women in the Old Testament

The Valiant Woman

The Bible was assembled by males who had little concern for the roles of women in society; their principal interests lay in the male dimensions of life, for example, worship, economy, warfare, governance, combat. Women, on the other hand, focused on household responsibilities, especially the maternal care of the children. Proverbs 31:10–31 is remarkable for its praise of the "ideal wife" (*'eset hayil*, "valiant woman") in biblical times, portraying her as almost superhuman. This eulogy has special meaning for the roles of resourceful women today. Bear in mind that Proverbs' encomium on women was composed centuries before the feminist movement. Even then, women were not merely submissive, nor simply the pawns of males—Proverbs states quite the opposite. To be sure, nowadays women's contributions to society far transcend domestic activities, as they rightly hold influential positions in a global economy.

In addition to her industry, courage, wisdom and kindness, this highly gifted woman is praised for her fear of Yahweh (*yir'at YHWH*), defined as a reverential fear and respect for Yahweh by reason of Yahweh's loving kindness (*hesed*) toward humanity. Herein lies the underpinning of religion. The bulk of this adulatory poem is dedicated to the wonderful deeds of the ideal woman, who provides for the needs (food and clothing) of her family; she acquires a field and plants a vineyard; she is a wise counselor and a prudent economist. These qualities, as well as her concern for the poor and less affluent, win the admiration of her husband, who has total confidence in his wife; her children, too, extol her (verses 11–28). What an appropriate tribute for Mother's Day and every other day of the year.

Women, as well as men, served as God's spokespersons. To appreciate fully the contribution of women in the Bible, one must understand the historical and social context in which these heroic women lived; the biblical world was patriarchal and androcentric. Among the many valiant women in the Old Testament are Miriam, Deborah, Huldah, Ruth, and Esther.

Miriam, Moses' Sister

Moses, Aaron, and their sister Miriam were the three leaders of the wilderness era, following the exodus from Egypt. When the basket bearing the infant Moses was floating on the river Nile,

Miriam suggested to the daughter of the Pharaoh that a woman among the daughters of the Israelites be found to care for the child. Coincidentally, Moses was reared by his own mother. Years later, to celebrate the crossing of the Red (Reed) sea, the prophet Miriam (the first woman to hold the title) led the women in a victory song and dance, accompanied with tambourines: "Sing to the Lord, for he is triumphed gloriously; horse and rider he has thrown into the sea" (Exodus 15:21).

When Moses married a Cushite (Ethiopian) woman, "Miriam [first named] and Aaron spoke against Moses because of the Cushite woman whom he had married" (Numbers 12:1). In reality, Miriam was rebelling against Moses' unique status as mediator between Yahweh and the people. Yahweh was so furious at Miriam's jealousy that she was afflicted with leprosy (not Hansen's disease), frequently a sign of God's displeasure.

The Cup of Miriam

Deborah is the prophet of war, Jeremiah the prophet of exile, and Miriam the prophet of water. The death of Miriam is recorded in Numbers 20; immediately following, it is noted that the Israelites in the wilderness had run out of drinking water (Numbers 20:2). The conjunction of these two events is the basis for the lovely legend about the well of fresh water that accompanied Miriam and the Israelites through the wilderness. Upon her death the fountain of living water dried up.

Today, this story has assumed new significance; at Passover rituals a cup of water is placed on the Seder table representing Miriam's well, to provide an opportunity to reflect upon Miriam's key role in the wilderness wanderings, as well as the contribution of women, in general, to the lives of ordinary people. In the course of this ritual, each woman at the Seder recounts the story of a woman whom she admires. Miriam's cup is a symbol of hope and renewal in the present life.

Deborah, Prophet and Judge

Deborah, one of the most remarkable women in the Old Testament, was both prophet and judge. She held court in Ephraim in a place known as Deborah's Palm Tree, where she reconciled disputes among the Israelites. Also, Deborah accompanied the warrior Barak into battle against the Canaanites. Deborah and Barak then sang a victory song over the Canaanites in the valley of Esdraelon (Greek form of "Jezreel"), designating the western section of the valleys and plains that separate Galilee from Samaria (Judges 5). "Praise of the Lord, the deliverer," is the recurring theme. The song of Deborah is one of the oldest poetic compositions in the Old Testament. After that battle, peace prevailed in the land for 40 years.

Huldah the Prophet

Huldah, a prophet living in Jerusalem during the time of King Josiah (640–609 BCE), was requested by the king to inquire of Yahweh on his behalf. She prophesied Jerusalem's destruction, which would happen only after the demise of Josiah. In that way he would be spared the national catastrophe (2 Kings 22:14).

Ruth, the Moabite Woman

Ruth, loving and selfless, was a Moabite by birth, hence a foreign woman. Elimelech of Bethlehem and his wife Naomi ("pleasant"), with their two sons, emigrated to Moab (plateau east of the Dead Sea bordered on the north by the Arnon River and on the south by the Zered) seeking fertile land after a severe famine broke out in Bethlehem of Judah. Elimelech died, and his two sons married Moabite women. Subsequently, the two sons died, leaving their widows, Orpah and Ruth; Orpah elected to remain in Moab, while Ruth left her own country, family, and faith to accompany her mother-in-law Naomi to Bethlehem. Her decision was courageous because as a widow without children, she put herself in a precarious position, not to mention her foreign status. Ruth expressed her ideal in-law relationship in these unforgettable words to Naomi: "Where you go, I will go; where you lodge, I will lodge; your people shall be my people, and your God my God" (Ruth 1:16). Ruth was a beautiful model of filial piety.

Boaz, a distant cousin, owned the field in Bethlehem where Ruth gleaned to provide food for Naomi, her mother-in-law, and herself. He was very generous to Ruth and her mother-in-law. Eventually, Boaz and Ruth married, and she bore a son Obed, who became the grandfather of King David.

One of the masterpieces of world literature, the Book of Ruth is a protest against narrow exclusiveness. Do not exclude foreigners, but accept them as family members. At a time when marriages are breaking up in large numbers, we can learn much from the loving kindness (*hesed*) of Ruth, the Moabite; *hesed* can be the glue that holds marriages together.

Esther, Queen in Persia

Esther (variant of the Babylonian goddess Ishtar) is the Persian name of the Jewish heroine Hadassah (from the feminine of *hadas*, "myrtle"), who became queen of King Ahasuerus (Xerxes I, 485–464 BCE) of Persia. She averted a pogrom, instigated by Haman, the king's jealous and ruthless advisor, by appealing to the king to save the Jewish community living in the Persian empire. The specific day of the planned genocide was determined by lots (*purim*), memorialized annually by the observance of the Jewish feast of Purim, accompanied with fun and frolic. The Book of Esther is a powerful reminder that divine providence watches over the Jewish people and all those who serve God faithfully, as well as those who reform their lives. In the uncertain atmosphere of today, not unlike that of Esther's day, God's saving presence is a source of unspeakable support.

Women in the New Testament

The New Testament also furnishes examples of profiles in courage among women in the Palestinian Jewish culture, one of the most patriarchal in the region of the Mediterranean Sea. By comparison, Jesus' interactions with women must have appeared revolutionary; he did not repudiate patriarchal society, he reformed it. By associating with the unclean, Jesus seems to have rejected many Levitical laws regarding clean and unclean. Clean describes the condition of being free from any physical, moral, or ritual contamination. For example, Jesus touched a corpse; one became unclean by contact with a corpse. He also stopped a funeral procession to assist a widowed mother who was burying her only son. Moved with pity upon seeing the bereaved mother, "Then he [Jesus] came forward and touched the bier, and the bearers stood still. And he said, 'Young man, I say to you, rise!' The dead man sat up and began to speak, and Jesus gave him to his mother" (Luke 7:14–15).

Women were both followers and traveling companions of Jesus.

Soon afterwards he went on through cities and villages, proclaiming and bringing the good news of the kingdom of God. The twelve were with him, as well as some women who had been cured of evil spirits and infirmities: Mary, called Magdalene, from whom seven demons had gone out, and Joanna, the wife of Herod's steward Chuza, and Susanna, and many others, who provided for them out of their resources. (Luke 8:1–3)

According to the gospel tradition, women were among the witnesses of Jesus' crucifixion, burial, empty tomb, and resurrection: "The women who had come with him [Jesus] from Galilee followed, and they saw the tomb and how his body was laid. Then they returned, and prepared spices and ointments" (Luke 23:55–56). "And returning from the tomb, they told all this to the eleven and to all the rest. Now it was Mary Magdalene, Joanna, Mary the mother of James, and the other women with them who told this to the apostles. But these words seemed to them an idle tale, and they did not believe them" (Luke 24:9–11).

Martha and Mary

Jesus also made clear that women should "listen and learn" (not a put-down) from him as his disciples, and not simply serve him in a woman's traditional role. The story of Martha and Mary illustrates the principle: When Jesus visited their home, Martha was preoccupied with the details of hospitality, while Mary "sat at the Lord's feet and listened to what he was saying." Martha complained to Jesus that her sister Mary had left the domestic chores to her. Jesus replied: "Martha, Martha, you are worried and distracted by many things; there is need of only one thing. Mary has chosen the better part which will not be taken away from her" (Luke 10:38–42).

Mary, the Mother of Jesus

The synoptic Gospels (Matthew, Mark, Luke) identify Mary as the mother of Jesus, but she is not as well known from the biblical perspective as she is from extrabiblical traditions, since we have only limited biographical information about her in the Gospels. This is not meant as a slight; simply, the intent of the New Testament is to portray Jesus, not Mary, who is not even named in John's Gospel. The author tells us the purpose of the Fourth Gospel: "These [signs] are written so that you may come to believe that Jesus is the Messiah, the Son of God, and that through believing you may have life in his name" (John 20:31). Mary is best honored when we accord her the dignity that is rightly hers in the New Testament, rather than indulging in "pious" exaltation.

To be sure, the New Testament communicates the essentials about Mary's role in the history of salvation, thereby portraying what is really important and deserving of our imitation. Matthew 1:18–25 and Luke 1:26–2:7 present different birth stories, but both attest to the virginal conception. Both Matthew and Luke identify Joseph as Mary's husband. John testifies to her presence at the marriage feast of Cana and at Jesus' crucifixion. Luke includes Mary among the women disciples praying in the upper room with the twelve after the ascension (Acts 1:14). Also, Mary received the Holy Spirit at Pentecost (Acts 2:1–4), as she did at Jesus' conception (Luke 1:35). From the cross, Jesus commended the beloved disciple (John) and Mary to each other

(John 19:26–27). The implication of this gesture is a matter of speculation among commentators, ranging from the literal to the symbolic; it may suggest a new and interdependent relationship between the two, or it may be conferring a new and elevated status on the beloved disciple among the apostles.

In the last analysis, the best insights into Mary's faith in God, her humility, and her familiarity with the Old Testament are best illustrated in the Magnificat (Latin, *magnificare*, "to magnify," "to extol"), Mary's marvelous hymn of praise reflecting Hannah's song at Samuel's birth (1 Samuel 2:1–10). The Magnificat (Luke 1:46–55) is Mary's expression of praise for God's extraordinary actions in her behalf. Mary's "lowliness" is contrasted with God's "might" (verse 48); what God has accomplished for Mary is extended to what God accomplishes for all those who fear God (verse 50). The lowly (the physically poor, the sick, the oppressed) are selected for God's blessings in place of the rich (the proud and arrogant), representing a reversal of the human condition (verses 52–53). The canticle closes with a remembrance of Yahweh's promises to Abraham and the ancestors; that is, the establishment of the covenant (Genesis 17:7; see Genesis 18:18; 22:17). The Magnificat is an important corrective to much Marian devotion. It is in happy contrast to her soft, socially indifferent image in sentimentalized devotions.

Mary Magdalene

Mary from Magdala, a town on the western side of the Sea of Galilee, is mentioned in first place on every listing of Jesus' female disciples. Let us be clear, Mary Magdalene is not to be identified with the woman of Luke 7:36–50, a sinner who bathed and anointed Jesus' feet in the course of a meal in the house of a Pharisee. According to the four Gospels, Mary Magdalene witnessed Jesus' death, the empty tomb, and the risen Christ; it was she who proclaimed the resurrection to the other disciples (John 20:11–18). Mary Magdalene had followed Jesus even to the foot of the cross while the male disciples fled. She was obviously a prominent person in the public ministry of Jesus.

In the Pauline Letters

In the Pauline community women assumed important roles: "The churches of Asia send greetings. Aquila and Prisca [wife of Aquila], together with the church in their house, greet you warmly in the Lord. All the brothers and sisters send greetings" (1 Corinthians 16:19–20). "Greet Prisca and Aquila, who work with me in Christ Jesus, and who risked their necks for my life" (Romans 16:3). Paul appeals to two women, Euodia and Syntyche in the church at Philippi, to reconcile their personal differences. "They have struggled beside me in the work of the gospel, together with Clement and the rest of my co-workers, whose names are in the book of life" (Philippians 4:2–3).

"There is no longer Jew or Greek, there is no longer slave or free, there is no longer male and female; for all of you are one in Christ Jesus" (Galatians 3:28). On the basis of context, Paul is speaking of the new relationship that comes through faith and Christian baptism. This "magna charta" of human equality amends the traditional prayer of a Jewish male who thanked God for not having been created a gentile, a slave, or a woman. Through baptism all are incorporated into Christ, and unity replaces prevailing social distinctions.

In Luke and Acts

Luke–Acts (Third Gospel and Acts of the Apostles) emphasize new roles for women, as well as the equality of women with men. Women exercise responsible positions in the community, such as hosting for house churches. "He [Peter] went to the house of Mary, the mother of John whose other name was Mark, where many had gathered and were praying" (Acts 12:12). Church meetings took place in the homes of women. "After leaving the prison they [Paul and Silas] went to Lydia's home; and when they had seen and encouraged the brothers and sisters there, they departed" (Acts 16:40). "All these [the eleven] were constantly devoting themselves to prayer, together with certain women, including Mary the mother of Jesus, as well as his brothers" (Acts 1:14). "Now in Joppa there was a disciple whose name was Tabitha, which in Greek is Dorcas [Greek for "gazelle"]. She was devoted to good works and acts of charity" (Acts 9:36). Some scholars conclude that women who owned these houses and provided hospitality also presided at the Eucharist.

The Gospel of Luke, renowned for its literary eloquence, shows an incomplete knowledge of Palestinian geography, customs, and practices, leading to the conclusion that the author of this Gospel was a non-Palestinian writing for a non-Palestinian audience, composed of gentile Christians. Along this same line, the author substitutes Greek names for Aramaic and Hebrew terms. This Gospel of mercy and compassion is principally interested in oppressed people, especially women and the indigent; Jesus was sometimes criticized for welcoming women.

The Fourth Gospel: *John*

In the Fourth Gospel, very different from the synoptics, John describes five episodes featuring women and their roles: the mother of Jesus at a wedding at Cana in Galilee (John 2:1); Jesus converses with a Samaritan woman (John 4:4–42); Martha and Mary (John 11:17–27); women (Jesus' mother, his mother's sister, the wife of Clopas, and Mary Magdalene) stood near the cross of Jesus (John 19:25–26); the appearance of Jesus to Mary Magdalene, the woman who experienced the first manifestation of the risen Lord (John 20:11–18).

The bulk of the material in John's Gospel appears here exclusively and not in the synoptics. The order of events in this Gospel is different from the synoptics; for example, the cleansing of the temple takes place early in Jesus' public ministry (John 2:13–22); in the synoptics it happens much closer to Jesus' passion and crucifixion.

Seven signs play a significant role in the first part (book of signs) of the Fourth Gospel; they are done to bring about belief in Jesus Christ (John 2–11). Note the relationship between "signs" and outright "miracles." If Jesus was interested only in performing miracles, he could have cured all the blind and the lame. The signs in John have a special meaning; they are not just meant to be displays of Jesus' miraculous powers.

The Gospel of Matthew

The Gospel of Matthew, intended primarily for an audience of Jewish followers of Jesus, is summarized in the golden rule—"In everything do to others as you would have them do to you; for this is the law and the prophets" (Matthew 7:12). The Gospel closes with the challenging commission: "Go therefore and make disciples of all nations, baptizing them in the name of the Father and of the Son and of the Holy Spirit, and teaching them to obey everything that I have commanded you" (Matthew 28:19–20). Then the final words of abiding encouragement: "Remember, I am with you always, to the end of the age" (Matthew 28:20). With that assurance, despite the inevitable hurdles in life, none is so high that it cannot be conquered.

The Gospel of Mark

Mark is the shortest of the four Gospels and probably the first to be compiled. Every Gospel is tailored to an anticipated audience; it seems that Mark's readership is predominantly gentiles because he translates Aramaic words and explains Jewish traditions. He also reveals a deficient grasp of Palestinian geography; Jesus travels northward (to Sidon), eastward, then southward to arrive at the Decapolis (10 cities of Hellenistic culture east of Samaria and Galilee) (Mark 7:31). Jesus may have had a reason for taking such a circuitous route, but the text does not explain.

Mark is disarming in his candor, relating how Jesus reprimands his disciples for their obtuseness: "Do you not understand this parable? Then how will you understand all the parables?" (Mark 4:13). After he stilled the storm at sea by rebuking the wind and the sea, Mark informs us that Jesus reproved the disciples: "Why are you afraid? Have you still no faith?" (Mark 4:40). Jesus may have been impatient with his companions, but, after all, the boat was being swamped, while he was in the stern asleep on the cushion. They awoke him in panic, charging accusatively: "Teacher, do you not care that we are perishing?" (Mark 4:38).

CHAPTER SEVEN

"Let Us Now Sing the Praises of Famous Men, Our Ancestors in Their Generations"

(SIRACH 44:1)

Men of the Old Testament

Moses, the Foremost Leader of the Israelites

"Beloved by God and people, Moses, whose memory is blessed" (Ben Sirach 45:1). The first great leader of the Hebrew people, Moses was also a preeminent lawgiver and prophet. "For his [Moses'] faithfulness and meekness God consecrated him, choosing him out of all mankind" (Sirach 45:4). The exodus event, so intimately connected with Moses, is remembered not only by the Israelites' descendants in the Jewish community but by all people striving for freedom until this very day.

One of the Israelites' most remarkable leaders and prophets, Moses was raised as an Egyptian. However, the turning point of his life came in the wilderness near Horeb (Sinai) when he observed that a "bush was blazing [burning], yet it was not consumed" (Exodus 3:2). Having removed his sandals out of respect for the holy ground, Moses received his call and commission to lead God's people out of Egypt.

Today, Jews commemorate the emigration from Egypt with the annual festival of *Pesach* (Passover), celebrated with a memorial meal called *seder* (in English, "order"). The *seder* is also known in the Christian tradition—the New Testament describes the last supper (the Lord's supper) of Jesus and his disciples as a Passover meal (in John' Gospel, Jesus' last meal is eaten before Passover).

The highlight of the Book of Exodus is the encounter of the Israelites with Yahweh (Exodus 19–24) when the Ten Commandments ("words"), a code of conduct endorsed by Jesus (Matthew 5:19; 19:18), were delivered (Exodus 20:1–17). The first four commandments, unique to Israel, concern the relationship between God and people; the remainder deal with human relationships, and appear in other ancient Near Eastern law collections, such as the Code of Hammurabi. The Ten Commandments are directives for the observance of the one great commandment of love. The deepest significance of the commandments is that God claims each of us for Godself. I have never forgotten the comment of my mentor, G. Ernest Wright, which I regularly quoted in class: "It would be well for us to be as candidly aware of our personal failure as the deuteronomists [editors of Deuteronomy] were of the national betrayal, and, at the same time, to be as serenely confident as they in the love of our God."[1]

In his farewell challenge, Moses exhorts the Israelites to choose life. "I [Yahweh] have set before you life and death, blessings and curses. Choose life so that you and your descendants may live, loving the Lord your God, obeying him, and holding fast to him" (Deuteronomy 30:19–20). This is Moses' last reminder of the necessity of faithfulness to God before the Israelites entered the Promised Land.

"Moses was one hundred twenty years old when he died; his sight was unimpaired and his vigor had not abated ... Never since has there arisen a prophet in Israel like Moses, whom the Lord knew face to face" (Deuteronomy 34:7, 10). It is well-known that Moses never crossed the Jordan into the Promised Land; the reason may not be so well-known. Three times in Deuteronomy (1:37; 3:26; 4:21) we are told that Moses bore the guilt of the people. "The Lord was angry with me [Moses] because of you, and he vowed that I should not cross the Jordan and that I should not enter the good land that the Lord your God is giving for your possession. For I am going to die in this land without crossing over the Jordan, and you are going to cross over to take possession of that good land" (Deuteronomy 4:21).

Joshua, the Successor of Moses

Joshua ("Yahweh saves"), Moses' apprentice, was appointed as leader of the Israelites upon Moses' death. Joshua would be invincible because God would be with him, according to the divine promise of assistance: "I hereby command you: Be strong and courageous; do not be frightened or dismayed, for the Lord your God is with you wherever you go" (Joshua 1:9). In the face of a herculean challenge, Joshua had the assurance of God's presence in the conquest of Canaan. The parallels between the life and deeds of Moses and of Joshua are notable: "Just as we obeyed Moses in all things, so we will obey you [Joshua]. Only may the Lord your God be with you, as he was with Moses" (Joshua 1:17). "The Lord said to Joshua, 'This day I will begin to exalt you in the sight of all Israel, so that they may know that I will be with you as I was with Moses'" (Joshua 3:7). As the Israelites approached the Jordan River, the waters parted, as they did for Moses at the Red (Reed) Sea. On the other hand, Joshua is mentioned only three times in the New Testament, compared to almost 80 times for Moses.

One of the highlights of Joshua's career was the momentous convocation at Shechem, in the hill country about 64 km (40 mi) north of Jerusalem. It was a reaffirmation and extension of the covenant ratified at Sinai. Joshua called the people to renew their commitment to the covenant. "Choose this day whom you will serve, whether the gods your ancestors served in the region beyond the River [Euphrates] or the gods of the Amorites in whose land you are living; but as for me and my household, we will serve the Lord" (Joshua 24:15). This treaty concludes with a series of blessings and curses to be experienced by anyone who either keeps or violates the covenant. This covenant renewal of the people makes Joshua 24 one of the most notable chapters in the Old Testament. Joshua's final meeting with the people of Israel occurred here at Shechem.

The books of Joshua and Judges appear to be dominated by terrorism, violence, and warfare. Like terrorism, violence, and warfare in our own day, they may seem to be a necessity, but at what a cost in lives and limbs, especially of young women and men! Against the background of the entire Bible, justice and love trump the tragedy of war and violence. Perhaps some governments may one day realize their downright futility.

Joseph, the Dreamer

Joseph, too, may be listed among the eminent figures in the Hebrew Bible; like Moses he was highly regarded. Whereas Moses lived 120 years, Joseph, 110; longevity was considered a divine blessing among people of the ancient Near East. His homeland was Canaan, but he spent most of his life in the unfamiliar land of Egypt. The Bible records nothing negative about Joseph, but like the rest of humanity he had his own foibles, outweighed by many virtues. In his youth he experienced sibling rivalry, some of it caused by his doting father Jacob who in a show of favoritism outfitted him in a "long tunic" (*ketonet passim*), described as a costly garment usually worn by great kings. And Joseph deliberately flaunted it before his brothers. Adolescent bragging about his dreams only enkindled the rivalry: "He [Joseph] said to them [his brothers], 'Listen to this dream that I dreamed. There we were, binding sheaves in the field. Suddenly my sheaf rose and stood upright; then your sheaves gathered around it, and bowed down to my sheaf'" (Genesis 37:6–7). After he described a similar dream to his brothers, "The sun, the moon and eleven stars were bowing down to me" (Genesis 37:9), they retaliated by selling Joseph into Egyptian slavery. When the wife of his master Potiphar tried to seduce him, ordering repeatedly, "Lie with me," he resisted. Nevertheless, Joseph, charged with rape, was cast into prison.

Eventually, Joseph became prime minister or vizier of Egypt. How to explain that a foreigner could attain such a lofty position!

When famine struck in the land of Canaan, "All the world came to Joseph in Egypt to buy grain, because the famine became severe throughout the world" (Genesis 41:57). When Joseph's brothers came down to Egypt to buy grain, they came into contact with Joseph, and then feared he would retaliate for the contemptible way they had treated him. Instead, he responded: "I am your brother, Joseph, whom you sold into Egypt. And now do not be distressed or angry with yourselves because you sold me here; for God sent me before you to preserve life" (Genesis 45:4–5). Such magnanimity! Joseph had undergone a radical transformation—from an egocentric adolescent to an altruistic savior.

The story of Joseph has meaning for today's society. Who cannot identify, at least to some degree, with these too-human events—family rivalry, deceit, seduction, slavery, imprisonment, envy, revenge? The Bible is a mirror of contemporary life.

Mass murder is macabre and revolting; but, to explain and not to excuse, we must keep in mind two considerations: first, those times and our times are very different; second, modern war is just as terrible.

Elijah and Elisha

Elijah ("My God is Yahweh") was a ninth century BCE Israelite prophet, whose ministry had a profound affect not only in the Old Testament but also in the New Testament. This passionate prophet was a fierce defender of Israel's God; his antagonist was King Ahab of Israel, along with his impudent queen, the Phoenician Jezebel. They promoted the worship of the idol Baal, the principal male god of the Canaanite religion, as well as symbol of fertility. The showdown came between Elijah and 450 prophets of Baal on Mount Carmel (in Haifa). The object was to prove whose god is the true God: each slaughtered a bull as a sacrifice, and each side called upon its god to consume it. The prophets of Baal invoked their deity with prayers, dances, and even self-mutilation, but to no avail; Yahweh, on the other hand, sent fire to incinerate the sacrificial bull. As a result, Elijah slaughtered the 450 prophets of Baal by the sword.

Fearful of Ahab retaliating, Elijah journeyed 40 days and 40 nights to Horeb (Sinai), the Mount of God. There, Yahweh directed him: "Go, return on your way to the wilderness of Damascus; when you arrive ... you shall anoint Elisha son of Shaphat ... as prophet in your place" (1 Kings 19:15–16). "As they [Elijah and Elisha] continued walking and talking, a chariot of fire and horses of fire separated the two of them, and Elijah ascended in a whirlwind into heaven. Elisha kept watching and crying out, 'Father, father! The chariots of Israel and its horsemen!'" (2 Kings 2:11–12).

In modern Judaism, Elijah is a symbolic guest at every *bris* (Yiddish for "circumcision"; Hebrew, *brit milah*: covenant of circumcision). Also, Elijah has a reserved seat at every *seder*. A special goblet is filled with wine and placed on the *seder* table for the prophet Elijah. At a certain point in the service the front door is opened to welcome Elijah. Elijah's cup symbolizes the ancient custom of welcoming strangers and others who have no *seder* of their own. No one should ever be alone for Passover!

The identification of Elijah with John the Baptist is evident: both were austere; in external appearance John evoked memories of the prophet Elijah. He wore a garment made of camels' hair with a leather belt around his waist; he ate locusts and wild honey (Mark 1:6; compare with 2 Kings 1:8).

The association of Elijah and Jesus in the New Testament is also striking. When Jesus inquired of his disciples: "Who do people say that the Son of Man is?" The answer: "Some say John the Baptist, but others Elijah, and still others Jeremiah or one of the prophets" (Matthew 16:13–14). On another occasion, "Jesus took with him Peter and James and his brother John and led them up a high mountain, by themselves. And he was transfigured [having a divine appearance] before them ... Suddenly there appeared to them Moses and Elijah, talking with him [Jesus]" (Matthew 17:1–3). The appearance of the threesome illustrates the continuity of Jesus the teacher with Moses the lawgiver and Elijah the prophet (Matthew 17:1–3).

In the early Christian community Elijah was regarded as the forerunner of the Messiah (Jesus). When King Herod (Antipas) heard about the ministry of the twelve, he was confused about who was spearheading this movement. "Some were saying, 'John the baptizer has been raised from the dead' ... But others said, 'It is Elijah'" (Mark 6:14–15). The Baptist was asked whether he was Elijah—"Why then are you baptizing if you are neither the Messiah, nor Elijah, nor the prophet?" (John 1:25).

Samuel the Prophet

Samuel held several positions of authority: judge (charismatic leader), prophet, priest, and military leader. Samuel was a transitional figure, providing leadership between the tribal existence under the Judges and the establishment of the monarchy. "The lamp of God had not yet gone out, and Samuel was lying down in the temple [at Shiloh] of the Lord, where the ark of God was ... So Samuel went and lay down in his place. Now the Lord came and stood there, calling as before 'Samuel! Samuel!' And Samuel said, 'Speak for your servant is listening'" (1 Samuel 3:3, 9–10).

Samuel made an annual circuit, passing through Bethel, Gilgal and Mizpah and judging Israel at each of these sanctuaries (1 Samuel 7:15–16).

He anointed Saul as Israel's first king. By failing to fight against the Amalekites until they were exterminated, Saul was guilty of disobeying Yahweh. Afterward Samuel was sent to Bethlehem to anoint David as king. Feminist interpretation of 1 Samuel moves away from the patriarchal reading, while placing emphasis on the roles of women.

Saul, Israel's First King

Saul, the first king of Israel, was anointed to deliver Israel from the oppressive power of the Philistines, but his brooding psyche deterred him from success in life. Saul was a very troubled person who suffered from clinical depression (a modern term), manifested in his outbursts of impatience, jealousy, rage, and rashness, especially evident in his conflicts with David and in war with the Philistines. "And Saul's servants said to him, 'See now, an evil spirit from God is tormenting you. Let our lord now command the servants who attend you to look for someone who is skillful in playing the lyre; and when the evil from God is upon you, he [David] will play it, and you will feel better'" (1 Samuel 16:15–16).

After David returned from slaying Goliath the Philistine, admiring women from surrounding cities came out to greet King Saul; singing and dancing, they played tambourines and sistrums; they sang: "Saul has killed his thousands, and David his ten thousands" (1 Samuel 18:7). Saul was angry and resentful at being diminished in this comparison with David, who was present, playing the lyre. Saul was holding his spear poised, planning to kill David, who evaded the spear.

On another occasion, after defeating the Amalekites (a nomadic people south of Judah), Saul retained some of the spoils, whereby God rejected him. In such wars of extermination, all persons and things were to be obliterated, and nothing preserved for private use.

Jonathan, the Beloved

Jonathan, the eldest son of Saul, was one of the magnanimous figures of the Old Testament—selfless, inspiring, loyal, courageous, and a devoted friend. What a contrast with his father, Saul! Jonathan and David made a covenant of friendship between them. Jonathan admonished David: "Do not be afraid; for the hand of my father Saul shall not find you; you shall be king over Israel, and I shall be second to you; my father Saul also knows that this is so" (1 Samuel 23:17). Saul was so overwhelmed by the might of the Philistines, he became disheartened. So desperate was Saul that he sought out a medium, even though they and fortune-tellers had been driven from the land. Disguising himself, he located the witch of Endor (north of Mount Gilboa), and asked that she conjure up the specter of Samuel for consultation. And the woman did so and saw "an old man is coming up; he is wrapped in a robe" (1 Samuel 28:14). Saul knew immediately from the garb that it was Samuel, who said: "The Lord will give Israel along with you into the hands of the Philistines; and tomorrow you and your sons shall be with me" (1 Samuel 28:19). Saul was extremely agitated by Samuel's prediction. The next day the Philistines slew Jonathan and his brothers on Mount Gilboa.

Pierced through the abdomen, "Saul took his own sword and fell upon it" (1 Samuel 31:4).

Shortly before his death, Saul expressed his remorse to David: "You are more righteous than I; for you have repaid me good, whereas I have repaid you evil" (1 Samuel 24:17). David's elegy for Saul and Jonathan is immortal:

Your glory, O Israel, lies slain upon your high places! How the mighty have fallen! ... From the blood of the slain, from the fat of the mighty, the bow of Jonathan did not turn back, nor the sword of Saul return empty. Saul and Jonathan, beloved and lovely! In life and in death they were not divided; they were swifter than eagles, they were stronger than lions ... How the mighty have fallen, and the weapons of war perished!" (2 Samuel 1:19, 22–23, 27).

The character traits of Saul, Jonathan, and David are present in each of us; all fit into the category of *humanitas*. As we reflect upon these episodes in the lives of ancient Israelites, we can put ourselves in the place of these three very human figures. It is not for us to judge, but to learn, and to decide how we would like to be portrayed. Their circumstances are different from ours, separated as we are in time and place, but the challenges are much the same. Each biblical character eventually recognizes his faults and defects, and ultimately is prepared to make amends, as difficult as that may be for every one of us.

David, King of Israel

David ("beloved"), Israel's second king, was a flawed hero, tragically human, a complex figure, whose life was filled with contradictions. He was multitalented: warrior, musician, poet, and statesman. The biblical writers convey a generally favorable impression of David as a person of integrity; at the same time, they do not condone his sins of lust and vanity, among others. David's adultery with Bathsheba, a tale of sin and repentance, besmirched his reputation. From the roof of his palace, he spied "a woman bathing; the woman was very beautiful" (2 Samuel 11:2). From that moment he craved her, lured her to the palace, and had intercourse with her. Learning that she had become pregnant, he tried to conceal the crime, plotting the death of Bathsheba's husband, Uriah, by placing him on the front line of the battlefield. "When the mourning was over, David sent and brought her to his house [palace], and she became his wife and bore him a son. But the thing that David had done displeased the Lord" (2 Samuel 11:27).

Nathan ("gift [of God]") the prophet confronted David, relating a parable about a rich man and a poor man. The rich man hosted a dinner for a wayfarer, but instead of taking from his own ample flocks and herds for the meal, he helped himself fraudulently to the sole ewe lamb cherished by the poor man and his children, and made a feast of it for the wayfarer. Upon hearing this, David was furious, and pronounced that the man who had done this unjust deed deserved death, thereby indicting himself for plotting the death of Uriah. Consider Nathan's immortal indictment: "You are the man (*'attah ha'ish*)" (2 Samuel 12:7). "David said to Nathan, 'I have sinned against the Lord.' Nathan said to David, 'Now the Lord has put away your sin; you shall not die'" (2 Samuel 12:13). David's repentance is praiseworthy.

David's heroism is no better illustrated than by his youthful slaying of the giant Goliath, a Philistine, who was six and a half feet (2 m) tall and armored from head to toe. He taunted the ranks of Israel: "Choose a man for yourselves, and let him come down to me. If he is able to fight with me and kill me, then we [Philistines] will be your servants; but if I prevail against him and kill him, then you [Israelites] shall be our servants and serve us" (1 Samuel 17:8–9). David approached Saul assuredly: "Let no one's heart fail because of him; your servant will go and fight with this Philistine" (1 Samuel 17:32). Everyone among us, from the oldest to the youngest, knows the outcome of that one-sided contest. Armorless, David ran quickly to the battle line, took out a stone from his bag, hurled it with the sling, striking Goliath on the forehead, who fell prostrate. David had struck the Philistine a mortal blow!

Amnon and Absalom, David's Sons

Amnon, the firstborn son of David, was obsessed with lascivious desire for his beautiful half-sister Tamar whom he enticed into his house, raped and then threw into the street. Absalom, the third son of David, ordered the murder of Amnon in retaliation for the rape of Tamar. Later, Absalom disloyally rebelled against David, likely over policies of tax administration, and made claims to the throne. While riding on a mule, Absalom's head was caught in a large terebinth. Joab, commander of David's army, dispatched him, and his body was tossed into a pit in the forest. When word reached David, he did not rejoice; rather he was disconsolate, saying as he wept, "O my son Absalom, my son, my son Absalom! Would I had died instead of you, O Absalom, my son, my son!" (2 Samuel 18:33).

"It was told to Joab, 'The king is weeping and mourning for Absalom.' So the victory that day was turned into mourning for all the troops; for the troops heard that day, 'The king is grieving for his son'" (2 Samuel 19:1–2). Then Joab reproached the king:

"Though they have saved your life today, and the lives of your sons and daughters ... you have put all your servants to shame today by *loving those who hate you and hating those who love you*" (emphasis added; 2 Samuel 19:6–7, New American Bible). These final words have remained with me for many years. The longer I live (83 years), the more keenly aware I am of the irony (and the truth) of Joab's indictment of David. I suspect most of us, in reviewing our lives, would find these unsettling words an accurate description of some of our own relationships. Is it that we take our friends for granted and never stop to appreciate what they really mean to us, while currying the favor of those who do not particularly like us?

David is immortalized in both Old Testament and New Testament. In the Old Testament, the prophets describe the Messiah (anointed one) promised by God as the Son of David. In the New Testament, this same title was bestowed on Jesus as he entered Jerusalem for the final time: "Hosanna to the Son of David! Blessed is the one who comes in the name of the Lord! Hosanna in the highest heaven!" (Matthew 21:9).

Men of the New Testament: The Disciples of Jesus

Certain figures play a prominent role in the New Testament as members of Jesus' inner circle; Peter, James, and John were closest to Jesus. The disciples were the first missionaries to proclaim the gospel of repentance and forgiveness, far and wide, by word and deed.

Peter the "Rock"

Peter stands out above all the rest; he was later recognized as the foremost leader of the early Church. He is the disciple most often mentioned in the Gospels, the first on every list of Jesus' disciples. "These are the names of the twelve apostles: first, Simon, also known as Peter" (Matthew 10:2).

Simon was nicknamed Cephas or *Peter* (Aramaic and Greek for "rock"). We know that Peter was married because he had a mother-in-law: "Now Simon's mother-in-law was in bed with a fever, and they [disciples] told him [Jesus] about her at once" (Mark 1:30).

Peter was a resident of Capernaum (town on the northwest shore of the sea of Galilee), which accounts for his Galilean accent. During Jesus' trial a servant girl announced to the bystanders, "This man [Peter] is one of them ... Certainly you are one of them; for you are a Galilean" (Mark 14:69–70). His accent betrayed him. During the principal events of Jesus' ministry, Peter was present. He was the first apostle to behold the risen Jesus (Luke 24:34). Peter was a spokesperson at the transfiguration: "Then Peter said to Jesus: 'Rabbi, it is good for us to be here; let us make three dwellings, one for you, one for Moses, and one for Elijah'" (Mark 9:5). During the last supper, Jesus began to wash and dry the disciples' feet; as he approached Peter, the disciple demurred, "You will never wash my feet" (John 13:8).

Jesus posed this question to his disciples, "Who do people say that the Son of Man is?" Then followed a more specific formulation, "Who do you say that I am?" Peter, acting for the disciples, answered, "You are the Messiah ("anointed one"; Hebrew, *mashiah*; Greek, *christos*), the Son of the living God!" (Matthew 16:13–16). On another occasion, Peter inquired of Jesus about the frequency of forgiveness: "Seven times [a round number]?" Jesus replied authoritatively: "Not seven times, but, I tell you, seventy times seven [an unlimited number]" (Matthew 18:21–22).

The synoptic Gospels (Matthew, Mark, Luke) do not spare Peter; they note his foibles and his sins, and occasionally Jesus had to rebuke him. Impetuosity was Peter's character fault that stands out. When Jesus informed the disciples of the suffering and rejection, and even death that lay ahead of him, Peter remonstrated with him. Jesus' reprimand followed immediately: "Get behind me, Satan! For you are setting your mind not on divine things but on human things" (Mark 8:33). Just before his arrest, Jesus said to his disciples: "You will all become deserters" (Mark 14:27). Peter retorted: "Even though all become deserters, I will not." Jesus' reply: "This very night, before the cock crows twice, you will deny me three times" (Mark 14:29–30).

When Jesus was praying in the garden of Gethsemane, he was accompanied by Peter, James, and John whom he ordered: "Remain here and stay awake." When he returned and found them asleep, he said to Peter: "Simon, are you asleep? Could you not keep awake one hour?" (Mark 14:37).

On another occasion, after the disciples had spent the whole night fishing without making a catch, Jesus directed Peter: "Put out into the deep water and let down your nets for a catch" (Luke 5:4). Peter and his mates were overwhelmed by the miraculous catch of fish. Peter fell at Jesus' knees, saying: "Go away from me, Lord, for I am a sinful man" (Luke 5:8).

Whenever Peter was rebuked for misunderstanding Jesus, it was principally because of Peter's fierce loyalty. Most of us, I reckon, can identify with the humanity of Peter; neither he nor we are stained-glass-window saints. In fact, sinners far outnumber saints in the Bible. We stand to learn so many lessons from the humanity of Peter—love, generosity, dedication, candor, willingness to acknowledge mistakes—the list is long!

Peter addressed Jesus: "We have left everything and followed you." He replied: "There is no one who has left house or brothers or sisters or mother or father or children or fields, for my sake and for the sake of the good news, who will not receive a hundredfold now in this age ... and in the age to come eternal life" (Mark 10:28–30).

We noted that Peter, despite his protestations to the contrary, denied Jesus three times. But recall, Jesus challenged Peter three times with the question: "Simon son of John, do you love me more than these?" Each time, more emphatically, Peter insisted: "Lord, you know that I love you" (John 21:15–17). Unconditional love!

Letters of John

The First Letter (exhortation) of John bears a striking resemblance to the Gospel of John, and is replete with references to the aphorism "God is love," meaning that love is God's very being, and is the source of love for one another (1 John 4:7–12). The word love is used 43 times in this letter. Recall there are three Greek words for "love": *philia*, or familial love; *eros*, passionate love (not found in New Testament); and *agape*, selfless love. Clearly, no New Testament author is associated with the concept of love more than John, especially in the First Letter of John. The message of this letter is summarized in terms of God's love for us and our love for one another. Through love for one another we can be certain that God dwells in us. To love God is to know God and to participate in God's life. "In this is love, not that we loved God but that he has loved us and sent his Son to be the atoning sacrifice for our sins" (1 John 4:10). The new emphasis here is on the divine initiative.

And the ultimate challenge: "Beloved, since God loved us so much, we also ought to love one another" (1 John 4:11). This is the work of a lifetime, but we must never stop striving. The practice of the love of neighbor is placed within the easy reach of everyone. "How does God's love abide in anyone who has the world's goods and sees a brother or sister in need and yet refuses help?" (1 John 3:17).

Our urban streets are filled with physically impaired and psychologically dysfunctional brothers and sisters. Do we ignore them or do we extend ourselves to them? The most meaningful compliment I ever received in my life came from a group of neighborhood friends who commented that my informal get-togethers with them as just another friend in a local coffee-house made a vast difference in their lives. In those daily gatherings over coffee I said little; I simply listened and learned.

Men of the New Testament: Paul the Apostle

Paul the apostle was born Saul of Tarsus (in southeastern Asia Minor, modern Turkey), a Jew and a zealous Pharisee. He is notable for his three missionary journeys to spread the gospel throughout the Roman Empire. Traveling the road to Damascus to persecute Christian believers, he had a conversion experience resulting in a radical change of life. His journeys through Asia Minor and Greece were far from luxurious; even today, to follow literally in the footsteps of Paul is formidable, despite limited amenities unheard of in Paul's time. Reading the Acts of the Apostles and Paul's Letters does not adequately convey a feel for the hardships involved—shipwreck, imprisonment, stoning, persecution, riots. Only by reliving, to the degree possible, Paul's horrendous experiences can we even vaguely appreciate what is entailed.

Paul's Epistles (Letters) were "occasional letters" addressed to particular churches about specific problems. Fourteen of the 21 Letters in the New Testament are traditionally considered as composed by Paul. Of all the Epistles in the New Testament, Christians regard Paul's Letter to the Romans as central to Christian faith. The pivotal theme is the relationship between Judaism and Christianity, a serious concern in the minds of the Roman Christians. The pattern of the letter may be summarized in these verses: "For I am not ashamed of the gospel; it is the power of God for salvation to everyone who has faith, to the Jew first and also to the Greek. For in it the righteousness of God is revealed through faith for faith; as it is written, 'The one who is righteous will live by faith'" (Romans 1:16–17).

The Letters to the Corinthians

Paul's two letters to the community at Corinth (in Greece), as well as the Letters to the Galatians and Ephesians (Greek cities, now part of Turkey) highlight the power of love. For a long time, people have found in these letters practical guidelines for life. Surprisingly, Paul composed his definition of love (1 Corinthians 13:1–8, 13), one of the most profound chapters in the New Testament, for the community at Corinth. The Corinthian community Paul addressed, however, should not be confused with the more ancient Corinth which was a seaport infamous for sexual promiscuity and prostitution.

In the earliest written account of the institution of Lord's supper (1 Corinthians 11:23–26), Paul comments on the words with which Jesus distributed the bread and the cup. The narrative underscores Jesus' action of self-giving expressed in the words over the bread and the cup.

The First Letter to the Corinthians contains the earliest formal instruction on Jesus' resurrection and its significance for Christian faith: "I [Paul] handed on to you as of first importance what I in turn had received: that Christ died for our sins in accordance with the scriptures, and that he was buried, and that he was raised on the third day ... and that he appeared to Cephas, then to the twelve ... Last of all, as to one untimely born, he appeared also to me" (1 Corinthians 15:3–8).

Letters to the Galatians and Ephesians

The Letter to the Galatian church, offering no thanksgiving for those addressed, is unusual for its harsh tone: "I [Paul] am astonished that you are so quickly deserting the one [God] who called you in the grace of Christ and are turning to a different gospel—not that there is another gospel" (Galatians 1:6–7).

The Letter to the Ephesians is concerned with the church as the household of God: "You are no longer strangers and aliens, but you are citizens with the saints [believers] and also members of the household of God" (Ephesians 2:19). Paul is concerned with maintaining unity in the body of Christ: "The gifts he gave were that some would be apostles, some prophets, some evangelists, some pastors and teachers, to equip the saints for the work of ministry, for building up the body of Christ, until all of us come to the unity of the faith and of the knowledge of the Son of God" (Ephesians 4:11–13).

The Letter to the Philippians

Philippi, in northeastern Greece, was a prominent city in the Roman province of Macedonia, and the Letter addressed to this community (Philippians) is one of Paul's most personal. Despite that Paul wrote it from prison in Rome (or Caesarea or Ephesus) while he awaited execution, the Letter resonates joy. Paul encourages unity among members of the community, and offers Jesus and himself as models of self-denial for the benefit of the whole. "Do nothing from selfish ambition or conceit, but in humility regard others as better than yourselves. Let each of you look not to your own interests, but to the interests of others. Let the same mind be in you that was in Christ Jesus" (Philippians 2:3–5).

Paul's Letters present us with a powerful example and at the same time with an enormous challenge. It is one thing to read these Letters piously; it is quite another to put them into practice. Philippians 2:3–5 (above) is at the heart of the gospel. Lest we become discouraged in our striving, bear in mind there were as many conflicts in the early church as today, and just as much weakness among us. Nonetheless, this is the goal to be achieved.

Letter to the Colossians

Much that had already been said was repeated in Paul's Letter to the community at Colossae (a city in Asia Minor). Special attention is given to the ideal Christian life in the world (Colossians 3:1–4:6), with emphasis on the renunciation of vices and the practice of virtues. The former are well known to us from personal experience; the latter are well worth our efforts. The following verses are guidelines for living a good life:

As God's chosen ones, holy and beloved, clothe yourselves with compassion, kindness, humility, meekness and patience. Bear with one another and, if anyone has a complaint against another, forgive each other; just as the Lord has forgiven you, so you also must forgive. Above all, clothe yourselves with love, which binds everything together in perfect harmony. (Colossians 3:12–14)

Bringing this section to a close with Paul's reflection on his impending death is appropriate:

As for me [Paul], I am already being poured out as a libation, and the time of my departure has come. I have fought the good fight, I have finished the race, I have kept the faith. From now on there is reserved for me the crown of righteousness, which the Lord, the righteous judge, will give me on that day, and not only to me but also to all who have longed for his appearing." (2 Timothy 4:6–8)

[1] G.E. Wright, "Book of Deuteronomy" in *Interpreter's Bible*, vol. 2 (New York: Abingdon Press, 1953), 309-537.

CHAPTER 8

Wisdom Literature

What Is Wisdom Literature?

The Old Testament may be divided into three sections: Torah (Pentateuch), Prophets, and Wisdom. Proverbs, Job, and Qoheleth (Ecclesiastes) are categorized as wisdom literature. The Wisdom of Solomon and Sirach (Ecclesiasticus) are classified under the Apocrypha (deuterocanonical books), found in the early Christian version of the Old Testament and which concentrate on the human condition as it is experienced in the here and now. They are ahistorical in that there is no special concern for the sacred traditions, such as the exodus from Egypt or the Sinai covenant.

Wisdom is a broad term, more easily described than defined. It is didactic literature whose principal interest is instruction in the appropriate ways of living. The objective is the good life characterized by longevity, prosperity, and preeminence. Wisdom, international in character, is also concerned with technical skills, as it describes one who excels in his/her own craft. When Solomon, whose name is associated with the wisdom literature, was offered (in a dream) any gift in the world of his own choosing, he preferred wisdom, much to the amazement of his people. They were certain he would request something to enhance himself and his position as king. Instead he asked for a wise and discerning mind (*leb shomea'*) to enable him to rule his people with righteousness (1 Kings 3:9, 12).

Proverbs, Job, and Qoheleth (Ecclesiastes) are concerned with the nature of retribution—the question of reward and punishment in a future life dependent upon one's conduct in this life. The theological term is "theodicy," derived from two Greek words: *theos* (God) and *dike* (justice), literally the justice of God. It deals with the problem of evil, specifically the attempt to reconcile the suffering of the innocent with the existence of a beneficent God. Because theodicy has a long history in the Bible, it is not easy to define. At the heart of the discussion is the answer to the nagging question Jeremiah posed to Yahweh—"Let me [Jeremiah] put my case to you. Why does the way of the guilty prosper? Why do all who are treacherous thrive?" (Jeremiah 12:1).

Book of Proverbs

Proverbs, one of the biblical books most frequently cited in literature, is an anthology of practical norms for ethical conduct (commonsense morality) if one is to enjoy everyday life. "The fear of the Lord is the beginning of wisdom, and the knowledge of the Holy One is insight" (Proverbs 9:10; see 1:7). This is the religious basis for the teaching of Proverbs, but it is frequently misunderstood. The reference here is not to a cringing fear before God, but a reverential respect on account of divine wisdom, justice, and love toward humanity. The principal purpose of Proverbs is to teach wisdom; it also presents the mainstream view of theodicy, dealing with secular concerns, as well as moral and religious truths. Proverbs attends to the poor and the needy; also the rights of widows and orphans.

The author embraces the concept of divine justice, whereby the righteous are rewarded and the wicked punished; for example, "The Lord's curse is on the house of the wicked, but he blesses the abode of the righteous" (Proverbs 3:33). A belief in the afterlife where some are rewarded and others are punished is not clearly elaborated in Proverbs.

Job, a Wealthy Chieftain

Job, an opulent oriental chieftain, was suddenly stripped of his daughters and his possessions. The well-known epithet "patient as Job" is not really accurate in view of Job 3 where he curses the day he was born. The problem of suffering is addressed in Job but remains unresolved. A fundamental issue of Job concerns the innocent person who suffers at Yahweh's hands; Job asks: "Why do the innocent suffer?" The main theme of Job is the problem of the righteous sufferer. Both Job and Qoheleth leave the issue of theodicy (divine justice) unanswered—there are no easy answers.

Ecclesiastes (Qoheleth)

The title Ecclesiastes is the Greek translation of the Hebrew Qoheleth, the literary name of the Book of Ecclesiastes, signifying teacher, preacher, or assembler; or it could be the pen name of the author who is not Solomon, despite the attribution in 1:1. Sometimes a famous name is attached to a book to lend prominence (or in our day, to promote sales). Concerned with the meaning and value of life, Qoheleth is a deeply human book, not to mention inherently ambiguous and enigmatic.

The theme of the entire book is succinctly stated in 1:2 [also 12:8]—"Vanity of vanities, says the Teacher [Qoheleth], vanity of vanities! All is vanity." Vanity translates the Hebrew *hebel*: "vapor" is a synonym, "substantial" is an antonym. Vanity of vanities is the Hebrew way of expressing the superlative; utter vanity has been proposed as synonymous. Vanity suggests that life is both transitory and futile.

In conjunction with the search for the meaning of life, Qoheleth is preoccupied with the question of divine justice, or theodicy, an issue left unresolved. He recognizes that virtue is not always rewarded and wickedness is not always punished. "In my vain life I [Qoheleth] have seen everything; there are righteous people who perish in their righteousness, and there are wicked people who prolong their life in their evildoing" (7:15).

In the final analysis, nothing in life makes much sense; life and its joys are fleeting. Death is the only certain thing in life; there is no concept of personal immortality. The human inability to fathom life and to control one's existence is classically summarized in 3:1–8:

For everything there is a season, and a time for every matter
   under heaven:
a time to be born, and a time to die;
a time to plant, and a time to pluck up what is planted;
a time to kill, and a time to heal;
a time to break down, and a time to build up;
a time to weep, and a time to laugh;
a time to mourn , and a time to dance;
a time to throw away stones, and a time to gather stones
   together;
a time to embrace, and a time to refrain from embracing;
a time to seek, and a time to lose;
a time to keep, and a time to throw away;

a time to tear, and a time to sew;

a time to keep silence, and a time to speak;

a time to love, and a time to hate;

a time for war, and a time for peace.

These antithetical pairs emphasize that everything is under inexorable law.

Book of Wisdom

The first part of the Book of Wisdom (chapters 1–6) treats the question of divine justice, notably the issue of the suffering of the righteous. The Book of Wisdom (also called the Wisdom of Solomon) was composed in Greek; furthermore the influence of Greek philosophy is evident, particularly regarding the doctrine of the immortality of the soul, which is a new emphasis in the Jewish tradition. "For though in the sight of others they were punished, their hope is full of immortality" (3:4); also, "For God created us for incorruption, and made us in the image of his own eternity" (2:23). Again, "But the righteous live forever, and their reward is with the Lord; the Most High takes care of them" (5:15). On the other hand, the Book of Wisdom does not refer to the resurrection of the body, although it does envision life after death.

Second Maccabees

The Second Book of Maccabees is well-known for its references to the resurrection:

He [Judas Maccabeus] also took up a collection, man by man, to the amount of two thousand drachmas of silver, and sent it to Jerusalem to provide for a sin offering. In doing this he acted very well and honorably, taking account of the resurrection. For if he were not expecting that those who had fallen would rise again, it would have been superfluous and foolish to pray for the dead. But if he was looking to the splendid reward that is laid up for those who fall asleep in godliness, it was a holy and pious thought. Therefore he made atonement for the dead, so that they might be delivered from their sin." (12:43–46)

The theological importance of the resurrection of the just on the last day is underscored repeatedly in 2 Maccabees: "And when he [one of the 'seven sons'] was at his last breath, he said, 'You [Antiochus IV Epiphanes] accursed wretch, you dismiss us from this present life, but the King of the universe will raise us up to an everlasting renewal of life, because we have died for his laws'" (7:9; see 7:11, 14, 23; 14:46). Conjoined to the concept of resurrection is the conviction that God's justice will reward the righteous and punish the sinner.

Book of Sirach (Ecclesiasticus)

The Book of Sirach derives its title from the name of the author. Because of the extensive use made of it in the early church, Sirach is also known as Ecclesiasticus, meaning church book; in Jewish tradition Sirach is known as Ben Sira. Sirach's views on future life do not go beyond those of Proverbs but share the traditional Old Testament position regarding sin, suffering, and retribution. Nor did he embrace the doctrine of body/soul dualism. Since life did not exist after death, retribution had to happen on this side of the grave. Afterward there was only Sheol, a biblical term for the abode of the dead in the Bible, where all the departed spirits would be on a par, whether righteous or unrighteous, and also judged according to their deeds.

"He [Yahweh] has placed before you fire and water; stretch out your hand for whichever you choose. Before each person are life and death, and whichever one chooses will be given" (Sirach 15:16–17; see Deuteronomy 30:15).

Book of Daniel

Daniel (chapters 7–12) is the only book in the Hebrew Bible that belongs to the genre of apocalypse, a literature characterized by arcane revelations disclosing a supernatural world and involving the judgment of the dead. Vision and symbolism figure prominently in apocalypse; angels and demons are also present. Daniel 12:1–3 encapsulates the doctrine of future life; Daniel 12:2 is one of the most notable verses in the entire book for its direct reference to resurrection, last judgment, and afterlife. "*Many* of those who sleep [euphemism, "are dead"] in the dust of the earth shall awake, *some* to everlasting life, and *some* to shame and everlasting contempt" (Daniel 12:2). In the Old Testament the concept of resurrection appears only in postexilic, apocalyptic literature. The doctrine of the resurrection became widespread in post-Old Testament Judaism, but opinions vary concerning who would rise—some/all the righteous, or both righteous and unrighteous.

CHAPTER NINE

Key Aspects of the Spiritual Life

"The Word of Our God Will Stand Forever" (Isaiah 40:8)

The Hebrew word *dabar* is most often translated as "word" in the Old Testament, just as the Greek word *logos* is rendered "word" in the New Testament; the meaning of these two words is essentially the same. In both Old Testament and New Testament "word" is that through which God expresses himself. In the Hebrew perspective, a word once uttered had a quasi-substantive existence of its own. In the ancient Near East, a spoken word was thought of as an entity fraught with power. The phrase "word of Yahweh" in the Hebrew Bible is employed most frequently to describe the medium of revelation. The idea of the divine word is central in the Bible, indicating that God speaks, reveals, and communicates. "By the word of the Lord the heavens were made, and all their host by the breath of his mouth" (Psalm 33:6).

The effectiveness of God's word is demonstrated in the following vibrant simile, using the comparison of rain and snow:

For as the rain and the snow come down from heaven,

and do not return there until they have watered the earth, making it bring forth and sprout, giving seed to the sower and bread to the eater, so shall my *word* be that goes out from my mouth; it shall not return to me empty, but it shall accomplish that which I purpose, and succeed in the thing for which I sent it. (Isaiah 55:10–11)

This passage reverberates in the opening passage of Isaiah 40:7–8—"The grass withers, the flower fades; but the *word* of our God will stand forever."

The prologue (verses 1–18) of John's Gospel encapsulates the gospel itself. John's Gospel begins with the affirmation that Jesus is the preexistent *logos* who was with God and was God from eternity (John 1:1). The Gospel of John states that without the divine Word nothing was made (John 1:3), and that the Word became flesh (an actual human being) in Jesus of Nazareth (John 1:14). This Gospel identifies *logos* with Jesus of Nazareth, and as the incarnate Savior. The person of Jesus Christ expresses God's all-powerful communication in the New Testament. Jesus speaks God's word and makes him known. "No one has ever seen God. It is God the only Son, who is close to the Father's heart, who has made him known" (John 1:18). "In these last days he [God] has spoken to us by a Son, whom he appointed heir of all things, through whom he also created the worlds" (Hebrews 1:2).

"For I Desire Steadfast Love and Not Sacrifice, the Knowledge of God Rather than Burnt Offerings" (Hosea 6:6)

The Hebrew *yada'* and the Greek *ginosko*, signifying knowledge/ knowing, are comprehensive terms embracing experience, emotion, and interpersonal relationship, as well as intellectual apprehension of reality. No simple definition suffices; it is not a purely intellectual process, but also includes a practical relationship. In the Old Testament, knowledge is a product of human experience. God is known because of self-revelation. In the New Testament, reflecting classical Greek influence, knowledge is equated with intellectual perception. At the same time, many of the characteristics of knowledge/knowing in the Old Testament are also found in the New Testament, where knowledge of God comes through Jesus Christ.

Knowledge in the New Testament can be empirical and relational as in the Old Testament. The heading of this section (from Hosea 6:6) is the motto of Hosea's message; it is also a key verse in the Book of Hosea. The prophet draws a prophetic parallel between *hesed* (steadfast love) and *da'at 'elohim* (knowledge of God), which far exceeds intellectual apprehension; it is the response of the whole person to God's love. To know God is to respond to him in faithful love. In the last analysis, knowledge of the heart, a personal relationship, is what the prophet has in mind.

To know God is to be in relationship with God. So, too, in everyday life: to know another human being is to have a relationship with that person. In both the Old Testament and New Testament sexual relations are described as "knowing"—"Now the man knew (*yada'*) his wife Eve, and she conceived and bore Cain, saying, 'I have produced a man with the help of the Lord'" (Genesis 4:1). "Mary said to the angel, 'How can this be since I do not know (*ginosko*) a man?'" (Luke 1:34).

"I [Yahweh] Will Take You [Israel] for My Wife in Faithfulness; and You Shall Know (*yada'at*) Yahweh" (Hosea 2:20 [Hebrew Bible 2:22])

Here again, the marital metaphor is used to express intimacy, going far beyond casual acquaintance or intellectual knowledge.

Knowledge of God (acknowledgment of God's ways) is a major theological theme in Hosea. "Hear the word of the Lord, O people of Israel ... There is no faithfulness or loyalty, and no knowledge of God in the land. Swearing, lying, and murder, and stealing and adultery break out [five of the ten commandments]; bloodshed follows bloodshed" (Hosea 4:1–2). Without knowing God (having personal knowledge of God's revealed law), violations of the commandments inevitably follow.

The true meaning of the knowledge of God is the living-out of that knowledge. "Whoever breaks one of the least of these commandments, and teaches others to do the same, will be called least in the kingdom of heaven" (Matthew 5:19).

"Those Who Love Me, I Will Deliver; I Will Protect Those Who Know (*yada'*) My Name" (Psalm 91:14)

"Knowing his name" points to the psalmist's intimate relationship with God, based on love and obedience. Loving God is synonymous with knowing his name (Exodus 3:13–15).

In ancient literature, to "know the name" was not simply having information about the person; rather the name represents both the person and the personality. For example, *nabal* means "fool," and the man Nabal was a fool. Abigail, wife of Nabal, addressed David: "My lord, do not take seriously this ill-natured fellow, Nabal; for as his name is, so is he; Nabal is his name, and folly is with him" (1 Samuel 25:25).

"My Presence Will Go with You, and I Will Give You Rest" (Exodus 33:14)

It has been said that Exodus 33 contains the most thorough struggle with the problem of presence in the entire Old Testament. Moses tried to cajole Yahweh to accompany the stiff-necked Israelites on their departure from Sinai, but he was reluctant because they had sinned gravely by fashioning a golden calf. The key verse is Exodus 33:14: Yahweh said, "My presence [literally, "my face"] will go with you, and I will give you rest." *Panim*, "face," is the most common Hebrew term for presence; in verse 18 it is designated "glory," and in verse 19 "goodness." "Presence," "glory," and "goodness" express the various modes of Yahweh's presence. The "presence of Yahweh" is the place of blessing in the Old Testament. Moses' face is covered while the glory of Yahweh passes.

In the New Testament the presence of Yahweh is made concrete by the incarnation, that God was made flesh in Jesus Christ. "Ever since the creation of the world his eternal power and divine nature, invisible though they are, have been understood and seen through the things he has made" (Romans 1:20; see 1 Peter 4:11). "And all of us, with unveiled faces, seeing the glory of the Lord as though reflected in a mirror, are being transformed into the same image from one degree of glory to another; for this comes from the Lord, the Spirit" (2 Corinthians 3:18). In John, the glorification of Jesus is his passion, death, and resurrection.

Kabod (glory), an intricate theological concept, describes God's active presence among the people of Israel. *Kebod YHWH* ("glory of Yahweh") is the most frequent expression for the manifestation of God's presence; in the Old Testament, the glory of Yahweh is closely related to Yahweh's self-revelation.

Glory is a cloud canopy over Israel—"Then the Lord will create over the whole site of Mount Zion and over its places of assembly a cloud by day and smoke and the shining of a flaming fire by night. Indeed over all the glory there will be a canopy" (Isaiah 4:5). The divine protection of Jerusalem is represented by imagery from the Exodus and wilderness traditions. The pillar of cloud and the pillar of fire are visible manifestations of Yahweh's presence and protection.

The ark, the visible sign of Yahweh's presence, was a portable chest of acacia wood, overlaid with gold inside and out, containing the two tablets of the Ten Commandments. Measuring 11.7 m x 6.9 m [3.9 ft x 2.3 ft], the ark was carried at the head of the column when the Israelites trekked through the wilderness (Numbers 10:33–34), and it accompanied them in warfare (Numbers 10:35–36).

The tent (tabernacle), a portable sanctuary, was the place of Yahweh's presence among the people of Israel during the wilderness period. It consisted of a rectangular enclosure measuring 43.5 meters x 21.6 m x 2.1 m [145 ft long, 72 ft wide, 7ft high]. The holy of holies within the tabernacle contained the ark of the covenant. The biblical tabernacle was an admixture of desert motifs and temple motifs.

"The Fear of the Lord is the Beginning of Knowledge" (Proverbs 1:7)

Fear, a central concept and a complex quality in biblical religion, has a wide semantic range extending from awe to terror. Fear of Yahweh is synonymous with reverential awe; it may also instill a feeling of terror, as when Adam and Eve fled from God in the Garden of Eden. To fear Yahweh connotes the rejection of competing deities to serve him exclusively. "The Lord your God you shall fear; him you shall serve, and by his name alone you shall swear" (Deuteronomy 6:13). To fear Yahweh is to recognize his supremacy; to fear Yahweh is to do his will. "You who fear the Lord, praise him! ... Stand in awe of him, all you offspring of Israel!" (Psalm 22:23). "He [an angel] said in a loud voice, 'Fear God and give him glory, for the hour of his judgment has come; and worship him who made heaven and earth, the sea and the springs of water'" (Revelation 14:7). The fear of Yahweh is an incentive to obedience and service; at the same time, it is to be understood in the context of covenant relationship with God. Fear of Yahweh is equivalent to Israelite faith in Yahweh. "Israel saw the great work that the Lord did against the Egyptians. So the people feared the Lord and believed in the Lord and in his servant Moses" (Exodus 14:31). "Now therefore revere the Lord, and serve him in sincerity and in faithfulness; put away the gods that your ancestors served beyond the River and in Egypt, and serve the Lord" (Joshua 24:14). "Fear God, and keep his commandments; for that is the whole duty of everyone. For God will bring every deed into judgment, including every secret thing, whether good or evil" (Ecclesiastes 12:13–14).

Love of God, the foundation of the fear of Yahweh, is analogous to Israelite faith in Yahweh. "Israel saw the great work that the Lord did against the Egyptians. So the people feared the Lord and believed in the Lord and in his servant Moses" (Exodus 14:31).

Only when we are afraid can we experience the significance of trust in God. "When I am afraid, I put my trust in you.

In God, whose word I praise, in God I trust; I am not afraid; what can flesh do to me?" (Psalm 56:3–4).

Psalm 112 celebrates the blessings bestowed on one who honors and remembers God. "They are not afraid of evil tidings; their hearts are firm, secure in the Lord. Their hearts are steady; they will not be afraid; in the end they will look in triumph on their foes" (verses 7–8).

In the New Testament, the concept of fear with its wide range of meanings offers notable parallels to those in the Old Testament. Examples are too numerous to cite, but a few may be in order.

During a treacherous windstorm at sea, the terrified disciples appealed to Jesus who was asleep in the boat. "Lord save us! We are perishing!" And Jesus' retort, "Why are you afraid, you of little faith?" (Matthew 8:25–26). Again, Jesus admonished his disciples, "But even the hairs of your head are all counted. Do not be afraid; you are of more value than many sparrows" (Luke 12:7).

Regarding the essence of the law, Jesus comments, "So, now, O Israel, what does the Lord your God require of you? Only to fear the Lord your God, to walk in all his ways, to love him, to serve the Lord your God with all your heart and with all your soul" (Deuteronomy 10:12). The antidote for fear is assurance that God is for us and with us.

The divine admonition to "fear not, for I am with you" is a pledge of tranquility and security. A few examples will suffice—"Do not fear, for I am with you, do not be afraid, for I am your God; I will strengthen you, I will help you, I will uphold you with my victorious right hand" (Isaiah 41:10). "But now thus says the Lord, ... Do not fear, for I have redeemed you; I have called you by name, you are mine" (Isaiah 43:1). "Do not be afraid of the king of Babylon, as you have been; do not be afraid of him, says the Lord, for I am with you, to save you and to rescue you from his hand" (Jeremiah 42:11).

Further examples from the New Testament: "When Zechariah saw him [an angel], he was terrified; and fear overwhelmed him. But the angel said to him, 'Do not be afraid, Zechariah, for your prayer has been heard. Your wife Elizabeth will bear you a son, and you will name him John'" (Luke 1:12–13). "When I [John] saw him [a vision of Christ], I fell at his feet as though dead. But he placed his right hand on me, saying, 'Do not be afraid; I am the first and the last'" (Revelation 1:17).

"Worship the Lord Your God and Serve Only Him" (Matthew 4:10)

The word "cult" today is usually applied pejoratively to fringe groups or to a contemporary religious movement. In the biblical sense, cult is a broader term than worship and includes rituals, prayers, pilgrimages, and sacrifices. It has a similar meaning in the Catholic church's "cult of saints." Cult may be defined as a formal means of expressing religious reverence. Hebrew has two basic words signifying the act of worship: *'abad*, to serve, and *hishtahawa*, to prostrate oneself. Just as one renders service to the king, it is incumbent upon a subject to pay homage to the deity. External gestures must be compatible with an internal attitude, both in accord with the proper service of God.

In his speech on fasting, the prophet Second Isaiah (chapters 40–66) defines authentic worship in terms of the biblical doctrine of righteousness. "Is not this the fast that I [Yahweh] choose: to loose the bonds of injustice, to undo the thongs of the yoke, to let the oppressed go free, and to break every yoke? Is it not to share your bread with the hungry, and bring the homeless poor into your house; when you see the naked, to cover them, and not to hide yourself from your own kin?" (Isaiah 58:6–7).

The altar was the exclusive domain of the Israelite priests. The principal Hebrew word for the altar is *mizbeah*, occurring 400 times in the Hebrew Bible. Derived from the root *zbh*, "to slaughter," "to sacrifice," the altar is the place where animal offerings were slain.

Hebrew worship incorporates religious feasts. The weekly observance of the sabbath, the seventh day of the week, commemorates both creation (Exodus 20:8–11) and Israel's liberation from slavery (Deuteronomy 5:12–15). The New Moon (*hodes*, Numbers 28:11–15) celebrates the first day of the lunar month. Like the sabbath, it was a day of rest and feasting.

Haggim (plural) designates the annual feasts of pilgrimage. Only three holy days are included among the *haggim*: the festival of unleavened bread, later combined with Passover (*Pesah*), the festival of weeks (*Shabu`ot*), and the festival of ingathering, also known as the festival of booths (*Sukkot*, Exodus 23:14–17). These feasts developed over time and became associated with major events in Israel's religious history; later they also became connected with Christian feasts.

The centrality of worship in the New Testament is summarized in the opening and closing of Luke's Gospel. "Once when he [Zechariah] was serving as priest before God and his section was on duty, he was chosen by lot, according to the custom of the priesthood, to enter the sanctuary of the Lord and offer incense" (Luke 1:8–9). "They worshiped him [the risen Jesus], and returned to Jerusalem with great joy; and they were continually in the temple blessing God" (Luke 24:52–53). Note that Luke's Gospel begins and ends in the temple.

Paul emphasizes the unique place of Christ Jesus in New Testament worship:

I give thanks to my God always for you [the church in Corinth] because of the grace of God that has been given you in Christ Jesus, for in every way you have been enriched in him, in speech and knowledge of every kind—just as the testimony of Christ has been strengthened among you—so that you are not lacking in any spiritual gift as you wait for the revealing of our Lord Jesus Christ. (1 Corinthians 1:4–7)

At the beginning of Paul's prayers of thanksgiving the words "through Jesus Christ" are prominent: for example, "First, I thank my God through Jesus Christ for all of you [the church of Rome], because your faith is proclaimed throughout the world" (Romans 1:8).

Therefore God also highly exalted him and gave him the name that is above every name, so that at the name of Jesus every knee should bend, in heaven and on earth and under the earth, and every tongue should confess that Jesus Christ is Lord (*kurios*), to the glory of God the Father. (Philippians 2:9–11)

This biblical citation (including verses 6–11), is one of the most elegant Christological passages in the New Testament. Apparently an early Christian hymn cited here by Paul, it consists of two principal parts: verses 6–8 where Christ is the subject of every verb, and verses 9–11, where God is the subject. In verse 11 "Jesus Christ is Lord" is an early Christian acclamation; compare Romans 10:9—"If you confess with your lips that Jesus is Lord and believe in your heart that God raised him from the dead, you will be saved."

The Jewish synagogue (from Greek, "assembly [of people]"), served three principal functions, all centering on Scripture: worship, prayer, and religious studies. Christian worship developed from Jewish synagogue worship; in its early forms Christian worship bore notable resemblance to Jewish worship. Jesus and his disciples were no strangers to the synagogues they frequented. "They [Jesus and his disciples] went to Capernaum; and when the sabbath came, he [Jesus] entered the synagogue and taught. They were astounded at his teaching, for he taught them as one having authority, and not as the scribes" (Mark 1:21–22).

On another occasion Jesus came to his hometown (Nazareth), and his disciples followed him. "On the sabbath he began to teach in the synagogue, and many who heard him were astounded" (Mark 6:2). "And he [Jesus] went throughout Galilee, proclaiming the message in their synagogues and casting out demons" (Mark 1:39).

"Then Jesus, filled with the power of the Spirit, returned to Galilee ... He began to teach in their synagogues and was praised by everyone" (Luke 4:14–15). Arriving in Nazareth, he went to the synagogue on the sabbath day, as was his custom. Then he stood up to read; unrolling the scroll of Isaiah, he proclaimed:

The Spirit of the Lord is upon me, because he has anointed me to bring good news to the poor. He has sent me to proclaim release to the captives and recovery of sight to the blind, to let the oppressed go free, to proclaim the year of the Lord's favor. (Luke 4:18–19; see Isaiah 61:1–4)

Only gradually did Christian worship supersede synagogue worship in the church. Christian worship in New Testament times was ordinarily offered to God as Father through Jesus Christ as Son. "First, I thank my God through Jesus Christ for all of you, because your faith is proclaimed throughout the world" (Romans 1:8).

The apostle Paul taught in synagogues in the course of his missionary journeys. "Every sabbath he [Paul] would argue in the synagogue and would try to convince Jews and Greeks" (Acts 18:4). "He [Paul] entered the synagogue and for three months spoke out boldly, and argued persuasively about the kingdom of God" (Acts 19:8).

Abram "Believed the Lord, and the Lord Reckoned It to Him as Righteousness" (Genesis 15:6)

God understood Abraham's unquestioning belief as a sign that Abraham wanted to be in a relationship of loving trust with Yahweh. The biblical concept of righteousness is a complex theological concept. Righteous acts are approved by God, whereby the doer manifests that he/she plans to be in a dependent relationship with God. "He [Abraham] believed the Lord; and the Lord reckoned it to him as righteousness" (Genesis 15:6). According to this verse, Abraham's faith was thought to be a righteous act.

Righteousness, the state of being in the right or being vindicated, is the basic theme in both Old Testament and New Testament. People are righteous when their personal conduct is in harmony with an established norm. In the Hebrew Bible righteousness entails conformity to the divine will. The range of righteousness far exceeds legal procedures and includes the entire covenant life of God's people.

Covenant love, the operative word in the present context, along with fidelity, judgment, and righteousness, are the attributes of the ideal ruler, according to the prophet Isaiah—"Then a throne shall be established in steadfast love in the tent of David, and on it shall sit in faithfulness a ruler who seeks justice and is swift to do what is right" (Isaiah 16:5). "Strive first for the kingdom of God and his righteousness, and all these things will be given to you as well" (Matthew 6:33). Balancing human needs with service to God demonstrates the disciple's confidence in God.

To consider the Old Testament as nothing more than a legalistic document is a misapprehension. Rather, righteousness is the fulfillment of the requirements of a relationship, whether with God or people. The relationships may be between the king and people, between priest and worshipers, or between the community and *gerim* (resident aliens). Each of these relationships involves specific demands, and their fulfillment establishes righteousness. The relationship is always the deciding factor. When God or a person conforms to the conditions imposed by a relationship, God or that person is, in Old Testament terms, righteous.

Hebrew *sedeq, sedeqa* and Greek *dikaiosyne* are the basic terms for righteousness; the adjectival forms are *saddiq* and *dikaios*. Their meaning is more easily grasped when applied to inanimate objects—a "righteous weight," that is, a weight that is what it is supposed to be (Deuteronomy 25:15). Also, "righteous paths" are paths that proceed in the right direction (Psalm 23:3). Saul said to David, "You are more righteous than I; for you have repaid me good, whereas I have repaid you evil" (1 Samuel 24:17). David was righteous (*saddiq*) because he was unwilling to kill Saul, with whom he shared a covenant relationship. Righteousness is the fulfillment of communal demands, and righteous judgments are those that restore community. "I [Moses] charged your judges at that time: 'Give the members of your community a fair hearing, and judge rightly (*sedeq*) between one person and another, whether citizen or resident alien (*ger*)'" (Deuteronomy 1:16).

One of the king's primary obligations was to support the Israelite community. Psalm 72, a prayer for the king, describes the peace and prosperity accomplished by the king who judges righteously. To achieve righteousness, it was incumbent upon Israel to fulfill the requirements of the relationship between Yahweh and the people.

The opening verses of Psalm 72 contain the words "justice" and "righteousness," each used twice. Second Samuel 8:15 is similar to Psalm 72: "So David reigned over all Israel; and David administered justice (*mispat*) and equity (*sedaqa*) to all his people." Also, *mispat* and *sedaqa* are often used together: "Because the Lord loved Israel forever, he has made you [Solomon] king to execute justice (*mispat*) and righteousness (*sedaqa*) (1 Kings 10:9). Just as ambiguity exists in these Hebrew words, so too in English. The fluidity of meaning among these concepts and their synonyms makes it difficult to grasp the subtle distinctions. Also, the differences between Eastern and Western thought patterns must be taken into consideration. To make the matter even more complex, the concepts of love and of judgment (which focus on the oppressed and the needy) must also be borne in mind. In sum, the purpose of these qualities is to make Israel holy as Yahweh is holy. Recall Yahweh's directive to the people of Israel via Moses: "You shall be holy, for I the Lord your God am holy" (Leviticus 19:2).

"Their delight is in the law of the Lord, and on his law they meditate day and night" (Psalm 1:2). Israel cherishes the law, but decrees have no meaning, aside from the covenant relationship between Yahweh and Israel.

In an announcement of future salvation, God's *sedeq* (righteousness) and salvation (expressed as the fulfillment of the promise to Abraham [Genesis 12:1–3]) are virtually synonymous (Isaiah 51:1–3). Regarding the reference to the Garden of Eden in verse 3, the time of salvation is often pictured in prophetic literature as restoration to the harmonious condition of paradise.

The practice of justice is incumbent on all members of the covenant community. To do justice means to advocate for the indigent and the downtrodden. "[God] has told you, O mortal, what is good; and what does the Lord require of you but to do justice (*mispat*), and to love kindness (*hesed*), and to walk humbly with your God?" (Micah 6:8).

As already stated, there is no single Hebrew word to express our concept of justice; what we understand by justice is incorporated in the concepts of judgment (*mispat*) and righteousness (*sedaqa*). In the Solomonic palace one of the public rooms was designated *'ulam hammispat* (the hall of judgment), where the king rendered judgments. Judges in Israel were appointed to maintain harmony among the people.

Likewise *mispat* has an assortment of meanings: justice, judgment, vindication, deliverance, and many more. In the last analysis, it is not conspicuous devoutness that Yahweh requires of us, but the practice of justice and righteousness: "Let justice (*mispat*) roll down like waters, and righteousness (*sedaqa*) like an everflowing stream" (Amos 5:24). Also, "The Lord judges the peoples; judge me, O Lord, according to my righteousness (*sedaqa*)" (Psalm 7:8).

Justice, founded in the being of God, is a primary divine attribute. The God of justice is the defender of the indigent and the oppressed. "Let those who boast boast in this, that they understand and know me [Yahweh], that I am the Lord; I act with steadfast love (*hesed*), justice (*mispat*), and righteousness (*sedaqa*) in the earth, for in these things I delight, says the Lord" (Jeremiah 9:23–24).

"So God Created Humankind in His Image, in the Image of God He Created Them" (Genesis 1:27)

Human sexuality is ultimately a mystery exceeding human understanding, as the author of Proverbs tells us, "Three things are too wonderful for me; four I do not understand: the way of an eagle in the sky, the way of a snake on a rock, the way of a ship on the high seas, and the way of a man with a girl [young woman]" (Proverbs 30:18–19).

The Bible teaches that sexuality is a constituent part of being human. Sexuality has been a component since creation; the Book of Genesis begins with not one but two accounts of creation. Some have the impression that the biblical view of sexuality is totally negative; not so—its view is quite positive. The consideration of sexuality in the Bible is an odd combination of candor and reticence. Nothing is more straightforward, for example, than the erotic dialogue between a loving man and a woman (companion) in the Song of Songs (Song of Solomon); it is basically an impassioned love song. Later, the Song was reinterpreted as an allegory describing God's love for Israel and Christ's love for the church.

Despite the many references to sex in the Bible, curiously the Bible has no single word for sexuality, but synonyms, euphemisms, ambiguities, and circumlocutions abound, produced especially by translators who have felt the need to sanitize the Bible. A classic case concerns the Hebrew verb *yada'*, "to know," used at times in the Hebrew Bible as a euphemism for the sexual act and denoting experiential and not primarily cognitive knowledge. *Yada'* is to be understood here in a sexual, personal sense. Other examples treat the hands, feet, and flesh as euphemisms for the male genitals. Since sex plays such a major role in the life of people, it is mentioned very often in the Bible. However, sexual relations take place therein principally for the procreation of children, especially male children to perform the intense labor required in agricultural communities.

The proper interpretation of a biblical text, as we have already noted, requires that it be situated in its historical, social, and cultural context; otherwise distortion will result. To know what the Bible *means*, one must first know what it *meant*. Also, with regard to sexuality one must not impose contemporary suppositions on an ancient culture. The modern understanding of human sexuality is far more developed than it was in the biblical era. In ancient Israel sexual intercourse was intended to build the community first and then to satisfy the individual's libido.

Through the generations the biblical view of human sexuality, especially as it concerns homosexuality, appears to have undergone striking development. Today the gay community, little by little, is gaining the respect that is the right of every human being, not to mention the requirements of the gospel, which directs each of us to relate with kindness and concern toward all people, for we are all sinners. It is hoped the time has passed when homosexuals were cruelly treated as pariahs, even by some Christian denominations. As one commentator said so well—"If homosexual persons are not welcome in the church, I will have to walk out the door along with them, leaving in the sanctuary only those entitled to cast the first stone."[2]

"Homosexuality," a word coined in the nineteenth century CE, has no equivalent in ancient Hebrew or Greek In fact, the Bible says remarkably little about homosexuality.

The New Testament records no word or action on the part of Jesus regarding homosexuality; he simply did not address the issue. Incidentally Jesus was particularly compassionate to those who had committed sexual sin. While Paul disapproves of homosexual acts, his "vice list" (a list of sinners) does not highlight this kind of behavior for explicit censure (1 Corinthians 6:9–10; 1 Timothy 1:9–10). For Paul, homosexual acts are not permissible among members of the church.

Nowadays several texts are erroneously invoked to condemn gay people, but the meaning of these texts is dubious or disputed. Additionally, words like "sexual orientation" and "homosexual" oversimplify the many-faceted human realities involved. Today homosexuality is a complex phenomenon, and it seems the same was true in biblical times. Consider the covenanted love between persons of the same sex; for example, the same-sex love relationship of David and Jonathan—"I [David] am distressed for you, my brother Jonathan; greatly beloved were you to me; your love to me was wonderful, passing the love of women" (2 Samuel 1:26). This passage expresses warm, personal affection between the two friends (also, there may be a political nuance intended). Such a relationship is not necessarily an "abomination" (wicked or unlawful conduct). We all know of similar covenanted friendships in our own time.

Let us consider briefly the few biblical texts, both Old Testament and New Testament, that may be enlisted as censuring homosexuality—Leviticus 18:22; 20:13; Romans 1:26–27; 1 Corinthians 6:9–10; 1 Timothy 1:10. Some of these texts seem not to address modern questions directly. Bear in mind that the background of the New Testament is Greco-Roman culture.

"You shall not lie with a male as with a woman; it is an abomination [a serious violation of purity]" (Leviticus 18:22). "If a man lies with a male as with a woman, both of them have committed an abomination" (Leviticus 20:13). This law is included in the Holiness Code (Leviticus 17–26), a collection of legal material reflecting the Israelites' concern for ethical and cultic purity, consonant with their unique relationship with God. The Holiness Code considers homoerotic activity between males an abomination. Lesbianism is not mentioned in the Hebrew Bible.

What does Paul say? "God gave them up to degrading passions. Their women exchanged natural intercourse for unnatural, and in the same way also the men, giving up natural intercourse with women, were consumed with passion for one another. Men committed shameless acts with men" (Romans 1:26–27). Joseph Fitzmyer notes: "The contrast between females and males (1:27) shows that the sexual perversion of which Paul speaks is homosexuality."[3] Paul considers same-sex intercourse a major example of the impurity characteristic of the gentiles (non-Jews) and reflects the Jewish tradition's strong aversion to homoeroticism. Modern considerations of homosexuality concern some or all of these passages, but the interpreters differ about the meaning and authority of these texts. Joseph

Fitzmyer's interpretation is worthy of serious consideration: "Paul is clearly referring here to the conduct of active male homosexual persons and is merely echoing the Old Testament abomination of such homosexual activity."[4]

In another place Paul refers to sodomites. "Do you not know that wrongdoers will not inherit the kingdom of God? Do not be deceived! Fornicators, idolaters, adulterers, male prostitutes, sodomites, thieves ... —none of these will inherit the kingdom of God" (1 Corinthians 6:9–10). The Bible defines the sin of the sodomites as something other than homosexual lust. Paul enumerates the sins that were common at Corinth as they came into his mind. The precise meaning of the ambiguous Greek words for "male prostitutes" (*malakoi*) and "sodomites" (*arsenokoitai*) is disputed. Whatever their exact meaning, they call to mind the biblical and Jewish condemnation of homoeroticism (compare with Romans 1:24–27).

"The law is laid down not for the innocent but for the lawless and the disobedient ... fornicators, sodomites, slave traders, liars, perjurers" (1 Timothy 1:9–10). The prime purpose of 1 Corinthians and 1 Timothy is not to teach about homosexual behavior (connoting deliberate acts of unrestrained desire). The authors of 1 Corinthians and 1 Timothy are arguing against a specific problem in the church; homosexuality and other objectionable activities are mentioned to support their thesis. "Paul singles out homosexual intercourse for special attention because he regards it as providing a particularly graphic image of the way in which human fallenness distorts God's created order."[5]

---

[1] Walter Brueggemann, *The Book of Exodus*, New Interpreter's Bible, vol. 1 (Nashville: Abingdon Press, 1994), 937.

[2] Richard Hays, *The Moral Vision of the New Testament* (San Franciso: Harper, 1996), 400.

[3] Joseph Fitzmyer, *Romans*, The Anchor Bible (Garden City, NY: Doubleday, 1992), 285.

[4] Joseph Fitzmyer, *Romans*, The Anchor Bible (Garden City, NY: Doubleday, 1992), 288.

[5] Richard Hays, *The Moral Vision of the New Testament* (San Franciso: Harper, 1996), 388.

Conclusion

WITH THE BIBLE AS OUR GUIDE, we are pilgrims, climbing mountains and descending valleys, on our way to the holy city Jerusalem. Some of us have been on the road longer than others, as all strive to reach the goal. The Bible illustrates for us the loving embrace of God, and shares with us the struggles of earlier pilgrims, men and women, some who have succeeded and others who have not.

Perhaps a closer reading of God's Word, clarified by *The Bible Is for Living*, in addition to countless biblical commentaries, will make the arduous journey just a little easier. It is written by one approaching the end of the road, who has experienced the ups-and-downs of life, who has struggled on the way, and who, in addition to the Bible, has found inspiration in the famous poem "The Hound of Heaven," by English poet Francis Thompson, who lived in poverty and suffered from addiction. It is so similar to the biblical story:

I fled Him, down the nights and down the days;
I fled Him, down the arches of the years;
I fled Him, down the labyrinthine ways
Of my own mind; and in the mist of tears
I hid from Him, and under running laughter.
Up vistaed hopes I sped;
And shot, precipitated,
Adown Titanic glooms of chasmed fears,
From those strong Feet that followed, followed after.

My own love of Scripture, fleshed out in *The Bible Is for Living*, has sustained me in this "valley of tears." Perhaps you, too, may gain from it some support along the tumultuous journey through life. If the reader finds this exposition by one biblical scholar as beneficial as did the writer, its purpose has been achieved. I have written several books, mostly technical, on the Bible and archaeology, but this is the book I really wanted to write. It is my last, and I am grateful to have lived long enough to bring it to completion. In the closing words of the Passover *seder*, *Le shana ha-ba'ah b'Yerushalayim* ("next year in Jerusalem").

Glossary

Amalekites: A people associated with the desert regions, inhabiting the territory assigned to Israel, Judah, and the Tranjordanian states.

Amorites: A Pre-Israelite tribe in Canaan, along with the Canaanites and Hittites.

Apocalyptic: A word of Greek origin, equivalent to "revelation." It is represented in the Bible principally by the Book of Daniel and is characterized by the presence of vision and symbolism.

Beatitudes: A literary form enumerating those who are blessed and associated with the pronouncements found in the Sermon on the Mount (Matthew and Luke).

Canon: An instrument of measure taken from the Greek word meaning "rule" or "standard." It connotes the list of religious writings considered authoritative.

Covenant: An agreement or treaty between two parties with each bound by certain obligations. The most significant example in the Bible is the treaty God makes with Israel at Sinai.

Decalogue: From the Greek meaning "ten words." It is a series of commands from God to the chosen people of Israel, mediated by Moses. It is frequently called the Ten Commandments.

Enuma elish: Literally "when above"; also called the Babylonian creation epic. Consists of seven tablets in praise of Marduk, the patron god of Babylon.

Eschatology: Based on the Greek term *eschaton*, meaning "end." Sometimes refers to the age to come and the kingdom of God.

Ephraim: Second son of the patriarch Joseph; also the name of a prominent Israelite tribe. Designates the whole of the Northern Kingdom comprising the central hill country of Palestine, from Bethel in the south to Shechem in the north.

Hermeneutics: Greek term meaning "interpretation." It deals with the interpretation of the Scriptures and the theories of interpretation.

Horeb, Mount: Sometimes used for Mount Sinai, "the mountain of God." The location of Sinai-Horeb is uncertain. It was the place of the apparition of the burning bush in Exodus 3:1 and the worship of the golden calf in Exodus 33:6.

Judah: Name of a region occupying the greater part of southern Palestine. It is used in three senses: as the son of Jacob and Leah; as one of the twelve tribes of Israel; and as the principal tribe of the Southern Kingdom, ruled by the Davidic dynasty. The region of Judah was later known as Judea.

Leprosy: A disorder affecting persons, fabrics, and houses. It is not to be confused with modern leprosy (Hansen's disease). It is impossible to determine the nature of this disease in the Bible.

Maccabees: A Hasmonean family supplying military and religious leaders for Judea during the second and first centuries BCE. The Hebrew word "Maccabees" means "hammer." It is the pseudonym of Judea, son of Mattathias, who led the Jewish insurrection against Antiochus Epiphanes (165–161 BCE).

Moab: Lot's son. Also a small Iron Age kingdom in Transjordan. The Moabite territory comprised the plateau east of the Dead Sea, bounded on the north by the Arnon River and on the south by the Zered (Wadi el-Hesa). It was the Moabites who refused to allow Israel to pass through their territory.

Northern Kingdom of Israel: Territory that split from Judah after the death of Solomon in the late tenth century BCE. It was an independent kingdom with its capital in Samaria until the Assyrian conquest in 722 BCE.

Philistines: A people of Aegean-Asian origin. It was one group of the Sea Peoples in the late second millennium BCE. Having failed to conquer the Egyptians, the Philistines settled on the southeast coast of the Mediterranean where they competed with Israel for control of Canaan. "Palestine" is derived from "Philistine." Historical evidence contradicts the derogatory connotation of Philistines as an unsophisticated people.

Prophet: From the Greek *prophetes*, meaning "one who speaks before others," and from the Hebrew *nabi'*, meaning "called by God." The prophet is an intermediary, carrying messages between the Deity and humankind.

Psalter: Another term for the Book of Psalms.

Rosh Hashanah: Hebrew for "head of the year." It is the Jewish New Year festival, commemorating the creation of the world. This holiday was well established by the fourth century BCE.

Septuagint: From the Greek word for the number 70. It is a Greek translation of the Hebrew Scriptures made 200 years after the Babylonian exile (586–538 BCE). According to legend, 72 men, six from each tribe, were sent from Jerusalem to Alexandria, Egypt, to make the translation.

Seraph: Its etymology suggests "fiery one." The seraph is an emissary of God, perhaps serpentine in form. According to Isaiah's vision of God (Isaiah 6) the seraphim have six wings and are the guardians before the divine throne.

Shechem: A city situated 65.6 km (41 mi) north of Jerusalem in a strategic pass between Mount Ebal to the north and Mount Gerizim to the south. It was a capital of the Northern Kingdom of Israel and the scene of the assembly when Joshua renewed the covenant between Yahweh and Israel (Joshua 24).

Sheol: Its etymology is uncertain, but it is the abyss into which the spirits of the dead passed, according to ancient Jewish belief. Its

Greek counterpart is Hades. The world was looked upon as a three-level structure: the heavens, the earth, and the underworld.

Sinai: The name given to a mountain and the surrounding desert. It is a wedge-shaped territory forming a land-bridge between Africa and Asia. It is the mountain on which God revealed himself to Moses and made the covenant with Israel.

Synagogue: A Greek word meaning "assembly of people," connoting a congregation of Jews who pray and read the Scriptures and also a place where the congregation assembles. Though its origin is unknown, the synagogue certainly existed by the first century CE. Unlike the temple, the synagogue is not an edifice where the Deity dwells, but rather a meetinghouse for prayer and study of Torah.

Syro-Ephramite War: The attack on Judah and Jerusalem by the Northern Kingdom of Israel and Aram (Syria) in 734 BCE in an attempt to pressure the Kingdom of Judah to join an anti-Assyrian alliance.

Tetragrammaton: From the Greek meaning "four letters" (*yhwh*) making up the personal name of God. It is vocalized in Christian translations as Yahweh. This name was too holy to be uttered, so Lord (Hebrew, *adonai*) was substituted when the name appeared in the text.

Theophany: Greek in origin, it means "appearance of God to humans."

Torah: A Hebrew word meaning "priestly instruction." It is not to be identified with legalism. It is the most general word for law in Judaism. Torah refers to the Pentateuch, the first five books of the Bible.

Ugarit: Ras-Shamra is the modern Arabic name of the ancient city Ugarit, which lies on the border of the Syrian coast of the Mediterranean sea. Ugaritic is a Semitic language closely related to Hebrew. The Ugaritic texts include many myths and epics that illuminate the Canaanite religion.

United Monarchy: During the tenth century BCE the ten northern tribes of Israel, along with the southern tribes of Judah and Benjamin, were united under the rule of David and his son Solomon. When Solomon died in 928 BCE the United Kingdom of Israel was divided into the Northern Kingdom of Israel and the Southern Kingdom of Judah.

Yom Kippur: The Jewish day of atonement. It is the holiest of Jewish holy days. The festival is observed ten days after the autumn new year.

Zion: A Hebrew word whose precise meaning is unknown. It is used to designate various parts of Jerusalem. Zion appears especially in poetic texts.

Bibliography

Adam, Peter. *Hearing God's Words: Exploring Biblical Spirituality*. Downers Grove, IL: InterVarsity Press, 2004.

Barton, Stephen C. *The Spirituality of the Gospels*. London: SPCK, 1992.

Bowe, Barbara Ellen. *Biblical Foundations of Spirituality: Touching a Finger to the Flame*. Lanham, MD: Rowman & Littlefield Publishers, 2003.

Burrows, Mark S. "To Taste with the Heart." In *Interpretation* 56, no. 2 (April 2002): 168–180.

Donahue, John R. "The Quest for Biblical Spirituality." In *Exploring Christian Spirituality, Essays in Honor of S. Schneiders*, ed. Bruce Lescher and Elizabeth Liebert, 73–97. New York: Paulist Press, 2006.

Endres, John. ""Psalms and Spirituality in the 21st Century." In *Interpretation* 56, no. 2 (April 2002): 143–154.

Green, Barbara. "The Old Testament in Christian Spirituality." In *Blackwell Companion to Christian Spirituality*, ed. Arthur Holder, 37–54. Malden, MA: Blackwell Pub., 2005.

Harrington, Wilfred J. *Seeking Spiritual Growth through the Bible.* New York: Paulist Press, 2002.

Larsen, David. *Biblical Spirituality: Discovering the Real Connection between the Bible and Life.* Grand Rapids, MI: Kregel Productions, 2001.

Powell, Mark A. *Loving Jesus.* Minneapolis, MN: Fortress Press, 2004.

Resseguie, James L. *Spiritual Landscape: Images of the Spiritual Life in the Gospel of Luke.* Peabody, MA: Hendrickson Publishers, 2004.

Ryrie, Alexander. *Silent Waiting: The Biblical Roots of Contemplative Spirituality.* Norwich, England: Canterbury Press, 1999.

Schneiders, Sandra. "The Foot Washing (John 13: 1-20): An Experiment in Hermeneutics." In *Catholic Biblical Quarterly* 43 (January 1981): 76–92.

_____. "Biblical Spirituality: Life, Literature, and Learning." In *Doors of Understanding: Conversations in Global Spirituality in Honor of Ewert Cousins,* ed. Steven Chase, 51–76. Qunicy, IL: Franciscan Press, 1997.

_____. *The Revelatory Text: Interpreting the New Testament as Sacred Scripture.* 2nd edition. Collegeville, MN: Liturgical Press, 1999.

_____. "Biblical Spirituality." In *Interpretation* 56, no. 2 (April 2002): 133–142.

_____. *Written That You May Believe: Encountering Jesus in the Fourth Gospel*. Revised and Expanded Edition with a Study Guide by John C. Wronski, S. J. New York: Crossroad, 2003.

_____. "The Resurrection (of the Body) in the Fourth Gospel: A Key to Johannine Spirituality." In *Life in Abundance: Stdies of John's Gospel in Tribute to Raymond E. Brown*, ed. John R. Donahue, 168–198. Collegeville, MN: Liturgical Press, 2005.

_____. "Biblical Foundations of Spirituality." In *Scripture as the Soul of Theology*, ed. Edward J. Mahoney, 1–22. Collegeville, MN: Liturgical Press, 2005.

_____. "The Gospels and the Reader." In *Cambridge Companion to the Gospels*, ed. Stephen C. Barton, 97–118. Cambridge, UK: Cambridge University Press, 2006.

_____. "Remaining in His Word: Faith to Faith by Way of the Text." In *What We Have Heard from the Beginning: The Past, Present, and Future of Johannine Studies*, ed. Tom Thatcher. Waco, TX: Baylor University Press, 2007.

Stevens, R. Paul. *Living the Story: Biblical Spirituality for Everyday Christians*. Grand Rapids, MI: William B. Eerdmans, 2003.

Young, Frances M. *Brokenness and Blessing: Towards a Biblical Spirituality*. Grand Rapids, MI: Baker Academic, 2007.

Theodosia

·ANNE COLVER·

THEODOSIA

Daughter of Aaron Burr

Holt, Rinehart and Winston

New York · Chicago · San Francisco

Revised Edition Published April, 1962
Second Printing, June, 1963
Third Printing, September, 1966

Library of Congress Catalog Card Number: 62-10213

91522-0312
Printed in the United States of America

THIS BOOK IS FOR
JEREMY HARRIS

Contents

Part One

· NEW YORK, 1783–1801 ·

· C H A P T E R 1 ·

The Parade

SCOTCH NANNY HAD made up her mind. And Scotch
Nanny had said her say. It was a raw, cold day in No-
vember with a damp wind blowing from the harbor of New
York and rattling the panes of the nursery windows angrily.
No sort of day, Nanny said, to be taking a wee baby outdoors
at all. Parade or no parade, Nanny added grimly, George
Washington or no George Washington, her baby Theodosia
was not leaving the house. And that was that.

Mrs. Burr, small Theodosia's mother, glanced down at
the dark curly head of her sleeping daughter. The baby, as
she lay in her crib between the two women, was peacefully
unconscious of any dispute. But a frown troubled her mother's
gentle face. "Her father will be very disappointed, Nanny,"
Mrs. Burr said. "You know he's given orders to have Theo
go with us. And Colonel Burr is not accustomed to having
his orders disobeyed. He says this is a historic occasion."

Nanny was unmoved. "Colonel Burr may know all about

3

historic occasions," she said. "He may be the cleverest law-yer in New York as some say—but I know my wee bonnie, and I'll not have her getting her death of pneumonia for all the generals of the Continental Army or the whole world for that matter."

Mrs. Burr's frown deepened. She dared not cross Nanny, for in spite of her fierce moods she was a devoted nurse to small Theodosia. Yet all the arrangements had been made to see the great procession when General Washington and his officers would make their triumphal entry into the newly freed city of New York. The Burr carriage had been ordered out and the two older boys, Frederic and John, were already waiting downstairs. Mrs. Burr made one more attempt. "I expect you're right about the weather, Nanny, but Colonel Burr is really quite determined. He feels that even the baby should have a part in such an important day as this. It's the beginning of her education, he says——"

"Education," Nanny echoed, and her Scotch voice gave the word a wicked twang. "It's stuff and nonsense to be talk-ing about education with a mite like this. What's more, edu-cation is for boys, not girls." She bent over the crib and touched the baby's rosy cheek. "Far better for her to grow up a bonnie lass than have her pretty head addled with notions of *education.*"

Mrs. Burr turned away, shaking her head gently. She closed the nursery door just in time to see her husband come up the stairs.

"Hello," Colonel Burr greeted her. "Is Theo ready?"

Mrs. Burr shook her head. "She's still sleeping, Aaron. Nanny says positively it would be most unwise to bring her out at all. Nanny says there's snow in the air. She feels it in her bones."

Mr. Burr's smile did not diminish as he paused to kiss his wife's cheek and moved swiftly past her. "So Nanny says that, does she?" he demanded cheerfully. "Well, we shall see what Nanny says to *me*."

What Nanny said, Mrs. Burr never knew, but before she finished putting on her cloak, there was a light tap on the door of her room.

"Your daughter, ma'am." Mr. Burr entered with a flourish, smiling broadly over baby Theo's head. She lay contentedly against his shoulder, bundled in woolly robe, with only her dark eyes visible, blinking and sleepy.

In the hallway beyond stood Nanny, a starched image of disapproval. But Nanny's opinions, however fierce, were kept to herself this time. Colonel Burr had spoken and Colonel Burr had a way about him that made a body say yes when she meant no. And that, Nanny reflected grimly, was that.

"Never fear, Nanny," Mr. Burr called back as he hurried down the stairs. "Your bonnie shall be on the steps of Trinity Church and hobnob with the most distinguished citizens of New York to watch the conquering hero. And if she should take cold—which I'll warrant she won't—I promise to sit up nights and rub her chest with camphor oil myself!"

So it was that baby Theodosia Burr was one of the cheering crowd that witnessed the triumphant march of General George Washington and his Continental officers along Broadway on that November afternoon in 1783.

It was a day of celebration and thanksgiving for the whole city. Eight long years New York had been held in the grip of war, its people divided, its commerce throttled. Two terrible fires had ravaged homes and businesses, and many buildings lay in ruins. But now the Revolutionary War was ended, and the last of the British redcoat troops had been evacuated. New York, capital of the new nation, was free.

As General Washington and his men passed the steps of old Trinity Church, a great shout went up from the close-pressed crowd. Hats were flung into the air, women waved their handkerchiefs and tossed flowers into the path of the soldiers.

Colonel Burr, standing beside his wife, with little Theo in his arms and the two boys at his side, watched quietly. These were the officers with whom he had served. His record in the army had been a brilliant one. For a while he had been, along with Alexander Hamilton, an aide to General Washington. Later he had been given command of the regiment, and his courage and military skill had made him one of the outstanding young officers in the long, bitter struggle. Until the last months of the war, he had fought shoulder to shoulder with the men who now rode past him. But a severe illness had brought an end to his military career.

Once or twice, as the parade passed, Mrs. Burr wondered whether her husband regretted not being among the officers in this hour of victory. But there was no expression on his handsome features to give a clue to his thoughts. For all the closeness of their devotion, there were moments like this when not even she could guess what lay behind the calm, inscrutable look in her husband's dark eyes.

Back in her nursery, later that afternoon, Theodosia proved herself a young lady of poise by taking her supper and falling asleep quite as amiably as if she had not begun her education by witnessing the historic entry of General Washington into New York. Nary a sniffle did she develop.

And that, as Nanny would have said, was that.

CHAPTER 2

Honey Cakes

I T WAS RAINING and it was teatime, and Theodosia stood between her two older half brothers at the front window of the tall, narrow house in Maiden Lane. The three children were making a game of guessing which carriage that came down the cobbled street below would be Papa's. Each time a rumble of wheels sounded, accompanied by the clop-clop of horses' feet, they waited, breathless, to see whether he had really come.

For three long weeks Mr. Burr had been away, trying a law case in Albany. Now at last he was coming home again —in time for tea, his letter had said. The table was ready, in the candlelit study, with tea and milk, bread and butter and jam. Best of all, Peggy had baked honey cakes as a treat.

A dozen times that day Theodosia had gone down to the kitchen in the basement. Enveloped in a huge apron to cover her frock, she had sat on a tall stool and watched Peggy, the cook, stuff an enormous turkey with a chestnut dressing that was Papa's special favorite. When Peggy had finished mixing the batter for the honey cakes, Theodosia had been given the wooden spoon and bowl to lick.

"But never tell Nanny I let you," Peggy had warned, and Theodosia had nodded solemnly, wiping a telltale dribble of batter carefully from her chin.

Even now, when Theo was a big girl past her fifth birthday, Nanny had all sorts of tiresome notions about things she mustn't do.

A sound in the room behind them made the children turn to see their mother. "Well, children." Mrs. Burr spoke in her quiet voice, but there was an excitement in her eyes that meant she was waiting as eagerly as they for Papa's arrival. "Let me see how you look."

They lined up, the two boys tall and straight, their cheeks still glowing from an afternoon ride in the rain. Theo was between them, freshly starched and shining, from the tips of her black, square-toed slippers to the top of her smooth curls.

"Very nice." Mama smiled approvingly. The next moment she raised her hand. "Listen—isn't that another carriage?" The children hurried to the window. There, sure enough, came a carriage and horses, splashed with mud as no city carriage would be. It must be—oh, yes, it was!

They reached the hall just as the door was flung wide, admitting a gust of slanting rain with the sharp wind. The door slammed shut and Mr. Burr stood in the hallway, shaking the raindrops from his heavy cloak and holding his arms wide.

"Papa—papa!" Theodosia hurled herself at him with an ardor that threatened to ruin her embroidered pinafore and send her parent flat upon his distinguished nose. "Papa *is* home," she cried, over and over. "Papa *is* home!"

Laughing, Mr. Burr stooped to gather up his little daughter. "Yes, my Theo, Papa is home," he echoed with amusement. Holding her against his shoulder, he managed to embrace his wife and the two boys. Although Frederic and John Prevost were his stepsons, being the children of Mrs. Burr by a former marriage, they were quite as dear to him as though they had been his own. "You all look well," he said approvingly.

"We've kept very well, Aaron," his wife answered. "But we *did* miss you. The boys and I struggled with lessons—and your poor Theo was quite heartbroken in your absence. She absolutely insisted that your place at table must be set each day."

"Do you know what Peggy made for tea, Papa?" Theodosia looked up at her father out of eager dark eyes so like his own. "Honey cakes! Just for you."

When tea was finished, and they had heard the details of Mr. Burr's law case in Albany, which had turned out successfully, the question of lessons was brought up.

"Now then, what about these troublesome studies your mama speaks of?" Mr. Burr asked. "Which of your subjects have tried your souls most particularly? Frederic, you first."

"It's Latin for me, sir. As usual." Frederic groaned in a heartfelt way and thumped his forehead as if to chastise his brains for their shortcomings. "The declensions just *don't* go right."

"And you, John?"

John, the younger, swallowed a last mouthful of honey cake with a hasty gulp. "Arithmetic," he answered thickly. "Mr. Barrows says I have the worst head for figures of any boy in the Western Hemisphere." He spoke with such an air of pride that they all laughed, but a moment later his stepfather shook his head soberly.

"It won't do, you know. If you boys expect to study law in my office, you'll have to come to me well prepared. Law is no profession for numbskulls these days. Most particularly as the firm of Burr & Sons will have the wit and eloquence of my friend Hamilton to contend with."

Young Alexander Hamilton rivaled Aaron Burr as the most promising and successful of New York lawyers.

Mr. Burr spoke lightly, but there was a sternness under his words that made the boys realize he meant what he said. For all his devotion as a father, Aaron Burr was a hard taskmaster. He had never spared himself, nor anyone else either, and even Theodosia had already learned the lesson of his iron discipline.

"And now, Miss"—Theo's father turned to her—"what report can you give of yourself? Have you improved your letters while I was away?"

"Mama says the last page in my copybook is the best yet," she said promptly, "all except the s's. They always twist the wrong way. But I've learned my numbers—and two new French songs from Mama."

"Excellent. I shall hear them tomorrow." Mr. Burr drew his chair nearer to the fire. A quiet peacefulness settled over the room. Only the sound of a baker's boy crying his wares sounded from the street outside. The lonely voice, half drowned by the splashing torrent of rain, made the room seem even cozier. The boys were bent over their books. Mrs. Burr took up her sewing.

Presently Theodosia climbed onto her father's knee. Her bright head rested against his safely encircling arm.

Papa was home once more. All was well.

·CHAPTER 3·

Richmond Hill

WHEN THE HEAT of summer descended on New York, bringing in its wake the annual scourge of yellow fever, the Burr family left for the country, where they stayed in a rambling farmhouse overlooking Long Island Sound at Pelham.

The children could roam through the woods and fields, and spend long hours on the beach, where the east breezes blew fresh and cool. They grew brown in the sun, and appetites that had waned languidly in the city became suddenly ravenous. Mr. Burr, journeying out from town as often as his busy law practice would allow, vowed he had never seen three young ones eat so much or grow so fast.

There were fishing trips and horses to ride and drives along winding country roads. Encouraged by the example of her sturdy brothers, Theodosia learned to fish and swim and climb trees in the old orchard, but she loved best the hours of riding a plump pony, Duchess, borrowed from a neighboring farm.

The last week before their return to New York was the happiest. Mr. Burr arranged his affairs in town so that he might spend the whole of it in Pelham, and for seven days he was on hand morning, noon, and night. He rode with the boys, led them on walks in the woods, and joined them for picnics on the shore.

In spite of the pleasure of summer, the three children had kept to their studies faithfully. Mr. Burr's system of education allowed for no vacations. Each morning and evening found the boys and Theodosia busily at work, reading, writing, parsing, and translating. Their brown fists clutched pens and pencils; their foreheads knotted industriously, sometimes despairingly, over phrases that would not construe and sums that refused to come right. But always they struggled on until the daily task, ordered by Papa, was done.

Copybooks must be neat and correct to show Mr. Burr, and carelessness was no more to be tolerated in the sunny schoolroom in Pelham than at the house in Maiden Lane.

When the morning of leave-taking came and the carriages, piled high with luggage, stood before the door ready for the journey back to town, the children made a farewell round of the farm. Each horse must be given a parting treat of carrots and sugar before the family climbed into the waiting carriage.

At noon they stopped beside a pleasant meadow to eat lunch. While Peggy unpacked hampers of cold chicken, bread and milk, and fresh-baked cookies, the children begged Papa for a story. Mr. Burr entertained them with their favorite account of how his uncle used to punish him.

Punishments, when Mr. Burr was a boy, had been taken

very seriously. But he maintained that his stern and puritanical uncle, with whom he had lived after the death of his parents, made an even more elaborate ceremony of chastising his nephew than did most parents of the time. Always, said Mr. Burr, there were three stages in the ordeal.

First would come the summons to his uncle's study, and there small Aaron would be lectured on his shortcomings in general and his most recent misbehavior.

Next, in the presence of the assembled family, there would be a prayer for the improvement and salvation of the young sinner.

After which came the third and final stage—the whipping.

"I could always tell," Mr. Burr concluded, "just how bad the whipping was going to be by counting how many minutes Uncle prayed over me."

It was by no means a happy or peaceful boyhood that Mr. Burr recalled, but it was typical of him to gloss over the loneliness and difficulties and tell only the cheerful parts. When he imitated his uncle's long face and pious despair over a wayward nephew, the children howled with laughter.

"All the same," Mr. Burr said, "it was good training Uncle gave me—though I didn't relish it at the time. After an old-fashioned Puritan raising, there's not much in life that can seem half so bad in comparison. Provided, of course," he added, laughing, "the child survives the bringing-up!"

There was plenty of excitement to be found in New York during the winter of 1789. The city enjoyed its brief period as capital of the new nation. With President and Mrs.

Washington in residence, the Congress in session, and hundreds of visitors, the narrow streets of the old city hummed with activity.

Theodosia was enchanted by the new sights. Hanging onto Nanny's arm, she would chatter about this and that as they walked along the water front at Battery Park to see the harbor crowded with vessels, or strolled in the Mall, that fashionable and exclusive section of Broadway near Trinity Church.

Often they saw the President or Mrs. Washington driving past, in their canary-colored coach, drawn by four glossy Virginia bays. Then Theodosia would squeeze Nanny's unresponsive arm with excitement and crane her head to catch a glimpse inside the carriage.

With the busy social life of New York, gossip was the order of the day. At tea parties and over dinner tables, all that winter, people talked about other people. In spite of its new importance, the city was still small enough so that nearly everyone knew everybody else. There were plenty of rivalries, political and social, and more than one ambitious career was neatly pulled to pieces in the fashionable drawing rooms.

A favorite topic of the gossips was Aaron Burr.

Mr. Burr, people said, was a brilliant man—no doubt about that. He had been a gallant and courageous officer and his law practice was still growing. But no man of thirty-three should spend as much money as Mr. Burr did. Some said they knew for a fact that in spite of his considerable income, he was head over heels in debt.

What was more, the gossips noted, Mr. Burr was beginning to dabble in politics. Not safe and sane politics—like Mr. Hamilton, who was a staunch Federalist and Secretary of the Treasury in Washington's Cabinet. Mr. Burr, if you please, was siding with the Antifederalists—which could only mean that his sympathies were with the rabble and not with the "best people," where any right-minded citizen would agree that proper sympathies belonged.

Yet if his debts and his political activities worried his critics, they certainly did not appear to trouble Mr. Burr himself. He went about his practice, and when the subject of his Antifederalist leanings came up, he merely smiled and answered amiably that he had always supposed all men were equal in a democracy, and he failed to see what difference it made whether one belonged to the party of the rich or of the poor.

It was at this point in Mr. Burr's career that a great many people began to disapprove of him. But disapprove as they might, they couldn't help liking him. Especially the ladies. He was so charming, so handsome and tactful—and clever, too. Oh, very clever. Make no mistake about that.

The following year Aaron Burr provided the gossips with a delectable new tidbit buying the elegant estate of Richmond Hill on the sloping bank of the Hudson River. Vice-president Adams and his family had been living there, and before that, during the war, the big house with its one hundred and sixty acres of land had been the headquarters for General Washington and his staff, and later for the British commander, when New York had fallen to the enemy. It was there that Burr and Hamilton had served together as aides to the commander in chief, George Washington.

Richmond Hill was a very handsome place indeed, with tall white columns, and broad green lawns that swept down to a fringe of willow trees along the river's edge. "Mr. Burr must have gone into debt for fair to buy such a house," the gossips assured each other. And as for running it, they agreed it would take a battery of servants and a princely income.

Even Mrs. Burr was troubled. "Debts frighten me, Aaron," she said. "I can't help but worry."

Mr. Burr smiled. "Debts," he said, "are something for the future. The future never worries me—so long as the present is good. Leave it to me, my dear. We'll manage."

The children, oblivious to anything so vague and remote as debts, plunged at once into plans for the new home. The boys promised to work like beavers. They would help with the grounds and stables and plant a garden for their mother. "We'll have our own stables now," Frederic said. "Why can't Theo have a pony of her own?"

"I know the place to get one," John put in. "A white Welsh one, very well trained and gentle. Would you like that, Theo-mio?"

Theodosia clasped her hands and gave a squeal of delight. "May I really have my own pony? May I, Papa? Cross your heart and hope to *die,* Papa?"

A few weeks later the family moved. If Mrs. Burr had any further doubts over the wisdom of her husband's undertaking, she kept them to herself in her wise and gentle way.

Before long, however, an unexpected development was to change the whole course of the Burrs' family life.

·CHAPTER 4·

Lonely Afternoon

F OR THEODOSIA THE change was an unhappy one, for it meant her beloved Papa must be away from home a great deal. At those times not even Snow Baby, her new pony, could console her.

Mr. Burr had been persuaded to leave his law practice for a time, and run for election to the United States Senate on the Antifederalist ticket. And his opponent for the office was General Schuyler, Hamilton's father-in-law.

Schuyler and Hamilton represented the thoroughly entrenched and conservative Federalist party. It seemed certain that Schuyler would win. After all, people said, Burr had no political experience, and no real party to back him—only the scattered, ragged ranks of the newly formed Antifederalists.

It was an exciting campaign and a bitter one. Only Mr. Burr seemed to keep his temper. He campaigned good-naturedly, neither slandering his opponents, nor concerning himself about their attacks on him. He was probably as much surprised as anyone to discover, when the election was over, that he had won.

Aaron Burr was the new Senator from New York. He had defeated General Schuyler and the Federalist forces of Alexander Hamilton. It was a victory that Hamilton never forgave him.

The bitter seeds of hate that led to the long feud between Burr and Hamilton were sown in the weeks of that campaign, and though the two men remained outwardly on friendly terms, they were enemies nonetheless from that day on.

And each, in his way, was a dangerous enemy.

Not even the Federalists mourned Mr. Burr's victory more than Theodosia. The capital had been moved from New York to Philadelphia. The two cities were a long journey apart by horse and carriage, and whenever Congress was in session, Mr. Burr, as Senator from New York, was obliged to stay in Philadelphia.

Without Papa's gay presence, Richmond Hill seemed suddenly too big to Theodosia—and much too lonely. Once her daily lessons were finished, there was nothing to do. She would roam from one quiet room to another, read a few pages from a book here, play half a dozen bars on the piano there, and then wander on, wishing desperately that something exciting would happen.

But nothing did.

On one particularly dismal winter's day, Theodosia sat at the desk in her room feeling miserable.

The whole house seemed heavy with silence. Mama was

resting and mustn't be disturbed, for she was feeling poorly. Frederic had gone to Philadelphia to be with Mr. Burr during the winter session of the Congress, and John was in the city for a fencing lesson. Ordinarily Theodosia would have accompanied John, but she had just recovered from the mumps. Now she had a wretched toothache to increase her misery and Mama had said she must not risk the long drive into town. So John had departed for the fencing lesson alone, leaving his sister to be poulticed by Peggy and to amuse herself as best she could. .

Theodosia sighed. She had read until her eyes ached, then she had written a letter to Frederic. Her tooth felt better, but it was too snowy to venture out for a ride on her pony. There was nothing, simply nothing left to do. Idly, she nibbled at the tip of her pen and glanced over the letter that still lay open on the desk before her.

Dear Brother:
I hope the mumps have left you. Mine left me a week ago.
Papa has been here and is gone again. . . . The day before Papa went, we had your good pig for diner.
Mr. Luet, an English music master, had an elegant forte-piano which Papa bought for me. It cost 33 Guineas, and it is just come home.
I am tired of affectionate, not of being it but of writing it, so I will leave it out; I am your sister,
Theodosia Burr

Theodosia folded the letter and heated a stick of red sealing wax over the candle flame. She wasn't altogether sure of her spelling in a few places, but Frederic wouldn't mind, not being nearly so critical as Papa in such matters. Stamping the seal firmly, she put the letter aside and got up to walk restlessly about the room.

It was hateful having the boys away, as well as Papa, and she worried about Mama being ill so often. Mr. Burr had talked of moving the whole family to Philadelphia for the winter but Mama's health had grown worse, and it was decided that she had best stay at Richmond Hill. It would be weeks now before Papa could come back for another visit. On the day he was expected, Theodosia must have her copybooks corrected and ready for his inspection. Her music would be well practiced and her best new frock ready to put on. If it were a good day, Theodosia would be allowed to ride down the Greenwich Road to meet his carriage. Snow Baby would be groomed until his white flanks gleamed, and there would be a blue satin bow on his forelock to grace the occasion. Theodosia could almost hear herself heralding the approach of his carriage with the joyful phrase she remembered from earliest babyhood: "Papa *is* home! Papa *is* home!"

But Papa *wasn't* home now. Theodosia turned impatiently toward the hall and started down the long passage that led to the servants' quarters. Maybe there, at least, she would find company.

Sure enough, a door was open at the end of the corridor. That was Lottie's room. Lottie was a young girl who had been in the Burr household only a short time, and at the sound of Theodosia's step she stood up quickly and greeted her young mistress with a curtsy.

"May I come in a minute, Lottie?" Theodosia asked. She crossed to the bed where the girl had been sitting and looked at a book that lay open on the neat white coverlet. "Were you reading this?"

Lottie shook her head. "Not rightly, Miss Theo. I was trying to make out words from the pictures, but I couldn't make the sense out. I never rightly learned to read."

There was a mournful note in the girl's voice that made Theodosia look up quickly. So, she thought, Lottie must have been feeling lonely and miserable, too. Theodosia perched herself at the edge of the bed. "Sit down, Lottie." She patted the place beside her invitingly. "Maybe I can help you a little. I do pretty well at reading now, except for the long words."

Lottie's gentle eyes shone. "I'd muchly like to learn, Miss Theo," she said softly. "If I could just write a little, maybe I could send a letter to my mother someday."

"Let's begin then." Theodosia settled the book between them firmly and drew a long breath. It was no easy undertaking for a nine-year-old, but she plunged earnestly into the task. Soon the two heads were bent together, and Lottie's shyness vanished as they struggled along, laughing over their mistakes.

"We'll do more tomorrow, Lottie," Theodosia promised. "You learn so quickly, it will be no time at all until you can write to your mother." She paused a moment, held by the wistfulness in Lottie's velvety glance. "Maybe," she offered, "you'd like me to write a letter for you now. You could tell me what you'd like to say."

"Oh, Miss Theo"—Lottie clasped her fingers eagerly—"if only you would. Just to let Mammy know I keep healthy and what good, kindly folks I'm with."

When, after heroic efforts, the letter was finished, Theodosia carried it to her mother's sitting room. Mrs. Burr was seated in a low armchair by the fire. She looked rested and refreshed, and a warm smile lighted her face as she heard Theodosia's account of the afternoon. Mrs. Burr shared her husband's firm belief in the right of every young person to be educated, and it was a household rule that every servant, whether free or slave, must be taught at least to read or write.

"You did very well, dear," Mrs. Burr said, when she had glanced through the blotted little message to Lottie's mother, concealing a smile here and there at oddly turned phrases and quaint misspellings. "I had meant to see to Lottie's instruction myself, as soon as I was able, but since you have begun the task so bravely, you may try the lesson each afternoon. Your papa will be pleased I know."

Peggy brought in buttered crumpets with tea, and Theodosia munched hungrily in spite of her afflicted jaw. By the time John came home from his fencing lesson, her spirits were remarkably revived. When he offered to show her the new fencing maneuver he had learned that afternoon, she lunged at him so eagerly that he drew back, looking quite alarmed.

"Slowly, Theo, slowly," he warned her. "We're not supposed to kill each other!"

·CHAPTER 5·

The Shadows Pass

THE NEXT SUMMER in Pelham was a quiet one for Theodosia. John was away a good deal, having begun his apprenticeship in reading law with Mr. Burr. Mrs. Burr grew gradually weaker and she spent the long days on the veranda, sewing or resting while she looked out over the orchard toward the sunlit shore.

To Theodosia and Frederic fell the responsibility of managing the household and the farm. Frederic took over the outdoor work while Theodosia helped to supervise the domestic affairs. Peggy and Anthony and the other servants found their young mistress surprisingly capable at planning meals, ordering supplies, and generally keeping track of the house.

Each week Theodosia drove into the village with Anthony to visit the shops, and by the end of the summer she was an expert marketer, able to select at a glance the best cut of beef, the freshest vegetables, and the plumpest chickens.

Shopkeepers who had treated her with patronizing indulgence at first, soon learned that their young customer had a sharp eye and no intention of being cheated, and before long they were striving as hard to please her critical taste as though she had been a grand lady instead of a little girl of ten.

When Papa came to stay, he found Theodosia able to give him a complete report on her mother's health. They talked a good deal together during the summer visits, taking long walks in the afternoons while Mrs. Burr napped. More and more Mr. Burr began to treat his daughter as an equal.

At the close of summer, it was decided that Frederic would remain at Pelham. Having tried to study law, and found it not to his taste, Frederic had decided to take up farming. So the Pelham house and the surrounding acres were formally deeded to him.

It was a sad wrench for them all when the time came to leave, and Frederic, his bronzed young face very sober, watched the carriage down the drive until a bend in the road hid the last glimpse of Theodosia's sunbonnet, waved in lingering farewell.

John was to be with Mr. Burr in Philadelphia for the winter, so only Mrs. Burr and Theodosia were left in Richmond Hill, and the big house seemed more empty and filled with echoes than ever.

But Theodosia had no long idle hours in which to contemplate her lonely state. There was responsibility to be shouldered, and Theodosia, feeling herself a young woman now, went at her tasks willingly. Papa depended on her—and she was determined not to fail him.

Instead of the playful little notes they had exchanged in

the preceding winter, Mr. Burr expected long, careful letters from Theodosia, giving reports of her mother, household news, and an account of her own activities and studies.

Mr. Burr answered with equal care. Never, on any account, he wrote, was *anything* to interfere with Theo's studies. On that point he was adamant. So Theodosia worked faithfully, and when she managed to bring her lessons up to his expectations, he gave her such generous praise and encouragement that she was fired with new ambition.

It was in March that Mrs. Burr's long illness became more grave. Less than a month later, when the willows that fringed the garden she loved so well had just begun to show the shadowy green of a new spring, she died.

Until the very end Mrs. Burr had refused to allow her illness to interfere with her husband's career. In spite of his frequent protests that he must resign from Congress to be at home with her, she had kept on so cheerfully, and endured her sufferings with such patience that he had yielded to her wishes and remained at his work.

It was typical of Aaron Burr's philosophy that, once the beloved presence of his wife had vanished from Richmond Hill, his letters to Theodosia made no reference to the loss. And so thoroughly had his daughter already been disciplined in his iron school of accepting the inevitable without lament that she also refrained from the slightest hint of grief in her answers. The letters that passed between them in the months following Mrs. Burr's death were full of news, affectionate pleasantries, and plans for the future, unshadowed by their knowledge that the close family circle, which had meant so much to them both, was now sadly shattered.

Nevertheless, the problem of his young daughter's loneliness concerned Mr. Burr deeply, and one day Theodosia was startled out of her mood of languid boredom by a letter from Papa which announced a new and charming plan.

A young French girl, Natalie de L'age, was to come to Pelham as Theodosia's guest for the summer. And, wrote Papa, Miss Theo would please to stir herself out of the doldrums and make every effort to make her guest's visit a pleasant one.

Nothing could have delighted Miss Theo more. Her natural good spirits returned with a rush, and by the time Natalie arrived her young hostess was waiting eagerly, with a dozen plans for picnics, horseback rides, and boating trips already arranged.

Natalie had been for some time a protégée of Mr. Burr. His theories about education had often led him to undertake the training and encouragement of youngsters who, by unusual talents and intelligence, attracted his attention. He had, indeed, a continual succession of boys and girls under his wing—and he contributed to their education with reckless generosity and his usual cheerful disregard of his already mountainous debts.

Natalie and Theodosia got on beautifully from the start. They were almost the same age and both girls liked riding and dancing and parties quite as much as they did reading and study. Before the summer was out they were dreading the time when they must separate, and great was their delight when Mr. Burr wrote that Mme. de L'age, who was returning to France for the winter, would allow Natalie to stay on at Richmond Hill.

As it turned out, Natalie's mother prolonged her stay in France for several years. So Natalie slipped easily into the family circle. The two girls were like sisters and Mr. Burr played papa to his pretty daughters with impartial devotion.

Soon Mr. Burr was bringing visitors home with him and the grace and liveliness of the two young hostesses of Richmond Hill charmed his most distinguished guests. There were luncheons and teas and dinner parties, and the big house that had been so long quiet rang once more with the laughter and voices of company.

Travelers from abroad came to dine frequently. M. Talleyrand was often there from France, and he was always delighted when the two girls chatted with him as easily and wittily in French as they did in English.

Jerome Bonaparte, the younger brother of Napoleon, was another guest from France. His darkly aristocratic good looks and elegant manners enchanted the girls.

"Mon Dieu," Natalie sighed to Theodosia after young Bonaparte's first visit, *"qu'il est beau, cet jeune homme!* Don't you wish, Theo, that we were older? Perhaps he might fall in love with one of us."

Theodosia smiled at Natalie, curled up in a big chair before the bedroom fire. "He is nice," she agreed. "All the same, I don't mean to fall in love with anyone."

Natalie sat up. "But what then, Theo? You surely don't want to be an old maid, do you?"

Theodosia shrugged. "I shouldn't mind so long as I can stay with Papa, and keep house for him. Later, he says, I can travel with him wherever he goes."

Natalie shook her head. "Papa won't want an old maid for a daughter, I can tell you that," she said wisely. "And for all your high and mighty airs, Theo-mio, you'll change your mind quickly enough when you meet the right young man." .

On one late spring day, Theodosia and Natalie learned that President Washington, who was visiting in New York, had accepted an invitation to dine at Richmond Hill. The girls threw themselves into a fever of preparation. The carriage was ordered out and Anthony drove them into the city to market. There they roamed from stall to stall, inspecting the delicacies with anxious eyes, while all about them the vendors hawked their wares, so that the air rang with a weird medley of raucous, singsong cries:

"Sweet potatoes! Carolina potatoes! Here's your sweet Carolinas!"

"Any oranges, lemons, or limes today? Very fine, very cheap."

"Oysters, oysters. Here's your beauties of oysters! Here's your fine fat, salt oysters!"

Their marketing was finished at last and when they came back to Richmond Hill with the carriage loaded, Theodosia went into long, earnest conference with Peggy over the menu. They would have two kinds of soup. Then shad fresh from the Hudson, broiled over a charcoal fire and served with butter and wine. A mammoth turkey, pickled cucumbers, and fresh peas. Four kinds of preserves, and, for dessert, one of Peggy's famous almond puddings.

When the last detail was arranged, Theodosia flew upstairs to find Natalie putting the last touches to a centerpiece of flowers on the long dining table. There were pink roses and mignonette with tall spears of blue larkspur.

"Do you like it, Theo?" Natalie tipped her head to one side. "I mixed pink and blue especially since M. Bonaparte will be here and pink and blue is very French."

"It's lovely," Theodosia nodded. "Oh, and Natalie—*did* we remember to tell Lottie to lay out fresh linen upstairs?"

"Of course we did," Natalie answered soothingly. "Now do calm yourself, Theo, or you will explode altogether and Papa will have to explain to the President that his charming daughter is in fragments."

Evening came at last and Lottie helped the girls dress in their frocks of white India muslin, embroidered and ruffled, with short puffed sleeves. Theodosia wore cherry-red velvet ribbon about her slender waist, while Natalie's sash was pale blue satin.

At the sound of carriage wheels in the driveway, they ran down the broad staircase to find Mr. Burr waiting in the dining room.

As Anthony swung open the door to admit the first guests, Natalie squeezed Theodosia's hand and whispered a last warning not to worry. Everything was certain to go off smoothly.

And indeed it did.

Mr. Burr was an excellent host, witty and charming. Politics were forgotten, or at least not mentioned, for the evening. Even Mr. Hamilton who arrived as a guest, with his pretty wife, seemed in excellent spirits. To see him standing next to his host, no observer would have guessed that these two handsome and urbane gentlemen, talking amiably over their cups of Madeira punch, were probably the bitterest rivals in all New York.

As for President Washington, he appeared to enjoy himself thoroughly. Silent and rather austere at first, he warmed to the charming gaiety of his young hostesses and told them stories of the days when he had lived in this house, dined at this table, and, on one nearly tragic occasion, had narrowly escaped being poisoned by a British spy who had obtained work in the kitchens.

Toward the end of dinner, under cover of the general laughter and talk, M. Bonaparte spoke quietly to Mr. Burr. "Forgive me for asking," he said, "but is it true that you are not, after all, to be the next ambassador to France? I had understood it was all arranged for you to go—but only this evening I learned that another man has been appointed instead. How can this be so?"

Mr. Burr toyed with his fork for a moment. "The plans were made, yes. The President himself had told me that I was chosen. But"—he paused—"other influences interfered at the last moment."

M. Bonaparte frowned. "What a pity. Your appointment would have been quite perfect, I assure you, and what a success your charming daughters would have been in Paris. If I am not too impertinent, what are these *other influences* that could spoil such an excellent plan?"

"My friend Hamilton had different plans," Mr. Burr said quietly. His cryptic glance rested on Mr. Hamilton seated farther down the long table. "You see, M. Bonaparte, I had the misfortune to spoil a plan of Mr. Hamilton's once."

"But that"—the Frenchman spread his hands—"is a

purely personal consideration. Surely the President would not allow himself to be moved because *one man* objected?"

Mr. Burr smiled. "When that one man is Hamilton," he said, "it might as well have been a thousand who objected to my appointment."

Late that evening, when the guests had gone, Natalie came into Theodosia's room. "Well, it was a success, our party, wasn't it, Theo? Papa says you must have charmed the President by magic, for he's never been known to talk as much or smile as often as he did for you. And I saw M. Bonaparte looking at you more than once, my Theo."

When Theodosia made no answer, Natalie added slyly, "But, of course, I might have told him not to waste his glances, since you never intend to fall in love anyway."

"Well, perhaps not *ever*," Theodosia admitted cautiously. "But certainly not for ages and ages. Papa says no woman ever knows her own mind before she's thirty, so I mean to wait until then at least."

"Thirty!" Natalie made a face of despair. *"Mon dieu!* At thirty one is already ancient. Papa must have been teasing."

"But listen, Natalie." Theodosia put down her brush. "Here's real news! Papa told me this evening that in the fall, when he goes to the Congress again, you and I are to go with him to Philadelphia. Just think, we'll be like real ladies with rooms of our own. What do you think of that?"

For the next hour the girls amused themselves by laying excited plans, punctuated by frequent bursts of smothered giggles, for the gay times they were to have as real young ladies in the capital.

CHAPTER 6

The People's Party

ALAS FOR ALL the plans.

When autumn came, Mr. Burr found that he must plead a law case in Albany, and another in Washington, which would keep him traveling continually between Philadelphia and these two cities. So the girls were left at Richmond Hill until the cases should be finished. Then, Papa promised, he would send for them at once.

Theodosia was badly disappointed. After her father's departure, she sulked unhappily, neglected her studies, and was generally so disagreeable that even Natalie's good humor was exhausted.

One morning the girls were riding the new saddle horses that Mr. Burr had given them. In spite of the golden sunshine and the bright October woods, Theodosia refused to break her moody silence. At length Natalie spoke out.

"You'd better be careful, Theo," she warned sharply, "or you'll have us both in trouble. I heard Mr. Leshlie complain that your lessons get worse every day. If Papa hears that news it will be *pfft—au revoir* for Theo."

Theodosia gave her reins an impatient flip. "Lessons," she said bitterly. "I don't believe Papa cares two pins for me, but only for my lessons. Greek, history, geography, mathematics, music, writing, fencing, dancing . . ." She checked them off on her fingers. "Sometimes I feel like nothing more than a walking copybook. I think perhaps," she added darkly, "that I shall marry young after all. At least a husband wouldn't forever be going off for months and months and leaving me nothing to amuse myself with but lessons."

Whether Mr. Leshlie complained to Mr. Burr, or whether hints of discontent crept into Theodosia's own letters, it wasn't long before Miss Theo received a communication from her busy father in which he took time to point out, in no uncertain terms, the deficiencies in her behavior:

> . . . I am sorry, very sorry, that you are obliged to submit to some reproof. Indeed, I am afraid that your want of attention and politeness require it. . . . A moment's reflection will convince you that this conduct will naturally be construed into arrogance; as if you felt that all attention was due to you, and as if you felt above showing the least to anybody. . . . I believe you will in the future avoid it. Observe how Natalie replies to the smallest civility offered to her. . . .
>
> Receive with calmness every reproof, whether made kindly or unkindly; whether just or unjust. Consider within yourself whether there has been no cause for it. If it has been groundless and unjust, nevertheless . . . we must learn to bear these things; and, let me tell you, that you will always feel much better, much happier, for having borne with serenity the spleen of anyone, than if you had returned spleen for spleen.
>
> You will, I am sure, my dear Theodosia, pardon such two grave pages from one who loves you, and whose happiness depends very much on yours. Read it over twice.

Make me no promises on the subject. On my return, I shall see in half an hour whether what I have written has been well or ill received. If well, it will have produced an effect.

. . . I cannot add anything sprightly to this dull letter. One dull thing you will hear me repeat without disgust that

I am your affectionate friend,
A. Burr

Thus reminded of her faults, Theodosia did credit to her training and had the grace to mend her ways. For a time, indeed, she was an altogether model pupil, and the very next letter from Papa showed that he was aware of her efforts:

Three hundred and ninety-five lines of Greek, all your exercises, and all your music. Go on, my dear girl, and you will become all I wish. . . .

On one of his trips to Albany that winter, Mr. Burr stopped off at a blacksmith's shop on a country road near Kingston. One of his horses had lost a shoe, and while the blacksmith worked, Mr. Burr strolled up the road. Returning a few minutes later, he was surprised to find, drawn on the stable door, a charcoal sketch of his own carriage and horses. He examined the picture with interest. Even in the hasty drawing there was a dash and spirit that made him wonder who the artist might be. Mr. Burr glanced around and saw a boy, thin and rather pale, but with an alert eager look.

Mr. Burr beckoned. "Boy, do you know who drew this?"
"I did it, sir."
"Indeed?" Mr. Burr eyed him thoughtfully. The lad

was dressed in a rough homespun shirt and trousers that dangled loosely about his thin legs. "And where did you learn to draw so well?"

"Nowhere, sir." The boy shook his head. "I live on a farm up the road a piece, and I'm apprenticed to the smithy here. But I like drawing pictures for fun—specially of horses."

Mr. Burr considered the sketch a moment longer, then he took a scrap of paper from his pocket and scribbled a few lines on it. "What's your name, boy?"

"John Vanderlyn."

"Very well, Vanderlyn." Mr. Burr handed over the paper with a smile. "Keep this. You're too bright a lad to be a blacksmith's apprentice forever. If the time comes when you'd like to see the world and learn to be a real artist, put a clean shirt in your pocket and come to this address I've written for you."

It was several months later that Mr. Burr, being home at Richmond Hill for a few days, was surprised at breakfast one morning by a small paper parcel that Anthony laid on the table before him.

"A boy brought this to the door, sir, and is waiting outside. He said you'd know when you opened it who he was."

Mr. Burr unwrapped the neat bundle and found a coarse, country-made, clean shirt inside, with a bit of paper tucked into the folds. It was the message, in his own handwriting, that he had given the blacksmith's boy on the country road near Kingston.

The lad was shown in at once, and welcomed. Within

a few days young Vanderlyn had been outfitted in city clothes, and was apprenticed to study drawing with one of Mr. Burr's artist friends in New York. So Mr. Burr had acquired still another protégé to educate, one whose talents and lively intelligence bade fair to make him a promising investment.

Even though the girls were left at Richmond Hill for the greater part of that year, there were still plenty of visitors.

One guest who was a great favorite was Dolley Madison. She had only recently been married to James Madison. Before that she had been a young widow with two small children and Mr. Burr had been the children's guardian.

"People may say unkind things about your papa sometimes," Mrs. Madison said to Theodosia one day. "I dare say sooner or later you'll begin to hear them. They say he's too extravagant—and always head over heels in debt. They may be right, but always remember, as I do, that much of his extravagance comes from helping other people. And he's as generous with his time and his friendship as he is with money. I shan't ever forget all his kindnesses to my children and me when we were left alone. He's the most unselfish friend I've ever had. I hope I may pay him back someday."

Theodosia and Natalie loved to listen to Dolley Madison's lively stories. "You wouldn't believe how different things were when I was growing up," she told the girls. "I was never allowed to dance or have music lessons, or so much as look at a boy. As for horseback riding or going on a picnic —such things would have been thought far too unladylike. My mother was so afraid the sun would ruin my complexion that she used to send me to school in long white cotton gloves with a muslin mask sewed under the brim of my sunbonnet to keep me from getting freckled."

"You must have looked like a little ghost," Theodosia said sympathetically. "Didn't you have any fun at all?"

"Well, not very much." Mrs. Madison shook her pretty head ruefully. "But I used to think when I grew up, and could do as I pleased, I'd learn to dance and play the piano and be the greatest flirt that ever lived." She laughed. "My husband says at least part of my wish has come true—though he'll never tell which part!"

In 1797, Mr. Burr's six-year term in the Senate came to an end. He ran for re-election, but was defeated. As usual he took his disappointment calmly. "After all," he observed to Theodosia on his return to Richmond Hill, "Heaven helps those who help themselves. With Hamilton exerting himself *against* my election so much more zealously than I worked *for* it—it's natural Heaven should have been on his side."

But although Mr. Burr was temporarily out of the political picture, he and Thomas Jefferson remained the leaders of the growing Democratic-Republican Party. The new party was the people's party and as they began to take a more and more active part in the government of their new nation, they rallied to the men who, they felt, represented them, rather than to the small and exclusive group of property owners who controlled the Federalist policies.

For years New York had been governed by a closed corporation of the best families—the Schuylers, the Clintons, the De Puysters, the Livingstons. Although Mr. Burr belonged with this group by birth and breeding and his own wealth and social position, his affiliation with the people's party threw him in direct opposition to those who had been his closest friends. There were those who felt that Aaron Burr's championing of the people's cause was nothing more than a trick for getting himself into high office. But Mr. Burr refused to take his political position too seriously. He went serenely on his way and never troubled to protest the charges of the Federalists, led by Hamilton, who called him a rabble-rouser.

Theodosia, however, was often troubled by the situation. She had always been a favorite with her father's friends, and they were the very people who now denounced Mr. Burr, even though they continued to invite his daughter to their homes and make a great pet of her. "It worries me, Papa," she complained one day, "to have people so kind to me when I know they're unkind to you."

Mr. Burr smiled. "They're not in the least unkind to me, dear Theo," he said easily. "They merely dislike some of my ideas. Which is no reason why they should dislike you, or you them. Treat them as your friends—which they are; avoid the subject of politics, and if they should happen to say something ill-natured about your papa, give them your most amiable smile and turn the conversation to the weather. In that way you will keep your own dignity, without, I assure you, harming mine in the slightest."

Talking to Natalie later, however, Theodosia sighed. "I do wish we could go on as we are now—with Papa just a plain lawyer again—and not have to worry about politics and people being rivals and hating each other."

"Perhaps you'll get your wish, Theo, but I doubt it."
Natalie shook her head. "John says he believes the new party
will win the next election, and if they do, Papa is quite likely
to be the President. So what would you think of that?"

"Oh, dear, I don't know." Theodosia sighed again and
ruffled her curls until they stood on end. "I'd be fearfully
proud of him, of course, and it *would* be fun living in the
President's house. But sometimes I think I'd rather belong
to a family without any ambitions at all."

The following year, Mr. Burr was elected to the New
York State Legislature. Once more the girls were left to keep
house at Richmond Hill while he attended the sessions in
Albany. But though political affairs and ambitions were
drawing him more and more into the public spotlight, Mr.
Burr always found time to be interested in the smallest details
of Theodosia's life at home. No matter how busy he was,
he managed to write to her by every post, long, detailed letters, in his most charming style, which commented on the
latest entries in her weekly journal, the progress of her studies,
her health, her household problems, and her amusements.

Those who regarded Aaron Burr as an ambitious
schemer, who cared for nothing in the world but his own
success, might have been surprised to read some of the letters
that went to Theodosia.

> Your being in the ballette charms me (*he wrote once*).
> If you are to practice on Wednesday evening, do not stay
> away for the expectation of receiving me. If you should
> be at the ballette, I will go forthwith to see you. *Adieu,*
> *chère fille.* . . .

·CHAPTER 7·

The Locket

O N THE MORNING of her seventeenth birthday, Theodosia wakened early. Lying still for a moment, she frowned at the unfamiliar sloping ceiling above her head . . . then she remembered. She was in Albany, of course. In a room at Witbeck's Tavern.

She and Natalie had arrived from Richmond Hill the night before for a visit. They had found the rooms pleasant and cheerful, with everything arranged for their comfort. There was a fire on the hearth, a maid appeared with jugs of hot water, and beside each place on the supper table they had found a nosegay of bright flowers and a note from Mr. Burr.

He was sorry not to welcome them in person, being detained by business, but would they be pleased to appear promptly at breakfast the next morning where he would be waiting to see them? In a postscript he added that a dancing party had been arranged for the evening following, in honor of Theodosia's birthday.

Theodosia pushed back the covers and rose to open the shutters. She drew a deep breath of the mild June air. In the town square, the old elms spread their green branches as though each leaf had taken on new freshness from the morning sun. Here and there, on the grass, cobwebs glistened like round, pale moons.

"Happy birthday, Theo," Natalie called from the doorway.

"Oh, Natalie"—Theodosia raised her arms to stretch delightedly—"isn't it a gorgeous day? Do you suppose we could get Papa to hire some horses and go riding with us after breakfast?"

"I shouldn't be surprised. But we'll have to hurry to meet Papa downstairs. Lottie just came to tell me that he is waiting. And, Theo, Lottie says Papa told her he has a young gentleman to take you to the party tonight, with John and me. His name is Vanderlyn."

"Vanderlyn?" Theodosia turned. "Oh, of course, the country boy who wanted to be an artist. He came to Richmond Hill one morning with a clean shirt done up in a paper parcel."

Natalie nodded. "Well, it seems the country boy is quite grown up and elegant now," she said. "He studied painting with Gilbert Stuart and then Papa sent him to Paris last winter. Lottie says she saw him last night and he's *very* handsome."

Mr. Burr greeted the girls in the dining room downstairs, then he inspected them with a critical eye. "You both look charming," he said, smiling. "The picture of health and the mirror of fashion. Here—sit down. I've sent the coffee out to be kept hot for you."

All through the meal the girls talked continually, interrupting each other to tell Mr. Burr the latest news and ask a dozen questions about the dancing party.

Presently Mr. Burr took a small, flat parcel from his pocket, and laid it next to Theodosia's plate.

"A little birthday gift for Theo," he said, "in the hope that she will wear it tonight and be as happy as her presence makes me."

He spoke lightly, but there was a look of tender pride in his eyes as he watched his daughter's pretty face bend eagerly over the package.

"Oh, Papa!" Theodosia opened the satin case. "Papa— it's *beautiful!*" She lifted a narrow black velvet ribbon from which hung a locket of delicate, chased gold, set with a filigree of pearls and emeralds. "See, Natalie, how well it will go with my new frock." She held the slender ribbon against her throat and looked up to meet her father's glance. "Papa, I do thank you a *thousand* times."

"One will be enough." Mr. Burr smiled. "It suits you very well, I think. I had Vanderlyn order it for me in Paris —and though he hasn't seen you since you were a little girl, my description of your devastating beauty must have been accurate—for he's chosen the very thing. Don't you agree, Natalie?"

Natalie nodded. She reached for the locket and opened the catch to show a small, glass-covered frame inside.

"What shall you put here, Theo?" she asked teasingly.

"It should be a lock of her true love's hair, shouldn't it, Papa?"

"And high time she had a true love, too," he agreed, still smiling. "Mind you find her one at the party tonight."

John came in, and there was another round of greetings.

"You've got fat, John," Theodosia eyed her brother critically. "That's what comes of reading too much law and not exercising enough."

"I follow Father's example," John said amiably, "and no one could accuse *him* of being plump!"

"Papa doesn't have your weakness for plum cakes and honey buns." Theodosia laughed. "But never fear, Natalie and I will take you in hand. To start things off, I propose a horseback ride this morning."

"No sooner said than done," John said. "I shall order the horses at once and select a particularly mean-tempered beast for you, Theo-mio, to pay you back for your remarks about my figure. You'll come with us, won't you, Father?"

Mr. Burr shook his head regretfully.

"I'm afraid not this time," he said, drawing out his watch. "There's an appointment I must keep. But I expect Vanderlyn will be happy to take my place."

"He certainly will," John agreed. "Poor Vanderlyn has heard so much about the fatal charms of these two young ladies that he's half smitten with them both sight unseen. I'll go and call him, and we'll meet in half an hour. . . . Mind you're prompt now," he called after Theodosia and Natalie as they hurried upstairs, "or Vanderlyn is likely to swoon away altogether with the strain of anticipation."

Later, as they guided their horses through the cobbled city streets and into a narrow lane that twisted and turned up the wooded hillside, they rode two and two. John and Natalie went ahead, and the sound of their voices drifted back through the clear, sunlit air as they chatted gaily.

For a while Theodosia and her companion rode in silence. Mr. Vanderlyn had grown from the awkward country boy she remembered into a quiet, serious sort of young man, not in the least given to the kind of nonsense that John was forever prattling. It was true, as Lottie had said, that Mr. Vanderlyn was handsome. Theodosia liked the way he rode, with an easy control of his horse.

Presently, turning to speak, Theodosia found her companion looking directly at her with a thoughtful expression in his eyes.

"You look very sober, Mr. Vanderlyn," she said. "Shall I offer you a sixpence for your thoughts?"

"I was just thinking how different you are from what I imagined, Miss Theodosia. I'd heard so much about you from your father—I really expected to be quite terrified by you. I thought you'd be most frightfully learned!"

Theodosia laughed. "I dare say Papa's descriptions make me sound awful, though I'm sure he means them well. He's spent so much time trying to make me a truly educated female that I suppose people expect me to be spouting Latin phrases and quoting obscure passages of Greek at every turn in the conversation. And instead——" She paused and shrugged.

"Instead, I find you very friendly and charming—and not in the least terrifying."

"Thank you, sir." Theodosia smiled at him with candid pleasure. "If another young man had said that, I should think it was only a pretty speech. But since you are a protégé of Papa's—and I know how thoroughly he detests flattery—I take you at your word, Mr. Vanderlyn."

"Good. I see there are even more advantages than I had thought in being one of your father's protégés. You know," he added soberly, after a moment, "there have been times when I've almost wished Mr. Burr hadn't as much faith in my talents as he appears to have. I'm no end grateful for all he's done for me, of course, but all the same it's a great responsibility. I feel that I *must* succeed in being a good painter, if only to show him that his encouragement hasn't been altogether misplaced. And yet I wonder sometimes if I ever can. He seems to expect so much of the people he believes in."

"Oh, I know," Theodosia said quickly. "I feel the same way often. I think the trouble is that Papa judges us all by himself. He thinks we should be as strong as he is, and he doesn't realize that sometimes we just aren't."

"It's odd, though, how hard we'll try," Vanderlyn said. "I remember talking to a young lawyer in your father's office one day. He said, 'I owe everything I have to Mr. Burr. He gave me my education and taught me all I know, but I'm most grateful for the way he's made me learn to depend on myself. *He made me iron.*' I suppose it's that quality in Mr. Burr that makes people either admire him so much or else mistrust him altogether."

"I suppose so," Theodosia agreed with a little sigh. "But I'm not altogether sure, Mr. Vanderlyn, that I *want* to be iron. It doesn't sound like a particularly comfortable thing to be."

When they came back for lunch, Vanderlyn helped Theodosia dismount and took her arm with a confidential smile.

"You won't tell your father that I may not turn out to be another Michelangelo after all, will you, Miss Theo?"

"Not a word, Mr. Vanderlyn. And you must never breathe to a soul that I didn't fire a single Latin phrase at you. Agreed?"

"On my solemn oath!"

They parted laughing, as Theodosia gathered up her long black skirt to run lightly up the steps after Natalie.

CHAPTER 8

The Third Waltz

WHEN THEODOSIA CAME down dressed for the party that evening, her dark curls were piled high on her head, and her bright coloring and slim, graceful figure were set off to perfection by the pale green of her watered-silk frock. At her throat she wore the new locket on its narrow black band, and Vanderlyn's smile lighted with pleasure as he saw it.

"How well the locket suits you, Miss Theodosia," he said. "You've no idea how I prowled through the shops in Paris trying to find just the very thing for you. I must admit I think I chose well."

Theodosia touched the locket lightly, and answered his look of frank admiration with a little curtsy. But Natalie, coming down just then, reached out to tap Vanderlyn's arm with her fan.

"Theodosia won't flirt with you, I warn you, M. Vanderlyn," she said. "So save your pretty speeches for a head more easily turned than hers."

"Like yours, for instance?" John asked.

Natalie nodded complacently, as she linked her arm in John's. She wore a frock of light yellow that brought out the delicate ivory tints of her skin, and in her dark hair she had pinned a cluster of tiny yellow rosebuds.

"Like mine," she agreed. "For you can be sure, M. Vanderlyn, that I get no overdose of compliments from John, who still scolds and teases me as if I were a naughty little girl in pigtails."

Coming into the candlelit, flower-decked rooms filled with people, Theodosia was instantly surrounded by friends, young and old. Their voices, gay and eager, rang about her, as, smiling, she greeted one after another.

"Theo, my dear, here's someone who's very anxious to meet you—a friend of your father's." Theodosia turned to find her hostess and a tall, broad-shouldered gentleman at her elbow.

"Mr. Joseph Alston," her hostess said, and, looking up, Theodosia found herself smiling into a pair of eyes, deep-set and extraordinarily blue. She felt her hand clasped for a moment in a warm, firm grip.

"Mr. Alston is from South Carolina," the hostess went on. "He's been in Albany on business, but now he claims he must go home again, which is altogether tiresome of him. See if you can't persuade him that there's far more to be said for a summer in the North than in the South, Miss Theodosia. If you succeed, I assure you every young lady in town will bless your name."

She turned away then and Theodosia found that she was still looking straight into Mr. Alston's eyes.

"It's rather a tall order I've been given, I'm afraid," she said. "But let's see—how shall I tempt you with the advantages of the North, Mr. Alston? Shall I tell you that we have excellent libraries? Or that our public parks are noted for their beauty? Or are you interested in birds, by any chance? Because if you are, we have some of the rarest specimens to be found——" She broke off suddenly with a laugh. "Really, Mr. Alston, I don't believe you're listening to me at all."

"Oh, but I am, Miss Burr. I was drinking in every word, but at the same time I was thinking of something that would tempt me more than libraries or parks or even rare specimens of birds." His blue eyes crinkled with amusement.

"Name it, Mr. Alston. If Albany possesses it, it shall be yours."

"I was thinking I should like very much to have a dance with you, Miss Burr. Unless the young gentleman you came in with has already claimed them all. In which case, I promise you, I shall set out for South Carolina this very instant, and I shouldn't be at all surprised if I drove so recklessly that I broke my neck."

"Oh, let's prevent that, by all means, Mr. Alston. Would the third waltz be sufficient to keep you from an untimely end, do you think? Or would you prefer a polka?"

"I'd prefer both," said Mr. Alston promptly.

Next morning at breakfast the talk was all of the party. Natalie and John exchanged opinions about this person and that, but Theodosia sat silent for the most part, breaking a piece of bread into a little heap of crumbs beside her plate.

"It's such a pity Mr. Alston must leave today, isn't it, Papa?" Natalie asked presently.

"You liked him then?"

"Oh, yes, ever so much. Didn't you, Theo?"

"Didn't I what, Natalie?" Theodosia looked up with a start.

Natalie laid down her fork. *"Didn't—you—like—Mr.— Alston?"* she repeated, exaggerating each syllable carefully.

"Oh"—Theodosia dropped her glance again—"why, yes —I thought he was very nice."

John and Natalie exchanged a quick glance, and Natalie shrugged lightly. "I think, Papa," she said, "that our Theo is in such a state of cloudy dreams this morning she seems scarcely able to recall meeting anyone."

As they were finishing their coffee, Lottie came into the dining room with a note for Theodosia. A man was waiting for an answer, she said.

Theodosia stared at her name written in a firm, slanting script as though she couldn't quite believe what she saw. Then she broke the seal. As she read, a curious change came over her face. She looked up with eyes grown oddly bright, and though she spoke quietly, there was a breath of eagerness beneath her words.

"Mr. Alston has changed his plans, Natalie. He won't be leaving today after all! He wants to know if we'll ride with him this morning. Shall I say yes?"

"Of course, if you like."

"Then I'll go." Theodosia jumped up. "And you'll go with us, won't you, Papa?"

When Mr. Burr shook his head, Theodosia made a little

pout of impatience. *"Please,* papa! we won't have half the fun without you, and Mr. Alston will be disappointed, I'm sure."

"I dare say Mr. Alston will survive his disappointment." Mr. Burr smiled pleasantly enough, but as he watched his daughter run quickly out to give her message, a curious look came into his eyes, as though something had suddenly surprised him, and the lines about his chin grew firm, even though he kept on smiling.

The last bright days of June melted into July and the Hudson Valley sweltered in the summer heat. Mr. Burr was detained in Albany from week to week, by his work and by a number of visitors who came to confer with him over the approaching elections.

For once Theodosia appeared not to mind the hot weather. She lingered on in the capital, saying merely that she would rather stay until her father's work was finished.

Somehow, mysteriously, Mr. Alston's business in Albany prolonged itself also. He, like Theodosia, seemed to thrive on the long hot days.

Most of Theodosia's friends had closed their houses and gone to the mountains or the seashore, but though there were no more parties, she and Natalie still found plenty to do. They rode in the early mornings now, through deep-shaded trails where the air was still cool and fresh from the dew that sparkled in the long grass beside the path. And in the evenings, there were picnics or sailing parties on the river.

Gradually Mr. Alston came to be included in their plans

as a matter of course. He rode well, cheerfully undertook a good share of the work on picnic suppers, and was an accomplished sailor. More and more his name began to be taken for granted in the family conversations.

Only Theodosia remained perversely silent on the subject of the tall, broad-shouldered young man with the deepset blue eyes.

On one Sunday morning in the middle of July, Mr. Burr had to visit a client in Schenectady. He suggested that the young people drive over with him. At the last moment Natalie developed a headache. So it happened that while Mr. Burr and John were at their client's house, Theodosia was left with Mr. Alston. It was a pleasantly cool day, and when they had finished dinner, they left the carriage at the inn and started out for a walk through the Sunday quiet of the elm-shaded streets.

They talked amiably enough of this and that, but presently there was a silence, and Theodosia looked up to find Mr. Alston smiling at her in a curious way.

"Do you realize, Miss Theodosia, that this is the first time you and I have been alone together since we've met?"

"Is it, Mr. Alston?"

"It is, Miss Theodosia. And what's more, I think you're quite as well aware of it as I."

"We've all been together so much——"

"Not so much but what you have plenty of time to talk with Vanderlyn."

"Mr. Vanderlyn likes to talk to me about his work."

"Oh! . . . Then I'm afraid you won't have very much to say to me, since I have no work to talk about."

Theodosia looked up seriously. "Don't you do anything at all, Mr. Alston?"

"Not very much. My father left me a great many rice fields, in South Carolina, but the plantation manager looks after those a good deal better than I could. Besides, I don't suppose you'd care to talk about rice fields; there isn't much to say about them except that they're damp and full of mosquitoes."

"I thought I heard Papa say one time that you'd taken a degree in law, Mr. Alston?"

"So I did." He nodded cheerfully. "But the law and I didn't seem to take to each other very well, so I haven't done much about it."

They walked in silence for a few minutes, then Mr. Alston asked curiously, "Is that why you disapprove of me, Miss Theodosia? Because I have no work to talk about?"

"I don't disapprove of you, Mr. Alston."

"But you don't approve of me either. And I approve of you so very much. You've no idea how many hours I've spent wondering what it was about me that didn't please you. Doesn't that make you feel a little sorry for me, Miss Theo?"

"Not in the least," she said, and they both laughed.

After a little they wandered into a park and sat down on a bench facing a pond where two white swans glided sedately about, nibbling at the shrubs and grass along the water's edge. Theodosia took off her wide-brimmed hat and let the light wind ruffle her curls.

"You know, Miss Theodosia," Mr. Alston went on after a few minutes, "I think you might at least tell me what it is you don't like about me."

"And what then, Mr. Alston?" Theodosia leaned down to scoop up a handful of pebbles and tossed them into the water, one by one. "Would you set about to change yourself?"

"Not at all," he said calmly. "I should merely try to convince you that they aren't such bad qualities after all."

"But I'm an extraordinarily difficult person to convince, Mr. Alston."

"And I'm extraordinarily persistent, Miss Theodosia."

Theodosia tossed the last pebble away and stood up.

"So I'm beginning to think," she said, and smiled as she took his arm.

As the days went on, Mr. Burr observed his daughter without comment. Never had he seen her looking prettier, nor in better spirits. But still she said nothing about Mr. Alston.

There was a night when they all went sailing on the river by the light of a full, bright moon. Suddenly a mutter of thunder rolled over the hills on the west bank, and within a few moments the moon was blacked out and a sharp wind whipped the river into gusty, squalling waves.

Mr. Alston shouted directions to John and Vanderlyn as they struggled with desperate haste to lower the canvas that cracked like pistol shots in the angry wind. Hurry as they might, they barely succeeded in lowering the last of the sails in time to prevent the gusts of wind from capsizing the boat.

They drifted on the black water, heaved this way and that by the waves, while flash after flash of lightning split the darkness and the thunder rolled and echoed between the riverbanks with deafening crashes.

When the storm was spent, and they were safe, the men managed to maneuver the limping, half water-logged boat to shore, and through a drenching rain the party climbed the hill from the landing back to town.

Mr. Alston walked beside Theodosia. His coat had been lost overboard, and his shirt was torn, leaving one shoulder half bare. He had had no chance to speak to Theodosia while they were in the boat, but now he looked down at her, drenched and shivering at his side.

"Are you all right, Miss Theo?"

She glanced up quickly. "Quite all right, Mr. Alston."

"You were so calm while we were out there. Tell me honestly, weren't you the least bit frightened?"

"Not particularly," she said.

"But most young ladies I know would have been terrified," he insisted. "They would have had hysterics, or fainted, or at the very least set up a howl because their frocks were ruined. Yet you and Miss Natalie were quite calm."

Theodosia laughed. "The young ladies you know weren't brought up by Aaron Burr, Mr. Alston. Ever since I can remember, Papa has taught us not to be afraid of things. Even when I was a little girl, and hated the dark, he'd never let Nanny leave a light in my room."

"Weren't you frightened of the dark just the same?"

"Oh, yes, more than ever. But I soon learned not to show it, for when I cried, Papa was disappointed in me and that was even worse. You mustn't think I'm especially brave, Mr. Alston, because I'm not. It's easy not to let yourself be frightened of thunderstorms and the dark and such things, but I *am* afraid sometimes of other things."

"What things, Miss Theodosia?" he asked gently.

She was silent for a moment, then shook her head without answering him. She couldn't explain, really, so anyone would understand, about the odd little corners of loneliness in her heart, where it seemed sometimes as if a tiny, faint bell were sounding, even in moments of happiness, a far-off note of warning. She couldn't explain how she was afraid sometimes for Papa—and the queer dread she had of leaving him, as though, if she weren't there, something terrible was sure to happen.

Theodosia sighed, and the sigh ended in a little shivering breath. In the darkness beside her, Mr. Alston said nothing. But she felt his hand on her arm, warm and sure and strong. And somehow understanding.

A few days later Mr. Burr's business was finished, and they prepared to leave at once for Pelham. Mr. Alston was leaving the same day, he said, to start south.

On the last evening in Albany they rode up into the hills for a farewell picnic supper. Sitting around the fire afterward, they felt a little sad, and the conversation kept lagging into silence, until at last Natalie jumped up and said that everybody was being altogether too mournful.

"Anyone would suppose," she said, "that we were all going to the ends of the earth and would never see each other again. I vote we play charades."

They played for an hour or so, laughing a good deal in the process. If anyone noticed that Theodosia's acting was less spirited than usual and that Mr. Alston looked strangely abstracted, they said nothing of it.

Nor did the others appear to notice how silent Theodosia and Mr. Alston were during the ride home under the twilight sky, where the first stars hung pale and faintly glimmering. But when they had said good-by to Vanderlyn and Mr. Alston, Mr. Burr came into the small sitting room and found Theodosia standing alone by the window.

"Theo——"

She turned quickly. "Yes, Papa?"

"You're not sad—or troubled, are you, Theo?"

For an answer, she drew her locket from beneath the high white muslin stock of her riding habit. Opening the catch, she showed him the little frame, still empty.

He looked down into the clear, dark eyes that met his glance so honestly. "When the time comes, Theo, you are to think of yourself and your own happiness—not of any misguided notion of duty toward *me*. Will you remember that?" There was a note of sternness in his voice, as if, somehow, he had sensed the vague, nameless misgivings Theodosia felt for him—and rejected them.

She snapped the locket shut, and the catch made a small sound of finality in the quiet room.

"I must remember for a long time, then," she said, laughing a little ruefully. "Because in spite of Natalie's warnings, you'll have to learn to be content with an old maid daughter—whether you like it or no."

·CHAPTER 9·

The Die Is Cast

B UT THEODOSIA HAD not reckoned on just *how* persistent
Joseph Alston could be.

For the rest of the summer, and the early weeks of
autumn, scarcely a post arrived from the South that didn't
bring her a packet of letters from Charleston.

Miss Theodosia need not think, wrote Mr. Alston, that
merely because they were now separated by a distance of
more than seven hundred miles, he was any the less determined to discover her objections to him, and to overcome
them.

Her objections, Miss Theodosia replied by the next post,
were not toward Mr. Alston, for whom she held the highest
regard, but toward the notion of marrying anyone, however
charming and however *persistent*.

Marriage, Mr. Alston wrote, is a noble estate.

True, admitted Theodosia, but an estate she had no
faintest intention of entering until she was of a sufficiently
mature age to grace its nobility.

And what, pray, demanded Mr. Alston, did she consider a sufficiently mature age?

Thirty, at least, Theodosia stated flatly.

Absurd, said Mr. Alston.

Not at all, retorted Theodosia with spirit. Papa agreed with her that no girl of seventeen was possibly to be considered capable of making up her own mind.

Then why not, Mr. Alston suggested, let him make it up for her?

Most certainly *not,* the haughty Miss Burr replied.

And as for quoting her Papa's opinion, Mr. Alston added, it was a mistake indeed to think *that* bore any weight. Had he not asked and received Mr. Burr's consent to the match? And not so much as a word had Mr. B. uttered, not a syllable, to the effect that he considered his daughter too young to be married.

Silence from Theodosia.

No more letters from Charleston.

Three weeks passed, and no word.

And as post after post arrived from the South and still no letter from Joseph, the strong-minded Miss Theodosia began to show certain signs of weakening.

It was observed in the Burr household that Theo appeared to be suffering from a mysterious loss of appetite. Frequent fits of dreamy absent-mindedness made her quite oblivious to the mundane matters of daily living, and before the arrival of each post she was thrown into the most curious agitation, only to be followed by equally unaccountable fits of gloom.

In short, as Natalie observed to Mr. Burr, it was plain to be seen that Theodosia was in love.

"But, oh dear, *why* did she have to be so horrid to poor Mr. Alston?" Natalie sighed. "Now she's made him angry, and though *she's* sorry, *he* doesn't know it—and they're both too proud to write and give in. Why *does* love have to be so complicated and why does it make everyone miserable, Papa?"

Mr. Burr shook his head. "Being miserable is only one of the peculiar fascinations of being in love," he said. "Don't worry too much, Natalie. They're a stubborn pair, but I think in the end each will learn to give in to the other a bit —and likely each will feel noble and virtuous in the bargain."

Nevertheless, when the time came for Mr. Burr to leave Richmond Hill to attend the legislature, he was not altogether at ease about the state of his daughter's heart.

It was the autumn of 1800, and, true to John's prediction, the growing sentiment in favor of the new party made it seem certain that an Antifederalist would win the coming presidential election.

Burr and Jefferson were the most popular leaders of the new party. One of them, it was clear, was sure to succeed John Adams as the next President of the United States.

Electoral votes were cast. The result was a tie between Jefferson and Burr.

The Senate, in Philadelphia, must vote now, to resolve the tie.

John wrote from Albany that the result was a foregone conclusion. People were saying everywhere that Aaron Burr would be chosen.

The household at Richmond Hill was thrown into the greatest excitement. *Papa* was going to be President! John said so. John said *everybody* said so! It must be so.

Theodosia overcame her prejudices against politics and was thrilled by the prospect. She planned with Natalie what sort of dresses they would have for the inaugural ball. She conferred with Peggy about the wonderful dinners they would serve to the new President and his Cabinet. She even forgot, for a time, to languish over the post which still brought no letters from Charleston.

But in the meantime Mr. Hamilton had heard the news also. He had heard that *everyone* was saying the Senate was sure to decide the tie in favor of Burr. And that, for Mr. Hamilton, was enough. He went straight to Philadephia and set out, virtually singlehanded, to keep the Senate from electing Aaron Burr.

Never in all the years he had opposed Burr had his attack been so furious as now. He was sincerely convinced that the election of Aaron Burr would ruin the country, and he used every ounce of his influence to convince the Senate that this was so. He denounced Burr on every conceivable ground: political, personal, and moral. If his charges were untrue, then why was not Mr. Burr present to deny them? Where, indeed, demanded Hamilton, *was* Mr. Burr at this most important crisis of his life?

Why, Mr. Burr was in Albany.

And in Albany Mr. Burr remained, serenely unper-

turbed while the battle raged. Not once did he make a move
to defend himself against the charges of Hamilton and the
other Federalists, and no entreaties from his friends could
move him from his policy of silence.

On the night when the news of the Senate's final vote
reached Albany, it was raining. William Van Ness, a friend
and loyal supporter of Mr. Burr, hurried to Witbeck's Tavern
as quickly as he could, and found Mr. Burr alone in his
sitting room.

"Mr. Burr," said Van Ness, "you have been defeated."

Mr. Burr looked up from his desk. "Have I?" he asked
mildly.

Van Ness flung himself into a chair and leaned his head
on his hands. "Jefferson is President," he said. "You'll be
Vice-president."

Mr. Burr looked thoughtful for a moment, then he
smiled.

"Don't take it too hard, Van Ness," he said. "Vice-
president is much better than nothing." Noticing the damp-
ness of his friend's coat, Mr. Burr said quickly, "Here, let
me take your coat before you get chilled through. I'll send
downstairs for a toddy for you."

Van Ness looked up. "Upon my word, Mr. Burr," he
said slowly, "I don't know whether you're the greatest hero
in this country—or the greatest fool."

The bland, enigmatic smile on Mr. Burr's face did not
change as he spread the coat before the fire to dry. "I hardly
think it likely," he said, "that I have the honor of being
either."

"But surely you must realize"—the younger man leaned

forward earnestly—"that Hamilton alone is responsible for this. That he deliberately kept you from the presidency by denouncing you, slandering you, accusing you of every corruption under the shining sun. And yet you've refused to so much as raise a hand in your own defense. Even now, with the damage already done, you don't appear to *care,* sir—or you would——"

"I would what?" Mr. Burr, seated at his desk again, glanced up quickly. "What would you have me do, Van Ness? Give way to bad temper and challenge my friend Hamilton?"

"Duels have been fought for a great deal less, Mr. Burr."

"I expect that's true," Mr. Burr nodded. He picked up a round glass paperweight and held it a moment in silence, as though he were testing its weight. Then, replacing it carefully, he drew a sheet of paper toward him, and asked if Van Ness would do him the favor of dropping two letters in the post on his way home.

"I'd like to send congratulations to Mr. Jefferson," he said, "and I must write a little note to Theodosia. This news will be a disappointment to her, I'm afraid." For the first time Mr. Burr's voice showed a trace of concern. "Though I expect," he added, smiling, as he began to write, "she'll go to the greatest pains to conceal that fact from me."

·CHAPTER 10·

Wedding Day

CHRISTMAS CAME AND WENT. Still there was no letter for Theodosia from Charleston.

Mr. Burr, home for the holidays, found his daughter in a mood that gave him fresh concern. Although she held to her stubborn pride and refused to mention the name of Joseph Alston, there was a new gentleness in her manner, and sometimes, as they sat around the study fire in the evenings, Mr. Burr observed that she was strangely silent, staring into the flames with a wistful longing in her eyes that went straight to his heart.

Meanwhile, in Charleston, Joseph was suffering precisely the same pangs of sadness and longing that plagued his Theodosia's lonely heart. It is hard to keep silent forever under such circumstances, pride or no pride, and Joseph wrote once again—a long, eloquent plea for the reconsideration of his cause that began, in peremptory and highhanded fashion: "Hear me, Miss Burr."

Because it was winter, and the roads were icy and travel-

ing difficult, the letter was a long while in reaching Theodosia. But there came a stormy evening, early in January,
when Mr. Burr looked up suddenly to find Theodosia staring
in silence at her dinner plate. He laid down his fork and
took a deep breath.

"You're not wearing your locket tonight, Theo."

"No, Papa." Theodosia's voice was low, but quick color
came into her cheeks. "I—put it away for a little while. It
hasn't seemed right, somehow, to wear the locket. As long
as it was empty, it was all right. But now . . ."

She paused and for a moment silence hung between
them, broken only by the sound of the crackling fire. There
was an odd expression on Mr. Burr's face; then, suddenly,
he smiled.

"I wish you'd wear it again, Theo," he said. "And be
happy."

Neither of them said anything more just then, but later
that evening Theodosia went to her room and lifted the
locket from its satin case. She watched the emeralds flash
in the candlelight. Then, slipping the velvet ribbon over
her head, she crossed quickly to the desk and sat down to
write:

> My dear Joseph:
>   I shall be very happy to see you whenever you choose;
> that, I suppose, is equivalent to very soon. . . . My fa-
> ther laughs at my impatience to see you, and says I am
> in love . . . *Adieu encore,*
>   Theodosia

Within a few hours after Theodosia's letter reached him,
Joseph Alston was on his way north, and he made the long,

difficult journey with such unprecedented speed that Mr. Burr declared he must have changed horses in every town along the way and driven the unhappy beasts into exhaustion in his impatience to reach Theodosia.

"And a good thing, too," Mr. Burr added. "For nothing in this world can change more quickly or unaccountably than a young lady's mind, Joseph—as you will doubtless have plenty of opportunities to learn."

But Theodosia, radiant and shining-eyed, showed not the slightest signs of wishing to change her mind again. She and Natalie plunged at once into plans for the wedding.

Everything had to be done quickly because both Theodosia and Joseph were anxious to be in Washington for the inauguration of Mr. Jefferson as President and Mr. Burr as Vice-president. It would be a small wedding, Theo decided. Natalie would be bridesmaid. In addition, only John and Frederic and Papa would be with them.

The night before the wedding the wind shifted to the west, and when Natalie came into Theodosia's room in the morning, she threw open the shutters to find that a heavy, silent snow was falling.

"Oh, Theo, do come and see how pretty it looks," Natalie said.

As the two girls stood together, arm in arm, looking out into the thickly swirling snow, Natalie turned suddenly. "Theo, whatever am I going to do without you?" she asked forlornly. "I've been so busy and excited about everything I hadn't stopped to think until this minute that you'll actually be gone. . . ."

"But not for long, Natalie," Theodosia answered quickly. "We'll all be together again in Washington in just a few weeks, and as soon as Joseph and I are settled in Charleston, you'll come to visit. Papa has promised to bring you, whenever he comes. And, Natalie"—for a moment the shining happiness in Theodosia's eyes clouded—"you *will* look after Papa, won't you? I . . ." She hesitated, leaving the words unfinished. Not even to Natalie could she speak of the vague, troubling fears for her father that haunted her so often.

There was a knock at the door, and Lottie came in with an armful of deep crimson roses. "Mr. Alston just brought these, Miss Theo," she said. Lottie was a grown woman now, tall and dignified, and very different from the gawky, lonely girl Theodosia had found in the little back room at Richmond Hill on a winter's afternoon long ago.

Taking the flowers, smiling into Lottie's eyes, Theodosia remembered that afternoon. And Lottie, looking back at the radiant face of her young mistress, remembered, too. "I do muchly hope you'll be very happy, Miss Theo," she said.

"Thank you, Lottie." Theodosia buried her face in the flowers, breathing the warm fragrance of the hothouse. "Oh, Lottie, I *am* so glad Papa says you can go south with Joseph and me. It'll seem like home to have you there."

She went to the bed where her wedding dress of creamy satin lay next to Natalie's rose-brocaded gown.

"See how lovely the roses look with our frocks, Natalie. We'll each carry an armful, and Joseph must have this one for his coat." She broke off a crimson bud and held the soft petals against her cheek for a moment.

It was a simple ceremony, and a pretty one. The curtains were drawn and lighted candles made a soft golden light over the greens and flowers banked before the fireplace where Joseph and Theodosia stood. Afterward there was a wedding breakfast, with champagne to toast the bride and groom, and when Theodosia started upstairs to change into her traveling suit, she paused for a minute on the stairs.

"Here," she cried. "The next bride must catch my bouquet." And she tossed the crimson roses straight into Natalie's arms.

When she said good-by to her father, Theodosia laid her cheek against the shoulder of his immaculate black coat, and for a moment she felt the quick, hot sting of tears.

"Papa—oh, Papa," she whispered.

Her father's arms held her gently. Then he drew back and touched the locket at her throat.

Instantly she straightened, and looked up with a smile as gallant and serene as his own.

"*Au revoir,* my Theo," he said.

"*Au revoir . . .*"

·CHAPTER 11·

The Inaugural

THE NEXT THREE weeks were a sort of triumphal tour
for the young Alstons. Traveling by easy stages, stopping here and there to visit friends on the way south, they
were received everywhere with the most cordial hospitality.
Dinners were given for them, balls and dances were arranged
in their honor, and all who met them were delighted by the
young couple who were so handsome, so gay, and so charmingly in love.

The days passed swiftly, in a round of visits and parties.
All Theodosia's friends were anxious to meet her husband,
and Joseph complained privately that he felt like a trained
seal on exhibition.

"But such a very nice, superior trained seal, Joseph,"
Theodosia laughed. "They do approve of you quite thoroughly, you know. Even Mrs. Livingston told me she could
almost understand my being willing to bury myself in the
wilds of Carolina for the sake of such a handsome and accomplished husband as Mr. Alston."

It was the last day of February when the Alstons reached Baltimore. There they went directly to the inn where Mr. Burr and Natalie were to join them, and a letter from Papa was waiting for Theodosia. She read it eagerly, not stopping even to take off her cloak, and when she had finished she looked up at Joseph with shining eyes.

"It's all right, Joseph, they're really on the way, and expect to be here by the day after tomorrow. Oh, dear," she sighed in relief, "I've been *so* afraid something might happen to delay them."

Joseph bent to kiss her cheek, still cold and bright with color from the long drive in the winter's air. "Goose," he said affectionately. "What could possibly happen to keep your father from being present at his own inauguration? To say nothing of the fact that he's probably pining to see how married life agrees with you."

"Oh, I know." Theodosia smiled quickly. "It's foolish of me to worry. But it's so hard for me to remember that I'm not still a little girl who has to stay home alone when Papa's business keeps him away."

The next day Mr. Burr and Natalie arrived and they all drove to Washington together. Theodosia had her first taste of being a celebrity's daughter. People crowded about the carriage, eager for a glimpse of the new Vice-president and his family, and at every stopping place on the journey they found themselves surrounded.

Excitement ran high over the coming inaugural. The time had come now, people felt, when *they* were actually going to have a voice in the government. The new party was the people's party, and Mr. Jefferson was a President after their own hearts. No closed carriages for *him*—none of your pomp and ceremony and standing on official dignity. Here was a President who would ride his own horse or even walk alone in the streets. A President you could walk right up to and shake hands with, if you had a mind to. A man who looked and dressed and acted precisely like themselves.

It was too late now for the Federalists to do more than wag their heads despairingly. For the democratic spirit had caught the public fancy, and Thomas Jefferson was the man of the hour. To him the people gave a full measure of confidence and loyalty.

The new Vice-president was scarcely less popular. Aaron Burr might be a rich man, from a fine family, yet he wore a plain black coat and shook hands with anyone who wanted a word with him.

As for Theodosia, her presence in Washington put the finishing touch of popularity on the new administration. From the moment she stepped out of the carriage in front of Dolley Madison's house in Washington, where she and Joseph were to stay, the people loved her.

It was late in the afternoon when they arrived, and a raw spring rain was falling. But no sooner had the carriage drawn up at the curb than passers-by, hearing that the Vice-president's daughter was inside, gathered about, shivering in the damp air, to see her.

Even Joseph was surprised by the success of his wife's first public appearance. As she stepped down, slim and graceful in her long fur cloak and with a little feathered bonnet perched fashionably on her dark curls, the circle drew back for a moment, awed by the elegance of her dress and manner.

Theodosia hesitated, aware that in that moment the friendliness of her welcome was in doubt. Then an old woman pushed her way to the front of the group and Theodosia suddenly knew what to do. With a quick smile, she reached out and shook the old woman's hand.

"How do you do?" she said. "It's very kind of you to stop in all this rain to greet us."

The woman bobbed a curtsy, beaming with toothless pleasure at the honor of being singled out. "You're a pretty lass," she said, "and you've a fine young husband. God bless you both, ma'am, and your father and the new President too."

From that moment Theodosia had no further doubts about her welcome. The people crowded around with a good will, and for the next few minutes she and Joseph were kept busy shaking hands, while the rain still fell and the feather on her bonnet lost its stylish curl and hung limp and draggled against the wet shoulder of her cloak.

Never, after that, was Theodosia afraid of the crowds that followed her through the days before the inauguration. Although she found it not always to her liking to answer the questions of total strangers, who sometimes insisted on examining the material of her gowns with curious fingers, she bore herself with an easy dignity that won her friends everywhere.

Since Mr. Jefferson was a widower, there was no "first lady" to catch the public eye. And to Theodosia fell the feminine honors of the inaugural entertainments. Her youth and beauty, her graceful manners and her wit, became the topics of popular conversation. At the inauguration ceremonies she had the seat of honor, and at the ball that night, in a gown of ivory velvet with white rosebuds in her hair, she led the cotillion on President Jefferson's arm.

When Joseph and Theodosia left for the south, Mr. Burr said good-by to his daughter as calmly as though they were parting for no more than a day or two.

"Mind you see that Theo keeps up her studies," Mr. Burr warned Joseph, as the two men shook hands. "I don't want to find her settled into an empty-headed little housewife next time we meet, interested in nothing but her marketing and a dozen babies."

"I'll make her study harder than ever, sir," Joseph promised. "And I shall send you reports on her progress and misdemeanors."

"And *I* shall fairly dazzle you with my wisdom when you come to visit, Papa." Theodosia laughed. But the next moment she leaned out of the carriage and her glance searched her father's face anxiously. "Papa, you *will* visit us? You promise?"

"Wild horses couldn't keep me from it," Mr. Burr said. And still smiling, he stepped back. Debonair and handsome, he stood with head held high as he waved farewell to the dearest treasure of his life.

Part Two

·CHARLESTON, 1801–1812·

·CHAPTER 12·

Peacocks on the Lawn

T HEODOSIA'S FIRST SIGHT of her new home was through
the late dusk of an April afternoon. For nearly three
weeks she and Joseph had been traveling over good roads
and bad, and on that last afternoon of the journey Theodosia observed with a sigh that she was so heartily tired
of being jounced about in a carriage that she meant, when
they got home, not to drive anywhere for at least a month.

But when they turned at last into the long avenue that
led to the Oaks, her weariness vanished and she leaned out
the window to exclaim with delight over the long, low house
of pink brick with tall white columns across the front.

"Joseph, it's *beautiful!*" Theodosia's eyes shone. "But
it's so very big. Shan't we feel quite lost in it, just the two
of us?"

She was leaning out for a second look. The cypress trees
that lined the drive were hung with long, misty gray strands
of Spanish moss that swung gently in the mild breeze, and
in the soft light the lawns on either side looked like wide

79

carpets of velvety green. Suddenly Theodosia clutched at her husband's hand.

"Joseph, there are two *peacocks!*" she exclaimed. "Do they belong to us?"

When he nodded, amused at her childish pleasure, Theodosia settled back beside him with a sigh of purest satisfaction. "Just wait until I write Natalie," she said, "and tell her there are peacocks on the lawn!" As they reached the end of the avenue and drew up before the broad front steps, she quickly smoothed her gloves and set her hat straight. "Do I look all right, Joseph?"

"You look very sweet, my Theo," Joseph said, smiling, "and about ten years old instead of a matronly and settled seventeen."

A few minutes later, when he led her through the door and down the line of household servants who stood in the big front hall to welcome their master and mistress in true plantation style, Joseph watched with pride the air of gentle grace with which his wife took possession of her new home. He saw the faces of the servants break into smiles of welcome as Theodosia paused for a word of greeting to each in turn.

Accustomed as she had always been to the well-staffed household at Richmond Hill, Theodosia nevertheless found herself bewildered at first by the elaborateness of life at the Oaks, and she wrote to Natalie that her greatest difficulty was in remembering just which of the servants to ask for when she wanted some specific task performed.

> Joseph assures me (she wrote) that we have no more servants than any well-regulated plantation—but with so many countenances surrounding me—all looking precisely

alike to my uninitiated eye—I feel like a duchess, and a
slightly confused duchess at that! There is a special boy
who has no other function in life but to black our boots,
another who shines silver night and day, one whose only
duty is to carry up vast tubs of hot water and still another
who spends all his waking hours (which are not many)
in feeding and tending the peacocks who roam on the
lawns. And woe be to Theo if I ask the boot-boy to fetch
me fresh candles, or the candle-slavy to polish my new
riding boots!

As the weeks went by, Theodosia forgot about such
small trials in the delights of her new life. The Alstons had
a town house in Charleston as well, and Theodosia found
Southern society very much to her liking. There were teas
and dinners, balls and theaters. The people were gay and
friendly, and they seemed quite as charmed with Joseph's
bride as she was with them. Indeed, it was no time at all
before young Mrs. Alston began to be regarded as the most
popular hostess in Charleston.

Theodosia wrote to her father with impatience. He *must*
arrange to visit soon. He must see her new home, Joseph's
family, and her friends, all of whom, she assured him, were
waiting with bated breath for the honor of entertaining the
Vice-president.

Mr. Burr replied that he would surely come. Twice he
even engaged passage on packet boats sailing for Charleston, but each time there were complications in his plans that
made it impossible for him to leave, and he sent, in his stead,
long, affectionate letters and parcels containing the most
charmingly extravagant gifts for Theodosia and Joseph.

Theodosia was disappointed, but not for long. It was

nearly summer now, and the lovely Southern spring was ending. Instead of mild balmy days, when Joseph and Theodosia rode together or strolled along the embankment in Charleston, the weather turned sultry and oppressive. The wind blew a hot, steady mist from the Carolina swamplands, carrying the threat of fevers and malaria.

Since he could not come to them, Mr. Burr wrote, why should not Theodosia and her husband travel north to join him for the summer months at Richmond Hill?

An excellent plan, said Joseph. And Theodosia agreed.

By the middle of June, the Alstons were traveling once more, and when they reached Richmond Hill, they found Mr. Burr and Natalie already there, and the big house open and ready.

It was the happiest of summers.

Since Congress was not in session, the Vice-president was not required to be in Washington, and Mr. Burr was free to devote himself to the entertainment of his guests. John was with them a good part of the time, and when, in August, Vanderlyn came to Richmond Hill to paint portraits of Natalie and Theodosia, the little group that had been such good companions the summer before was once more united.

Again there were picnics and rides and sailing parties to fill the long bright hours of the summer days and on weekends they often took the big coach and drove far up through the Westchester hills and stopped for the night at some country inn.

Toward the end of August, Mr. Burr left for Washington, and Joseph suggested that he and Theodosia might take a trip across the state that would include a visit to Niagara

Falls. On the return journey, when they had stopped over-
night in Buffalo, their breakfast was interrupted by a startled
servingmaid who informed them that "a naked Indian"
was outside and said he had a letter for Mrs. Alston.

Joseph looked up from his coffee in astonishment. "Upon
my word, Theo," he said. "Have you taken to corresponding with savages?"

He went to see what was wanted, and came back to
report that the Indian was, fortunately, *not* naked, and that
the letter was from Chief Joseph Brant of the Mohawk tribe,
who had often been a guest at Richmond Hill.

Chief Brant had learned that Theodosia was in Buffalo
and wished, he said, to request the honor of a visit from her
and her husband. Would they come and stay at his camp
for a few days, and allow him, in some small measure, to
repay the hospitality that Miss Burr had so kindly offered
to him at her father's house.

They sent the messenger back to say that they would
accept with pleasure, and on the following morning a guide
appeared to lead the way to the Mohawk encampment.
Chief Brant was waiting to receive them, looking more imposing than ever, in his native dress, as he bowed low over
Theodosia's hand.

Joseph was pleased at the opportunity of meeting the
famous chief, and the two men spent a great deal of time in
conversation during the next three days, while Theodosia
visited the Indian women in their homes. She watched them
making pottery and grinding the late summer harvest of
corn, and amused the children vastly by allowing them to
investigate the contents of her handbag. The whole settle-

ment seemed charmed by the visitors, and all the tribe, from the tallest and fiercest-looking elder to the smallest toddling infant, showed the guests every possible courtesy.

When the Alstons were ready to leave, the camp gathered around to see them off, and nearly every one insisted on presenting the "Graceful One" and the "Handsome One" with a parting gift.

The Alstons stopped for a few days at Richmond Hill before beginning the long journey home to Charleston. Although Mr. Burr was able to join them there, and they had a last pleasant visit together, the easy, carefree spell of summer seemed to have vanished. There was frost in the September nights that touched the Palisades with red and gold, and a haze of autumn hung over the last stray blooms that lingered in the gardens.

Natalie was planning a trip to France to visit her mother, and since Mr. Burr was to be in Washington for the winter, it had been decided that Richmond Hill was to be closed.

On the last day before her departure, Theodosia wandered from room to room in the big house. The furniture, shrouded in dust covers, already had a forlorn and deserted look.

"Oh, dear," Theo sighed, "I do *wish* you weren't going to France, Natalie. It makes me feel homesick already to think of Richmond Hill being left alone and empty."

"I know." Natalie nodded soberly. "I'm afraid I shall be most desperately homesick myself. We've been so happy here." She broke off suddenly, as a shadow of a frown crossed

Theodosia's face. "Theo, you aren't worrying about Papa for any reason, are you?"

Theodosia said slowly, "I don't know. He seems very well, I think, though he works too hard, and is tired sometimes. But that's not what troubles me, Natalie. It's the things people keep saying about him. That he's too ambitious—and all the long trouble with Mr. Hamilton."

"Ah, yes, Mr. Hamilton." Natalie sighed. "If only that dreadful business with Hamilton had never started. It's silly for grown men to act so! Hamilton determined to make Papa angry—and Papa equally determined not to *be* angry. Sometimes"—she whisked a handful of silver out of the chest she was packing and rattled it briskly—"I feel like *shaking* the two of them!"

Theodosia smiled at that, but after a moment she went on soberly, "Of course I'd never dare speak to Papa about any of it. He'd be furious, I know, for he'll never admit that the slightest thing is wrong. But sometimes I wonder if he doesn't try to carry too much alone. Joseph says he doesn't believe any man can keep the self-control Papa does forever. He says he's afraid someday it might break, and then" —Theodosia spread her hands—"I don't know what might happen."

John and Vanderlyn had already gone, and Joseph had driven into the city. Mr. Burr and the two girls had their supper in front of the study hearth that evening, since the dining-room things were packed away. Peggy sent up platters of cold turkey, bread and pickles and cheese, and a big pot of hot, rich chocolate. Sitting before the fire, they were very cozy and contented. It was like old times, Natalie said. Yet it wasn't quite like old times, for Natalie's thoughts were already of her journey to France, and Theodosia kept listening for Joseph's carriage and jumping up to look out the window each time she thought she heard it.

Only Mr. Burr was the same. He was in excellent spirits, and as he talked on about his life in Washington, amusing them with stories about the people he had met there, Theodosia watched his face, dark and handsome in the firelight, and wondered whether perhaps her fears and doubts were foolish, after all.

They had nearly finished supper when the door opened suddenly and Joseph came into the room. He still wore his cloak, and in one hand he carried a folded newspaper, which he handed at once to Mr. Burr.

"I'm sorry to burst in like this, sir," Joseph said, "but I think you ought to see this right away." He pointed to an article on the front page. "It's a new attack on you, and a thoroughly contemptible one."

Joseph's face was grave as he waited for Mr. Burr to comment.

But, having glanced through the article, Mr. Burr merely laid aside the paper without comment.

"What is it, Papa?" Theodosia reached for the paper.

Mr. Burr shrugged. "Nothing much," he said. "Only some anonymous writer airing his views about the Vice-president."

"But this is different, sir." Joseph set his chin stubbornly. "This writer claims that you are actually plotting to overthrow Jefferson and take the presidency for yourself. Even though the whole thing is a preposterous lie, it's causing a tremendous stir, I assure you. The whole city is talking about nothing else. It's bound to get back to Mr. Jefferson, and unless you deny the charges and give proof, there are certain people, even in your own party, who will believe these things."

"Will they?" Mr. Burr asked calmly. He poured a cup of chocolate and handed it to Joseph with a smile.

Joseph shook his head impatiently. "I'm aware, of course," he said, "that you expect to have enemies. So does any man in public life. But I think you're going too far when you allow these vicious and unfounded lies to go undefended."

"You forget one thing, Joseph." Mr. Burr leaned back in his chair. "To defend oneself is to admit that there is a charge worth denying. To defend oneself against an enemy is meaningless. Against my friend Hamilton"—he paused, with a shrug—"it's hopeless."

A silence followed his words.

Theodosia glanced at her husband's face. She had seldom seen Joseph as near to anger as he was now. In her heart she believed Joseph was right, and she longed to say so—to beg her father, just this once, to take Joseph's advice and defend himself against Mr. Hamilton's attacks. She might have spoken, but a warning flashed to her from the bland, impassive depths of her father's eyes and she felt the words die in her throat.

"Trust me, Theodosia," his look seemed to say. "Trust me—believe only in me."

She looked down, still silent.

"Come, Joseph." Mr. Burr stood up. "We've upset Theo by all this talk. We'll say no more about it. As for this"—he picked up the newspaper and walked to the fireplace—"we can dispose of it quite easily." He tossed the crumpled pages into the flames.

"How shall we amuse ourselves this last evening?" Mr. Burr asked. "A game of cards?" He walked over to put his hand affectionately on the young man's shoulder. "I know you mean well, Joseph, but please believe me, I know best how to deal with these things."

"It's for you to decide, of course, sir." Joseph nodded.

Theodosia was relieved to see that the anger had died out of Joseph's blue eyes. And as she and Natalie rose to fetch the cards, she passed the fireplace and noticed that the last fragments of paper had vanished, leaving only a bed of coals that burned bright and steady on the hearth.

·CHAPTER 13·

Little Gampy

IT WAS MID-OCTOBER when the Alstons reached South Carolina again, and Theodosia was soon caught up once more
in the affairs of her two households and the pleasant round of
social events.

But, although she and Joseph continued to entertain and
be entertained, Theodosia was not content to become entirely absorbed by the round of teas and dinners. The habit
of studying, instilled by years of training, was not easily forgotten, and she still reported faithfully to her father. From
him she received encouragement and suggestions. Once, being pleased by a pretty turn of phrase in one of her letters,
he observed: ". . . Your letters contain now and then a spark
of Promethean fire: a spark, mind ye; don't be vain." Another time he advised that it would be "better to lose your
head than your habits of study."

The example of Theodosia's industry made its mark on
Joseph. Encouraged by her, and by occasional advice from
Mr. Burr, Joseph began to take his plans for a career in poli-

tics more seriously. He ran for the state legislature and was elected. Before long his keen judgment and enthusiastic interest in public affairs established him as one of the rising young statesmen of the South.

Theodosia was delighted by her husband's success, and as she became more and more engrossed by his career and the pleasant diversions of her own life, the old days at Richmond Hill faded gradually into the background. There was no time to think on the past; no place in her full, happy days for homesickness.

Natalie, too, seemed to have been caught up in such a whirl of new experiences that she had no regrets for the old days she had left behind. Her letters to Theodosia were filled with accounts of good times and pleasant friends in Paris, and in particular of a certain Mr. Thomas Sumpter whom she had met.

"Our Natalie is in love," Theodosia observed at breakfast one morning. "And a very good thing too. Papa says Mr. Sumpter will be a splendid husband for her."

"Upon my word, what a pair of matchmakers you and your papa are." Joseph laughed. "You have Natalie's future all settled between you before she's so much as breathed a word about it herself. Can this be the same Theo who used to argue with me over the folly of any woman marrying before she was in her dotage? How you have changed, my dear."

Theodosia buttered a toasted scone and nibbled at the corner of it thoughtfully. "If you weren't such an utterly misguided male, Mr. Alston," she said, "you might take my attitude as a very pretty compliment for yourself. But since

I must be plain about it, I'll confess that having tried married life and found it *very much* to my liking, I'm naturally anxious for everyone else to enter into the same state of bliss. As for Natalie—just wait, and you'll see that I was right."

Surely enough, a few days after the bells of St. Michael's Church had rung the New Year into Charleston, a letter came from Paris saying that Natalie was engaged and would soon be married. "My mother thoroughly approves of the match and is charmed with Mr. Sumpter, whom," she added ingenuously, "you may recall my having spoken of once or twice before. As for myself, I am deliriously happy, a state that none can understand more completely than you, dear Theo."

"So you see, Joseph," Theodosia said, "I *was* right."

And Joseph was content merely to shake his head wonderingly and kiss the tip of his wife's pretty nose.

In the late spring of that year, it was at last arranged for Mr. Burr to visit Charleston. The Congress having adjourned early, he was able to leave Washington on the first of May, and wrote that he was "proceeding south with the speed of lightning."

For days in advance Theodosia was busy preparing for her father's arrival, and her friends were so anxious to show the Vice-president every hospitality that dinners, dances, luncheons, and even breakfast parties were arranged in his honor. Joseph must bring him to a hunt breakfast—and, of course, without fail, he must go to St. Michael's on Sunday morning and sit in the celebrities' pew where General Washington had sat.

Mr. Burr was charmed by everything. He made himself such an agreeable and entertaining guest that, by the end of his stay, someone observed that "half of Charleston is entirely infatuated with the Vice-president, and the other half is furious over not having had the chance to entertain him!"

The real event of his visit, however, did not take place until the end of June. That was the birth of a little son to Joseph and Theodosia.

Never was a baby more enthusiastically welcomed. Mr. Burr, quite as much as the young parents, threw himself into preparations for the event with a frenzy of plans, anticipations, and general to-do.

For days in advance everything was in readiness at the Oaks. Mr. Burr had commissioned Natalie to buy the most beautiful cradle obtainable in Paris. Joseph's mother had sent the faithful Mammy who had cared for her own children when they were babies. The doctor in attendance was personally instructed, by the Vice-president, as to his solemn responsibility in ushering the new Alston into existence. Every detail of Theodosia's welfare and health was supervised with such scrupulous care by her husband and father that she declared at last that she felt as if the future of the whole human race might well depend on her ability to produce a satisfactory infant.

On the twenty-ninth of June, Aaron Burr Alston was born.

He was a healthy, handsome, entirely charming baby, and he so delighted his father and grandfather that by the time Theodosia was up and about again, she complained, with some justice, that it was no longer possible to have a conversation with Joseph or her father that did not center on the perfections of her remarkable son.

"A finely shaped head," Mr. Burr declared solemnly. "See how rounded his brow is, a sure sign of intellect and good judgment."

"He has his mother's eyes, don't you think?" Joseph put in. "And obviously a good wit, too. This morning he smiled very plainly when I showed him a new rattle. Mammy says he shows far more sense than any of us did at the same age."

Mammy said much else besides. She complained bitterly to Theodosia that it was quite impossible to bring up a baby properly with two great men constantly underfoot, cluttering up the nursery with enough toys for fifty babies, and hanging over her honey lamb at all hours.

Mr. Burr stayed at the Oaks until the middle of July, unwilling to tear himself away from the fascinating spectacle of his grandson. When it at last became apparent that the Vice-president had obligations besides being the most devoted and attentive grandpapa ever seen, he left for Washington. But it was arranged before his departure that as soon as Theodosia and the baby were able, Joseph would bring them for a visit to New York, where Mr. Burr promised to open Richmond Hill especially for them.

By Christmas the three Alstons were back in Charleston, and from that time on the letters from Theodosia to her father were filled with accounts of the behavior and accomplishments of little Aaron. As soon as he could talk, she taught him to say "Grandpa," which he twisted into *Gampy,* and for a while that became the baby's own nickname.

In every letter Mr. Burr demanded "more of Gampy's doings." Before the boy had passed his first birthday, Mr. Burr had already laid out elaborate plans for his training and education, and meanwhile he delighted in sending most extravagant gifts to the whole family. Little suits of embroidered linen, patent-leather boots, and dozens of toys for Gampy. The latest bonnets, gloves from Paris, laces, scent, and furs for Theodosia; and for Joseph, books from England and France. When Theodosia wrote that they were remodeling the big pink-brick plantation house, Mr. Burr immediately commissioned Natalie to buy a whole suite of French furniture for Theodosia's sitting room. And once, when Theo complained of the scarcity of good cooks in the South, Mr. Burr lost no time in locating one in New York and dispatching her to Charleston on the next packet, with his compliments.

In the spring of 1803, Theodosia fell ill with malaria. For nearly four weeks the fever raged, and in spite of all the medical advice and care that her distracted husband could summon, her recovery was slow and difficult. She was depressed and miserable. She worried about herself, about her husband, and her boy. Most of all she was troubled about her father. The old fears, never quite forgotten, came back to plague her restless nights and weary days, until at last Mr. Burr became alarmed by the gloomy cast of her letters and insisted that Joseph leave his work as soon as possible and bring her north.

Joseph was only too glad to do anything that might bring back his wife's health and high spirits, and on the eve of

Theodosia's birthday, they arrived in New York by boat and were driven straight to Richmond Hill.

But not even the welcome that awaited her there, nor all the loving care and attention her husband and father gave her throughout the quiet summer, seemed quite to restore Theodosia. When autumn came, and she was still pale and languid, Mr. Burr talked long and earnestly with Joseph.

It was plain to be seen, he said, that the Southern climate had not agreed with Theodosia. Why not stay in New York, instead of taking her back to the danger of more fevers from the swamplands of Carolina? Joseph could take up politics in New York, quite as well as in the South. Mr. Burr would see to it that he met the right people, made the proper connections. . . .

But Joseph, for all his unbounded devotion to Theodosia, could be firm. He would *not,* he said, trade on his father-in-law's prominence. He had begun his career by his own efforts in the South, and there he would continue it. Charleston was his home, and Theodosia's home and, for better or for worse, they would return to Charleston.

And return they did.

If Theodosia regretted her husband's decision, she was too much her father's daughter ever to show her disappointment, and at every stopping place on the return journey she sent back little notes to her father designed to reassure him of her health and good spirits.

The Alstons stopped a few days in Washington, and from there Theodosia sent Mr. Burr a long letter telling of the people they had seen. Dolley Madison had come to call at once, and had been charmed with little Gampy. They were entertained by various of Mr. Burr's friends in the capital, but, strangely, no invitation came to them from the President.

Mr. Jefferson could scarcely have failed to know that the Vice-president's daughter was in Washington, yet he sent no word of greeting. And although Theodosia made no comment to her father on the omission, she was more than ever disturbed by the persistent rumors of the ill feeling between the President and Mr. Burr.

On the last morning of their stay, a chambermaid brought the morning tray, and being disposed to gossip, she lingered while Theodosia had her breakfast.

"We don't like seeing you go, ma'am, and that's the truth," the girl said. "It's all about town that Mr. Burr is a gentleman not to be trusted—and folks here were near ready to believe it until you came with Mr. Alston and the little boy. But it doesn't appear likely, as I was saying myself this morning in the kitchen, that any gentleman connected with *you,* ma'am, could be the sort of rapscallion they talk of Mr. Burr's being. That it doesn't."

Theodosia put down her cup slowly. Ordinarily she would have been impatient of such gossip, but now she wondered.

"What sort of things do they say of my father?" she asked.

"Oh"—the girl folded her arms under her apron—"it's more a question of what *don't* they say, ma'am. The tales we hear about the plots and deviltries our Vice-president is up to. Some say he's trying to be President himself."

Theodosia glanced up quickly, and a little shiver of

fear went through her as she saw the girl's eyes, pale and credulous, fastened eagerly on hers. Then, remembering herself, she forced a smile.

"I don't think those things are true," Theodosia said quietly. "I really don't."

"Nor do I, ma'am." The girl shook her head. "But all the same it's a pity more people who talk so against Mr. Burr can't know *you*, ma'am. They'd stop then." She nodded her head with decision. "I know they would!"

Over and over, on the long journey home, Theodosia kept hearing again the singsong voice of the chambermaid. Leaning back in the carriage, her eyes closed against the dull ache of fatigue that pounded in her head with every jolt over the dusty, rutted roads, she kept wondering whether perhaps the girl had been right.

Would it really make a difference if she were with her father more? If, instead of being so much alone, he had the stabilizing influence of a family—of herself, and Joseph, and little Aaron? Was it true that Mr. Jefferson no longer trusted her father, that even his friends were beginning to suspect him of plots and schemes?

The questions circled in her mind until they seemed to mingle with the rumble of the wheels and the monotonous swaying of the carriage, and Theodosia pressed her hands against her ears as if to shut them out forever. Then, suddenly, she seemed to hear her father speak, as he had long ago when she was a child and frightened of something. "Courage," she seemed to hear him whisper. "Courage, Theodosia."

·CHAPTER 14·

The Gathering Clouds

O N A BRIGHT summer's morning Theodosia and Natalie sat side by side on the veranda steps of the Alstons' summer cabin in the Carolina mountains. A fortnight past, Natalie and her husband and their little daughter had landed in New York from abroad. There Mr. Sumpter learned that he would be required to make a business trip to Charleston, so he had brought his family south with him, and while he stayed in the city to complete his work, Natalie and her little girl visited Theodosia.

The mountain air was crystal clear and pleasantly cool, and a light breeze whispered through the tall pines now and then, gently ruffling the curls of the two children who played together near the steps.

For the first few days of the visit, Theodosia and Natalie had talked almost without stopping. There had been so much to tell, so many questions to be asked and answered, after their long separation. Now, sitting together in the peaceful silence of the morning sunshine, they watched the children.

"How well they play together, don't they, Theo?" Natalie asked presently, smiling to see how her fair-haired little girl, named for Theodosia, insisted on giving her favorite doll to Gampy.

Theodosia nodded. "I'm afraid your young Theo will spoil my young Aaron, though," she said. "She gives him all her best toys, and last night at supper she refused to eat a bite until she had fed Gampy all the nicest bits of chicken from her plate. Joseph says it's plainly a case of love at first sight."

"Oh, it's *so* good to be here, Theo," Natalie said. "I used to wonder sometimes, when we were in France, whether we'd ever really be together again. And now to have this lovely visit, and to find you and Joseph so well . . ." She smiled. "You know, Theo, I had no idea what a success Joseph was making. They even talk of his running for governor of the state."

"I know." There was pride in Theodosia's voice. "He deserves to succeed, Natalie, he's worked so hard and faithfully." She paused. "Natalie, Papa *was* all right when you saw him in New York, wasn't he? You've told me so little about him."

Natalie did not reply at once. Leaning down, she scooped up a handful of pine needles, and let them trickle slowly through her fingers. "There wasn't much to tell," she said guardedly. "He seemed in good spirits. But . . ."

"But what, Natalie?"

Natalie tossed away the pine needles and brushed the soft dust from her fingers, frowning a little.

"I know I oughtn't to trouble you, Theo, but all the while Thomas and I were in New York, we kept hearing the most fantastic rumors. It seemed as if, wherever we went, people talked of nothing but *Burr—Burr—Burr*. All the old stories, you know"—she paused and sighed—"about his debts, and the fact that he and Mr. Jefferson had quarreled, and that Jefferson accuses him of trying to split the party and turn his friends against the President. It seems that Mr. Hamilton has been more bitter than ever against Papa. I don't understand it very well, Theo, but I'll admit that the stories troubled me, though Papa himself only laughed when Thomas tried to talk to him. He said that the rumors were nothing more than fancies spread by Hamilton and Clinton and the other Federalists. I wonder sometimes, Theo, whether so much bitterness and distrust hasn't changed Papa, and made *him* bitter and distrustful of others, I mean, even though he'll never admit it."

"I know," Theodosia answered soberly. She bent down to smooth her little son's dark head as he climbed up the step to lay a pine cone in her lap. "Oh, Natalie, if only that old quarrel with Mr. Hamilton could die. I've so hoped and prayed it might."

Natalie shook her head. "There's one comfort at least, Theo. The old quarrel has gone on for so many years that it's hardly likely now that anything will ever come of it. And whatever happens, Theo—whatever people may say against Papa—I'll always trust him."

"So shall I," Theodosia said. "As long as I live."

That was the morning of June 17 , 1804.

In the afternoon of that same day, William Van Ness presented himself at the town house of Mr. Hamilton in New York.

He delivered a letter to Hamilton from Aaron Burr, and a copy of a newspaper with two sentences underlined. One said that Mr. Hamilton considered Burr a dangerous man, not to be trusted with the reins of government. The other that there was "a still more despicable opinion which General Hamilton has expressed of Mr. Burr."

In the letter which Van Ness carried, Mr. Burr called Hamilton's attention to the marked passages, and demanded "a prompt and unqualified acknowledgment or denial."

Mr. Hamilton was astonished. He had not, he said, seen the statements until this moment. He must have time to consider them, and Mr. Burr's note, before he could give an answer.

When, after two days, he did reply, it was to state at length that he could make neither the acknowledgment nor the denial that Burr had demanded. He could not consent to be questioned as to the justice of the *inferences* of things he had said of an opponent during fifteen years' competition. He trusted that Colonel Burr, upon further reflection, would see the matter in the same light. If not, he could only regret the fact, and accept the consequences.

During the next few days, several more letters were exchanged, and it became clear that the long battle between the two men had at last reached a climax. Neither would yield an inch. There was only one means left to settle the matter.

Burr challenged Hamilton to a duel, and Hamilton accepted the challenge.

On the twenty-third of June, Van Ness and Mr. Hamilton's second, Mr. Pendleton, met to decide the final details. The duel would take place on July eleventh, at seven in the morning: the place, Weehawken; the weapons, pistols; the distance, ten full paces.

That was all.

The twenty-third of June chanced also to be Theodosia's twenty-first birthday, and in the evening Mr. Burr entertained some friends for dinner at Richmond Hill. Writing to Theodosia the next morning, he said nothing of the coming duel, but he was careful to tell her about the party the evening before. They had, Mr. Burr said, "laughed an hour, and danced an hour, and drunk her health." He had brought her picture to the dinner table and put it in the place where she usually sat.

In the last days before the duel, both Mr. Burr and Mr. Hamilton went about their businesses quite as usual. No one except themselves and their seconds knew what was to take place.

Under the code of the times, Hamilton had had no choice but to accept Burr's challenge. Dueling was still the accepted custom in settling disputes between gentlemen, and there were few men in public life who had not taken part in a duel for one reason or another. Both Burr and Hamilton had fought before. Three years earlier Mr. Hamilton's son Philip had been shot and killed on the dueling field. That two men who had been such long and bitter enemies should fight was in no way surprising. The only surprising part was that Burr, who had borne in stubborn silence so many injuries and insults from Mr. Hamilton, should now suddenly, without warning, demand the ultimate revenge for a comparatively mild and insignificant slur.

What moved Burr to break his years of stoical silence, no one was ever to know. For in this moment as in all others, Mr. Burr kept his own counsel.

·CHAPTER 15·

The Distance: Ten Full Paces

THE NIGHT BEFORE the duel Mr. Burr dined alone at
Richmond Hill. Later he went to his study, and there
he sat before his desk for a long while, writing, arranging his
affairs with methodical care. At last the desk was clear of
papers, and everything was done. All was finished, except
for one last thing. To write two letters.

Mr. Burr drew a fresh sheet of paper, and paused for a
moment staring at the blank white square. Then he dipped
his pen, and began to write:

"My dear Joseph . . ."

It was very still in the room. Outside the open windows
the summer night lay dark. Now and then a faint breeze
sent the candle flames flickering. Only the far-off sound of
the crickets' chirping and the steady scratching of the pen
broke the silence, as Mr. Burr wrote:

> . . . If it should be my lot to fall, yet I shall live in you
> and Theodosia and your son. I commit to you all that is
> most dear to me—my reputation and my daughter. . . .

Let me entreat you to stimulate and aid Theodosia in
the cultivation of her mind. It is indispensable to her
happiness, and essential to yours. . . . She will richly compensate your trouble. . . .

The letter done, and sealed, Mr. Burr laid it aside and
bent once more over the desk.

"My dearest Theodosia . . ."

This was a longer letter. It held no bitterness, no regrets,
no explanation of what was to take place on the morrow.
Only calm, dispassionate directions for the disposition of his
affairs. To Theodosia he committed all his belongings, his
letters, and what property might remain when his estate
was settled.

. . . Tell my dear Natalie that I have not left her anything, for the very good reason that I had nothing to leave
to anyone. My estate will just about pay my debts and no
more. . . . Give her one of the pictures of me. There
are three in this house; one by Stuart, and two by Vanderlyn. . . .

John and Frederic were to have his clothes, a seal of
General Washington was to be saved for Gampy, and he
begged Theodosia to see that the faithful servants at Richmond Hill were provided for, and, if possible, kept on in the
Alstons' service.

That was all, but for a last few lines:

. . . I am indebted to you, my dearest Theodosia, for a
very great portion of the happiness which I have enjoyed
in this life. You have completely satisfied all that my
heart and affections had hoped or even wished. With a
little more perseverance, determination, and industry, you
will obtain all that ambition or vanity had fondly imag-

ined. Let your son have occasion to be proud that he had a mother. Adieu. Adieu.

A. Burr

It was scarcely daybreak when Van Ness came into the room and wakened Mr. Burr. Everything was ready, he said. The boat was waiting at the river landing. As they walked together down the path to the water's edge, a fresh breeze blew from the west and light, fluffy clouds scudded across the sky. Mr. Burr climbed quickly into the boat, and sat in the stern, his eye fixed on the line of the Jersey shore while Van Ness rowed steadily across the river and tied the boat to the trunk of a young tree by the shallow water.

In silence the two men made their way up from the shore to a place where they emerged into a flat, open clearing. There they laid aside their coats, and while Van Ness got out the pistols and examined them, Mr. Burr stood looking through the trees toward the broad river that sparkled and glittered in the morning sun.

"It's a quarter to seven, Mr. Burr," Van Ness said. "Are you ready?"

Aaron Burr nodded.

There was a sound of footsteps. Three men came into the clearing. Mr. Hamilton, his fine face as composed as Burr's; Mr. Pendleton; and Dr. Hosack, a physician.

The principals and seconds exchanged the customary word of greeting. Then, saying no more, they made their final preparations. Ten full paces were measured; the two men took their places.

When Pendleton handed Mr. Hamilton his pistol, he asked if he should set the hairspring.

Without turning his head, Mr. Hamilton said in a quiet voice, "Not this time, Pendleton."

The seconds withdrew, the men stood waiting.

"Are you ready?"

Both nodded.

Van Ness spoke the word. "Present."

Each raised his arm, and Burr took quiet, deliberate aim and fired.

Somewhere above Mr. Hamilton's head a bird had been singing, a sweet cadence of notes that fell upon the sunlit air. As the sound of the shot shattered the stillness of the woods, the bird's song ceased and there was a startled whir of wings as it sprang up and away from the low bough.

Silence for a split second—then another shot. Hamilton's finger had closed on the trigger and in the instant before he crumpled to the ground, his wild shot struck a branch high above Burr's head.

Pendleton and the doctor sprang forward to where General Hamilton lay motionless. Burr moved toward him also, but before he had taken more than a step, Van Ness was at his side, urging him to come down to the boat at once.

On the trip back, Mr. Burr sat again in the stern. Everything in the calm scene was as before. The two men were as silent, the sky as blue, the clouds as white, and the broad waters of the Hudson still flashing clear beneath the morning sun—all was as before—except that somewhere, hidden among the trees on the receding shore, a man lay mortally wounded.

And a bird, his song cut short, had flown away.

·CHAPTER 16·

"Hang Burr!"

BY MIDMORNING THE streets of lower New York were milling with people. They came out of shops and offices, up from the docks and out of their homes, shocked by the news that spread through the city like wildfire.

At the house to which General Hamilton had been carried, a crowd gathered, silent and tense, waiting for the bulletins that came each hour. Mrs. Hamilton, with her children, had hurried into the room where, behind drawn shutters, her husband lay dying.

Handbills, hastily printed, appeared on the street corners. Everywhere, on every tongue, the news was discussed with indignation and horror.

"Burr has murdered Hamilton!"

"Burr has escaped . . ."

"It was a fair duel, fairly fought . . ."

"Burr provoked it . . ."

"No, Hamilton provoked it . . ."

"They say Burr has disappeared . . ."

"Pendleton swears that Hamilton intended deliberately to fire into the air. He says Hamilton refused to have the hairspring set for his first shot."

"If Hamilton dies, this will ruin Burr, no matter who was to blame."

Through the crowds, from lip to lip, the rumors flew—confused and contradictory. But always they came back to the same verdict. The Vice-president had *murdered* General Hamilton, and in the swelling tide of public anger and grief, it was forgotten that the two men had met under fair and honorable conditions, according to the accepted rules of dueling.

Shortly after noon, a young man rode up Broadway and stopped his horse at the corner of Wall Street, to dismount in the midst of a group gathered by the steps of Trinity Church. Puzzled by the crowds and excitement, he inquired of a passer-by what had happened.

The stranger stared at him curiously.

"You haven't heard? Why, the Vice-president met General Hamilton in a duel this morning, and Hamilton was wounded and is dying. They say Burr has already escaped. He's disappeared, they say, and——"

An expression of blankest astonishment and disbelief came over the young man's face as he shook his head. "There must be some mistake. I've just come from breakfast with Colonel Burr. He is my uncle. He said nothing of a duel." Still bewildered, the young man turned to where the poster blazoned the news in bold, unmistakable letters. Then, without another word, or a glance for the crowd that still muttered angrily around him, he mounted and wheeled his horse back toward the Greenwich Road.

Mr. Burr was in his study when the young man rushed in breathlessly. Seated at his desk, he was engaged in writing a letter, but when he looked up to see his nephew's distraught countenance, Mr. Burr laid down his pen with an air of courteous surprise. "What brings you back so soon, Edward?" he asked. "Has something happened?"

For a full moment the young man stood speechless. Then, flinging himself into a chair, he launched into an account of what was happening in the streets of the city. The angry crowds—the rumors—the printed bulletins crying the news of the duel from every corner.

Mr. Burr listened calmly. "All this is very surprising," he said. "It is true that I met General Hamilton in a duel this morning. It's also true that it was I who challenged. But everyone knows that I had far more than ample grounds for challenging. For fifteen years Hamilton has provoked me, insulted me, libeled my name, and deliberately attempted to ruin me at every turn. A dozen times before I might have challenged him. Indeed, I've been advised to do so more than once. And we met fairly. General Hamilton had precisely the same chance as I this morning——"

"I know, Uncle. But, I tell you, no one is considering that now. They say you killed him deliberately. There's even talk of hanging you for *murder*. If Hamilton dies, they say——" He stopped short, startled by a move from Mr. Burr.

"They say," Mr. Burr repeated, in a voice of bitterest

scorn. Leaning forward across the desk, he faced his nephew with blazing anger in his dark eyes. "Be kind enough not to speak those odious words to me again. Do you think I care a rap for what *they say?*" With a gesture of rare violence, he brought his hand down sharply on the polished mahogany desk. "Name me a critic, and I'll answer him. Name me a hundred, I'll answer them all—gladly. But I cannot, and will not, listen to what *they say.*"

"I'm sorry, Uncle, truly." The young man drew back. "I only meant to warn you—to ask what you are planning to do now?"

Mr. Burr sat back in his chair and, as if all emotion had been erased from his features with a sponge, he eyed his nephew with his usual impassive composure.

"Do?" Mr. Burr inquired calmly. "I don't propose to do anything."

"But, Uncle, surely, in view of the general feeling, it would be better if you were to go away for at least a few days, until things have settled down."

"I scarcely think," Mr. Burr said quietly, "that it would do my cause any good to run away. No man has even been hanged for taking part in a fair duel. Believe me, Edward, the choice was not mine. It was Hamilton who chose to make me his enemy—not I him."

The young man rose.

"Just as you say, sir, of course. But if they should carry out their threat of indicting you for murder . . ."

"Then," said Mr. Burr, "they will at least be spared the trouble of having to hunt me out. If I'm wanted, I shall be right here—waiting."

"And is there anything you want me to do in the meanwhile, sir?"

Mr. Burr glanced up kindly.

"You might stay for luncheon with me, if you will."

It was an afternoon ten days later when Theodosia heard the news of the duel. She and Natalie had driven down from the mountains to do some shopping in Charleston. The bundles were being piled into the back of their carriage when Theodosia remembered a certain small stuffed kitty she had intended to buy and take back to Gampy.

"Wait for me here," she called to Natalie. "There's one thing more that I'd forgotten."

A few minutes passed, while Natalie sat in the carriage, idly watching the people who came and went along the embankment on the water front. A packet boat was just in the harbor from New York.

Suddenly her eye was caught by the figure of a young man standing near the dock. There was something familiar about the set of his shoulders and the way he held his tall beaver hat tucked under one arm. He turned just then, and with a cry of surprise, Natalie was out of the carriage and running toward him.

"Mr. Vanderlyn," she called, nearly tripping over her full muslin skirts in her eagerness. "Mr. Vanderlyn. . . ."

He turned quickly, and for a moment his sober face lighted. "Oh, Miss Natalie, it's good to see you." He took her hand in his.

"But this is wonderful. We hadn't a notion that you were in Charleston, Mr. Vanderlyn. Did you just get here?

Theodosia will be delighted, I know. She'll be along in just a minute."

"Miss Natalie, wait." He held fast to her hand as she drew him toward the carriage. "I must speak to you first. There's bad news, I'm afraid. Mr. Burr sent me down by the first boat because he feared that otherwise Theodosia might be alarmed by the rumors that are being spread about him. . . ."

As briefly as possible, Vanderlyn told her what had happened. Of General Hamilton's death on the day following the duel, and of the unexpected and wholly unprecedented tide of public fury that had been roused against Mr. Burr. A fury that had reached its culmination on the afternoon of the funeral, when Mrs. Hamilton and her children had stood beside the coffin on the steps of Trinity Church, and the whole city had gone into mourning. All day the boats in the harbor had boomed their solemn salute of guns, and from every steeple the bells tolled through the melancholy streets below.

"There's never been anything like it, Miss Natalie," Vanderlyn said, his face strained and grave. "General Hamilton was a popular man—even a great man—but I think no one could have foreseen the way his death affected people. They could talk of nothing else, think of nothing else, and everything that had led up to the duel was forgotten. There wasn't any thought of justice or fair play in anyone's mind, only loyalty to the fallen hero and a hatred against the man who had the ironic good fortune to escape from the duel alive."

Natalie shook her head slowly. "I can't believe it," she said in a stunned voice. "I can't believe that Papa—after all those years when he'd never say one word to defend himself against Mr. Hamilton—would suddenly change like that." She turned quickly. "Oh, what ever made him do it, Mr. Vanderlyn?"

"No one knows," he said. "Mr. Burr says nothing—only that what is done is done. Even now he won't defend his action, no matter how his friends try to persuade him. I think he must have been as surprised as anyone by the people's attitude, yet he won't admit it. You know how he can be— stubborn as iron, on the surface, and never letting you see for an instant what he's really feeling——" He stopped short, as he looked up to see Theodosia coming out of the shop door.

She walked quickly toward the carriage, the stuffed kitty in one hand, and in the other a long-legged rag doll she had found for Natalie's little girl. Her face was shaded prettily by a broad-brimmed leghorn hat. Catching sight of Vanderlyn, Theodosia's eyes lighted with pleasure, but her gay greeting died on her lips as she saw his grave expression and Natalie's white face.

"Mr. Vanderlyn, has something happened to my father?" Theodosia asked.

As gently as possible, he told her. When he had finished, she was silent for a moment. Then, with a queer, choked cry, she covered her face with her hands.

"Oh, poor Mrs. Hamilton," she said. "What a terrible thing for her."

Theodosia's slender body swayed, but as Vanderlyn and Natalie moved to steady her, she straightened quickly and looked up, her eyes clear and strangely calm.

"And my father?" she asked quietly. "Where is he, Mr. Vanderlyn?"

Her father was quite safe, Vanderlyn assured her. He explained how Mr. Burr had insisted on remaining at Richmond Hill, stubbornly refusing to listen to the counsel of his friends who advised him to leave. His only concern, Vanderlyn said, was the fear that Theodosia would be alarmed by the wild rumors that were being published and circulated.

"He asked me to come straight to you, Miss Theodosia, and to say that he is well, and quite safe. As soon as he is able, he'll let you know his immediate plans, and in the meantime, he said I was to give you one special message."

"What was it, Mr. Vanderlyn?"

"He said, 'Tell Theodosia to remember just one word—*courage.*'"

In the days that followed, lengthening miserably into weeks, Theodosia had more than one occasion to summon her father's message to her mind. The news came that her father had been indicted for murder by the state of New Jersey. Then came a burst of rumors and speculation: that Mr. Burr had escaped, and was in hiding; that there had been attempts to assassinate him; that he was threatened with impeachment; that President Jefferson had refused to intercede in Burr's defense.

Through it all Theodosia waited for some word from her father. And while she waited she wrote to him—long letters in which she told him the news of herself, and Joseph's work, and little Gampy. Cheerful letters, and never a word of reproach for what he had done. Never a single question, nor a hint of what she was suffering in the long nights when she lay awake, listening to the wind in the pines, and haunted always by the memory of Mrs. Hamilton with her sweetly gentle ways.

Whether her letters were reaching their destination, Theodosia could not know. But at last, on an afternoon in August when the mountain air was filled with a mellow, golden haze, Joseph drove up from Charleston and went directly to Theodosia's sitting room to hand her a letter.

In silence she read the few lines—undated, brief. They explained nothing, told her only that her father had left Richmond Hill, and that he was well.

> . . . I shall journey somewhere within a few days, but whither is not yet decided. My heart will travel southward, and repose on the hills of Carolina. Adieu, my dear child . . .

A few days later came another letter, this time dated from Philadelphia. Two of Theodosia's letters had been forwarded to him, and he was pleased to find in one of them an account of some little incident involving Gampy. Still there was no word of his plans, no hint of remorse or regret for what had happened, except for one passage near the end. "Don't let me have the idea that you are dissatisfied with me for a moment," Aaron Burr had written. "I can't just now endure it."

That was all.

Shortly before the time when the Alstons were to leave the mountains, more news came. Mr. Burr wrote that he expected to travel for a while before the opening of Congress made it necessary for him to return to Washington. There was no cause for alarm. The indictment for murder, still pending against him, had been a mere gesture, an expression of hysterical protest, and the action would doubtless come to nothing and be forgotten. For the present it was considered advisable for Mr. Burr to drop out of the public eye, and he proposed, therefore, to go south. Would it be possible for Theodosia to meet him at some village in the mountains near her house?

Theodosia carried the letter to her husband and handed it to him in silence. When he had read it, he looked up and nodded.

"We'll go, of course," he said. "We can arrange to take Gampy with us."

"But, Joseph, how can you, my dear? With everyone crying out against my father and calling him a murderer, it might ruin your career if you went with me to meet him."

Joseph looked into her anxious eyes, smiling a little. "Very well then," he said, without hesitation, "my career will be ruined."

"But, Joseph . . ." She stopped, silenced by her husband's fingers laid gently across her lips.

"Do you think for one moment, Theo, I'd let you go alone? You know," he went on slowly, "that there are some things about your father I've never altogether understood. I don't suppose anyone understands why he chose to do this frightful thing. Certainly I don't. But that's hardly the question now. What's done is done, and you and I will weather together whatever comes, Theo."

Theodosia looked up at him, tall and straight and steady. She saw the tenderness and loyalty that shone in his eyes.

"Oh, Joseph . . ." She stepped closer, and felt his arms close warm and strong about her. There was no need then of words between them.

The meeting with Mr. Burr was arranged after a good deal of difficulty and delay. Nothing could have made Theodosia realize more sharply the terrible change in her father's life than the pitiful subterfuges that were necessary in planning the visit. It was best, he wrote, that they should meet quietly, in some small town where none of them would be recognized. He had established himself in comfortable obscurity at a certain house in Statesburgh and would await their arrival.

They went at once, traveling the short distance in a carriage driven by Joseph himself. Little Gampy, sitting between them, was greatly excited over the prospect of a visit with Big Gampy. On the way he asked a thousand questions. Would Big Gampy tell him stories? Would he remember to bring the red-painted wagon he had promised he would?

But when they reached the house, Gampy hung back suddenly. Clutching at his mother's skirt, he peered about the dingy, close-smelling hall.

"Mummy"—Gampy's voice rose in a wail—"I don't *like* this place."

For a moment Theodosia's heart failed her. Standing in the dusty, poorly lighted corridor, so strangely out of place in her fashionably cut gown and stylish bonnet, she had a sudden impulse to turn and run away, as if from some horrid, unbelievable dream. Surely her father couldn't be waiting here—in this mean and sordid little place. Her fastidious, proud father, who was never satisfied with anything but the most luxurious and tasteful surroundings. In that moment she had a vision of the long ago evening when she and Natalie had reached the tavern in Albany. The fire on the hearth, and the supper Papa had ordered, the bright nosegay beside each plate and a note to tell them of the dancing party that had been planned for Theodosia's birthday.

"Mummy . . ." The boy tugged at her skirt. "I want to go 'way, Mummy. Big Gampy isn't *here!*"

Quickly Theodosia bent to take the small hand in her own. "Come, darling," she said. Her voice was calm and reassuring as she led him up the narrow, uncarpeted stairs. "We must find Big Gampy."

At the top of the steps a door opened, and Mr. Burr stepped out. He was smiling; his head was high. As he embraced his daughter, then lifted the boy in his arms, Theodosia felt the uncertainty and fear ebbing gradually from her heart. This was her father, as courteous, as composed, as self-possessed as ever. He was talking easily, telling Gampy what a big boy he had grown to be, saying how charming Theodosia looked. No dramatics, no apologies for the mean, shabby little bedroom into which he led them.

Theodosia was aware that beneath the casual manner of his greeting, her father was reaching out to her, seeking to ease her over the difficulty of this meeting. He was telling her, in his own way, not to mind the shabbiness of their surroundings, not to think of all that had happened since they last met, but only of the fact that they were together again. With perfect dignity and grace he was refusing to let this moment he spoiled by any shadow of sorrow or disgrace. But she knew better than to put her gratitude and pride into words.

Instead, kneeling to unfasten the buttons of little Gampy's jacket, she smiled up at her father over the boy's head.

"The rooms seem very nice, Papa," was all she said. But she saw the quick approval that lighted his dark eyes, and she knew that he understood.

When Joseph came up, he found Mr. Burr seated on the floor with little Gampy beside him, while Theodosia looked on, smiling at the boy's raptures over the presents his grandfather had brought.

"Look, Papa—just *look!*" Gampy jumped up to run and take his father's hand. "Big Gampy *did* bring the wagon. And it has wheels that go round; and he brought me a horsy that I can *ride!*"

·CHAPTER 17·

High Treason

THE FEW DAYS of the visit passed quickly and pleasantly.
Mr. Burr devoted himself to Gampy, and kept the boy
in such a state of delight with his stories and songs and won-
derfully exciting new games that Theodosia declared he was
the most superior nursemaid she had ever beheld.

Of his plans for the future Mr. Burr spoke little, but always cheerfully. Even the fact that Richmond Hill was now
gone, having been seized by his creditors, and sold to John
Jacob Astor for twenty-five thousand dollars, to cover a portion of his debts, seemed to dismay him not at all. Richmond
Hill was really too large a place for a lonesome bachelor, he
said. His only regret was that his books had been taken by
the creditors along with all the other furnishings.

"But then," he added, "since it seems fairly certain that
I shall find myself without occupation after the coming
elections, I expect I shall have time and to spare to set about
collecting a new library."

That a new vice-president would be chosen to run with Jefferson for the second term was now a foregone conclusion. And to add one last drop of bitterness to the cup, the new vice-president would be George Clinton of New York, Hamilton's great friend and a lifelong enemy of Burr. The political career of Aaron Burr was ended, people said. He would never again be able to show his face in New York. His law practice was destroyed, for surely no clients would trust themselves to be defended by a man who had been indicted as a murderer. His friends, all but a faithful few, were gone, and his fortune, too—seized by his creditors. There was not a person in New York but believed that Aaron Burr was finished, disgraced, and done forever.

Not a person, that is, but one. Aaron Burr himself.

He might be poor, homeless, and without occupation, but he was never for a moment shaken from his conviction that fortune's wheel would take another turn. When he returned to Washington, he took up his official duties for his few remaining weeks as vice-president as serenely as though nothing had happened. With unperturbed dignity he presided over the Senate. A Washington newspaper reported:

> On Saturday, the 2d of March, Mr. Burr took leave of the Senate. It was said to be one of the most dignified and impressive speeches ever uttered.

Mr. Burr left the Senate with expressions of personal respect, and with prayers and good wishes.

So simple and affecting was the speech that "cheers rang for twenty minutes in the Senate chamber when he had finished speaking, and more than half the audience was in tears." A resolution was at once drawn up, and passed unanimously, "That the thanks of the Senate be presented to Aaron Burr, in testimony of the impartiality, dignity, and ability with which he had ever presided over their deliberations. . . ."

As always, no matter what the public attitude toward him might be, those closest to Burr found much to admire in him. So, without bitterness on either side, he left the Senate chamber that afternoon, having bid a last farewell to his career in public life.

The days following his retirement as vice-president were probably the most crucial in the life of Aaron Burr. Which way would he turn now? What would he do?

There were still a few who believed that he might yet re-establish himself in a position of honor and trust in the public eye. One who clung pathetically to this slim hope was Theodosia. But even though his letters to her in those weeks were full of good cheer, she, reading them, was not altogether deceived. As time went on, it began to be plain even to her tender and loyal heart that her father had flaunted public opinion once too often. All his charm, wit, and imperturbable poise would not, for many a day to come, be likely to blot out the shadow of Hamilton's death.

Even Mr. Burr admitted that to return to his law practice in New York was for the present impossible. He had greatly underestimated the length of public memory, and feeling against him was still so strong that, as he wrote to Joseph:

In New York I am to be disenfranchised, and in New Jersey hanged. Having substantial objections to both, I shall not, for the present, hazard either, but shall seek a new country. . . .

But what country, and where?

What does the irresistible force do when confronted by an immovable object? Why, the force simply takes a new direction.

To Theodosia, Mr. Burr wrote of his plans. Immediately after the fourth of March he would leave Washington and go to Pittsburgh, there to embark on a curiously bizarre journey. He would board a houseboat, which he had had specially constructed, and he would travel southwest, following the course of the Ohio River into the Mississippi, and thence to New Orleans. The prospect of this trip seemed to please him. It would give him an opportunity to see a new section of the country, and he expected to stop frequently and visit various friends who were now settled along the river.

But Theodosia remained anxious and troubled. What, she wondered, was the object of this strange pilgrimage? Her father did not say. And who were the friends he spoke of visiting? His letters mentioned them vaguely, naming only Andrew Jackson and General Wilkinson, a gentleman of not altogether savory reputation who was in charge of the American forces in the Southwest, and who was suspected by many of being secretly in the employ of Spain.

To make matters worse, the newspapers, which ever since the duel had reviled and slandered the name of Burr, treated this latest venture to reams of contemptuous comment, not unmixed with amusement. There was a distinct flavor of comic opera in the spectacle of the former vice-president setting out on a houseboat, to float splendidly down a thousand miles of waterway, and in the accounts of the strange cavalcade of Burr and his entourage, the erstwhile villain appeared now as merely a figure of fun.

To Theodosia and Joseph this ridicule was the hardest thing they had yet been called upon to bear. To hold up one's head under tragedy and disgrace is one thing; laughter is quite another.

One morning, over breakfast in the paneled dining room at the Oaks, Joseph flung down his newspaper in disgust.

"Upon my word, Theo," he said, "your father has gone beyond all bounds with this nonsensical voyage. If it's true, as some people think, that he's hatched some sort of plot for gaining political power in the Southwest, then heaven help him. It would be just the chance Jefferson has been waiting for to discredit your father entirely. The Federalists have always hated him. Now with his own party against him, he'd find himself without a single friend in court."

Theodosia made no answer. She turned a fork in her hand, over and over. It was a heavy silver fork—one that her father had given her from Richmond Hill, engraved with the Burr crest.

"God knows, I've tried to understand your father," Joseph went on. "I've admired and respected him—not because he's your father—but because I honestly believed in him. In the Hamilton affair I thought, and still think, that Hamilton was more at fault. I even pitied your father for the accident of circumstances that made everyone turn against him after the duel. But now . . ." He paused and shrugged.

"But now you pity him no longer. Is that it?" Theodosia asked.

"I don't know," Joseph said slowly. "It's hard to pity a man who can never admit he's been mistaken. Your father has so much to make him a great man, Theo. He has brilliance and ambition and energy. And magnificent courage. But he has more pride than any man is entitled to in this world."

Theodosia's hand closed over the fork with its deeply graven crest. "Pride can be a lonely thing, Joseph," she said. "I think if I pity my father for anything, it's for his pride."

But as more time passed, and no new developments came of Mr. Burr's affairs, Theodosia's anxieties grew less. The Alstons' life settled back into untroubled ways. Joseph's work was going well, and as they became more and more engrossed in the busy, pleasant round of days in Charleston, the figure of Aaron Burr faded gradually into the background.

Now, when summer came, there were no more trips to New York. Instead, Joseph took Theodosia and the boy to the mountains again, or to Debordieu Island, where the cool trade winds blew steadily from the sea. Natalie came often to visit, bringing her little Theo to play with Gampy. Then there were long, pleasant days on the beach, while the children built sand castles and paddled in the shallow water, growing brown and sturdy as two young Indians.

They were happy hours for Theodosia, but sometimes, when they all sat together before the blazing pine logs in the cool evenings, a faraway look would come into her eyes and she would watch the flames that leaped and crackled on the hearth. She wondered, then, about her father: when and where they were destined to meet again, and by whose fireside he sat that night.

For many months there was little news from Mr. Burr. Letters came occasionally, but these were mostly comments and instructions to Theodosia for Gampy's first lessons. Now and then a bulky parcel would arrive, with gifts for them all. Feathered Indian headdresses for the boy, and laces and embroideries for Theodosia from the French convents in New Orleans.

Of his own plans and activities he wrote always cheerfully, but in vague terms. By the autumn of 1806 he was on his way north again, traveling by land this time, as he retraced his journey through Tennessee, Kentucky, and Ohio. Again he spoke of visiting friends along the way, and in particular he mentioned a certain Mr. Blennerhassett at whose home, on an island in the Ohio River near Marietta, he had spent a good deal of time.

Joseph frowned over this latest development. But he said nothing to Theodosia of disturbing rumors he had heard in Charleston recently. Rumors of a conspiracy in the Southwest, something about a fantastic plan to conquer Mexico and set up a rival nation on the border of the United States. Rumors in which the names of General Wilkinson and

Blennerhassett figured. Supposing, Joseph thought, Mr. Burr should somehow become involved in this mad scheme? Supposing . . .

There came a day, late that winter, when it was no longer possible for Joseph to keep silent.

It had been a mild afternoon, and Theodosia had driven out in the open carriage, taking young Aaron with her.

As the carriage drew up before the broad front steps of the Oaks, Theodosia gave the boy's shoulder a little pat. "Here we are, Aaron," she said cheerfully. "Out you go, and in to Mammy. We're late for your supper, and I expect we'll both be scolded."

It was not Mammy, but Lottie, who came out the front door and ran down the steps to lift Aaron from the carriage.

"Mr. Alston is in the library, Miss Theodosia," Lottie said. "He says will you come in, please, right away."

Theodosia got out of the carriage quickly. It was odd, she thought, hurrying through the hall and past the dining room. Odd that Joseph should send such a message instead of coming out to meet them himself. She pushed open the library door.

"Joseph . . . ?"

He turned from the window and came straight to her. Then, as if he could not bring himself to speak, he thrust a paper into her hands. "Read this," he said.

She barely glanced at the paper, bewildered by the jumble of strange legal terms.

"I can't understand this, Joseph. Tell me what's happened."

"Your father was arrested, Theo, two weeks ago, by

federal officers, on a charge of high treason. They're bringing him to Richmond for trial. The news just reached
Charleston this morning. I can't find out any more than
what is printed in the papers, though I've been trying all
day."

Theodosia walked over to a sofa and sat down. Slowly,
very carefully, she began to draw off her gloves. Papa had
sent her these gloves for her birthday last year, she thought.
Joseph was talking, trying to explain this puzzling, dreadful
thing.

Her father and Mr. Blennerhassett were accused, Joseph
was saying, of a plot to separate the southwestern states from
the Union. They had raised an armed force in secret, and
their plan had been to take possession of Kentucky, Tennessee, and Louisiana and establish the territory as an independent nation. Later they were to invade and conquer Mexico, and there, it was said, Mr. Burr had intended to set himself up as an emperor.

Suddenly, as the meaning of Joseph's words reached
her, Theodosia flung aside her gloves and stood up.

"Joseph, *stop!*" Her face was white, but she faced him
bravely. "I—I can't let you say these things, Joseph. *Treason
. . . traitor . . .* these words have nothing to do with my
father. My father loves his country, whatever his faults may
be. You must know that. You must *believe* it, Joseph."

"Theo, my dearest girl"—Joseph put his hands on her
shoulders and looked down into the desperate pleading of
her eyes—"I don't know yet what to believe. We can't know
the truth until your father has had a chance to explain and
defend himself. I'm only trying to tell you what's happened,

Theo. To explain how serious these charges are. God knows," he said gently, "I'd give anything I own to spare you this. Even yet, it may come out all right. Your father will have to prove his innocence, though with the trial in Virginia, Mr. Jefferson's own home state, I wonder——"

"Mr. Jefferson," Theodosia broke in eagerly. "Why, don't you see, Joseph? Mr. Jefferson can help Papa. Surely, if I write him, he'll know best how to straighten out this horrible mistake. I'll write to him, and explain everything . . ."

She crossed to the desk and searched hastily for paper and pen. But before she could begin to write, Joseph's hand closed over hers.

"It's no use, Theo." He drew the pen from her fingers and laid it gently aside. "The order for your father's arrest was signed by President Jefferson."

·CHAPTER 18·

If It Please the Court

THE TRIAL OF Aaron Burr for treason was a national sensation. For days, before the arrival of the prisoner, Richmond was seething with excitement. From miles around, people gathered, anxious for a glimpse of this villain who had dared to attempt the most flagrant plot ever uncovered against the United States.

Zachary Taylor was there, and Winfield Scott. Young Washington Irving, who had once been an apprentice in the law office of Mr. Burr, had been sent by a New York newspaper to write articles covering the trial. And General Andrew Jackson came up from Tennessee, to stamp about the corridors of the Old Eagle Tavern in his rough boots and startle the courtly Virginians by proclaiming loudly that his friend Burr had been the victim of trumped-up evidence, manufactured by General Wilkinson and basely used by Jefferson in an attempt to discredit the former Vice-president.

A few voices, here and there, were heard to agree with

Jackson's. But only a few. In general, people were ready to condemn Burr.

"Let's hang the traitor and be done with it," they said angrily.

Probably no man on trial for his life ever walked into a more thoroughly hostile atmosphere than Aaron Burr did on the spring afternoon when he was escorted into the Old Eagle Tavern. But he carried off the moment in true Burr style.

Stepping out of the carriage, he paused to survey the angry, threatening faces that pressed around him. For an instant Mr. Burr hesitated, then, raising his hat, he made a gracious bow and smiled pleasantly.

The crowd shifted uneasily. A current of uncertainty passed through them. This was not what they'd expected at all. They had been prepared for a villain, and here was a man who smiled and bowed and didn't look in the least villainous.

He was small and slight, and it was plain to see he was a gentleman. There was something surprisingly likable about the way he held his head up and looked straight at them.

There was a sudden stir near the tavern door, and General Jackson came out, shouldering his way through the crowd to thrust out a long arm and shake Mr. Burr's hand vigorously.

"Come along inside, sir. Don't let these gawping folk trouble you," Jackson's voice boomed out as he turned to glare at the crowd from under bristling red eyebrows. "They've only come to rubber at the newest curiosity. And don't be worrying about this trial. Three days before any fair court, and I'll guarantee you'll show up the whole thing for what it's worth. A mean, ornery plot against you, cooked up by Jefferson——"

"Take it calmly, Jackson," Mr. Burr's voice broke in with easy good humor. "Save your breath for the jury. I have a presentiment we may need it." With a last amiable nod for the spectators, Mr. Burr turned to follow his guards, and disappeared through the tavern door.

From that day public sentiment toward the prisoner was divided. To many, it still seemed that Burr was guilty. But guilty or no, there was a likable quality about Burr that couldn't be denied. More and more, as days went on, people felt more kindly toward him. He was quiet, he was well-behaved, and no matter how Mr. Hay, the prosecuting attorney, thundered his charges, Mr. Burr only smiled. And the longer the trial dragged on the less serious the charges against him appeared.

The main reason for the delay, which was so fortunate to Burr's cause, was the failure of General Wilkinson to appear in Richmond. He was the chief witness against Burr. The trial could not proceed without him, for it was Wilkinson who had informed Jefferson of the conspiracy, and on his statement depended the proof of Burr's guilty intentions.

And where, people asked of one another, *was* this mysterious Wilkinson? Why wasn't he present in Richmond?

This was the question that dominated the first sessions before the Grand Jury.

Chief Justice John Marshall of the Supreme Court presided over the small courtroom in the State Capitol. It was a little like a circus, those first few days. The room was packed and jammed to overflowing. People stood on chairs and tables, craned over other people's heads and shoulders for a glimpse of the prisoner who sat, with his counsel, at a bench near the rostrum. The Chief Justice had all he could do to maintain decent order. He struck his gavel, again and again, but the crowd simply would not be silent.

Sitting between Edmund Randolph and John Wickham, the lawyers engaged for his defense, Mr. Burr watched the proceedings with a detached and courteous interest. Now and then, when some point of dispute arose, the prisoner would rise, bow politely to Chief Justice Marshall, and offer a suggestion or motion.

There was the increasingly embarrassing absence of General Wilkinson. Again and again, when some point of evidence arose that involved the testimony of the missing Wilkinson, Mr. Burr would inquire, with ironic surprise, *why* Wilkinson was not yet present in Richmond.

Had he not been subpoenaed? He most certainly had.

Had not the prosecution had ample time to fetch their star witness? They most certainly had.

Well, then, Mr. Burr would suggest in his smoothest, most deferential tone, perhaps Mr. Jefferson might know the whereabouts of General Wilkinson.

The point never failed to score.

Gradually the trial began to take on more and more the aspect of a farce. Here was the court, here was the Grand Jury, here was the prisoner. But where was the evidence against him?

Time passed. The trial had been called for early April.

Nearly two months passed.

Still no Wilkinson.

Frantic communications passed between Prosecutor Hay and President Jefferson in Washington. How, Mr. Hay demanded, could the President expect him to convict this man Burr when the chief witness and informer against him could not be produced?

At last, on the thirteenth of June, General Wilkinson arrived. But it was too late for the prosecution to work up much confidence in their witness. He blustered and thundered, contradicted himself on a dozen points, and shook his fist accusingly in the direction of the smiling, composed prisoner.

Never had Mr. Burr's natural manner of easy detachment stood him in better stead than now. In contrast to General Wilkinson, Burr's quiet voice, his thorough knowledge of the legal points, made an impression in his favor.

Not that people in general believed Burr to be innocent. It seemed plain enough that he had actually plotted with his friend Blennerhassett to raise an armed force with which they would ultimately march into Mexico and take possession of that territory. Indeed, Mr. Burr himself admitted this. The point of difference between Burr and his accusers lay in the distinction as to just *who* was to profit by his schemes of empire?

Said his accusers: Burr wished to establish himself as dictator of an empire in the Southwest.

Said Burr: Why, no such thing. He had merely meant to acquire the Mexican territory *for* the United States.

Wilkinson's testimony served only to discredit himself, for his own part in the alleged conspiracy was so hopelessly confused that he appeared a fool as well as a rogue. Whereas Mr. Burr was certainly no fool.

Mr. Hay did his best with the case, but the cards were badly stacked against him. Although, eleven days after Wilkinson's appearance, the Grand Jury formally indicted Burr on two counts, treason and misdemeanor, nobody, least of all Mr. Burr himself, took the indictment seriously.

On the morning when it was handed down, and Justice Marshall ordered that the prisoner should now be removed from his comfortable quarters at the Eagle Tavern and confined to the penitentiary, Mr. Burr emerged from the court with his customary smile and bow for the curious crowd, and contented himself by observing, as he stepped into the carriage, that now he was moving to jail, his friends would always find him at home.

So the lengthy trial proceeded again. More visitors than ever arrived in Richmond. The array of witnesses lent a carnival air to the quiet, genteel city. There were raftsmen from the Ohio River barges, planters and politicians from Kentucky and Tennessee, Spaniards from New Orleans, whose swarthy complexions looked fiercely out of place in the mild Virginia landscape.

Justice Marshall, dignified and impartial, presided in the packed courtroom. In spite of his efforts, there was a continual buzz of conversation, particularly from the gallery where the fashionably gowned ladies peered around each others bonnets for a glimpse of the prisoner, and whispered to one another.

"Which one is Burr?"

"The dark one, at the table there. With the black coat and white stock."

"Oh! . . . Very *handsome,* isn't he? I suppose that's Wilkinson, the gray-haired one with the shifty eye. Revolting-looking creature."

"Shh, listen. Burr is getting up to say something."

In the midst of the trial Mr. Burr produced his greatest surprise. If it please the court, Mr. Burr asked permission to subpoena one more witness in his own defense.

Justice Marshall nodded. Who was it the defendant wish to call?

Mr. Burr would like to subpoena Thomas Jefferson, President of the United States, and demand that he produce, as material evidence, certain papers, now in his possession, relating directly to General Wilkinson's part in the alleged conspiracy for which Mr. Burr was being tried.

There was a gasp of astonishment from the spectators. Then a burst of excited comment. Fancy Burr daring to ask that the President be called in *defense* of the prisoner.

Mr. Hay was on his feet at once, protesting angrily that Mr. Burr's request was brazen impudence, and deserved a rebuke as such.

But Justice Marshall, rapping sternly for order, leaned across the desk to ask a question. Was Mr. Burr reliably informed that these papers were actually in the possession of Mr. Jefferson?

Mr. Burr was. He was likewise positive that they bore directly upon the case in hand, and would shed considerable light on the value of General Wilkinson's testimony.

A pause, while the Justice considered. Then in a sober, unemotional voice, Marshall gave his decision. Under the circumstances, he could see no reason why the President should not be served with a subpoena, and ordered to produce the papers in question.

Further sensation among the spectators. This was amazing, truly—and wholly without precedent.

Mr. Hay, his face very red, sat down. He was heard by those near him to observe bitterly, "Burr must be inspired by the devil himself to know about those papers!"

Whatever his inspiration, Mr. Burr proved to be right. Jefferson was duly subpoenaed, and although he was excused from appearing in person at the trial, he was compelled to send the papers as evidence. And quite as Burr had asserted, they shed a new and unfavorable light on the reliability of Wilkinson's testimony.

Mr. Burr's defense of his own actions was simple, and disarmingly candid. He had purchased a good deal of land in Louisiana, during his visit in New Orleans. He freely admitted that he had conferred with his friend Blennerhassett on the possibility of organizing a group of men to settle this land. The two men, encouraged by General Wilkinson, had discussed the possibility of mobilizing their settlers into a sort of private army, for the purpose of taking over a portion of Mexico, now belonging to Spain.

But—and here Mr. Burr was very emphatic—they had at no time considered or even mentioned any plan to sever any states from the Union.

A fantastic, storybook sort of explanation, to be sure. But still it *was* an explanation. Any way you looked at it, people said, the Mexican venture had been a thoroughly wild scheme. And when it was brought out in evidence that the total armed forces which the defendant had mustered consisted of some fifty-odd adventurers, owning, among them, a dozen rifles, the whole thing appeared more ridiculous than ever.

As for Wilkinson, it was now plain to be seen that his reasons for disclosing the alleged plot to Jefferson had been prompted by nothing more than his own dissatisfaction with the share of the "proceeds" allotted to him by Burr.

So the weeks passed, each day's evidence establishing more and more surely the fact that neither the accusers nor the accused deserved any particular respect, and that Jefferson—the great Jefferson—had been fooled by the rascally Wilkinson.

Except for Justice Marshall and the unfortunate Mr. Hay, no one took anything pertaining to the trial very seriously any more. Certainly, the prisoner, after the first tense weeks, appeared to be rather enjoying himself.

CHAPTER 19

The Hour of Noon

BUT TO THEODOSIA, in Charleston, the weeks that passed so quickly and in such excitement in Richmond were a different story. She had only two sources of information as to how the trial progressed: the newspapers, with their lurid accounts of the proceedings at Richmond, and her father's letters.

These, to be sure, were cheerful enough. But then he was always cheerful, and she knew from long and bitter experience that his efforts to minimize anything unfavorable to himself were by no means always to be trusted. Letters, such as the one in which he described his new "lodgings" in the Richmond jail, brought her small comfort, for all the lightheartedness of his tone:

> I have three rooms in the third floor of the penitentiary [he wrote] making an extent of one hundred feet. My jailer is quite a polite and civil man—altogether unlike the idea one would form of a jailer. You would have laughed to hear our compliments the first evening.

Jailer: I hope, sir, it would not be disagreeable to you if I should lock this door after dark.

Burr: By no means, sir; I should prefer it, to keep out intruders.

Jailer: It is our custom, sir, to extinguish all lights at nine o'clock; I hope, sir, you will have no objection to conform to that.

Burr: That, sir, I am sorry to say, is impossible; for I never go to bed till twelve, and always burn two candles.

Jailer: Very well, sir, just as you please. I should have been glad if it had been otherwise; but, as you please, sir.

While I have been writing different servants have arrived with messages, notes, and inquiries, bringing oranges, lemons, pineapples, raspberries, apricots, cream, butter, ice and some ordinary articles.

That Mr. Burr was aware of the sober side of this proceeding, and of the pain and anxiety Theodosia was suffering, was shown in a briefer and quite different passage written to her a few days later.

He had urged her to come to Richmond and be present at the trial. She had hesitated. He guessed that the reason for her reluctance was her dread of seeing him in a position of humiliation—the accused prisoner before the court. Very kindly and understandingly, he let her know that she need fear no such painful spectacle.

. . . I should never invite anyone, much less those so dear to me, to witness my disgrace. . . . I cannot be humiliated or disgraced. If absent, you will suffer great solicitude. In my presence you will feel none. . . .

Nevertheless, Theodosia continued to feel bitterly the shame of the position in which her father now found himself. That he, who had served his country as a soldier of the

Revolution, who had only a few years ago narrowly missed being elected to the presidency itself, should now be brought before a court and charged with high treason was the cruelest blow she had ever suffered. To see her father who had had such a wealth of opportunities before him—who might, if only fate and his own nature had varied *ever so slightly,* have attained the greatest honor and dignity—reduced to hoping at best for a dubious victory, following a shamefully shabby trial, cut her to the heart.

Finally it was arranged that Joseph should visit Mr. Burr in Richmond. He returned a few weeks later to report to Theodosia that her father's health and spirits were excellent.

"On my word, Theo," Joseph said, in an odd mixture of despair and amusement, "your father is the hero of Richmond. His rooms in the penitentiary are a great deal more like a fashionable apartment than a jail. Visitors come and go all day. The best families in Richmond send their servants with baskets of flowers, and hampers of home-cooked foods. You never saw such an assortment. Roasted birds, cakes and pies, and so many bottles of the choicest wines that your father says he'll soon have to petition the jailer for the use of the cellar to store them in."

Theodosia shook her head with a sigh. "I don't like it, Joseph," she said.

"Nor do I," Joseph answered soberly. "I couldn't help but admire his courage. But a man can defy his fate just so far. I've wondered sometimes whether perhaps the shock of the duel and all the trouble that followed may not have changed your father more than he realizes."

"Sometimes," Theodosia said slowly, "I've wondered, too." She was silent for a moment. "If only we could do something to help him, to bring him back to himself . . ."

"I think, perhaps, if you would be willing to go to Richmond . . ." Joseph hesitated, seeing the quick look of distress in his wife's eyes. "I know it's asking a great deal of you, Theo. But still, your father is on trial for his life."

Theodosia looked up. "I do want to go, Joseph," she said quietly. "It's been selfish of me to refuse, simply because I dreaded to see my father a prisoner. If he needs me, I shan't hesitate any longer."

Within a few days they were packing to leave for Richmond. It was arranged that Natalie should come and stay at the Oaks while they were gone. It was the first time Theodosia had really been separated from her son, and she pressed a thousand anxious directions on Natalie.

"You *will* be careful about his food, won't you, Natalie?" Theodosia said for the twentieth time. "He's always been dreadfully susceptible to fevers. Oh, dear, if I could only divide myself in half, and send one part to Richmond while the other half stayed here."

Natalie was comfortingly certain that all would be well. "Since you must remain all in one piece, Theo, it's Papa who needs you just now far more than young Aaron. And, Theo, you won't forget to give Papa my dearest love? And write me exactly how things are going?"

The night before the Alstons reached Richmond, they stopped at an inn in Fayetteville. Theodosia found a note from her father waiting.

Under no circumstances, her father wrote, was she to allow herself the slightest twinge of sentimental pity or concern on his account:

> . . . I beg and expect it of you that you will conduct yourself as becomes my daughter, and that you manifest no signs of weakness or alarm. Remember, no agitations, no complaints, no fears and anxieties on the road, or I renounce thee.

Just as on that other occasion, in the dingy little inn at Statesburgh, Theodosia resolved to met him with the dignity he required of her. When they arrived next afternoon in Richmond, and drove directly to the penitentiary, her head was lifted proudly. There was in her manner no slightest hint that she looked forward to the meeting with anything but pleasant anticipation.

John Prevost was at the door to greet them. "It's good to see you, Theo-mio." John's round, cheerful face shone with brotherly affection. "And, my word, how handsome you look. Come along upstairs. Papa is in the greatest wax of impatience, waiting for your arrival. He's sent me down at least a dozen times in the last hour to watch for your carriage."

"John, how is he?" A shadow came into Theodosia's eyes.

"Never better," John said quickly. He tucked her hand beneath his arm and turned to lead her up the steps and into the gray stone corridor. "Only one thing has troubled him, and that's been his concern for you. But one glance will be enough to show him that his Theo hasn't the slightest intention of pining away."

If one thing more had been needed to sway the balance of popular opinion in favor of Mr. Burr, the appearance of Theodosia in Richmond accomplished it. Already people were disposed to *like* the prisoner. For Theodosia they went one step further: they *trusted* her completely. Her appearances in the courtroom, where she sat quietly in the gallery, observing the proceedings with an air of gentle dignity, did more for her father's cause than all the array of witnesses who were called to testify in his behalf.

But for the most part she wisely refrained from attending the hearings. While Joseph went each morning, to sit with Mr. Burr and his attorneys, Theodosia was busy attending to her borrowed household. Daily she visited her father's rooms in what he called his "town house" and saw that everything there was arranged for his comfort. Nearly every evening she and Joseph and John were permitted to dine with Mr. Burr, and in the pleasant companionship of the little family circle they seemed to forget that barred windows cast a grim shadow of doubt over the future.

Never for one moment did Mr. Burr allow that shadow to depress them. Theodosia wrote to Natalie that her father had seldom been in better spirits. How much of his good humor was assumed for their sakes, she added, even she couldn't guess.

On the morning of Tuesday, the first of September, Theodosia was in her small first-floor sitting room. The day before, Justice Marshall had directed the jury to retire and consider its verdict on the guilt or innocence of Aaron **Burr.**

It was a fair morning, bright with a warm sun that streamed in the front windows and shone across the desk where Theodosia sat writing to her brother Frederic and his wife. She was alone. Joseph had gone to court as usual.

"You must go, of course, Joseph," Theodosia had insisted. "If the decision is favorable, I'm quite willing to wait a little longer for the good news. And if the verdict should go against Papa"—she paused—"he'll need you far more than I."

She sat now, writing steadily, while the small gilt clock on the mantel ticked away the minutes in the quiet room. The outcome, she wrote, was as yet unknown, but whatever it might be, she believed that somehow, in some place, her father's name would still be freed from the shadow of the word "traitor." As for herself and Joseph and John, they were all well. People in Richmond had been kindness itself, showing her "the most delicate attentions and sympathy."

The clock whirred, making ready to strike the hour of noon. Any moment now, she thought, the word might come. The last chiming note died into silence, and there was a loud knock at the door.

Theodosia rose. From the back of the house she could hear a servant coming to answer the door, but she did not wait. The silk folds of her skirt rustled lightly as she hurried into the hall.

A strange youth, standing on the doorstep, looked up at her curiously.

"Mrs. Alston?"

"Yes."

"A message for you, ma'am. From Mr. Burr."

She took the paper and opened it with steady fingers. In her father's meticulous hand, was written:

The jury has brought in a verdict. Not guilty. God bless thee.

A. Burr

·CHAPTER 20·

Farewell

O N THEIR RETURN to Charleston, the Alstons found
that young Aaron had been ill for ten days before
their arrival. It was nothing serious, Natalie assured them.
She'd called Dr. Logan at once, and he had said it was the
fever again, and put the boy to bed on a diet of thin gruel
and barley water.

Fevers, after all, were to be expected in this season.
Scarcely a child in the South escaped them, and parents
learned to accept philosophically the sight of plump, rosy
cheeks turned pale, and small bodies grown thin and languid.

Nevertheless, Theodosia and Joseph were alarmed, and
for the first few days after their home-coming they had no
thought for anything but their son. Little by little he began
to improve.

"Tell me about Big Gampy, Mum," he asked one day.
"Why didn't he come home with you?"

"Because he had to go north, dear. On business. But he

148

sent you all sorts of messages and a wonderful surprise I've been keeping until you felt stronger."

Theodosia went to fetch a box of lead soldiers, gaily painted, and began to set them up on the bed.

"See how fine and brave they look, Aaron." She smiled, remembering the day her father had left the courtroom after his acquittal, and how he had driven, the first thing, to a shop in Richmond to hunt out a gift for his grandson. "These soldiers on horseback are the cavalry, and this one in the cocked hat is their colonel."

"Like my grandfather was in the war," Aaron said eagerly. He propped himself up on one thin elbow to examine the little lead officer in his blue-painted coat. "Will Big Gampy be coming to visit later, Mum? When his business is finished?"

"I hope so, dear. But it may not be right away. He's thinking of taking a long trip. To England, perhaps, and France, where Natalie used to live."

"Oh!" The boy dropped back against the pillow. "France is awfully far away. Natalie says it took days and days to come from there."

"Yes, I know. But wherever Gampy is, no matter how far away, he's always thinking of us, Aaron. You must remember that."

By the time winter came Aaron was quite well. Dr. Logan assured Theodosia that she had no more cause to worry about him. "Let the boy start riding next week," he advised, "and keep him outdoors as much as you can. We'll soon have him as good as new again."

In the late spring Theodosia learned that her father was to sail for England within the month. All his friends advised him, and he agreed, that it was best for him to be out of the country for the time being. How long he might be absent, he could not say. But he must go.

Theodosia began at once to make plans for a trip to New York. Although her father had carefully refrained from asking her to come, she sensed, for the first time, a certain loneliness in him. And she felt that they must have the comfort of one last brief visit together before he set out on the long journey.

Joseph agreed. But since his work would keep him in the legislature, Theodosia sailed alone from Charleston. Six days later she was in New York.

She soon discovered the extent of the bitter humiliation her father had endured since the September afternoon when they had parted in Richmond. Even though the court had acquitted him, the shadow of disgrace still hung over him. And though he remained self-possessed and calm as ever, she saw in their first meeting that his old bravado was shaken.

Joseph had once said, "A man can defy his fate just so far." Now, it seemed, the fate that Aaron Burr had for so long refused to admit or accept had caught up with him at last. No man can live without making mistakes, but Mr. Burr, for all his brilliance and ability, had chosen his mistakes with peculiarly disastrous genius. The very qualities which had once made him strong—his stubborn independence, his reckless scorn for public opinion, above all, his fatal pride— had made him seem almost invulnerable. But there had been no provision in his iron code for the possibility of defeat, and now that defeat had come it was too late to change.

Again, Theodosia reflected sadly, it was Joseph who had said, "It's hard to pity a man who can never admit he's been mistaken." Long ago Aaron Burr had chosen to walk alone. And now, except for a handful of friends who remained loyal, he must be content to travel his way—alone.

The debts which he had accumulated over the years, with such a blandly cheerful disregard for the day of reckoning, now rose up like angry ghosts to torment him. Even though it was commonly known that he was financially ruined, his harrying creditors pursued him, determined, at least, that he shouldn't escape the country a free man.

Because of these creditors, and their relentless efforts to throw her father into the debtor's court, Theodosia was forced to meet him secretly—here for an hour, there for a few minutes—always at night and under a cover of mystery and subterfuge that grieved and dismayed her.

Early in June the packet boat *Clarissa* lay at anchor in the Narrows of New York harbor, awaiting a fair wind to set sail for England. A passage had been engaged in the name of Mr. G. H. Edwards, for a gentleman who was to share a modest cabin with three strangers.

Late on the night of June sixth, a skiff was rowed out from the Long Island shore to where the *Clarissa* rode the quiet sea under a calm, starlit sky. A rather small man, something over middle age, to judge from his appearance, left the skiff and came aboard the *Clarissa* where he was met, as prearranged, by the captain.

"Mr. Edwards?"

"Yes."

"Good evening, sir. Everything has been arranged, I hope to your satisfaction."

"I'm very grateful, captain." The small man bowed. "My wants will be very simple, I assure you."

"Your instructions have been carefully followed. No one but myself has been informed of your presence."

"Excellent. When do you plan to sail, captain?"

"At dawn, if the wind holds. Is there anything I can do to make you comfortable before you go to your cabin, Mr. Edwards?"

"Only one favor, if it's not too much trouble." The small man drew a letter from his pocket. "I should be very grateful if this could be sent ashore by the pilot boat in the morning. It's to go to Mrs. Joseph Alston. The address is noted."

On the morning of June seventh, Theodosia woke early. She rose at once and went to the window that faced south, across the trees and promenade of Battery Park to the harbor dotted with ships. Anxiously, her eyes searched the horizon for the spot where, for the past week, the *Clarissa* had been visible. There was nothing there now. Only an empty stretch of blue water glittered beneath the early summer sun. "Farewell, Papa," Theodosia whispered softly. "Farewell."

Then she dressed quickly, and went to the desk where a package of folded papers lay. The evening before, her father had given them to her, with instructions. They were notes and accounts representing various sums of money due him.

"Contrary to the general opinion," he had said with an

odd smile, "I not only borrowed considerable money, but also, on occasion, lent it. You'll find the notes here, duly signed and witnessed. Also a number of uncollected fees from my formerly grateful law clients. If you can manage to raise any portion of the cash, and forward it to me, it will be useful. I'm asking you to do it, instead of John or Van Ness, because the people who owe me are mostly your friends. No lawyer would stand a ghost of a chance of collecting the money, with me out of the country. But an appeal from you, I think, they will scarcely dare to refuse. Believe me, Theo," he had added, "I dislike asking such a disagreeable favor of you, but, at present, it seems that fate leaves me little choice in anything."

Selecting two or three of the more promising accounts, Theodosia rose from the desk. She had slept poorly, and a dull, nagging ache throbbed miserably behind her eyes. Nevertheless, she put on her best mantle of blue silk, and adjusted a small velvet-trimmed hat to just the proper tilt.

At the first office, that of a prominent judge who, in years past, had often dined at Richmond Hill, Theodosia was asked to wait in the dim, walnut-paneled anteroom. This wasn't going to be too bad, after all, she thought. There couldn't be anything very terrifying, surely, in talking to the judge, whom she remembered as a kindly, whiskered gentleman interested in horses and sailing.

When the clerk came back, she stood up quickly.

But instead of showing her in, the young man began to speak rapidly, his pale eyes never quite meeting hers. He was extremely sorry, it was *most* unfortunate that the judge hap-

pened to be, on this particular morning, unusually pressed
for time. He sent his warmest compliments to Mrs. Alston.
In the meantime, if there were anything the clerk might do
. . . or if she cared to leave a message . . .

Theodosia took up her gloves and handbag. She was
grateful for the judge's kindness, but there was no message.

The young man leaped to open the door for her, and
bowed with effusive, nervous politeness as she walked swiftly
past him and down the worn, wooden steps.

Once in the street, she stood for a moment as if uncertain
which way to turn. All about her, people moved with quick,
purposeful steps, intent upon the business that carried them
in and out of the red-brick office buildings that lined Wall
Street. Though the sun was high now and waves of heat rose
shimmeringly from the cobbled pavement, Theodosia felt
a shiver pass through her and drew the light silk of her
mantle closer.

Then, opening her handbag, she glanced at the address
on the second paper. It was a number in Maiden Lane.

For days Theodosia continued to make her weary
rounds. In one anteroom after another she waited, with
patient dignity, for some young clerk to return with a message. Occasionally the men she sought would see her. They
would greet her with friendly courtesy, and talk cordially
enough until she broached the subject of her father's accounts. Then their smiles would grow thin, or vanish altogether, and they would speak vaguely of troubled times, and
many commitments which, to their regret, made any im-

mediate action quite impossible. Perhaps, if Mrs. Alston would return some time in the future . . .

Toward the end of the month, Theodosia left the city and went to visit Frederic and his wife in Pelham. There, in the cool quiet of the country, where the water lapped peacefully along the curving shore, she could forget for a while the long procession of dim, paneled office anterooms and the apologetic faces of pale young clerks.

But Frederic was alarmed by the deep shadows of weariness that ringed her eyes.

"You've got to stop this, Theo," he said firmly when she told him what she had been attempting to do. "Father would a thousand times rather starve—though you may be sure it won't come to that—than have you wearing yourself out on his account."

"But I must try a little longer, Frederic. I shall write some letters while I'm here. Perhaps that's a better plan than calling in person. And it isn't as if I were asking favors. These people owe Papa money. Every one of them."

Frederic shook his head and sighed. "Just now," he said slowly, "anything connected with the name of Burr is a doomed cause. The sooner you realize that the better. Besides, you'll make yourself ill going on like this. Already you look as dragged out as a drowned kitten."

"Oh, surely, Frederic, not that bad." She smiled. "I'm not ill, only tired. And I think, for the first time in my life, a little homesick."

The letters over which she worked so long and patiently brought no better results. At length, worn out with strain and discouragement, and desperately lonely for Joseph and Aaron, she began to feel feverish and miserable. Writing to her father one day, she was forced to admit that all her efforts to collect his money had utterly failed.

> Except myself, all your friends are well. But the world begins to cool terribly around me. You would be surprised how many I supposed attached to me have abandoned the sorry, losing game of disinterested friendship. Frederic and John alone, however, are worth a host. Adieu once more . . .

Only John came to see Theodosia off on the morning when she sailed from New York. Looking back to where he stood on the pier, waving his hat, she could hear him calling to her cheerfully above the clanging confusion of harbor sounds.

"Good-by, Theo-mio. Get well soon, and my love to young Aaron. Don't forget."

"Good-by, dear John."

Tears of weakness were in her eyes as she stood by the rail later, watching the shore line of New York gradually recede. It seemed almost a strange city to her now, somehow different. Yet nothing had really changed at all. The spire of old Trinity still rose, straight and slim, above the peaked roofs, and somewhere, just out of sight beyond the curving shore, the green lawns of Richmond Hill still sloped down to the fringe of willows that bordered on the broad, blue river.

A fair wind was with them nearly all the way to Charleston. It was late afternoon, getting on toward dusk, when they dropped anchor in the harbor and the passengers gathered on deck to look for familiar faces among those who waited on the dock. None searched more eagerly than Theodosia.

Suddenly she leaned over the rail to wave excitedly, and the other passengers, who had observed her during the voyage, always alone, reading or looking sadly out to sea, were surprised now to see how very young and pretty she looked.

A few minutes later Theodosia was going down the gangplank. Joseph hurried toward her and young Aaron, in a new blue suit and sailor hat, hurled himself upon his mother with a joyful shout.

"Oh, Aaron, *darling,* how huge you look! You must have grown inches while I was gone. And Joseph . . ." Theodosia straightened and turned, smiling with all her heart, as his arms, strong and sure, held her close.

"Oh, Joseph—Joseph," she whispered against his shoulder. "You can't possibly know how *good* it is to come home."

·CHAPTER 21·

Christmas Eve

I T WAS CHRISTMAS EVE in Charleston, and a light, wet snow was falling. Down through the gaunt, black cypress trees it drifted, frosting the strands of Spanish moss until they sparkled like lace in the light of a misty moon.

On a hill, just outside the town, stood the Orphanage where the boys and girls, who were young Dr. Logan's special charges, were in the midst of a Christmas feast. The bare dining room, with its long wooden tables, had been trimmed with bright festoons of holly, and each of the small guests wore a gay paper hat that contrasted oddly with the plain gray stuff of the little boys' suits and the girls' sober frocks of serviceable brown cambric.

At the head table, next to Dr. Logan, Theodosia sat smiling down the long line of happy, well-scrubbed faces. Small fists were busily stuffing away quantities of roast turkey.

"I do wish Joseph could be here to see the children," Theodosia said. "He sent especially to the plantation for the turkeys. But at the last minute some visitors arrived from Washington on business, and he had to receive them."

"It was good of you to come and bring Aaron." The doctor smiled. "I was afraid my young ones might be shy with him at first, but from the looks of things he seems to have made friends without much trouble."

Theodosia glanced down the table to where her son was devouring his dinner as eagerly as any, talking meanwhile, through a mouthful of turkey, to a little girl beside him.

"There's one thing to be said for Aaron," she said laughingly. "He's never at a loss for words. I expect that's what comes of having a father and a grandfather in politics, not to mention all his ancestors who were preachers."

After supper they trimmed the Christmas tree. Whatever shyness the children might still have felt in the presence of the visitors vanished entirely at the sight of the huge hampers, crammed with good things, that Theodosia knelt down to unpack. There were figs and dates, walnuts and cinnamon sticks, and enough striped peppermints, Theodosia said, to guarantee a hundred stomach-aches the following morning.

Each child, from the tallest, gangling boy to one baby girl who could scarcely walk, had a turn at putting his own bit of decoration on the tree. When they had finished, the broad green branches had all but disappeared beneath garlands of strung popcorn and scarlet cranberries.

There were games for another hour, and while the children romped and shouted through Blind Man's Bluff and

London Bridge Is Falling Down, Theodosia and the doctor stood together near the big fireplace where the pine logs crackled.

After a few minutes, Theodosia spoke hesitantly. "I have one more surprise for the children, Dr. Logan, but first I wanted to ask your approval. Some weeks ago I wrote to my father, and happened to mention the Orphanage, and the work you were doing with the children here. Yesterday I had an answer from him, written from Paris, and enclosing a check. He said it would make him very happy if you would divide it among the children, so that each one would have a little pocket money of his own to spend as he chooses. I"— she paused uncertainly, and then went on, her voice very low—"I don't know what sort of things you may have heard of my father, but I've brought the check—in case you care to accept it."

Dr. Logan took the slip of paper. "People say many things about Mr. Burr," he said slowly, "but nothing I hear in the future will ever make me forget this. I can guess what it meant to him to send this gift. Most of these children have never had a penny of their own to spend. I dare say your father guessed that. Shall I tell them who sent the money, Mrs. Alston?"

Theodosia shook her head. "Just say it came from someone very far away," she said.

On the way home that night Theodosia and Aaron heard the bells of St. Michael's chiming the hour as they turned into King Street where the damp snow had clung to the iron grillwork on the balconies of the tall brick houses, making them look like patterns of spun sugar.

"Ten o'clock," Theodosia said. "It's quite scandalously late for you to be out, sir. But I hope you had a good time."

Aaron wriggled comfortably under the fur rug beside her. "I had three helps of turkey, Mum, but that wasn't the most. One of the other boys had four. I wish I could play up there every day. I like the children much better than the ones I know."

"I like them, too. Suppose we ask Dr. Logan to bring some of the boys and girls to the house someday soon. And later, in the spring, we might have a picnic at the Oaks for all of them. Do you know"—she looked out the carriage window—"it almost looks as if we might have a white Christmas as we used to in New York. Then we had sleighs instead of carriages, and the horses had bells on their harnesses so the whole city would sound like a jingling music box. When I was a little girl I'd stay awake just to listen to them. My nurse was always cross about it. She said sleigh bells were nonsense. But then"—she laughed—"Nanny always thought things that were fun were nonsense."

"I guess all nurses are the same." Aaron sighed. "I'm awfully glad I'm almost nine now, and don't have to have Mammy any more. I always liked you and Papa much better than I liked Mammy."

"Did you, Aaron?"

"Oh, yes." After a moment he added. "You always let me have more sweets, you see."

When Aaron had been put to bed, Theodosia went into

her sitting room across the hall. Joseph was still busy with the visitors downstairs. She could hear their voices as she crossed the landing.

She paused by the desk, half intending to write her father a description of the Christmas supper at the Orphanage, telling him how gratefully Dr. Logan had received his gift for the children. Instead she went to the window and stood looking out across the low rooftops to the harbor, black and still beneath a starless sky.

Since the night her father had boarded the *Clarissa,* she had had letters from England, Sweden, Germany, and now from Paris. Cheerful letters for the most part, telling of his travels, of the people he had met, and the houses where he had been entertained. When he mentioned, rarely, the difficulties of being an exile in strange countries, perpetually embarrassed by lack of money, it was always in a light vein, twisting the stories so as to make them into amusing anecdotes for her.

She had one comfort in the fact that Vanderlyn was also abroad, and spent much of his time with Mr. Burr. And from Vanderlyn's letters she drew a much clearer picture of her father's actual existence. It was true that he was obliged to live in the most meager style, Vanderlyn replied to her anxious query. But poverty, he assured her, was by no means an unfashionable state in Paris. Mr. Burr had kept his health and good spirits. Indeed, he had made so many friends that wherever one went in Paris one was more than likely to find "Monsieur le Colonel Burr" surrounded by an affectionate and admiring circle.

Vanderlyn himself was having a considerable success.

His painting, "The Ruins of Carthage," exhibited in the Salon of 1808, was awarded the highest of all honors, the gold medal of the Emperor Napoleon, who took occasion to compliment the artist in person.

Theodosia smiled, a trifle ruefully, over this news, remembering the first afternoon when she and Vanderlyn had met, and his troubled confession of his doubts that he should ever live up to Mr. Burr's expectations. Now he had justified his patron's faith brilliantly, but fortune had twisted things about so oddly that the first proceeds of Vanderlyn's success went to buy a supply of firewood, rice, potatoes, as well as other food and a much-needed greatcoat, for Mr. Burr, who had once done so much for him.

So long as Vanderlyn and his other friends in Paris were near, Theodosia was confident that her father would be looked after as faithfully and generously as his pride would allow. But still she grieved for him. The thought of his exile and the disgrace that prevented his return to America was the one blight in the peaceful contentment of her life.

Looking out now over the dark waters of the harbor, she heard the church bells toll the hour of eleven. One hour more, and it would be Christmas. A message, unspoken, went from her heart across the lonely black ocean.

"Merry Christmas, Papa—Merry Christmas."

"Theo . . ."

Theodosia turned to see Joseph. "What's happened?" she asked curiously. "You look as if you were fairly bursting with news of some sort."

"Do I?" Joseph laughed, but the next minute a sober

expression came into his deep-blue eyes. "Theo, those men came direct from Washington. They say there's no doubt about it. We shall be at war with England before the new year is out. Things can't go on as they are now. Our ships are being raided constantly, and the crews and cargoes interned. I've dreaded the thought of war. But if it comes, our country must be united, and prepared to defend itself." He paused. "Theo . . ."

"Yes?"

"They came tonight to ask me to run for governor of the state."

"What did you tell them, Joseph?"

"I said I would."

Theodosia looked up at him, pride and tenderness shining in her dark eyes.

Late that night Theodosia lay awake. Outside the wind had shifted, turning the wet snow into rain that pattered gently against the windows. So Aaron wouldn't wake up to see his first white Christmas, after all.

Lying very still, Theodosia thought of what Joseph had told her. If war was really coming, perhaps, at last, the bitterness against her father would be forgotten, pushed aside by the confusion of a thousand more pressing concerns. If only she could help him to come home before the war began. . . . There must be *something* she could do. There must be someone she could appeal to, someone who would understand and help her. Someone, somewhere, who would know how to break down the barriers that still kept her father from coming back to America.

It was three o'clock on Christmas morning when Theodosia rose and went into the sitting room to light a candle on the desk. She shivered a little, drawing her warm robe closer, as she dipped her pen.

She hesitated at first, wondering how to begin the letter. It had been years since she had had a word from Dolley Madison. James Madison was President now, and the cheerful, friendly Dolley lived in the White House, surrounded by all the dignity and caution of being the President's wife. But Dolley had spoken once, on a morning long ago in Richmond Hill. "I shan't ever forget all your father's kindnesses. . . . I hope I may pay him back someday," she had said.

Theodosia dipped her pen again and commenced to write:

Madam:

   You may perhaps be surprised at receiving a letter from one with whom you have had so little intercourse in the past years. But your surprise will cease when you recall that my father, once your friend, is now in exile. . . .

·CHAPTER 22·

A Gold Watch

DOLLEY MADISON HAD not forgotten.

And the first lady, moreover, knew a thing or two about getting her way with "the little Madison." To Theodosia's long, touchingly humble, and eloquent letter, she made no direct reply, perhaps because she had been warned that Joseph knew nothing of Theodosia's plea. Whatever may have been the means of persuasion employed upon the President, they had their effect.

A few weeks after Theodosia had written, wheels were set in motion to provide a passport for Mr. Burr, and a guarantee that no further legal action would be taken against him upon his return.

But the wheels moved slowly. And weary lengths of red tape had to be unwound before the day when, at last, the American ambassador in Paris delivered the final necessary paper into the hands of Mr. Burr.

Even then, there were more delays and difficulties to be faced. First, the perpetually vexing problem of money.

"And the problem of money," said Mr. Burr to Vander-lyn, "is that there *is* no money."

He must raise the money needed for his passage home. He sold nearly all of his books; Vanderlyn was willing to contribute as much as his slender treasury would allow, but still there was not enough. At the last moment Mr. Burr offered for sale a small gold watch. A very fine watch, in a case most beautifully chased. Engraved inside were the words: *For Aaron Burr Alston, with his grandfather's love.*

During the long months in Paris, Mr. Burr had more than once scrimped on his dinner, or shivered in his room without a fire, for the sake of adding a few more sous to the fund he was saving toward the little watch. On the day it was sold he wrote to Theodosia:

> . . . I have raised the money by the sale of all my little possessions and loose property. Among others, alas! my dear Gamp's watch. . . . After turning it over, and looking at it, and opening it, and putting it to my ear like a baby, and begging you a thousand pardons, the beautiful little watch—was sold.

But though her father grieved over the loss of his treasure, to Theodosia only one thing counted now. Her father was coming home.

She had word that he would sail for Boston in the last week of September. More than a month passed, a month of joyful anticipation while she waited for the news of his arrival. Then a letter came, not from Boston, but England.

His ship had been overtaken by a British frigate two days after sailing, and put back into a British port where the passengers and crew were unceremoniously dumped.

Now there were fresh reams of red tape to be waded through. Permissions, passports, and papers had to be granted all over again. And new passage money must be raised. The last treasures held in reserve for Theodosia, must be sold. Mr. Burr wrote:

> Got some things out of my trunk to sell . . . a length of velvet which I had sealed up for you, and resolved to keep through thick and thin. But everything visible must go, or I shall lose the opportunity of the ship. . . . Found some ribbons I had bought for you at the Palais Royal. After gazing at them, and painting to myself the pleasure they would give, I reluctantly resolved to sell them. . . . Thus I am obliged to plunder you and Gampillo to the last article.

In March, 1812, Mr. Burr finally sailed from Liverpool on the ship *Aurora*. After five stormy weeks, he landed in Boston. A few days later he had sold his last precious half-dozen books to Dr. Kirkland, the president of Harvard University, and was on his way to New York, where he arrived one bright June morning, exactly four years from the night the *Clarissa* had sailed from the harbor.

It was, however, a very different city to which he now returned.

War was in the air and with the whole populace united to arm itself, there was no time for old grudges. The grievances against Mr. Burr, which had once seemed so important, faded before more pressing concerns. Indeed, it was felt by many that Burr had, perhaps, been *too* harshly treated, after all. Time had passed, tempers had cooled. Here was a man who, no matter what his faults, had taken his punishment bravely. Let him be forgiven, and no hard feelings.

Nothing, probably, could have surprised Mr. Burr more than such a mellow reception. But he accepted good fortune with precisely the same philosophic good temper with which he had borne the years of disgrace.

"If it takes a war to make people change their minds about me," Mr. Burr told a friend, "I suppose I should be grateful to heaven for providing one at this particular moment. But the main thing is that I want to go to work again. If you'd care to do me one service, I'd be very grateful. You see, my funds right now are a trifle limited. Limited, in fact, to exactly twelve cents. If you could advance me a little capital, say, ten dollars . . . ?"

"Oh, but surely, sir, you must take more than that," his friend, Robert Troup said. "It's only fair, considering that I owe you everything I have. If you hadn't helped me through my law work, and bought me all my books, as well as food and clothes and——"

"Please, Robert"—Mr. Burr shook his head, laughing—"spare me a catalogue of my good deeds. They're forgotten, I hope, as completely as my bad ones. Ten dollars will be quite enough, I promise you. I shall rent an office immediately. And then," he finished with a shrug, "we shall see if I have any clients left."

That same afternoon a single room in a modest building at Number 23, Nassau Street, was engaged by a slight, unassuming gentleman in a shabby blue coat.

"A queer sort of chap, he seems," the landlady confided later to her husband. "Quiet-like, not too young, but lively as a cricket, he was, sweeping out the place himself and wheedling an old table and chair for furnishings."

She went to the window and looked down curiously. The "lively little chap" was just then engaged in tacking a small painted sign outside the door. He had scarcely driven the last tack before his first client came knocking. And there was a steady stream to follow.

With the advent of war, there was a bumper crop of law business in New York that year, and plenty of people recalled that Aaron Burr had once had the reputation of never losing a case.

If anyone bothered to recall that Mr. Burr had once been in prison, they only shrugged and echoed the words of his landlady. "Let bygones be bygones."

Soon the small room at 23 Nassau Street was crowded with clients. The rickety table and chair were replaced by newer furniture. There were lawbooks on the shelves now and, in one corner, a leather couch on which Mr. Burr slept.

If, his landlady observed, he slept at all, which she doubted, as she never looked in at the door but what she found him still bent over his books in the candlelight.

Once, being up late herself because of a toothache, she stopped in to offer Mr. Burr a hot cup of tea. He seemed very pleased, pushing his spectacles up on his forehead and leaning back in his chair to chat as politely as you please while he drank. She noticed over the fireplace a picture of a pretty young lady, very elegant and fine, with dark curly hair and a handsome white dress. When she asked Mr. Burr who the lady was, a queer look came into his dark eyes, that usually looked sharp as gimlets, for all their merry twinkling.

"That is my daughter, madam," he said after a minute.

She was surprised to think such a plain little man would have a daughter who looked like a great lady.

To Theodosia nothing could have been sweeter news than the reports of her father's reception and occupation in New York.

"You remember," she said to Joseph one evening, "Papa used to say then that if fortune's wheel turned down, it was only a question of time before it would turn up again. And he was right, for it really has, at last."

"I had a letter from him today," Joseph said, "full of all sorts of advice about running for governor."

They were out on the piazza, watching the last rays of the June twilight fade gently over the gardens. Even with the sun gone, there was little relief from the sweltering heat and the faint breeze from the south brought only the heaviness of swamp vapors.

"I do wish the wind would change." Theodosia sighed. "Dr. Logan says there's always more fever when the swamp winds blow, and it makes the mosquitoes worse than ever." She brushed at one that buzzed persistently about her head. "Do you think there's any chance of our getting away to the island fairly soon, Joseph?"

"You and Aaron can go at once if you like. In fact, I'd feel easier if you would. But I'll have to stay until we have some definite news from Washington about the war, and heaven only knows when that will come."

Presently young Aaron wandered up the path from the paddock and sat down on the piazza steps. His dark hair clung damply about his flushed cheeks, and there was a beading of moisture on his upper lip.

"Aaron, dear"—Theodosia leaned forward anxiously—"you look dreadfully hot. Surely you haven't been riding on an evening like this?"

"Oh, just a few turns around the paddock." As his mother reached out to touch his forehead, he drew away impatiently. "I'm all *right,* Mum." He turned to Joseph. "Is it true we're going to declare war most any day now, Father?"

"I'm afraid so, Aaron."

"Pete says he's going to be a sailor, if we do. I wish I could go with him. Pete says they're building a new schooner in Charleston, and that's the one he wants to be on. It's going to be named the *Saucy Jack,* and it'll have sixteen guns, Pete says. Is that *true,* Father?"

Joseph nodded. "You can't go to war just yet, Aaron," he said, "but, if you like, I'll arrange for you to be taken aboard the day they launch the *Jack."*

"Honestly, father?" The boy jumped up, his dark eyes shining with eager excitement. "And, Father, do you think if I asked, very specially, they might let me wear one of those caps the sailors have? You know, with letters on the ribbon?"

"I shouldn't be surprised," Joseph said, "if you were to ask *very* specially."

CHAPTER 23

Success to the Saucy Jack

T HE NEXT MORNING the long-awaited word came from Washington.

All day the harbor thundered with the salute of booming guns, and at noon the South Battery was thronged with people who gathered round to hear the sheriff read President Madison's formal proclamation of war.

From all over Charleston young men hurried to enlist, and the highways leading into town swarmed with carts and wagons, bringing planters eager to volunteer against the enemy that had for so long plundered their cargoes of rice and corn and indigo, and throttled the commerce of the once thriving port. One young fellow shook his fist toward the harbor where, just out of sight, the British vessels lay in wait.

"Just let 'em wait," he cried, above the cheers of the crowd and the sound of rolling drums. "They'll jolly well find out that England doesn't own *our* ocean!"

It was after dusk when Joseph got home that evening.

The candles burned quietly in their tall brackets on either side of the wide hall, but oddly there was no sign of Theodosia.

Joseph went upstairs, his footsteps echoing in the silence of the house. Then, as he paused on the upper landing, the door of Aaron's bedroom opened, and Theodosia came out to meet him.

"Joseph"—she spoke quietly, but her eyes were dark and tragic—"oh, Joseph!" She slipped into his arms with a quivering breath. "I'm so glad you've come. Aaron's ill and I'm so frightened."

It was the fever again.

Shortly after breakfast Aaron had been taken with a chill. Dr. Logan had been sent for. He was with Aaron now, sitting beside the bed in the darkened room where the boy lay.

"He says there's nothing more we can do now, Joseph, except to wait," Theodosia whispered. "But I was afraid—terribly afraid—until you came."

For four days and nights all life in the big house seemed suspended. The servants spoke in hushed voices, tiptoeing about through the silent rooms. Then, a little after twilight on the last day of June, the boy's thin body gave up its gallant fight to live. Dr. Logan, his young face drawn and weary, looked across the bed to Theodosia and Joseph.

"I'm sorry," he said, in a queer, gruff voice. "I—did the best I could."

Late that evening a man knocked at the broad front door of the Oaks. He had a message for Mr. Alston. Very urgent.

The servant tried to turn him away, but there was a step in the hall, and Joseph came to the door.

"What is it you want?"

"I have a message, Mr. Alston. You've just been appointed commander of the militia for the state of South Carolina. You're wanted at headquarters, sir, just as soon as possible . . ." The man hesitated, sensing something strange in the silence. "I—I'm sorry to've disturbed you, sir, only they said I mustn't fail to tell you tonight. And they say, sir"— he paused again, turning his hat uncertainly—"that this means you're sure to be elected governor."

Joseph still said nothing for a moment. Then he lifted his shoulders. "If you'll be good enough to wait," he said, "I'll have a horse saddled and ride back to town with you. Only first"—he turned slowly back toward the stairs—"I must tell my wife."

It was a winter's day, mild and bright, when Joseph took the oath of office as Governor of South Carolina. Riding beside him in the open carriage drawn by four white horses, Theodosia looked out at the people who lined the flag-draped streets leading to the Capitol steps. Many of them had known Joseph during his years in the legislature, and as the carriage passed they called out greetings. Joseph, his dark head bare in the winter sunlight, bowed to this side and that.

As they moved slowly along, Theodosia sat very still. Her hand rested quietly on her husband's arm, while she smiled at the lines of cheering people. Only once, when the carriage halted briefly at a crowded corner, she leaned forward suddenly, to look at a boy who stood on the edge of the curb waving a small silk flag. He was a merry-looking lad, about ten years old, but there was nothing about his freckled face to attract particular attention. Nothing—except that he wore a sailor's cap, jauntily tipped on his head, and written in bright gold letters on the ribbon band were the words "Success to the *Saucy Jack.*"

For just a moment then, the smile faltered on Theodosia's lips. The memory of her lost son stabbed her like a knife.

The carriage moved forward, and she turned quickly to Joseph. There was nothing in his expression to show that he had seen, but for an instant his hand closed over hers. She felt the gentle pressure of his fingers.

"All right, Theo?"

"All right, Joseph," she whispered back. And her smile, as she looked up into his blue eyes, was steady once more.

A few days after the inauguration the Alstons returned to Charleston. Ever since Mr. Burr's return to New York, it had been planned that they were to go north for a visit with him as soon as the trip could be arranged. But with Joseph's doubly important duties as governor and commander of the state militia, there was no telling when he might be able to go.

Why not then, Mr. Burr had written, have Theodosia come alone?

Joseph was doubtful. He agreed with Mr. Burr that the visit and a change of climate would be the best possible tonic for his wife. But the trip by land was long and fatiguing, and not considered safe for a woman alone. And sea travel, with the country at war, was none too certain either. Finally it was suggested that Dr. Timothy Greene, an old friend of Mr. Burr, would go to Charleston and accompany Theodosia, and to this plan Joseph gave his consent.

Dr. Greene arrived, preparations for the journey were made, and on the last day of December, Theodosia and Lottie, escorted by the kindly, gray-haired physician, boarded the schooner *Patriot*.

Theodosia's spirits had revived amazingly with the prospect of the trip. At the dock, where Joseph and Natalie had come to see her off, she bade them good-by cheerfully and, for the first time in many months, there was color in her cheeks and a sparkle of eagerness in her dark eyes.

Natalie had brought a parcel of new books and a woolen muffler for Mr. Burr.

"You won't forget to tell Papa I knitted the muffler myself," she said anxiously, "so he'll excuse the lumps in it. And be sure to give him my dearest love, Theo—and John and Frederic, too."

"Of course I will." Theodosia kissed her cheek. "You must keep an eye on Joseph for me. See that he doesn't work too hard, and don't let his head be turned altogether by too many ladies casting sheep's eyes at the handsome new governor."

"Don't worry. I shall guard him like a dragon," Natalie promised.

Theodosia turned to her husband for one last moment.

"I do wish you were going too, Joseph," she said, her voice suddenly forlorn. "But I shall come home soon, you know—quite soon."

·CHAPTER 24·

New Year's Eve

I<small>T WAS A</small> little after ten o'clock that night when the storm broke.

All up and down the Carolina coast the sea raged, driven by the fury of the wind. Great waves, rolling inward over the long sand bars outside Currituck and Pamlico sounds, dashed themselves against the lonely beaches with a thunder that mingled with the high drone of the wind.

It was New Year's Eve.

In the houses of Charleston people were celebrating. Safe from the storm that shuddered and thundered outside, they raised their glasses to toast health and good fortune as the stroke of midnight was tolled. The bells of old St. Michael's rang loudest, their bronze voices pitched deep and clear against the sound of thunder.

"Victory," the toast was given. "Victory to the United States."

Somewhere off the Carolina coast, making its way through the black sea, was a small schooner pilot boat. In the lighted dining saloon the passengers huddled together, seeking comfort from the storm in each other's presence. There, too, glasses were raised at the stroke of midnight and a toast was given.

"To the New Year—and a safe journey."

North of the Carolinas, along the sand bars that lay off the treacherous coast, there were settlements of a strange, half-wild people called *"bankers."* Descendants of the fierce and bold pirates who had for years roamed the coastal waters, these ragged, long-haired derelicts no longer sailed the seas, but were content to wait, like vultures, for ships that might founder along the shoal waters on such a night as this, delivering their victims of the storm into the bankers' plundering and murderous hands.

Under cover of the black, wild night, the bankers lay in wait for disaster. Along the sand bars of Kitty Hawk and Nags Head, they led an old horse up and down the shore, a lantern tied about its neck, so the bobbing, wavering beam of light might lure passing ships to a false haven from the angry sea. Up and down, up and down, through the driving fury of the night, the old nag stumbled along the uneven shore.

Only one passenger was missing from the little company in the schooner's dining room. A young woman, dressed in gray, who had come aboard just before they sailed. She had slipped away quietly, a little after dinner, and no one appeared to notice her absence. But shortly after midnight an elderly gentleman left the group and made his way to the second deck where he tapped at a cabin door.

"Come in."

Dr. Greene entered.

Theodosia was sitting alone in the small, lighted cabin, her hands folded in her lap. "I expect you've come to tell me I ought to go to bed, Doctor," she said, "and so I shall— presently. I didn't mean to alarm you by coming off alone. I'm quite all right, truly."

The doctor steadied himself as the ship gave a sudden heave, her timbers groaning before the angry buffeting of the sea.

"I thought perhaps the storm had frightened you."

She shook her head. "Not very much. Poor Lottie was wretched with a headache. I sent her to bed an hour ago. I've been thinking . . ." She paused, looking up. "You know, Doctor, it seems as if I'd never had so many things to think about. A great deal has happened to me lately. So much, really, that I hadn't stopped to realize it all until tonight. Some things have been good, and some . . ." She paused again, and let the words trail away. "But it will be wonderful to see my father. It's been a long while, you know, and we shall have so much to say. That's what I was thinking of mostly."

"I'll leave you to your thoughts then." The doctor turned away, but at the door he looked back. "Only mind, you mustn't sit up too late."

"I won't. I promise."

"Good night, then." He closed the cabin door on his last sight of her. She was looking up at him, the lamplight shining softly on the dark waves of her hair and catching a gleam of gold from a locket that hung at the throat of her plain gray gown. Sitting there, serene and smiling, she might have been in her own bedroom at home, instead of in a cramped, close cabin, on a small boat, in the twisting fury of a black and storm-swept sea.

A full week passed after the dawn of the New Year, but still the schooner *Patriot* had not reached New York. The boat must have been delayed—thrown off her course, perhaps, by the storm. Or she might have been overtaken by a British boat and forced to land her passengers at some port along the way. Surely, in a few days more, there would be news. . . .

Another week passed, and then another—and still no word.

Frantic messages passed from Mr. Burr in New York to Joseph in Charleston. "Have you had no news?" . . . "No, none." Nothing was known, nothing had been heard since the December afternoon when the *Patriot* sailed out of Charleston harbor.

Rumors began to come then. Rumors of a wreck, of a crew that had mutinied, and plundered and burned the ship, forcing the passengers to walk the plank. Rumors that the ship had foundered off the Carolina coast and fallen into the evil hands of the bankers. Rumors that the ship had been sunk by the British because she was carrying a cargo of contraband.

But they were only rumors. Gradually, as time passed, they died away into the mist of doubt from which they had come. With their death the last lingering hope died, too. There was nothing to wait for now. No answer to heart-broken questions came from the silent, restless sea which alone knew the end of the lost schooner *Patriot* and all her passengers and crew.

Theodosia was gone. None of those who loved her and waited for her ever knew her fate.

Sometimes, on a winter's afternoon, the gentleman at Number 23, Nassau Street, would leave his busy office for an hour and walk down to Battery Park. There, among the fashionable ladies and gentlemen who strolled along, arm in arm, he would be seen standing alone by the embankment rail, looking down the Narrows to the sea. He would seem, for a time, to be watching for someone, with a curious, expectant look in his dark eyes.

After a while, the gentleman would turn and walk quickly away. . . .

Anne Colver was thirteen when she first heard of Theodosia Burr, and decided someday to write her biography. The author has had eighteen books published, but *Theodosia* remains a favorite of hers because the idea was her first for a book.

She attended Friends school in Washington, D.C. and Pine Manor Junior College, then graduated from Whitman College in Washington state. After writing five mysteries, she turned to historical fiction. The Early American period, the era of the Burr family, is one of her specialities.

Anne Colver lives in Irvington-on-Hudson, New York, with her husband, a lawyer and writer, and their daughter, Kate.